Comprehensive
Preventive Dentistry

Comprehensive Preventive Dentistry

Edited by

Hardy Limeback

WILEY-BLACKWELL

A John Wiley & Sons, Ltd., Publication

This edition first published 2012 © 2012 by John Wiley & Sons, Ltd.

Wiley-Blackwell is an imprint of John Wiley & Sons, formed by the merger of Wiley's global Scientific, Technical and Medical business with Blackwell Publishing.

Editorial Offices
2121 State Avenue, Ames, Iowa 50014-8300, USA
The Atrium, Southern Gate, Chichester, West Sussex, PO19 8SQ, UK
9600 Garsington Road, Oxford, OX4 2DQ, UK

For details of our global editorial offices, for customer services and for information about how to apply for permission to reuse the copyright material in this book please see our website at www.wiley.com/wiley-blackwell.

Library of Congress Cataloging-in-Publication Data

Comprehensive preventive dentistry / edited by Hardy Limeback.
      p. ; cm.
   Includes bibliographical references and index.
   ISBN 978-0-8138-2168-9 (pbk. : alk. paper)
   I. Limeback, Hardy.
   [DNLM: 1. Tooth Diseases–prevention & control.   2. Comprehensive Dental Care–methods.
3. Preventive Dentistry–methods.   4. Tooth Diseases–diagnosis. WU 166]
   617.6′3–dc23
                                        2011050621

A catalogue record for this book is available from the British Library.

Wiley also publishes its books in a variety of electronic formats. Some content that appears in print may not be available in electronic books.

Set in 10.5/12.5pt Minion Pro by SPi Publisher Services, Pondicherry, India
Printed and bound in Singapore by Markono Print Media Pte Ltd

Disclaimer

1   2012

Contents

List of Contributors

Editor

Hardy Limeback, BSc, PhD, DDS
Professor and Head, Preventive Dentistry
Faculty of Dentistry, University of Toronto
Toronto, Ontario, Canada

Contributors

Amir Azarpazhooh, DDS, MSc, PhD, FRCD(C)
Assistant Professor, Faculty of Dentistry
Department of Biological and Diagnostic Sciences
Discipline of Dental Public Health
Department of Clinical Sciences
Discipline of Endodontics
University of Toronto
Toronto, Ontario, Canada

Donna Bowes, RDH, BHA
Dental Supervisor
Halton Region's Health Department
Oakville, Ontario, Canada

Grace Bradley, DDS, MSc
Associate Professor
Oral Pathology and Oral Medicine
Faculty of Dentistry
University of Toronto
Toronto, Ontario, Canada

**Ann-Marie C. DePalma, CDA, RDH,
MEd, FADIA, FAADH**
Private Practice
Stoneham, Massachusetts, USA

Shirley Gutkowski, RDH, BSDH
Clinical Advisor American Association for Long Term
Care Nursing
Cross Link Presentations
Sun Prairie, Wisconsin, USA

W. Peter Holbrook, BDS, PhD, FDSRCSE
Professor, Faculty of Odontology
University of Iceland
Reykjavík, Iceland

Ferne Kraglund DDS, MSc, FRCD(C)
Assistant Professor, Dental Public Health
Faculty of Dentistry
Dalhousie University
Halifax, Nova Scotia, Canada

**Gajanan Vishwanath (Kiran) Kulkarni, BDS, LLB,
MSc, PhD, FRCD(C)**
Associate Professor
Pediatric and Preventive Dentistry
Faculty of Dentistry
Toronto, Ontario, Canada

Jim Yuan Lai, DMD, MSc(Perio), FRCD(C)
Assistant Professor and Discipline Head, Periodontology
Faculty of Dentistry
Toronto, Ontario, Canada

Iona Leong, BScHons, BDS., MSc, FRCD(C)
Assistant Professor
Department of Oral Pathology and Oral Medicine
Faculty of Dentistry
University of Toronto
Toronto, Ontario, Canada

David Locker, BDS, PhD, DSc, FCAHS (Deceased)
Professor of Dental Public Health
Faculty of Dentistry, University of Toronto
Toronto, Ontario, Canada

Kiet A. Ly, MD, MPH
Clinical Assistant Professor
Northwest Center to Reduce Oral Health Disparities
Department of Oral Health Sciences
University of Washington
Seattle, Washington, USA

Peter Milgrom, DDS
Professor, Department of Oral Health Sciences
Adjunct Professor of Pediatric Dentistry and Health
Services
Northwest Center to Reduce Oral Health Disparities
University of Washington
Seattle, Washington, USA

Paula Moynihan, BSc, PhD, RPHNutr, SRD
Professor of Nutrition and Oral Health
Institute for Ageing and Health
School of Dental Sciences
Newcastle University
Newcastle Upon Tyne, United Kingdom

Hien Ngo, BDS, MDS, PhD, FADI, FICD, FPFA
Professor and Chair of General Dental Practice
School of Dentistry
University of Queensland
Brisbane, Australia

Ross Perry
President, CHX Technologies
Toronto, Ontario, Canada

Iain A. Pretty, BDS(Hons), MSc, PhD, MFDSRCS (Ed)
Professor of Public Health Dentistry
Colgate Palmolive Dental Health Unit
School of Dentistry
University of Manchester Upon Tyne
Manchester, United Kingdom

Fran Richardson, RDH, BScD, MEd, MTS
Registrar/Chief Administrative Officer
College of Dental Hygienist of Ontario
Toronto, Ontario, Canada

Colin Robinson, PhD
Professor Emeritus, Dental Institute
University of Leeds
Leeds, United Kingdom

W. Kim Seow, BDS (Adel), MDSc (Qld), PhD (Qld), DDSc (Qld), FRACDS, FICD, FADI
Professor and Director, Centre for Paediatric Dentistry
Research and Training
School of Dentistry
University of Queensland
Brisbane, Australia

Prakeshkumar S. Shah, MBBS (India), MD (India), MSc (Toronto), DCH (UK), MRCP (UK), FRCPC
Associate Professor, Department of Paediatrics
University of Toronto
Staff Neonatologist, Mount Sinai Hospital
Toronto, Ontario, Canada

Eva Söderling, MSc, PhD
Adjunct Professor, Institute of Dentistry
University of Turku
Turku, Finland

Mary-Lou van der Horst, RN, BScN, MScN, MBA
Project Consult Seniors Health
Conestoga College-Research Institute for Aging-
Schlegel Villages School of Health, Life Sciences and
Community Services
Kitchener, Ontario, Canada
Nursing and Knowledge Consultant in Older Adult
Care Regional Geriatric Program - Central Hamilton
Health Sciences - St. Peter's Hospital - SJuravinski
Reserach Centre
Hamilton, Ontario, Canada

Laurence J. Walsh, BDSc, PhD (Qld), DDSc (Qld), GCE d, FFOP(RCPA), FICD, FADI, FPFA
Professor and Head
School of Dentistry, University of Queensland
Brisbane, Australia

Preface

Who should read this book?

This textbook has been written for the practicing dentist, dental hygienist, dental assistant, and those students who aspire to enter the rewarding profession of dentistry. It is also meant to be a resource for dental educators. It is written in such a way that even patients interested in learning more about preventive dentistry should be able to easily understand this book: it is not a research text or complicated clinical manual. As with most clinical textbooks in dentistry, however, the current literature has been reviewed and cited. Each chapter discusses the current state of knowledge, with numerous practical suggestions for the private practice setting and discussions as to which products have been successfully used in preventive dentistry. A public health approach to managing dental disease in the population as a whole is occasionally mentioned in this book, but this is not its focus. Nevertheless, community dentistry students and Public Health Dentists would find this a useful text to learn about preventive procedures that might be adapted from the private practice setting to a public health setting. The main goal of the book is to bring to the reader new concepts not covered in other texts in dentistry and introduce the reader to new approaches to preventing dental diseases, especially dental caries.

What is preventive dentistry?

Preventive dentistry has its roots from the Latin terms 'praevenire', which means 'to anticipate' and 'dens', which is the word for tooth. Dentists and their team members strive every working day to 'anticipate' what could happen to their patients' teeth and supporting structures. To predict whether a subject under observation will end up with damaged or diseased oral tissues, diagnosing the presence or absence of disease and then assessing risk for future disease, is required. These topics are discussed in Chapters 2 and 15, respectively.

In Chapter 1, the introduction chapter, we discuss the various levels of prevention. This book endeavors to review the best methods for primary prevention of dental disease: through primary prevention it is possible with intervention to 'anticipate' disease and prevent it altogether. Comprehensive preventive dentistry also includes intervening early, when the disease is just starting, and returning the subject to good health. This is secondary

prevention. A new branch of dentistry has emerged called Minimal Intervention Dentistry, and some consider this to be part of preventive dentistry. Others, however, feel that this still represents restorative dentistry, but patients are treated using a more conservative approach, with minimal removal of tooth structure. True preventive dentistry means not having to remove ANY tooth structure. This book's focus is to review the approaches that can be used before Minimal Intervention Dentistry is required.

There is actually very little evidence in the literature on what is really effective in protecting people from developing soft tissue diseases such as periodontal disease and oral cancer. Of course there are journals and texts in periodontics or oral pathology describing the management of these diseases once they develop. When an 8-mm periodontal pocket has formed, there has already been tissue damage. Similarly, when cancer is detected in the mouth and confirmed microscopically after a biopsy is taken, the cancer has already started. The cornerstone for the prevention of periodontal disease has been to control the biofilm that leads to tissue destruction. This can be achieved mechanically or with the aid of antimicrobials. To prevent oral cancer, alternatives to biopsies used for early detection and surgical removal are only now being explored. These include various molecular-based diagnostic markers. Since smoking is a risk factor for all oral diseases, smoking cessation education and motivation should be provided in each dental office. Dental insurance plans lag far behind new developments in providing preventive services, and it takes a long time for third-party insurers to recognize their values. Patients are not reimbursed for preventive services that would be considered 'new'. Thus, dentists are slow to adopt modern preventive services, especially in soft tissue disease prevention. It is not surprising, then, that this book's primary focus is prevention of hard tissue destruction. It is what dentists have been most familiar with during the twentieth century. The new millennium will witness a massive expansion of products and techniques for the early detection and prevention of dental diseases.

Client versus patient

Because this book is written for the preventive dentistry team, dental hygienists will want to apply what they can learn from this book in clinical practice to treat their 'clients'. There is a trend in North America for the dental hygiene profession to refer to their patients as 'clients.' The reason being is that the term 'patient' is derived from the Latin verb '*patior*,' meaning 'I am suffering.' For literally centuries health care providers have considered those who receive their services as 'patients.' But some people are in perfect health and are not 'suffering' from any illness or malady. These people seek the services of health care professionals to prevent illness. Although the term 'client' can be used to infer that the person is not ill or has any dental disease, it really is a term meant to describe a person involved in a business transaction receiving commerce goods and services. Lawyers, consultants, accountants, and hairdressers provide services to 'clients.' It may be an appropriate term for someone receiving 'preventive dental care' by a dental hygienist. Still, people accessing the services of most health care professionals prefer to be called 'patients' (Wing 1997).

To many in dentistry, it has become second nature for the dental hygiene profession to refer to those who receive their service as 'clients.' Within the same setting of a dental office with dentists and dental hygienists working together, the customer is sometimes called a client and sometimes called a patient. It would be ideal to have a term that everyone could be comfortable using.

Clinical researchers have traditionally avoided this relatively recent dichotomy of terms by calling the people in their clinical trials 'subjects.' This term is used throughout the book as well where appropriate.

Is preventive dentistry still needed?

As discussed in Chapters 1, 3, and 4, dental diseases are still widespread problems worldwide. Researchers have estimated the total expenditures on dental treatment and compared them to the costs of some medical diseases, and it might astound the reader to know that more money is spent in dentistry on treating patients than treating all cancer patients combined (Baldota and Leake

2004). The cost of treating patients with dental problems is only second to the cost associated with cardiovascular diseases. The cost of treating patients' dental problems continues to increase annually. As decay rates decline, dentists turn their interest to previously underutilized therapies such as cosmetic dentistry, orthodontics, third molar extractions, implant dentistry, and so on. Despite approximately half of children growing up these days free of dental decay, there is still a huge demand for preventive dentistry. With more children undergoing orthodontics, there needs to be improved preventive care. People are keeping most of their teeth into old age and living longer, which means that preventing root caries, periodontal disease, and oral cancer will be even more important than before. The frail elderly is the fastest growing segment of the population, and they will need even more preventive care because of their increased risk for disease. We dedicate Chapter 19 to the frail elderly in the long-term care setting.

Although some dentists prefer to provide only cosmetic dentistry, or only orthodontics, most dental offices provide all-encompassing general dentistry services using teams to provide comprehensive preventive therapy. Dental hygienists and dental assistants are important members of the preventive team. The team approach is discussed in Chapter 21.

We have attempted to cover as many topics as possible in preventive dentistry in this textbook. I trust the title *Comprehensive Preventive Dentistry* best describes the contents of this book.

Dr. Hardy Limeback, BSc, PhD, DDS
Professor and Head, Preventive Dentistry
University of Toronto

Baldota, K.K. and Leake, J.L. (2004). A macroeconomic review of dentistry in Canada in the 1990s. *Journal of the Canadian Dental Association*, 70, 604–609.

Wing, P.C. (1997). Patient of client? If in doubt, ask. Canadian Medical Association Journal, 157, 287–289.

Acknowledgments

This book started with a visit to our dental school in Toronto on May 7, 2008, by Sophia Joyce, Senior Commissioning Editor for dentistry books at Wiley-Blackwell in Oxford, UK. I was honored to be asked by such a well-known publisher of dentistry texts to edit a textbook. I was initially also assisted by Shelby Allen, Senior Editorial Assistant for Wiley-Blackwell in Ames, Iowa, and then Melissa Wahl, Wiley-Blackwell Editorial Assistant for Dentistry and Nursing in Ames, Iowa, who took over and provided me with expert guidance. Her cheerful emails and patience made the book editing process surprisingly pleasant.

This book is dedicated to my wife Lynne whose love, tolerance, and support made the project possible. I would like to thank my two sons for providing artistic direction. Many of the figures in my chapters were created by my youngest, Kevin, whose illustrations had visual beauty in their simplicity. My eldest son, Kurt, oversaw the design of the text front and back covers and provided crucial feedback throughout the whole process.

I could not have taken on this project without being a 'wet-fingered' dentist. For this, and for some of the clinical photos, I am grateful to my patients. My wife Lynne, my two loyal dental assistants Kellie and Tonia Bogle, and my part-time dental hygienists Susan Sung-Li and Samantha Campbell kept the dental office running while I spent all my spare time at the keyboard.

Several practicing dentists took the time to forward me clinical photographs for this textbook, and their contributions are gratefully recognized and noted throughout the text. By taking a 6-month sabbatical and relying on Assistant Professor Shaheen Husain in our department to take on some of my teaching duties, I was able to focus more on editing the text. I am particularly grateful to the preventive discipline's administrative assistant, Bruna Valela, for taking on more duties while this text was being written.

I was honored by the willingness of recognized experts from far and wide with international reputations to provide full chapters for the book. We have authors from Finland, the UK, Iceland, Canada, the USA, and Australia. This text should therefore appeal to an international audience. These authors all lead such busy lives, but they gave their time generously to enhance the quality of this text. Without their contributions, I doubt this text would ever have been completed. Thank you very much chapter authors.

Hardy Limeback

1

A brief introduction to oral diseases: caries, periodontal disease, and oral cancer

Hardy Limeback, Jim Yuan Lai, Grace Bradley, and Colin Robinson

Introduction

By the late 1990s, treating dental disorders cost more than it did to treat mental disorders, digestive disorders, respiratory diseases, and cancer, at least in Canada (Leake 2006). The only group of disorders that exceeded dental treatment in terms of direct cost of illness was cardiovascular disorders (Leake 2006). In dealing with disease, "prevention is better than a cure." Dental disorders are an enormous burden to society, especially when one now considers the connection between poor oral health and systemic illness, which is a topic that is becoming increasingly important and a focus of other scholarly books. Papananou and Behle (2009) describe the mechanisms linking periodontitis to systemic disease. Dentistry in the past has been treatment oriented, but we are witnessing an unprecedented interest in prevention. It is obviously better to prevent the disease in the first place, than treat it once it has taken hold. This is quite true for most diseases in medicine.

The three general disease categories of focus in dentistry are dental decay, periodontal disease, and oral cancer. In the case of oral cancer, associated with a high degree of mortality, preventive dentistry even saves lives. Figure 1-1 summarizes the general hierarchy of prevention in dentistry.

The goals of preventive dentistry are to avoid disease altogether. Maintaining a disease-free state (green) can result from primary prevention. When lifestyle changes are made early on, the risk for developing dental disease are minimized. Secondary prevention and early intervention (yellow) can be used to reverse the initiation of disease. An outcome of good health can still be achieved

when incipient enamel lesions are reversed before cavities form, when gingivitis is reversed before periodontitis sets in, when dysplasia is found and excised before cancer develops, thus returning to good health and controlling dental disease is possible. Far too often though, dentists spend most of their time treating dental disease in an endless cycle of repeat restorations and surgery (red), which leads to tooth loss, and in the case of cancer, disfigurement and even death.

No one would disagree that it would be better to maintain oral health throughout life, never to have had any kind of dental disease. This is the goal of primary prevention (green area in Figure 1-1). Throughout the book we have used a 'traffic light' color system: "green is good," "yellow means caution," and red means "stop! fix the problem." A similar theme has been used commercially in buffering capacity tests and in risk assessment (Ngo and Gaffney 2005).

Primary prevention for dental diseases such as dental caries and periodontal disease could include eating a healthy diet, maintaining low intake of fermentable carbohydrates, practicing meticulous oral hygiene throughout life, and reducing the other risk factors, such as smoking, that would normally lead to dental disease. In the case of oral cancer, primary prevention might include successful smoking cessation counseling, where a patient has been smoking for quite some time. Obviously it would be better for the patient not to have smoked at all.

Secondary prevention ('caution') suggests that the disease has started but can be reversed, and good health can still be achieved. For example, incipient carious lesions (white spot enamel lesions) can be arrested and reversed using appropriate 'preventive' measures so that

Comprehensive Preventive Dentistry, First Edition. Edited by Hardy Limeback.
© 2012 John Wiley & Sons, Ltd. Published 2012 by John Wiley & Sons, Ltd.

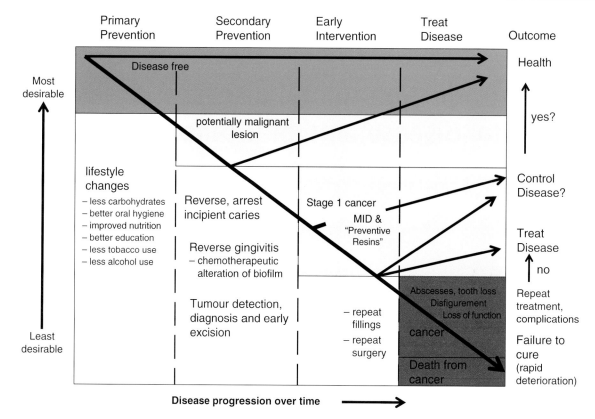

Figure 1-1 A hierarchy of prevention and treatment of oral diseases.

a full-blown carious lesion never develops. It was well established that frequent oral hygiene reinforcement by dental professionals can prevent caries, gingivitis, and periodontal disease (Axelsson and Lindhe 1978).

Secondary periodontal disease prevention might include other strategies such as the chemical elimination of bacteria known to initiate periodontal disease. Secondary prevention of oral cancer could include identification of dysplastic tissue and its removal as well as stopping the irritation that leads to the dysplasia.

It will be obvious to the reader that this book has attempted to be all-inclusive: a comprehensive text on prevention of oral diseases. Despite this ambitious goal, there is a heavy concentration and discussion around dental decay. It is important to realize that the literature on prevention of caries is quite extensive, compared to the prevention of periodontitis or oral cancer. If the reader is interested in the *treatment* of periodontal disease and oral cancer, it is suggested that the reader turn to more comprehensive reading material on the management of these diseases once they have developed. For example, two resources that are excellent reading material are books by Dibart and Ditrich (2009) and Tobia and Hochhauser (2010). Nevertheless, at least some approaches that have been successful in preventing periodontal disease and oral cancers are reviewed in this text.

The global burden of oral diseases

The World Health Organization's definition of health is "a state of complete physical, mental and social well-being and not merely the absence of disease or infirmity" (World Health Organization 1946). One of the true indicators of a good quality of life, of true physical, mental, and social well-being, includes being in good general health. Oral health is an integral part of good general health. Unfortunately, it is the poor and socially disadvantaged that carry most of the burden of poor oral health (Karim *et al.* 2008). Table 1-1 summarizes some of the general overall risk factors known to be associated with oral diseases, the diseases that result, and their consequences.

People in poverty in developing counties face an overwhelming burden of chronic and severe caries, periodontal disease, tooth loss, oral cancer, and other oral disorders. These have detrimental effects on health and create negative behavioral situations that simply contribute more to the cycle of social deprivation. Perhaps only by improving the socio-economic status, education and literacy, oral education, and access to affordable dental care can the cycle of poor oral health be broken.

In most developing countries there are relatively few organized public health programs. If they exist, there

Table 1-1 Risk factors associated with oral diseases and their consequences

Risk factors	Oral disease	Consequences
• Malnutrition	• Rampant dental decay • Periodontal disease	• Pain and tooth loss • Compromised chewing with further nutritional deficiencies • Social isolation
• Poor oral hygiene • Lack of dental care	• Dental caries • Periodontal disease	• Pain and tooth loss • Compromised chewing with further nutritional deficiencies • Social isolation
• Poor quality drinking water	• Disturbed tooth development (e.g., fluorosis)	• Mottled teeth • Social isolation
• Tobacco products and alcohol in excess	• Caries in children • Periodontal disease • Oral cancer	• Pain and tooth loss • Disfigurement • Death
• Poverty • Illiteracy • Lack of access to dental care • Serious systemic illnesses (e.g., HIV AIDS)	• Dental caries • Periodontal disease • Oral cancer • Oral infections • Oral cancer	• Pain and tooth loss • Continued social isolation, poverty • Inability to thrive • Death

is an uneven distribution of these dental services (concentration of dentists in urban centers) and a lack of modern dental services. Clearly, as poor nations begin to improve their standard of living, they will be able to afford to spend money on dental disease prevention.

Dental decay (dental caries): global patterns

Most countries have seen a dramatic decline in oral diseases and are entering the new millennium with less oral disease to manage than in the previous century. Figure 1-2 shows how the prevalence of caries has changed over the decades. In nearly every developed country, there has been a steady decline in dental decay. It is interesting to note, however, that there was a period of extreme shortage of sugar during World War II resulting in an almost elimination of caries. As the supply of sugar returned, so did the caries. This observation was made not only in Japan but also Norway. The decline of caries started many years before the introduction of fluoride and may be related to numerous other factors, such as the introduction of penicillin, the increased use of sugar substitutes, and improved nutrition (which includes better access to calcium and Vitamin D). Experts believe, however, that it was primarily the introduction of fluoride therapies after the 1960s that had a huge impact on dental decay rates (Bratthall *et al.* 1996).

The reason for the decline in caries worldwide in most developed countries is multifactorial. Other factors may have had an influence on the caries rates. Sucrose has traditionally been used to make preserves of fruit when in season. The introduction of the electric refrigerator likely increased the consumption of fresh fruit and vegetables as well as fresh milk. Penicillin and Vitamin D-fortified milk were introduced during World War II (WWII). Both could have affected caries—penicillin, because it is effective against streptococci, and Vitamin D because its deficiency can lead to caries susceptibility, especially in those countries where there is little sunlight during the year (the northern countries). The first non-cariogenic sweetener (cyclamate) was introduced shortly after WWII, and then fluoridation and fluoridated toothpaste made their impact. The effects of fluoride were striking, according to researchers even today, but caries may have already been on the decline. Chlorhexidine, xylitol, and fissure sealants also had their role to play in reducing caries in the post-fluoride era. Separate chapters are dedicated to these agents in this book. The result is that cases of caries are now at an all time low throughout the developed world.

In 2003, Dr. Poul Erik Petersen, Responsible Officer for Oral Health, World Health Organization (WHO) in Geneva, reported on the oral health status of nations worldwide (Petersen 2003). The distribution of dental

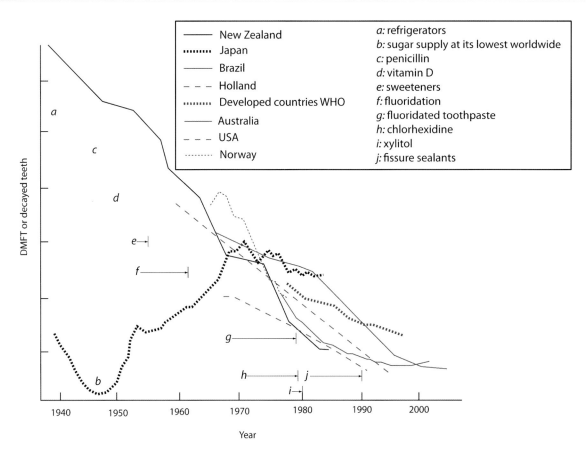

Figure 1-2 Global prevalence of caries from World War II to present. The relative (not to scale) decline in caries, represented by reported caries or DMFT (decayed, missing, filled teeth) are compared in this diagram from the start of World War II to the end of the twentieth century (each country, or countries, represented by different lines as shown). Also labeled are other factors that have contributed to the decline in caries worldwide (labeled **a** to **j**) and the approximate periods that they were introduced, represented by the horizontal arrows following the letters.
Sources:
New Zealand: Colquhoun (1997)
Japan: Miyazaki and Morimoto (1996)
Brazil: Cury *et al.* (2004)
Holland: Marthaler (2004)
Developed countries: The World Health Organization
Australia: Armfield and Spencer (2008)
USA: US Center for Disease Control
Norway: Von der Fehr and Haugejorden (1997)

decay throughout the world for children and adults is shown in a world map (Figure 1-3).

Despite this lowering of caries rates in children in most developed countries, the rate of edentulism remains quite high in the >65-year age group (Peterson 2003). The inevitable loss of teeth because of caries and periodontal disease is something that half of the population worldwide, on average, expects even today. The caries-free status of the younger population has been increasing however. As the younger population ages, dental professionals will witness a change in their dental practice profiles where their caries-free children, who grew up in the post-fluoride era, become adult and start raising

another generation of children with very few caries. In the next 30 years, there will be at least two generations of adults where at least half of them are caries and filling free. The annual increment of caries in any given population and age group can be measured, and the projected caries for a certain age can be estimated. For example, in New Zealand, a cohort of children was followed from the time of their birth in 1972–1973, and their caries experience recorded until age 30 (Broadbent *et al.* 2008). This study appears to be the only dental study that followed a group from birth to adulthood. Based on the findings, one can conclude that, out of the 932 participants who consented to dental examinations from birth to age 32,

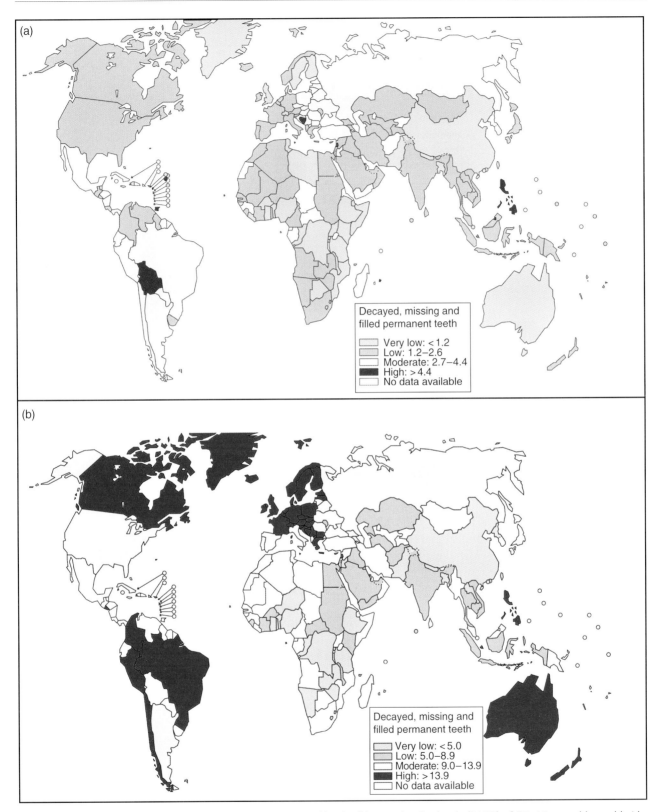

Figure 1-3 (a) Dental caries levels (DMFT) of 12-year-olds worldwide. (b) Dental caries levels (DMFT) of 35–44-year-olds worldwide. Reprinted from Petersen 2003, with permission from John Wiley & Sons, Inc.

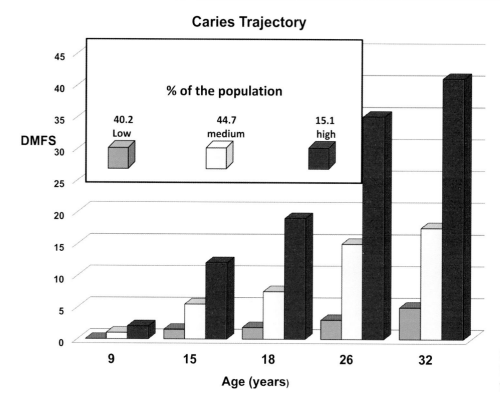

Figure 1-4 New Zealand caries incidence in a long-term clinical trial.

the trajectory of the caries is a linear one, with a minority of subjects (15.1%) experiencing a high increment of caries, 44.7% experiencing a moderate level of caries, and 40.2% experiencing a very low level of caries (Figure 1-4).

Nearly 1,000 patients were followed from birth to adulthood in this prospective clinical trial (no interventions). Approximately 15% of the population had the highest decay rates (red). The rest of the population was nearly equally divided between the low (green) and moderate (yellow) caries active patients.

By the end of the last century the edentulism rate from caries and periodontal disease was still high (see previous discussion). It is anticipated that as the current cohort of 30 year olds age toward their senior years, they can fully expect to keep their teeth. The rate of edentulism will decline dramatically as did the caries rates. Until that happens, a typical profile of the average dental office might include young adults with very little dental restorations and some older patients who have experienced extensive restorations and tooth loss (Figure 1-5).

Caries prevention: how far we have come in one century!

If one considers that the terminal stage of caries is the loss of a tooth, then early intervention (minimal intervention dentistry) is obviously desirable. When the

disease has progressed significantly and more drastic measures are required (surgical intervention such as root canal therapy), one is still 'preventing' tooth loss. This was the goal in the early days of dentistry more than a century ago when Dr. G.V. Black proposed the "Extension for Prevention" concept during the restoration of teeth (see Figure 1-6) (Black 1875; Jokstad 1989).

It has taken over a century for dentistry to advance from the pioneering "extension for prevention" concepts proposed by Dr. G.V. Black. By removing a significant proportion of tooth structure so that only the easily cleansed tooth surfaces remained, there was a reduction in the need for further operative treatment. As dental decay rates began to fall worldwide in industrialized countries after WWII, a new concept of operative dentistry began to take hold. It is called minimal intervention dentistry, or MID (Mount and Ngo 2000).

Minimal intervention dentistry, as the term suggests, refers to a principle of treatment in dentistry in which early intervention minimizes tooth destruction because the disease is diagnosed prior to cavitation, and steps are taken to remineralize the enamel and arrest the decay. However, more than that, it is a whole philosophy of managing caries. Chalmers (2006) summed it up:

"The main components of MID are assessment of the risk of disease, with a focus on early detection and prevention;

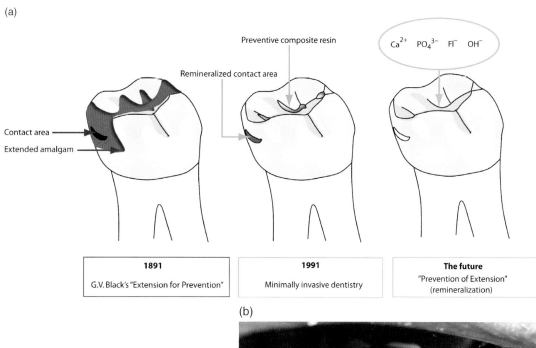

Increasing Caries Experience	DMFS = 0 No restorations
	DMFS = 8 preventive composite restorations only
	DMFS > 60 Fillings, terminally decayed teeth, missing teeth
	Complete tooth loss (four implants and dentures)

Figure 1-5 Radiographic profile of representative adult patients in a typical dental office in North America today. Most young adults will be either caries free (top, green) or have a select few fillings, many of them preventive resins, indicating a moderate risk for caries (middle, yellow). However, there is still a significant percentage of patients whose caries activity is extremely severe (red) leading to multiple root canals, extractions, and finally total tooth loss with teeth replaced with dentures or implant-supported prostheses (bottom). Radiographic images courtesy of Dr. Ray Voller of Pittsburgh, PA.

(a)

Preventive composite resin

Ca^{2+} PO_4^{3-} Fl^- OH^-

Remineralized contact area

Contact area

Extended amalgam

1891	**1991**	**The future**
G.V. Black's "Extension for Prevention"	Minimally invasive dentistry	"Prevention of Extension" (remineralization)

(b)

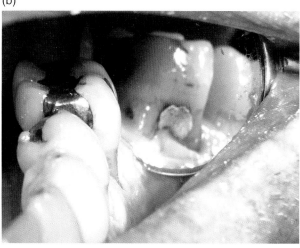

Figure 1-6 A century of caries prevention: (a) Illustration of the major changes in preventive dentistry. Left: G.V. Black's 'extension for prevention' showing a typical class II amalgam restoration. Middle: Minimally Invasive Dentistry 100 years later. Somewhat smaller restorations have been placed in a patient at moderate risk (yellow) for caries. Right: The latest concept in remineralization therapy in low-risk patients (green) ensures that the minerals are returned to the enamel before caries lesions start. (b) A clinical image of a typical class II amalgam restoration showing 'extension for prevention' as well as an amalgam restoration in the furcation area of the exposed root. Photo courtesy of Dr. Aaron Fenton, University of Toronto.

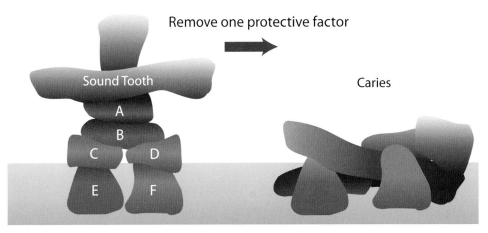

A: Protective saliva (flow, buffering, pH, anti-bacterial proteins)
B: Adequate remineralization capacity (salivary Ca^{2+}, PO_4^{3-}, F^-, alkali)
C: Good oral hygiene (bacterial flora—low *S. mutans*, *Lactobacillus*)
D: Ideal diet (calcium, protein, less frequent refined carbohydrates)
E: Good tooth resistance (morphology, no crowding or enamel defects, fluorapatite)
F: Ideal dentistry (alternative orthodontic therapy, gold restorations)

Figure 1-7 An illustration of how protective factors maintain sound tooth structure. This is an illustration of an Inuit Innunguat, a human figure made of stone by the native peoples who live in the arctic. The component rocks of the arctic stone figure are in delicate balance. Each protective factor (each stone) plays its part in keeping the human figure together. If any one of the parts is removed (loss of a protective factor), the structure collapses (caries results).

external and internal remineralization; use of a range of restorations, dental materials and equipment; and surgical intervention only when required and only after disease has been controlled."

Assessing caries risk can be done in several ways using many different approaches (see Chapter, Caries Risk Assessment). A popular approach is using Caries Management By Risk Assessment, or CAMBRA (Featherstone 2004) or Ngo and Gaffney's Traffic Light system (Ngo and Gaffney 2005), which has been adopted in this text.

A thorough analysis of patient history (social, medical, and dental), followed by a careful extra- and intra-oral examination will provide the necessary background for assessing caries risk in order to determine the most appropriate preventive therapy. Changing dietary patterns, controlling the cariogenicity of the oral microflora, and providing a healthy environment for remineralization are primary goals of MID.

Humans have developed several defense mechanisms that are in balance with each other and protect teeth against damage. If any of these protective factors are disturbed, the balance is disturbed and caries will result.

In Figure 1-7 an Inuit Innunguat representing a human figure standing alone and precariously against the elements, illustrates how caries is in delicate balance. Each protective factor (each stone) plays its part in keeping the human figure (tooth) together. If any one of the

parts is removed (loss of a protective factor), the structure collapses (caries results).

This is a convenient analogy to understand and is an offshoot of the classic Venn diagram (Figure 1-8) first introduced by Keyes (1962).

Caries results when all of the factors that contribute to caries overlap. One must have a tooth, plaque bacteria, fermentable carbohydrate, saliva, and enough time in order for a carious lesion to develop (red color, center). Several factors influencing each component, listed in the diagram, affect the rate and severity of the caries.

Dental professionals provide the initial care, reversing caries, but then they need to guide patients to maintain the good habits at home. A recognition that early enamel lesions can actually be arrested or reversed with various therapies (some practitioners go so far as to use the term 'healed'), has taken the MID concept to its ultimate level, where enamel, and even dentin, demineralization can be reversed with appropriate chemical therapy, resulting in carious lesions that have either been arrested or reversed. "Prevention before extension," a reversal of Dr. G.V. Black's idiom (Wesolowski 2008) has not yet found its way into the English dental literature, but it should be the goal of every dentist. Working together with the dental hygienist, prevention should be the primary focus of each dental office. Although in many dental offices, providing the preventive services is the sole responsibility of the dental hygiene team, 'prevention before extension' can only be achieved if the dentist

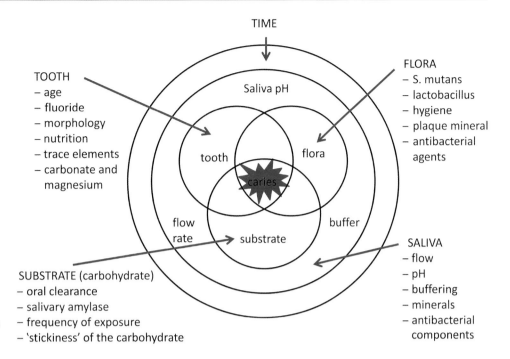

Figure 1-8 The classic Venne diagram of caries.

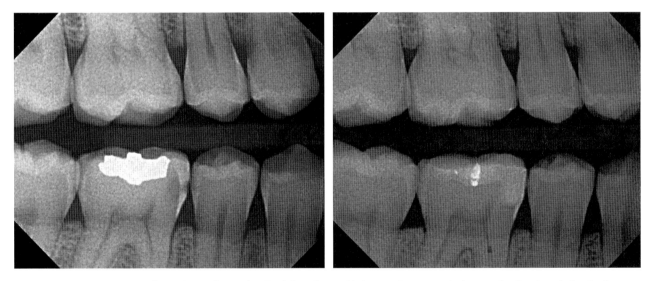

Figure 1-9 Caries as seen on bite wing radiographs. The left radiographic image shows a typical approximal carious lesion in the mandibular right first molar that has progressed into the dentin. The radiographic image of the same tooth on the right shows most of the previous amalgam removed and the caries treated with a posterior composite resin.

recognizes the value of providing this service. There is every reason to believe that, in modern times, each and every person should be able to expect to achieve a caries-free status.

An introduction to dental decay

Figure 1-9 shows a bitewing radiograph using a digital system identifying an interproximal carious lesion and the composite restoration that replaced the class I amalgam and repaired the carious dentin/enamel. Early carious lesions into enamel can be reversed. In this section we introduce the biochemistry and microbiology that leads to carious lesions.

Caries as an infectious disease

Dental caries does not occur in a sterile mouth. However, no mouth can ever be made sterile. The conditions in the oral cavity are ideal for the growth of bacteria that metabolize sugar to acids. The oral cavity is generally a warm place, at body temperature (37°C) encouraging the growth of bacteria.

Table 1-2 Salivary components and their role in caries

Classification of component	Ingredient	Function
Inorganic	Water (99%)	Dilutes and clears acid, wets teeth and mucosa, the vehicle for other ingredients
Inorganic, organic	Carbonate, phosphate, protein	Buffers acid
Organic	Amylase, lipase, protease, pyrophosphatase, lysozyme	Antibacterial
Organic	Mucins	Lubricant, calcium binding
Organic	IgA	Antibacterial

Caries is an infectious disease that is actually transmissible, usually when the mother, infected with *S. mutans*, infects her infant when the child's first teeth appear in the oral cavity (Kulkarni *et al.* 1989). In fact, it has been shown that the caries rates of the offspring can be reduced if the parents' *S. mutans* are reduced and the child is not colonized by *S. mutans* until after age 2 (Isokangas *et al.* 2000).

The role of saliva

Saliva contains antibacterial proteins, electrolytes for remineralization but also the essential nutrients for bacteria to grow. However, it is the food that is ingested by the host that provides the dietary carbohydrates that are easily converted to energy and acids by the bacteria that leads to dissolution of dental hard tissues.

The main components of saliva and their function are shown in Table 1-2.

Because of its buffering capacity and ability to neutralize acids, a simple intervention such as stimulating the saliva with chewing gum can arrest white spot lesions and prevent cavities from forming (Stookey 2008).

The role of dietary sugars

Not all sugars are cariogenic. In a chart of cariogenicity (Figure 1-10), the more common dietary sugars are presented.

The disaccharide sucrose and the monosaccharide glucose, a component of sucrose, are most cariogenic and, with frequent ingestion, can cause severe damage to the tooth (Paes-Leme *et al.* 2006). Other dissacharides are less cariogenic, and the sugar alcohols are nearly

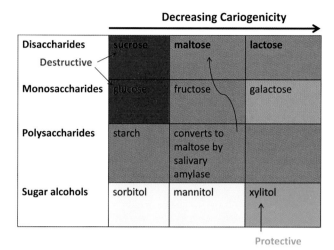

	Decreasing Cariogenicity →		
Disaccharides *Destructive*	sucrose	maltose	lactose
Monosaccharides	glucose	fructose	galactose
Polysaccharides	starch	converts to maltose by salivary amylase	
Sugar alcohols	sorbitol	mannitol	xylitol

Protective

Figure 1-10 Cariogenic potential of carbohydrates. This chart summarizes the cariogenic potential (cariogenicity) of various carbohydrates. The sugars with the most cariogenicity are sucrose and glucose (red). Other carbohydrates (maltose, lactose, fructose, and starch) are less cariogenic. The sugar alcohols, such as sorbitol and mannitol, are the least cariogenic (yellow), and xylitol has even been shown to be anticariogenic (green).

neutral in their cariogenicity. Xylitol stands out as an anti-caries sugar, and more about this sugar will be discussed in Chapter 9.

One of the strategies in prevention of caries is to limit access to the more cariogenic sugars and substitute them with the anti-cariogentic ones. As we saw in our discussion of the global patterns of caries, when the sugar supplies dried up during WWII, caries rates declined to almost nil. There is no question that carbohydrates are the main etiological reason for the development of caries. Not only does their conversion to acid result in enamel dissolution, but they also encourage the growth of more virulent cariogenic bacteria.

Plaque biofilms and their role in caries and periodontal disease

Biofilms responsible for caries and periodontal disease might occur in the same location (interproximally, at the margins of fillings, and at the gingival margins). The supragingival bacteria are dominated with streptococci and lactobacilli that can lower the plaque pH and induce decalcifications (white post lesions). Below the gingival margin and in the gingival sulcus, periodontal pathogens start to grow. They induce the formation of calculus and cause host immune responses that is initially inflammation, but as the bacteria migrate deeper into the periodontal pocket, the more virulent species cause host reactions that lead to the destruction of the periodontal attachment apparatus. In Figure 1-11, three different methods were used to visualize plaque.

(a)

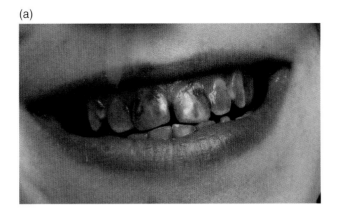

(b)

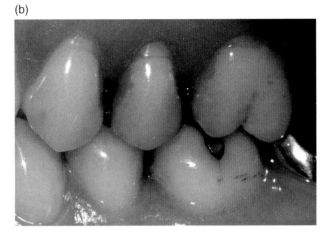

(c)

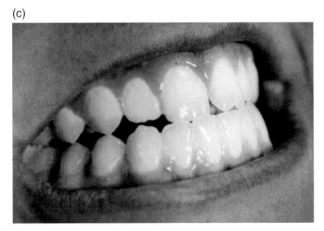

Figure 1-11 Three plaque disclosing methods: (a) 2-Tone. Plaque on a teenager revealed with Young's cherry-flavored 2-Tone Disclosing Solution. New plaque is stained red, and old plaque is stained blue to identify areas continually missed. (b) Red-Cote. Plaque revealed on adult teeth with Red Cote (Butler G.U.M.) disclosing solution. Chewable tablets produce the same effect. (c) Plak-Check. The plaque on this 16-year-old patient is revealed with Plak Check (Sunstar Butler G.U.M.), a sodium fluorescein dye, made more visible with a blue-filtered light source.

Disclosing agents such as 2-Tone (Young Dental Manufacturing) can reveal very thick, old plaque (blue color) and recently formed plaque (pink) (Pretty *et al.*

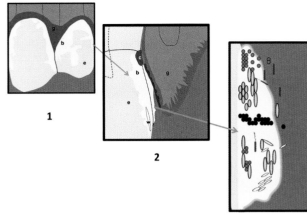

Figure 1-12 Illustration of plaque: (1) Plaque stained with sodium fluorescein: the enamel (e) has plaque biofilm (b) growing at the border of the inflamed gingival (g). (2) Same plaque as in 1 but a closer look. There is a 'white spot' lesion (w) developing at the margin of the gingiva, and brown calculus (c) developing in the sulcus attached to the tooth. (3) Close-up view of plaque. Sodium fluorescien not only stained the plaque biofilm bacteria, which consists of several species of bacteria (cocci, rods, motile spirochetes), but also the organic material (salivary proteins) and organic matter secreted by the bacteria (yellow-stained matter between bacteria depicted in 3).

2005). Sodium fluorescein (Plak Lite, Butler) uses a blue filter and bright light to highlight plaque, which glows fluorescent yellow (Lang *et al.* 1972; Gillings 1977). With this technique there is no messy cleanup. The third method is the more common one and uses erythrosine dye (Butler Red Cote) (Gillings 1977). Erythrosine stains more plaque than sodium fluorescein (Gillings 1977).

Figure 1-12 shows an illustration of dental plaque at the gingival margin.

In this example, plaque is growing at the gingival margin attaching to the tooth surface and growing below the gingival margin as well (usually where tooth brushing is inefficient). The bacteria that are associated with caries differ from those that are associated with periodontal disease. The pathogens involved in periodontal disease are geographically located deep in the sulcus, and are different species with different metabolisms. The plaque that is responsible for caries is generally located supragingivally and is acidogenic.

Dental plaque is quite complex in composition and extremely dynamic (Marsh and Bradshaw 1999; Filoche *et al.* 2010). Early colonizers attach to the enamel pellicle, the salivary organic film that forms immediately on freshly cleaned enamel surface. This allows the attachment of other bacteria, and eventually several communities of bacteria form that adhere to each other and

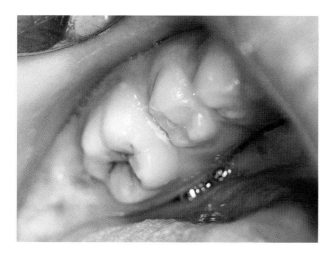

Figure 1-13 The enamel white spot lesion. This is a representative enamel white spot lesion at the mesial contact zone of the first maxillary right molar after exfoliation of the primary second molar. The premolar can be seen erupting into contact with the molar. These white-spot lesions are sometimes filled by dentists but can be remineralized.

interact with each other. People who consume sugars frequently in their diet increase the levels of streptococci and lactobacilli, the two bacteria species thought to be responsible for caries. These bacteria can be stimulated to grow in the right conditions, and they continue to thrive as the pH drops. If the plaque is not removed, eventually, the enamel starts to decalcify and an incipient 'white spot' lesion ensues, as shown in Figure 1-13.

The microflora associated with periodontal disease is really much more complicated, and researchers have been studying the virulent species for decades. It has been known for some time now which bacteria start to grow in unhealthy periodontal pockets. The main bacteria in health and disease are listed in Table 1-3, which shows a brief list of bacteria associated with dental disease. There are literally hundreds of microorganisms that are known to grow in unhealthy periodontal pockets (Listgarten 1994; Kumar *et al.* 2006).

Table 1-3 Bacterial species associated with dental disease

	Bacteria associated with health	Bacteria associated with disease
Caries	Normal flora	*S. mutans* and other low-pH streptococci (*Streptococcus oralis, Streptococcus mitis, Streptococcus anginosus*), *Rothia, Actinomyces, Lactobacilli Bifidobacterium* spp., *Candida albicans* Source: Filoche *et al.* 2010
Periodontal disease	*Streptococcus sanguis, Streptococcus mitis, Veillonella parvula, Actinomyces naeslundii, Actinomyces viscosus, Rothia dentocariosa.* Also *Veillonella* spp. oral clone X042 (Kumar *et al.* 2006), *Deferribacteres* clone W090, and clone BU063 from *Bacteroides, Atopobium rimae,* and *Atopobium parvulum*	*Porphyromonas gingivalis, Treponema denticola*
Gingivitis		*Actinomyces* species, *Streptococcus* species, *Veillonella* species, *Fasobacterium* species, *Treponema* species, *Prevotella intermedia*
Chronic periodontitis		*Treponema* species, *Prevotella intermedia Porphyromonas gingivalis, Candida* species, *Tannerella forsythia Peptostreptococcus micros, Campylobacter rectus, Aggregatibacter actinomycetemcomitans, Eikenella corrodens, Fusobacterium* species, *Selenomonas* species, *Eubacterium* species
Localized aggressive periodontitis		*Aggregatibacter actinomycetemcomitans*
Generalized aggressive periodontitis		*Aggregatibacter actinomycetemcomitans, Porphyromonas gingivalis, Tannerella forsythia Campylobacter rectus, Eikenella corrodens*
Chronic/aggressive periodontitis		*Aggregatibacter actinomycetemcomitans, Porphyromonas gingivalis, Prevotella intermedia, Tannerella forsythia Campylobacter rectus, Peptostreptococcus micros*

Data from
P.D. Marsh, Microbial Ecology of Dental Plaque and its significance in Health and Disease *ADR* 1994 8:263

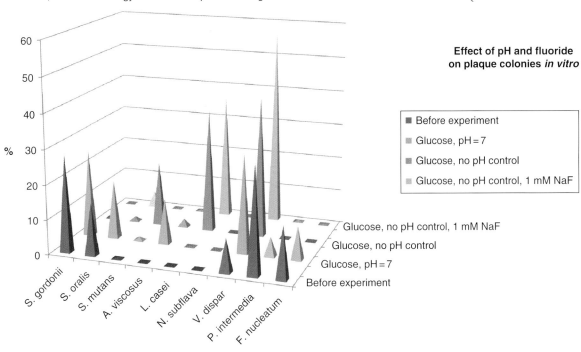

- Repeated glucose rinses encourages SM and LB growth when plaque acid is not controlled
- At low pH periodontal micro-organisms do not thrive; there is an ecological shift to cariogenic flora
- Fluoride at high concentrations inhibits SM but not LB

Figure 1-14 Changes in oral flora under controlled culture conditions.

In a series of elegant experiments, Marsh (1994) was able to show, at least in well-controlled chemostat cultures, that feeding mixtures of bacteria a meal of glucose can encourage the growth of cariogenic bacteria and suppress the growth of periodontal pathogens when the pH is allowed to drop (see Figure 1-14).

Nine different oral bacteria were cultured together in controlled conditions. Glucose rinses (second row) at neutral pH encouraged *A. viscosis* and *V. dispar* growth, but if the pH is not controlled and allowed to drop, the acidic conditions encourage the growth of *S. mutans* and *L. casei* but inhibit the growth of periodontal pathogens. There is an ecological shift to cariogenic flora. Fluoride at high concentrations inhibits SM but not LB.

In their experiments, the cultures were pulsed daily with glucose. To simulate a healthy mouth, the pH was maintained at neutral pH in some bacterial mixtures. In other mixtures the pH was allowed to fall as acid was produced from the glucose. As the pH dropped, the *S. mutans* were encouraged to grow. *In vivo, S. mutans* is able to secure sucrose and make an extra-cellular coat of glucan that favors its attachment to enamel and rapid growth. It can also tolerate low pH. *S. Mutans*

thrives at low pH. The others don't do well at low pH. Thus, a cariogenic flora is encouraged to grow. Fluoride has to be at mM concentrations to significantly inhibit *S. mutans,* and it has no effect on lactobacilli. In separate experiments Marsh's group was able to show xylitol had inhibitory properties for both cariogenic and periodontal bacteria. These observations were made by other researchers as well (Ccahuana-Vasquez *et al.* 2007).

The demineralization–remineralization balance in caries

As plaque thickens *in vivo,* and becomes dominated by cariogenic bacteria, it can effectively keep the saliva from reaching the enamel surface. In addition, the more plaque there is, the more acid is produced. These acids have a longer time to penetrate into the enamel under thick biofilm. If the saliva reaches the acids they are washed away and neutralized by the salivary buffers. This allows the tooth to remineralize. The cycle repeats itself over and over with every sweet snack and meal containing fermentable sugars (Figure 1-15).

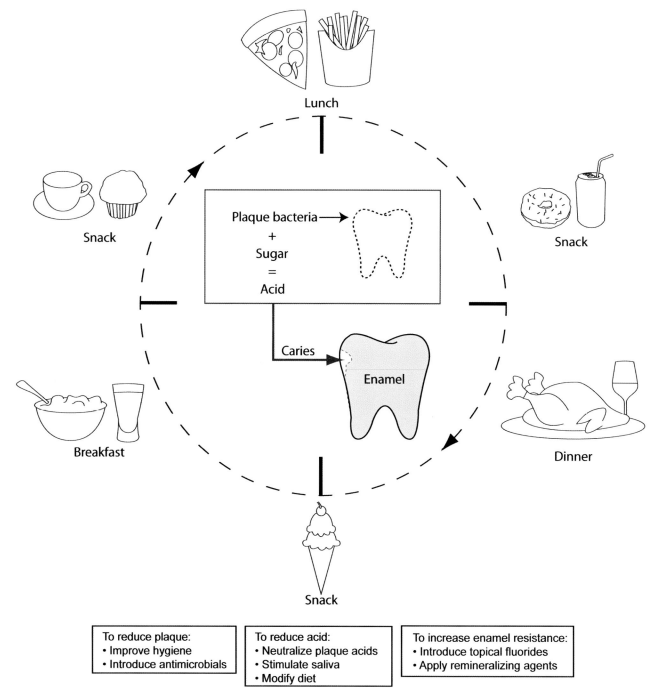

Figure 1-15 The repeated cycle of 'sugar attacks.'

Caries occurs when the frequency of sugar exposure during the day is high. There are many strategies in preventive dentistry to reduce the risk for caries from this frequent exposure to carbohydrates. One can limit how much plaque is on the tooth surface through better hygiene and antimicrobials, reduce plaque acids by introducing buffers, increase salivary flow, modify the diet (changing to less cariogenic foods), and increase the resistance of the tooth structure with topical fluorides and remineralizing agents.

Preventive interventions aim to modify the steps in the repeat demineralization and remineralization cycles.

1. Neutralize the plaque acids: This can be done by adding base or adding buffers such as sodium

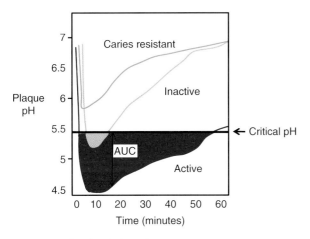

Figure 1-16 The classical Stephan Curve.

bicarbonate (baking soda) to the saliva to boost its ability to neutralize acids.

2. Improve hygiene: With bacterial levels low, less acid is produced. Also, plaque layers don't have a chance to grow thick; saliva can penetrate better to the enamel surface through thin layers of plaque.

3. Introduce antimicrobials: Since caries is a disease caused by bacteria, simply eliminating the bacteria or controlling their growth would go far to reduce the caries incidence. Chlorhexidine, xylitol, ozone, even experimental antibodies, have been used to control bacterial growth.

4. Stimulate saliva: Saliva contains numerous components that fight tooth decay (buffers, remineralizing minerals, antimicrobial enzymes, antibodies).

5. Topical fluorides: Fluoride added to the remineralizing incipient lesion increases the enamel crystals' resistance to dissolution by plaque acids.

6. Remineralizing strategies: Remineralization can be promoted with the use of calcium-phosphate complexes such and ACP-CPP.

The pH of dental plaque in response to glucose has been studied using the classic Stephan curve (Stephan and Miller 1943) (Figure 1-16).

This diagram illustrates the plaque pH response curves that have been obtained from patients with different risks for caries. A high-risk individual, when given a glucose rinse at time zero, will experience a dramatic drop in the plaque pH well below the critical pH of 5.5. The recovery to neutral pH in the high risk individual will be slow. The area under the pH-time curve (AUC) representing the time spend at pH lower than the critical pH is a better measure of total caries risk. The AUC for a high risk individual (red) will be very large. For a more moderate risk individual (yellow), the initial pH drop may only be a little lower than the critical pH, and the

AUC will be much less. For a caries-resistant person (green), the initial pH drop of that person's plaque may not even reach the critical pH, and the recovery will be very quick.

In these experiments, the pH of plaque is monitored after a patient is given a glucose rinse. The degree to which the pH drops will depend on several factors and is governed by how quickly the acids are eliminated and neutralized. It can depend on how thick the plaque is and how deep the sugar penetrates into plaque. A theoretical model was even developed to demonstrate this (Dawes and Dibdin 1986). Some people are caries prone, others are caries resistant. In caries-resistant people, the pH drop in response to a rinse with glucose does not fall below pH 5.5, a pH thought to be a 'critical pH.' The concept of 'critical pH,' where there is net loss of calcium and phosphate from the enamel (Ericsson 1949), is actually a 'moving target' and is not the same for every person. The critical pH can be different for different people. If salivary phosphate and calcium levels are low, the critical pH, the pH when there is net loss of mineral, can be as high as 6.5. People that tend to have very high calcium and phosphate levels in their saliva (and plaque fluid) may have a lower critical pH, such as 5.1 (Dawes 2003).

What is crucial, really, is the time that the enamel surface is exposed to acid. This is quantified as the area under the curve (AUC) in the classic Stephan graphs. If this area is large, one can expect that more calcium and phosphate would have escaped from the enamel. If this is repeated on a daily basis several times (i.e., because the subject is constantly snacking on cariogenic foods or beverages) then the 'red' AUCs combine during the day, and there will undoubtedly be a net mineral loss. This is demonstrated in Figure 1-17.

In this hypothetical comparison, the person at low risk (green) may not snack at all and has three meals of low cariogenicity spread apart during the day to allow remineralization to occur. The person with moderate (yellow) caries risk might have three meals and one snack of moderate cariogenic potential on a daily basis, and the combined AUCs below the critical pH might result in a net loss of mineral. At this stage, remineralization strategies might work. The person with a high risk for caries (red) snacks frequently during the day, and the total AUCs clearly are excessive and will not allow remineralization to occur. If that daily trend continues, the person will undoubtedly experience dental decay.

Researchers have determined that it is not only the frequency of ingestion that is important, but it is also the type of fermentable carbohydrate that is ingested. (We discuss these issues more in Chapter 6, on diet and

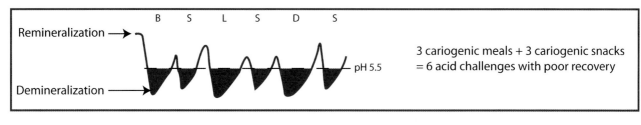

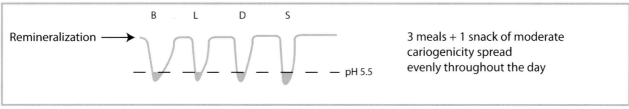

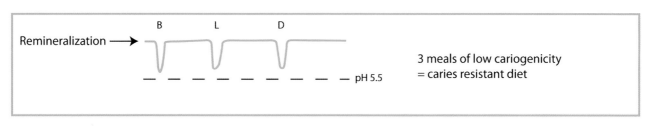

Figure 1-17 Daily repeat Stephan curves in low to severe risk individuals. Top: A high-risk individual (red) is exposed to several repeated acid challenges each day because of the many cariogenic snacks and meals that consumed in one day. The AUCs, which are large to begin with, all combine to add up to a net demineralization of tooth structure. Middle: An individual with moderate risk will have fewer daily cariogenic challenges, with less severe pH drops in the plaque, and may have enough time under remineralization conditions to allow for 'repair' of the enamel that could have lost some mineral. Bottom: The individual that is caries resistant is likely to be one who does not eat cariogenic meals or snacks more than three times a day. This person may never reach a plaque pH that risks the loss of mineral from the enamel.

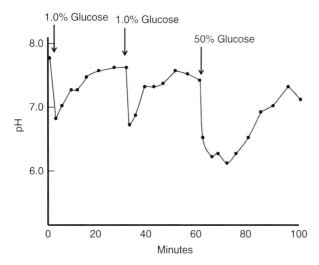

Figure 1-18 Plaque pH is dose dependent. Reprinted from Kleinberg *et al.* 1982, with permission from SAGE Publications.

caries.) For example Kleinberg *et al.* (1982) determined that increasing glucose concentrations results in lower pH drops (Figure 1-18).

In these experiments, it was shown that exposure to dilute glucose solutions lowered plaque pH but not too far for the saliva to neutralize the acid and return the plaque to neutral pH. However, when a concentrated solution of glucose is used, the plaque pH drops further and stays in the acidic range longer. This suggests that caries also depends on the concentration of sugar in the cariogenic foods.

Lingström *et al.* (1993) showed that the indwelling electrode was the most sensitive method for producing Stephan curves and discovered that potato chips were more cariogenic than soft white bread, which was more cariogenic than starch solutions or glucose solutions. This could reflect the fact that food impaction into pits and fissures as well as interproximal contact areas would prolong the retention of sold starches. The solid starches are then slowly converted to maltose by salivary amylases. The areas under the pH curve are more pronounced for retained solid foods.

Coronal versus root caries

Thus far we have discussed the general principles of enamel caries. Most of the coronal caries in modern times occur on the pits and fissures, making them ideal hiding places for bacteria since they are not easily

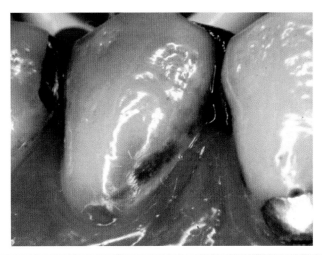

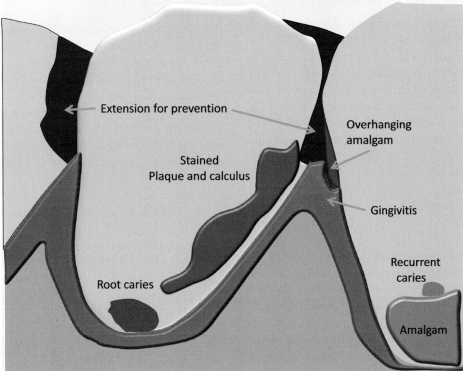

Figure 1-19 Example of root caries. This clinical image of a mandicular right first premolar demonstrates the start of cavitation at the demento-enamel junction at the gingival margin at the cervical region of the crown. Two brown stain areas are present but the most apical lesion is cavitated and an active root caries lesion. The illustration shows the various landmarks of this image.

disturbed with tooth brushing, and in the contact areas between the teeth where the plaque is sometimes left undisturbed for days because the toothbrush does not reach that area. It is only with flossing that the interproximal areas are disturbed.

Another form of caries is the caries that forms at the root surface that has been exposed due to gingival recession or periodontal disease (see the next section). The same bacteria are believed to be responsible for the decay of dentin (*S. mutans, Lactobacillus*), but *Actinomyces*

species that are able to metabolize starch to sugars are also involved (Chen *et al.* 2001).

Root caries usually starts at the weakest point. The cement-enamel junction at the exposed root surface may or may not be hidden by plaque (Figure 1-19).

Cavitation occurs much more quickly; dentin has no critical pH and dissolves more quickly at low pH because the dentin tubules allow bacterial invasion, and the dentin crystals are smaller and readily dissolved at low pH.

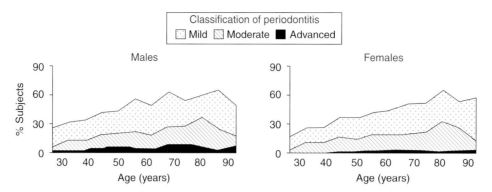

Figure 1-20 Percentage of individuals with advanced, moderate, or mild periodontitis among US adults examined from 1988 to 1994 by age and gender. Reprinted from Albandar, Brunelle and Kingman 1999, with permission from the American Academy of Periodontology.

Current patterns of periodontal disease

The prevalence of periodontal disease in the US has been monitored in a large-scale clinical study called the National Health and Nutrition Examination Survey (NHANES III). Mild periodontal disease is generalized, moderate periodontal disease is less prevalent, and severe periodontal disease is not very common. The prevalence increases with age in the adult population. A little more than one-third of the adult population has periodontal disease with 22% having mild periodontal disease and 12.6% having moderate to severe periodontal disease (as defined by pocket depths ≥3 mm and bone loss). The results showed that at the time of the NHANES III study (1988–1994), 21 million people had at least one site with ≥5 mm probing depth and 35.7 million persons had periodontal disease (Figure 1-20).

The World Health Organization developed a community periodontal index to measure the prevalence of periodontal disease in several countries. Gingival bleeding, periodontal pocketing, and loss of bone attachment were measured. Gingivitis, or gingival bleeding, was prevalent in all regions of the world. Severe periodontal disease (>6 mm pockets) is generally found in 10 to 15% of adults worldwide. The WHO identified periodontal disease risk factors that included poor oral hygiene, tobacco and alcohol use, stress, and diabetes. It proposed several preventive strategies to lower the risk for periodontal disease, and these were obviously aimed at reducing the risk factors (Petersen 2005).

Caries versus periodontal disease

Caries and periodontal disease are infections. They are caused by bacteria that can infect the oral cavity or by bacteria that are already present that become virulent. These bacteria reside in communities, sometimes in harmony, living in a symbiotic relationship, other times in conflict, competing for the same nutrients or resisting conditions that would result in their demise. On surfaces such as teeth, microorganisms usually live in communities called biofilms. It is now known that these biofilms change in their composition, properties, and adherence and that their inhabitants can change from being dominated by passive bystanders to those that over-run the biofilm and become aggressive pathogens. Commensal microorganisms, defined as those bacteria that live symbiotically with others, providing a benefit to themselves or the host, without affecting other organisms negatively, allow the body to function normally. It is estimated that there are 10^{14} cells in the human body and only 10% of them are mammalian (Sanders and Sanders 1984).

So many factors can disrupt this balance, and this can result in the host infection and pathological responses. Environment factors that affect the metabolism and numbers of active bacteria include, but are not limited to, oxygen tension, pH, energy supply, inorganic and organic chemical changes, inflammatory host response to foreign proteins/objects, and anti-bacterial agents (both intrinsic and extrinsic).

There are numerous surfaces in the oral cavity to which biofiolms adhere, each with their own unique characteristic. The mucosa of the inner lip, vestibule, attached gingival, tongue, and palate all have different families of resident bacteria that at any time can change in composition. The biofilms attached to the mineralized tissues (enamel, dentin, cementum) have bacteria with the ability to adhere to the salivary pellicle, a layer of proteins, lipids, and inorganic molecules derived from the saliva that make adherence to the mineralized tissue possible. This microflora is dominated by the facultatively anaerobic gram-positive bacteria, especially streptococci. There are more than 500 taxa of microbes normally found in the oral cavity, and these appear to be unique to the oral cavity since only about 29 of them end up in the feces (Moore and Moore 1994).

The bacteria in the gingival crevicular crevice are bathed not only in saliva but in crevicular fluid, a serum-like exudate from the sulcus of the periodontium. Both are rich in protein, are neutral in pH, and are warm, perfect conditions to encourage bacteria to grow. As inflammation occurs, the crevicular fluid flow increases. Redox potentials change, and anaerobic bacteria start to grow, many of which produce proteolytic enzymes that breakdown host cells and soft tissue matrices and feed on the breakdown products. The gram-negative anaerobes such as *Prevotella, Porphyromonas, Fusobacterium*, and *Treponema* are found in the periodontal pockets where there is attachment loss (Moore and Moore 1994). It is suspected that the pathogens for both caries and periodontal disease can be transmitted from person to person, but disease emerges because quiescent pathogens that have always been present in small numbers in health oral flora are allowed to proliferate and dominate the plaque as a result of certain stresses and stimuli. Clearly, preventive strategies would seek to eliminate the stresses (Marsh 2003). Changes in redox potentials and pH in the plaque can favor the growth of periodontal pathogens. *P. Gingivalis,* for example, grows better when the pH is alkaline and haem-containing proteins (blood proteins such as haemaglobin) are available as a substrate (McDermid *et al.* 1988).

Periodontal disease etiology

'Periodontal disease' is an all-encompassing term that refers to a number of diseases of the periodontium. These include gingivitis, chronic periodontitis and aggressive periodontitis. The bacteria involved in these periodontal disease states were introduced in Table 1-3. How these bacteria come to dominate the sulcus is based, in part, on the *in vitro* experiments by Marsh and others (2003) in the previous section.

The pathogenesis of gingivitis

Gingivitis occurs when the gingival margin becomes red and edematous, and bleeds easily on palpation or probing. There are changes to the anatomy (usually puffiness or swelling), loss of adaptation to the tooth, and increased gingival crevicular fluid. Histologically, the tissue responds to local plaque bacteria in three ways (Payne *et al.* 1975). First, there is an acute inflammatory response with infiltration of neutrophils. Second, a chronic inflammatory infiltrate dominated by T and B lymphocytes is accompanied by collagen breakdown and proliferation of junctional epithelium. Third, progression through the acute phase of inflammation is followed by a chronic inflammation and progressive destruction of gingival tissue. Many systemic conditions predispose the gingiva to this inflammatory response. These include the conditions that affect vascular changes (leukemia, hemophilia, diabetes, Addison's disease),

immunodeficiency conditions (HIV), hormonal changes (puberty, pregnancy, steroid therapy), and abnormal responses to drugs (seizure therapy, anti-rejection drugs) (Research Science and Therapy Committee of the America Academy of Periodontology 1999).

The pathogenesis of periodontal disease

Periodontal disease is characterized by attachment loss where the periodontium (gingival, periodontal ligament, and bone) fail to remain attached to the tooth and its root surfaces. Most sites of periodontal attachment loss start with inflammation, or gingivitis, but this is not always the case. The factors that lead to the initiation of periodontitis are not well known. It has been observed that periodontitis with attachment loss can be sporadic, acute, or chronic (Jeffcoat and Reddy 1991). In young adults loss of attachment can start in the proximal sites of the posterior molars (Thompson *et al.* 2006) where one expects poor oral hygiene. In susceptible patients, however, the disease can be quite aggressive and rapid and not be associated with gingivitis. The invasion and proliferation of virulent pathogens in the crevicular sulcus can lead to destruction of periodontal tissues because some of the periodontal pathogens produce enzymes especially dangerous to the integrity of the periodontium. Organisms such as *P. Gingivalis* can produce proteolytic enzymes (proteases, collagenase, fibrolysin) that degrade collagen and noncollagenous proteins. Metabolic byproducts such as hydrogen sulfide and ammonia can be toxic to mammalian cells, and lipopolysaccarrhides (LPS) can induce bone resorption (Hausmann 1970).

Once established in a periodontal pocket that has progressed (e.g., >6 mm), host-mediated destructive processes are initiated after the barrier of an intact periodontium is breached. Under normal circumstances, polymorphonuclear leucocytes are usually effective in staving off invading bacteria, but in the periodontium, they are overwhelmed trying to phagocytose the invading bacteria and the LPSs, releasing destructive enzymes in the extracellular environment. More collagen and basement membrane destruction ensues. The host response mechanism is believed to involve prostaglandin E_2 (PGE_2) and arachadonic acid, which promote the local release of matrix metalloproteinases, enzymes that lead to further destruction of the host tissues. Inflammatory mediators (also include the interleukins (interleukin 1 or IL-1; interleukin-6 or IL-6; interleukin 8 or IL-8) and tumour necrosis factor (TNF-α).

The biofilm in deep pockets responds to changes in oxygen tension, and anaerobic bacteria begin to dominate away from the influence of the saliva and in the

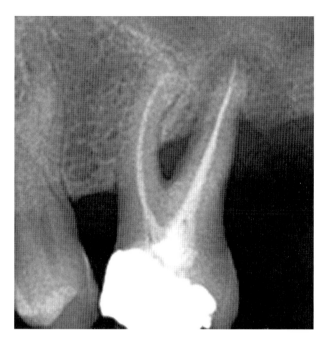

Figure 1-21 Radiograph of a tooth with periodontal bone loss. This periapical view of the maxillary right left first molar indicates significant bone loss and furcation involvement. Notice the large amalgam filling and the root canal treatment. Despite efforts to save this tooth through conventional restorative procedures from previous extensive caries, this tooth will be lost to periodontal disease.

deeper depths of the pockets. Advanced periodontitis is now an established anaerobic, gram-negative infection. Obvious treatment strategies include oxidizing agents, but at this point the disease has already been established. Our interest lies in preventing attachment loss, not treating the infection after the fact or intervening surgically—that is a topic for other textbooks. When the tooth has progressed to the point of major bone loss (Figure 1-21), it is obviously too late.

Oral cancer

Squamous cell carcinoma arising from the oral mucosa is the most common malignant tumor of the oral cavity, constituting more than 90% of all oral malignancies (Neville and Day 2002). In this book, the term 'oral cancer' will be used synonymously with oral squamous cell carcinoma. The oral mucosa is structurally similar, although not identical, to the mucosa of the oropharynx, hypopharynx, and larynx, and all of these mucosal surfaces are subject to the carcinogenic effects of smoking and alcohol. Many epidemiologic studies have been reported for 'head and neck cancer' and primarily refer to carcinoma of the oral cavity, oropharynx, hypopharynx, and larynx (Curado and Hashibe 2009). Data on the oral cavity will be presented where these have been reported separately; otherwise the discussion will be based on data on these sites studied as a group.

Oral cancer causes destruction of local tissues resulting in pain, inability to chew, swallow, and speak, and altered facial appearance. Metastasis to lymph nodes of the neck occurs frequently, and the metastatic malignant cells can invade vital tissues of the neck such as major nerves and blood vessels. The two major treatment modalities for oral cancer are surgical resection with neck dissection and radiation therapy to a field that includes the primary site and regional lymph nodes with evidence of metastases. The need to eliminate the entire malignant tumor often leads to extensive loss or damage to orofacial tissues. Despite surgery and/or radiation therapy, oral cancer can recur at the primary site or in the neck. The 5-year survival rate is only about 55% overall, but survival is much better for small localized lesions (stage I disease) where the 5-year survival is above 80% (Neville and Day 2002; Jemal et al. 2010).

The morbidity and mortality from oral cancer can be reduced through prevention. Primary prevention is achieved by reduction or elimination of risk factors due to lifestyle or habits, thus avoiding the development of disease. Oral cancer is strongly associated with tobacco use and alcohol drinking. In a global analysis of cancer mortality that can be attributed to behavioural and environmental risk factors, 52% of deaths from oral and oropharyngeal cancer (163,000 deaths/year) are attributable to smoking and alcohol use. When high-income countries and low- and middle-income countries are separately analyzed, 80% of oral and oropharyngeal cancer deaths (32,000 deaths/year) in high-income countries are attributable to these risk factors (Danaei et al. 2005). Better education of health care professionals and the public about the risk of oral cancer from tobacco and alcohol can curtail these habits and reduce the incidence of oral cancer and the burden of treatment.

Secondary prevention is achieved by treatment of incipient or early lesions to stop progression of disease and to promote a return to health. The oral mucosa is accessible to regular examination with simple equipment, so monitoring, detection, and treatment of early disease are highly feasible. Oral cancer may be preceded by a clinically identifiable premalignant lesion, which is typically a white or red patch, called leukoplakia and erythroplakia, respectively. Premalignant oral lesions and early oral cancer are often subtle and asymptomatic, but they can be detected by clinical oral examination by a health care professional who is familiar with the clinical features of these lesions. Secondary prevention also requires effective treatment of premalignant lesions and early cancer (Neville and Day 2002).

Secondary prevention complements primary prevention by intercepting disease that develops in the absence of known or controllable risk factors or after the exposure to carcinogenic agents has ceased. Early intervention increases the chance of success of treatment with minimal side effects and complications.

Why do people get dental decay, periodontal disease, and cancer?

It would be important for the dental practitioner to identify those patients who are at high risk for dental disease. Some people just seem prone to disease. Some, despite all effects of optimal dental hygiene and healthy diets struggle to avoid dental decay and periodontal disease, and are worried about oral cancer. We discuss more in detail throughout the book what the risk factors are that increase a person's risk to dental disease. It seems that genetic susceptibility, poor oral hygiene, poor diets, and lifestyle choices all combine to increase the risk for poor oral health outcomes.

Poor oral hygiene

Poor oral hygiene is an obvious risk factor for dental diseases, primarily dental caries and periodontal disease. Although some people manage to remain dental disease free with minimal daily hygiene, mouth care remains one of the best preventive measures for controlling the onset of dental disease. It is the mainstay of primary prevention.

Lifestyle choices

A smoker who indulges in frequent snacks containing sugar will undoubtedly struggle with not only coronal caries but with root caries as he develops deep periodontal pockets. The outcome is early tooth loss, and a compromise in his ability to eat healthy foods. This creates a spiral of deteriorating poor oral health. Changing one's lifestyle is difficult, no question. However, when a dentist or hygienist is successful in influencing a patient's lifestyle choices, and that person changes for the better with obvious improved oral health, there is a sense of satisfaction for both patient and dental practitioner.

Diet and preventing oral cancer

Oral cancer rates can also be influenced by the diet. Although counter-intuitive, some researchers have found that a diet rich in animal protein may be protective (Carley *et al.* 1994; Morse *et al.* 2000), while others found higher intake of fruits protective (Winn 1995; Horn-Ross *et al.* 1997).

Smoking: an addiction that increases the risk for all three dental diseases

Caries

The evidence that smoking is an independent risk factor for caries in children is accumulating. For example, a study by Leroy *et al.* (2007) indicated that passive smoke was a risk factor for caries in children even after other known risk factors were taken into account. One study *in vitro* may have uncovered a mechanism to explain this increased risk for caries (Baboni *et al.* 2010).

Periodontal disease

The more adults smoke, the greater their risk for periodontal disease (Haber *et al.* 1993; Martinez-Canut *et al.* 1995). Smoking affects periodontal tissue vasculature, promotes proliferation of periodontal pathogens, and reduces the immune response to invading periodontal bacteria. Smoking cessation benefits patients with periodontal disease (Dietrich *et al.* 2007). Thus, long-term smoking makes it difficult to treat periodontitis. Indeed, a subset of refractory periodontitis patients is smokers (Schenkein *et al.* 1995).

Oral cancer

The link between tobacco use and oral cancer has been established (US Department of Health and Human Services 2004). It is a global problem, and the effects of tobacco consumption can be worse in some countries than others according to Professor Newell Johnson (2001):

> "Taken together, the effects of tobacco use, heavy alcohol consumption, and poor diet probably explain over 90 percent of cases of head and neck cancer."

Getting patients to change their habits and reduce excessive tobacco use and alcohol consumption would obviously go a long way to prevent oral cancer. One approach would be education since very few people know the risks for oral cancer (Horowitz, *et al.* 1995).

Based on Gelskey (1999) and a general knowledge of the caries and oral cancer literature, a summary table of causation could be developed (Table 1-4). There are still unanswered questions as to the role of cigarette smoke contributing to the etiology of caries, periodontal disease, and oral cancer. However, it can be concluded from this table that smoking is a major risk factor in the development of all three major oral diseases.

Can dental professionals prevent oral diseases before they occur?

A common thread of prevention attempts to tie these three main oral diseases together. Clearly their etiologies are different. Caries results from opportunistic bacteria that produce acids from dietary sugars. Periodontitis results from the growth of proteolytic bacteria deep in the gingival crevice in conditions of low oxygen tension and protein nutrient supply. Oral cancers result from the uncontrolled growth of dysplastic host cells as a result of carcinogenic stimuli. Each dental disease requires separate preventive strategies. Preventing these diseases on a population basis will require public health strategies

Table 1-4 Smoking—a risk factor for all three dental diseases

Criteria of causation	What is needed	Caries	Periodontal Disease	Oral cancer
strength of association	Does the association produce high odds ratios (after regression analysis)?	yes	yes	yes
consistency	Do other studies looking at the same association find similar results?	yes	yes	yes
specificity	Does the disease increase when the cause is introduced (or decrease when taken away)?	Some evidence	yes	yes
temporality	Does the cause precede the disease?	?	yes	yes
biological gradient	Is there a dose response?	ND	yes	yes
biological plausibility	Does the biological mechanism make sense?	mechanism unknown	yes	yes
coherence	Is the cause not in conflict with the natural history of the disease?	yes	yes	?
analogy	Is the cause associated with other diseases of similar etiology?	yes	yes	yes
experimental evidence	Do clinical trials prove causality?	None available, may be unethical to test	None available, may be unethical to test	None available, may be unethical to test

that mostly involve increasing the standard of living, better education, and improved access to professional care. These are lofty goals for some third world countries with limited resources. The more developed countries have managed to do this by making oral health an important part of overall general health and spending a higher proportion of their health care budgets on oral diseases. Their populations therefore experience relatively low oral disease prevalence despite engaging in high risk activities, such as the consumption of sugar-rich processed foods, excess alcohol ingestion, regular tobacco use, and neglect of the oral cavity. The WHO is attempting to reduce the risk of oral diseases by promoting healthy lifestyles, encouraging public health programs, improving education, and encouraging the control of chronic diseases such as diabetes (Petersen and Ogawa 2005; Petersen 2009).

This textbook is not meant to be comprehensive in terms of public health solutions to these diseases. Nor is it comprehensive in terms of providing advice on how to manage diseases once they have taken root. The reader of this text will find strategies to prevent dental diseases in clinical practice. The reader might be a dentist, dental hygienist, a dental student, a dental hygiene student, a dental therapist or dental assistant, or any person working, or seeking to work, in an auxiliary position in a dental or dental hygiene clinic. Some dental public health programs now provide direct professional care in government-sponsored dental clinics or subsidized nongovernmental organiza-

tions. Such an organization is the Head Start program in the US that partners with private practitioners (From: http://www.aapd.org/headstart/information.asp).

Final remarks

In this text, with a heavy focus on caries, the reader will be able to gain some insight on how to identify patients at risk for dental disease, how to introduce therapies that are known to reduce the risk, how to prevent caries or reverse caries, how to diagnose and prevent periodontal disease, and how to help those patients at risk for oral cancers. Education and guidance is paramount in a clinical practice setting in an attempt to achieve better oral health for the patient. Restorative dentistry can only be successful when the disease is under control. To quote the founder of "Your Teeth for a Lifetime," Dr. William Hettenhausen, who dedicated his career to preventive dentistry and nutrition, "You don't call the carpenter when your house is on fire."

References

Albandar, J.M., Brunelle, J.A., Kingman, A. (1999) Destructive periodontal disease in adults 30 years of age and older in the United Stated, 1988–1992. *Journal of Periodontology,* 70, 13–29.

Armfield, J. and Spencer, A.J. (2008) Quarter of a century of change: caries experience in Australian children, 1977–2002. *Australian Dental Journal,* 53, 151–159.

Axelsson, P. and Lindhe J. (1978) Effect of controlled oral hygiene procedures on caries and periodontal disease in adults. *Journal of Clinical Periodontology,* 5, 133–151.

Baboni, F.B., Guariza Filho, O., Moreno, A.N., *et al.* (2010) Influence of cigarette smoke condensate on cariogenic and candidal biofilm formation on orthodontic materials. *American Journal of Orthodontics and Dentofacial Orthopedics*, 138, 427–434.

Black, G.V. (1875) Probabilities. *American Journal of Dental Science*, 8, 241.

Bratthall, D., Hansel-Petersson, G., Sundherg, H. (1996) Reasons for the caries decline: what do the experts believe? *European Journal of Oral Science*, 104, 416–422.

Broadbent, J.M., Thomson, W.M., Poulton, R. (2008) Trajectory patterns of dental caries experience in the permanent dentition to the fourth decade of life. *Journal of Dental Research*, 87, 69–72.

Carley, K.W, Puttaiah, R., Alvarez, J.O., *et al.* (1994) Diet and oral pre-malignancy in female south Indian tobacco and betel chewers: a case-control study. *Nutrition and Cancer*, 22, 73–84.

Ccahuana-Vásquez, R.A., Tabchoury, C.P., Tenuta, L.M., *et al.* (2007) Effect of frequency of sucrose exposure on dental biofilm composition and enamel demineralization in the presence of fluoride. *Caries Research*, 41, 9–15.

Chalmers, J. (2006) Minimal Intervention Dentistry: Part 1. Strategies for addressing the new caries challenge in older patients. *Journal of the Canadian Dental Association*, 72, 427–433.

Chen, L., Ma, L., Park, N.H., *et al.* (2001) Cariogenic actinomyces identified with a beta-glucosidase-dependent green color reaction to Gardenia jasminoides extract. *Journal of Clinical Microbiology*, 39, 3009–3012.

Colquhoun, J. (1997) Why I changed my mind about water fluoridation. *Perspectives in Biology and Medicine*, 41, 29–44.

Curado, M.P. and Hashibe, M. (2009) Recent changes in the epidemiology of head and neck cancer. *Current Opinions in Oncology*, 21, 194–200.

Cury, J.A., Andaló Tenuta, L.M., Ribeiro, C.C.C., *et al.* (2004) The importance of fluoride dentifrices to the current dental caries prevalence in Brazil. *Brazilian Dental Journal*, 15, 167–174.

Danaei, G., Vander Hoorn, S., Lopez, A.D., *et al.* (2005) Comparative Risk Assessment collaborating group (Cancers). Causes of cancer in the world: comparative risk assessment of nine behavioural and environmental risk factors. *Lancet*, 366(9499), 1784–1793.

Dawes, C. (2003) What is the critical pH and why does a tooth dissolve in acid? *Journal of the Canadian Dental Association*, 69, 722–734.

Dawes, C. and Dibdin, G.H. (1986) A theoretical analysis of the effects of plaque thickness and initial salivary sucrose concentration on diffusion of sucrose into dental plaque and its conversion to acid during salivary clearance. *Journal of Dental Research*, 65, 89–94.

Dibart, S. and Dietrich, T. (2009) *Practical Periodontal Diagnosis and Treatment Planning*, Wiley-Blackwell, Iowa, USA.

Dietrich, T., Maserejian, N.N., Joshipura, K.J., *et al.* (2007) Tobacco use and incidence of tooth loss among US male health professionals. *Journal of Dental Research*, 86, 373–377.

Ericsson, Y. (1949) Enamel-apatite solubility. Investigations into the calcium phosphate equilibrium between enamel and saliva and its relation to dental caries. *Acta Odontologica Scandinavica*, 8 (Suppl 3), 1–139.

Eriksen, H.M., Grytten, J., Holst, D. (1991) Is there a long-term caries-preventive effect of sugar restrictions during World War II? *Acta Odontologica Scandinavia*, 49, 163–167.

Featherstone, J.D. (2004) The caries balance: the basis for caries management by risk assessment. *Oral Health and Preventive Dentistry*, 2 Suppl 1, 259–264.

Filoche, S., Wong, L., Sissons, C.H. (2010) Oral biofilms: emerging concepts in microbial ecology. *Journal of Dental Research*, 89, 8–18.

Gelskey, S.C. (1999) Cigarette smoking and periodontitis: methodology to assess the strength of evidence in support of a causal association. *Community Dentistry and Oral Epidemiology*, 27, 16–24.

Gillings, B.R. (1977) Recent developments in dental plaque disclosants. *Australian Dental Journal*, 22, 260–266.

Haber, J., Wattles, J., Crowley, M., *et al.* (1993) Evidence for cigarette smoking as a major risk factor for periodontitis. *Journal of Periodontology*, 64, 16–23.

Hausmann, E., Raisz, L.G., Miller, W.A. (1970) Endotoxin: stimulation of bone resorption in tissue culture. *Science*, 168(933), 862–864.

Horn-Ross, P.L., Morrow, M., Ljung, B.M. (1997) Diet and the risk of salivary gland cancer. *American Journal of Epidemiology*, 146, 171–176.

Horowitz, A.M., Nourjah, P., Gift, H.C. (1995) U.S. adult knowledge of risk factors and signs of oral cancers: 1990. *Journal of the American Dental Association*, 126, 39–45.

Isokangas, P., Söderling, E., Pienihakkinen, K., *et al.* (2000) Occurrence of dental decay in children after maternal consumption of xylitol chewing gum, a follow-up from 0–5 years of age. *Journal of Dental Research*, 79, 1885–1889.

Jeffcoat, M.K. and Reddy, M.S. (1991) Progression of probing attachment loss in adult periodontitis. *Journal of Periodontology*, 62, 185–189.

Jemal, A., Center, M.M., DeSantis, C., *et al.* (2010) Global patterns of cancer incidence and mortality rates and trends. *Cancer Epidemiology Biomarkers and Prevention*, 19, 1893–1907.

Johnson N. (2001) Tobacco use and oral cancer: a global perspective. *Journal of Dental Education*, 65, 328–339.

Jokstad, A. (1989) The dimensions of everyday class-II cavity preparations for amalgam. *Acta Odontologica Scandinvavica*, 47, 89–99.

Karim, A., Mascarinhas, A.M., Dharamsi, S. (2008) A global oral health course: Isn't it time? *Journal of Dental Education*, 72, 1238–1246.

Keyes, P.H. (1962) Recent advances in caries research. Bacteriology. *International Dental Journal*, 12, 443–464.

Kleinberg, I., Jenkins, G.N., Chatterjee, R., *et al.* (1982). The antimony pH electrode and its role in the assessment and interpretation of dental plaque pH. *Journal of Dental Research*, 61, 1139–1147.

Kulkarni, G.V., Chan, K.H., Sandham, H.J. (1989) An investigation into the use of restriction endonuclease analysis for the study of transmission of Mutans Streptococci. *Journal of Dental Research*, 68, 1155–1161.

Kumar, P.S., Leys, E., Bryk, J.M., *et al.* (2006) Changes in periodontal health status are associated with bacterial community shifts as assessed by quantitative 16S cloning and sequencing. *Journal of Microbiology*, 44, 3665–3673.

Lang, N.P., Ostergaard, E., Löe, H. (1972) A fluorescent plaque disclosing agent. *Journal of Periodontal Research*, 7, 59–67.

Leake, J.L. (2006) Why do we need an oral health care policy in Canada? *Journal of the Canadian Dental Association*, 72, 317.

Leroy, R., Hoppenbrouwers, K., Jara, A., *et al.* (2008). Parental smoking behaviour and caries experience in preschool children. *Community Dentistry and Oral Epidemiology*, 36, 249–257.

Lingstrôm, P., Imfeld, T., Birkhed, D. (1993) Comparison of three different methods for measurement of plaque-pH in humans after consumption of soft bread and potato chips. *Journal of Dental Research*, 72, 865–870.

Listgarten, M.A. (1994) The structure of dental plaque. *Periodontology 2000*, 5, 52–65.

Marsh, P.D. (2003) Are dental diseases examples of ecological catastrophes? *Microbiology*, 149, 279–294.

Marsh, P.D. (1994) Microbial ecology of dental plaque and its significance in health and disease. *Advances in Dental Research*, 8, 263–271.

Marsh, P.D. and Bradshaw, D.J. (1999) Microbial community aspects of dental plaque. In: *Dental Plaque Revisited*, pp. 237–253. Eds. Newman, H.N., M. Wilson, M. Cardiff: BioLine.

Marthaler, T.M. (2004) Changes in dental caries 1953–2003. *Caries Research*, 38, 173–181.

Martinez-Canut, P., Lorca, A., Magán, R. (1995) Smoking and periodontal disease severity. *Journal of Clinical Periodontology*, 22, 743–749.

McDermid, A.S., McKee, A.S., Marsh, P.D. (1988) Effect of environmental pH on enzyme activity and growth of Bacteroides gingivalis W50. *Infections and Immunity*, 56, 1096–1100.

Miyazaki, H. and Morimoto, M. (1996) Changes in caries prevalence in Japan, *European Journal of Oral Science*, 104, 452–458.

Moore, W.E.C. and Moore, L.V.H. (1994) The bacteria of periodontal diseases. *Periodontology 2000*, 5, 66–77.

Morse, D.E., Pendrys, D.G., Katz, R.V., *et al.* (2000) Food group intake and the risk of oral epithelial dysplasia in a United States population. *Cancer Causes and Control,* 11, 713–720.

Mount, G.J. and Ngo, H. (2000) Minimal intervention: a new concept for operative dentistry. *Quintessence*, 31, 527–533.

Neville, B.W. and Day, T.A. (2002) Oral cancer and precancerous lesions. CA: A Cancer Journal for Clinicians, 52, 195–215.

Ngo, H. and Gaffney, S. (2005) Risk Assessment in the Diagnosis and Management of Caries. In: *Preservation and Restoration of Tooth Structure* (Eds. G.J. Mount and W.R. Hume, 2nd edn. pp. 61–82. Knowledge Books and Software. Brighton Queensland AU).

Paes-Leme, A.F., Koo, H., Bellato, C.M., *et al.* (2006) The role of sucrose in cariogenic dental biofilm formation—new insight. *Journal of Dental Research,* 85, 878–887.

Papapanou, P.N. and Behle, J.H. (2009) Mechanisms linking periodontitis to systemic disease. In: *Periodontal Medicine and Systems Biology*. Henderson, B., Curtis, M., Seymour, R., *et al.,* Eds. Wiley-Blackwell, pp. 97–116.

Petersen, P.E. and Ogawa H. (2005) Strengthening the prevention of periodontal disease: The WHO approach. *Journal of Periodontology*, 76, 2187–2193.

Petersen, P.E. (2003) The World Oral Health Report 2003: Continuous improvement of oral health in the 21st century—the approach of the WHO Global Oral Health Programme. *Community Dentistry and Oral Epidemiology*, 31, 3–24.

Pretty, I.A., Edgar, W.M., Smith, P.W., *et al.* (2005) Quantification of dental plaque in the research environment. *Journal of Dentistry*, 33, 193–207.

Research Science and Therapy Committee of the American Academy of Periodontology. (1999) Pathogenisis of Periodontal disease. *Journal of Periodontology*, 70, 457–470.

Sanders, W.E. and Sanders, C.C. (1984) Modification of normal flora by antibiotics: effects on individuals and the environment. In: *New Dimensions in Antimicrobial Chemotherapy*, (Eds. R.K. Koot and M.A. Sande), pp. 217–241. Churchill Livingston, New York.

Schenkein, H.A., Gunsolley, J.C., Koertge, T.E., *et al.* (1995) Smoking and its effects on early-onset periodontitis. *Journal of the American Dental Association*, 126, 1107–1113.

Stephan, R.M. and Miller, B.F. (1943) A Quantitative Method for Evaluating Physical and Chemical Agents which Modify Production of Acid in Bacterial Plaques on Human Teeth. *Journal of Dental Research*, 22, 45–51.

Stookey, G.H. (2008) The effect of saliva on dental caries. *Journal of the American Dental Association*, 139, 11S–17S.

The World Health Organization. (1946) Preamble to the Constitution of the World Health Organization as adopted by the International Health Conference, New York, 19–22 June, 1946.

Thomson, W.M., Broadbent, J.M., Poulton, R., *et al.* (2006) Changes in periodontal disease experience from 26 to 32 years of age in a birth cohort. *Journal of Periodontology*, 77, 947–954.

Tobias, J. and Hochhauser, D. (2010) *Cancer and its Management*. 6th edn. Wiley-Blackwell, Iowa, USA.

US Department of Health and Human Services. (2004) Oral cavity and pharyngeal cancers, congenital malformations, infant mortality and child physical and cognitive development, and dental diseases. In: *The health consequences of smoking: a report of the Surgeon General*. pp. 63–115, 577–610, 732–766. Washington, DC.

Von der Fehr, F.R. and Haugejorden, O. (1997) The start of caries decline and related fluoride use in Norway. *European Journal of Oral Science,* 105, 21–26.

Wesolowski, M. (2008) Extension for prevention? Prevention before extension! *Dentalzeitung*, 3, 34–36.

Winn, D.M. (1995) Diet and nutrition in the etiology of oral cancer. *American Journal of Clinical Nutrition*, 61, 437S–445S.

2

Caries detection and diagnosis

Iain A. Pretty

Portions of this work have previously appeared in "Caries detection and diagnosis: novel technologies. *J Dent*, 34 2006(10), 727–739."

Summary of chapter

Recent years have seen an increase in research activity surrounding diagnostic methods, particularly in the assessment of early caries lesions. The drive for this has come from two disparate directions. The first is from the dentifrice industry, which is keen to develop techniques that would permit caries clinical trials (CCT) to be reduced in duration and subject numbers to permit the investigation of novel new anti-caries activities. The second is from clinicians who, armed with the therapies to remineralize early lesions are now seeking methods to reliably detect such demineralized areas and implement true preventative dentistry. This review examines novel technologies and the research supporting their use. Techniques based on visual, optical, radiographic, and some emerging technologies are discussed. Each has its benefits although systems based on the auto-fluorescence (such as quantitative light-induced fluorescence [QLF]) of teeth and electrical resistance (such as electrical conductance measurement [ECM]) seem to offer the most hope for achieving reliable, accurate detection of the earliest stages of enamel demineralization.

Introduction

There has been a developing paradigm shift in dentistry—one moving away from a surgical model of treatment to one based on the prevention of disease. As with many disease entities, prevention is at its most effective when detection is early within the natural history of the disease. Our understanding of the caries process has continued to advance, with the vast majority of evidence supporting a dynamic process that is affected by numerous modifiers tending to push the mineral equilibrium in one direction or another, that is, toward remineralization or demineralization (Holt 2001). All of these interactions are taking place in the complex biofilm overlaying the tooth surface that comprises the pellicle as well as the oral microflora of the plaque (Featherstone 2004). The modifiers of this system are well known and are summarized in Table 2-1. Figure 2-1 presents an overview of the dynamics of the caries process (Featherstone 2004).

With this greater understanding of the disease comes an opportunity to promote 'preventive' therapies that encourage the remineralization of non-cavitated lesions resulting in inactive lesions and the preservation of tooth structure, function, and aesthetics. Central to this vision is the ability to detect caries lesions at an early stage and correctly quantify the degree of mineral loss, ensuring that the correct intervention is instigated (al-Khateeb *et al.* 1997; Amaechi and Higham 2001). The failure to detect early caries, leaving those detectable only at the deep enamel, or cavitated stage, has resulted in poor results and outcomes for remineralization therapies. It can also be argued that practitioners have often failed to embrace prevention because its efficacy cannot be easily monitored. Therefore, the ability to monitor early lesions and determine if they have indeed arrested or stabilized is also key to ensuring that effective prevention can become commonplace in general dentistry.

Table 2.1 Risk and modifying factors for caries

Primary risk factors

Saliva

1. ability of minor salivary glands to produce saliva
2. consistency of unstimulated (resting) saliva
3. pH of unstimulated saliva
4. stimulated salivary flow rate
5. buffering capacity of stimulated saliva

Diet

6. number of sugar exposures per day
7. number of acid exposures per day

Fluoride

8. past and current exposure

Oral biofilm

9. differential staining
10. composition
11. activity

Modifying factors

12. past and current dental status
13. past and current medical status
14. compliance with oral hygiene and dietary advice
15. lifestyle
16. socioeconomic status

A range of new detection and monitoring systems have been developed and are either currently available to practitioners or will be shortly. Such technologies are combined with more rigorous visual examination techniques, and there is considerable interest in the International Caries Detection and Assessment System (ICDAS) (Ismail *et al.* 2007; Ismail *et al.* 2008).

It is a crucial distinction that the systems described within this chapter are correctly classified as caries *detection* systems, rather than diagnostic systems. Diagnosis is a decision process that rests with the clinician and is informed by, initially, detection of a lesion and should be followed by an assessment of the patient's caries risk, which may include the number of new caries lesions, past caries experience, diet, presence or absence of favorable or unfavorable modifying factors (salivary flow, mutans streptococci counts, oral hygiene), and qualitative aspects of the disease such as color and anatomical location (Kidd 1998). These detection systems are therefore aimed at augmenting the diagnostic process by facilitating either earlier detection of the disease or enabling it to be quantified in an objective manner. Visual inspection, the most ubiquitous caries detection system, is subjective. Assessment of features such as color and texture are qualitative in nature. These assessments provide some information on the severity of the disease but fall short of true quantification (Maupomé and Pretty 2004a). They are also limited in their detection threshold, and their ability to detect early, noncavitated lesions restricted to enamel is poor. It is this

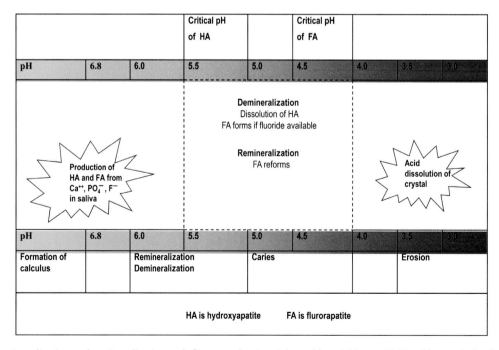

Figure 2-1 Demineralization and remineralization cycle for enamel caries. Adapted from McIntyre 2005, with permission from Knowledge Books and Software.

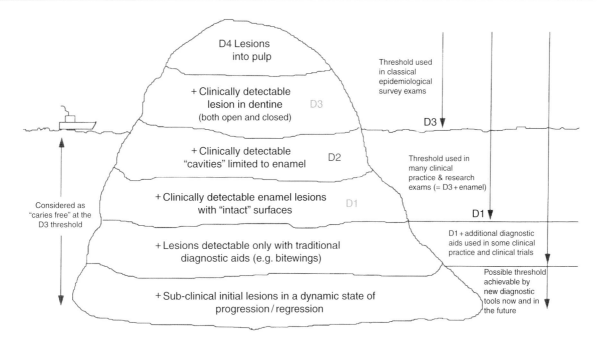

Figure 2-2 The 'iceberg' of caries and the influence of detection system. Modified from Pitts 2001, with permission from the American Dental Education Association.

ability to quantify and/or detect lesions earlier that the novel diagnostic systems offer to the clinician.

Pitts provides a useful visual description of the benefits of early caries detection (Pitts 2001). Using the metaphor of an iceberg, it can be seen that traditional methods of caries detection result in a vast quantity of undetected lesions (Figure 2-2). There is a clinical argument about the significance of these lesions, with some authors believing that only a small percentage will progress to more severe disease, however, it is a undisputed fact that all cavitated lesions with extension in pulp began their natural history as an early lesion.

From this it can be seen that as the sensitivity of the detection device increases so does the number of lesions detected. It can also be seen that the new detection tools are required to identify those lesions that would be amenable to remineralizing therapies (Pitts 1997).

When assessing the effectiveness of such methods, the preferred reporting metrics are those of traditional diagnostic science; namely specificity, sensitivity, area under the ROC curve, and the correlation with the truth (the true state of the disease, established using a gold standard). The reliability or reproducibility of the test can be established using either intra-class correlation or kappa co-efficients depending on the nature of the metric output, that is, either continuous or ordinal (Pretty and Maupomé 2004a; Pretty anbd Maupomé 2004b).

Novel diagnostic systems are based upon the measurement of a physical signal; these are surrogate measures of the caries process. Examples of the physical signals that can be used in this way include X-rays, visible light, laser light, electronic current, ultrasound, and possibly surface roughness (Verdonschot 2003). For a caries-detection device to function it must be capable of initiating and receiving the signal as well as being able to interpret the strength of the signal in a meaningful way. Table 2-2 demonstrates the physical principles and the

Table 2-2 Methods of caries detection based on their underlying physical principles. Modified from (Angmar-Mansson, al-Khateeb *et al.* 1998)

Physical principle	Application in caries detection
X-rays	Digital subtraction radiography
	Digital image enhancement
Visible light	Fibre optic transillumination (FOTI)
	Quantitative light-induced fluorescence (QLF)
	Digital image fibre optic transillumination (DiFOTI)
Laser light	Laser fluorescence measurement (DIAGNOdent)
Electrical current	Electrical conductance measurement (ECM)
	Electrical impedance measurement
Ultrasound	Ultrasonic caries detector

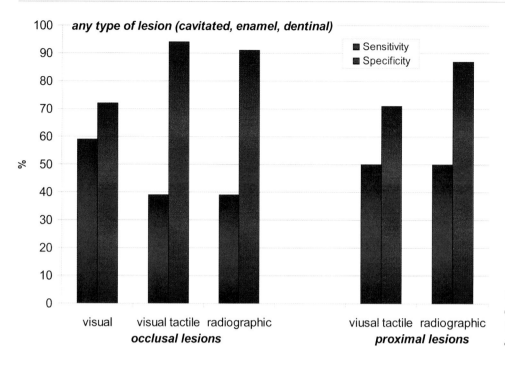

Figure 2-3 Effectiveness of traditional caries detection systems based on lesions of any severity, after Bader *et al.* 2001.

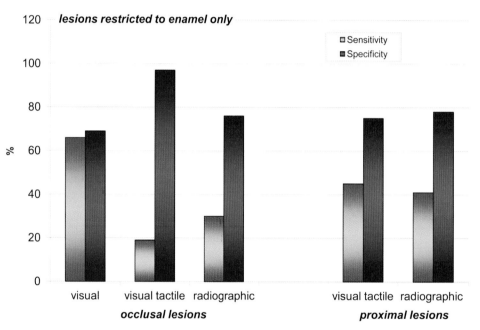

Figure 2-4 Effectiveness of traditional caries detection systems based on lesions restricted to enamel only, after Bader *et al.* 2001.

detection systems that have taken advantage of them (Verdonschot 2003).

It is worthwhile to take an overview of the performance of the traditional caries detection systems, and these are shown, in terms of sensitivity and specificity in Figures 2-3 and 2-4. Figure 2-3 demonstrates the methods' performance irrespective of the severity of the lesion, with Figure 2-4 presenting the same data for lesions confined to enamel.

These data are based on the excellent systematic review by Bader (Bader *et al.* 2001), who restricted his assessment of studies to those that employed histological validation. This, therefore, indicates that while the 'true' diagnostic outcome is not in doubt, these studies were conducted *in vitro*, and hence the actual values in clinical practice are likely to be poorer. A scant assessment of the figures indicates that while specificity is adequate, the sensitivity scores of the traditional methods are poor, with many being significantly less than chance. That is, a guess would provide the same or a better result in many cases. These figures serve to illustrate the need for detection devices that are objective, quantitative, sensitive, and enable early lesions to be monitored over time. This longitudinal monitoring is especially important when one considers the treatment of early caries lesions.

The following sections describe those systems that have potential to meet the aims of clinicians and researchers for enhanced sensitivity and objective, metric, continuous measures of mineralization status.

Detection systems based on purely visual examinations

Although much of this chapter is concerned with technological advances in caries detection, it should not be forgotten that the vast majority of carious lesions are detected by dentists using visual methods. The use of accompanying tactile examination, while popular in the United States, is not recommended because rigorous probing of lesions can lead to cavitation. The use of a blunt probe, ideally a periodontal probe, can be used to detect differences in surface roughness.

In the early 2000s, a group of caries experts felt that there was a need to develop a new visual index for caries, one that could be used in a range of settings, from epidemiology through to general practice. From the development of the index, the proposal was to develop a caries management system where care pathways were linked to lesion status and patient risk factors. A number of consensus meetings were held, and the International Caries Detection and Assessment System (ICDAS) was developed (Pitts 2004). The current iteration of the system is known as ICDAS II and has codes for smooth surface and occlusal lesions.

The ICDAS system is one that advocates a careful and thorough assessment of the dentition following cleaning and drying (although Code 1 and Code 2 lesions require examination wet and dry in order to discriminate between them). Early lesions are categorized in Codes 1–3, and these are the lesion types that would be most amenable to preventive intervention (Ismail *et al.* 2007; Ismail *et al.* 2008). The ICDAS foundation has undertaken considerable work to promote the system, and there is an online training system that is free to access. The Web site provides examples of each of the lesion types and offers a training course in four languages. Readers are encouraged to access the site and learn more about the system at http://icdas.smile-on.com/.

There is developing evidence that ICDAS can prove to be a useful and reliable system in detecting early lesions (Braga *et al.* 2009a; Braga *et al.* 2009b; Diniz *et al.* 2009; Agustsdottir *et al.* 2010). Work is ongoing to implement this within a general practice setting, and the development of the care pathways linked to lesion codes is currently under way. However, within the introduction to this chapter, it was recognized that there are two components of systems for caries detection that are required within a general practice setting—The first is the ability to detect lesions, and the second is to be able to monitor them over time. Currently there are insufficient data to determine if the ICDAS codes are sensitive enough to support effective lesion monitoring. For example, is it possible for a lesion to double in size (or severity) and yet remain within the same code? Research is being undertaken in this area, and efforts have been made to combine ICDAS examinations with other caries detection technologies. Despite this limitation, the ICDAS methodology has a great deal to offer practitioners in terms of developing a rigorous approach to caries examination as part of their patient examinations (Ferreira Zandoná *et al.* 2010).

Detection systems based on electrical current measurement

Every material possesses its own electrical signature. For example, when a current is passed through the substance the properties of the material dictate the degree to which that current is conducted. Conditions in which the material is stored or physical changes to the structure of the material will have an effect on this conductance. Biological materials are no exception, and the concentration of fluids and electrolytes contained within such materials largely govern their conductivity (Ekstrand *et al.* 1998). For example, dentine is more conductive than enamel. In dental systems there is generally a probe, from which the current is passed; a substrate, typically the tooth; and a contra-electrode, usually a metal bar held in the patient's hand. Measurements can be taken either from enamel or exposed dentine surfaces (Verdonschot *et al.* 1995).

In its simplest form caries can be described as a process resulting in an increase in porosity of the tissue, be it enamel or dentine. This increased porosity results in a higher fluid content than sound tissue, and this difference can be detected by electrical measurement by decreased electrical resistance or impedance.

Electronic Caries Monitor (ECM)

The ECM device employs a single, fixed-frequency alternating current, which attempts to measure the 'bulk resistance' of tooth tissue (Longbottom and Huysmans 2004). See Figure 2-5.

This can be undertaken at either a site or surface level. When measuring the electrical properties of a particular *site* on a tooth, the ECM probe is directly applied to the site, typically a fissure, and the site measured. During the five-second measurement cycle, compressed air is expressed from the tip of the probe, and this results in a collection of data over the measurement period, described as a drying

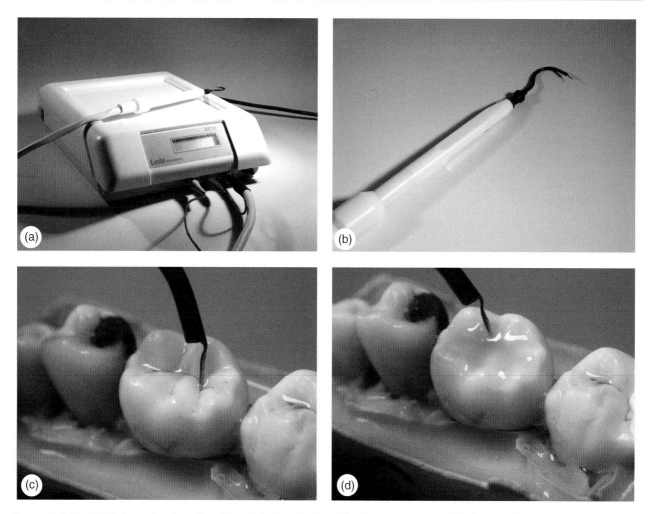

Figure 2-5 The ECM device (version 4) and its clinical application: (a) The ECM machine; (b) The ECM handpiece; (c) Site-specific measurement technique; (d) Surface-specific measurement technique.

profile, that can provide useful information for characterizing the lesion. An example of this is shown in Figure 2-6.

Although it is generally accepted that the increase in porosity associated with caries is responsible for the mechanism of action for ECM (Longbottom and Huysmans 2004), there are some points to consider:

1. Do electrical measurements of carious lesions measure the volume of the pores, and if so, is it the total pore volume or just a portion, perhaps the superficial portion, that is measured?
2. Do electrical measurements measure pore depth? If this is the case, what happens during remineralization where the superficial layer may remineralize, leaving a pore beneath?
3. Is the morphological complexity of the pores a factor in the measurement of conductivity?

A number of physical factors also will affect ECM results. These include such things as the temperature of

the tooth, the thickness of the tissue, the hydration of the material (that is, one shouldn't dry the teeth prior to use), and the surface area (Huysmans *et al.* 2000; Longbottom and Huysmans 2004).

An excellent review of the performance of ECM was undertaken in 2000 by Huysmans (2000) who collated information from a variety of validation studies. She was unable to perform a meta-analysis of these data, stating that aspects of the studies such as version of equipment, storage medium, cut-offs, and tooth type prevented direct comparisons. A summary of her findings is presented in Table 2-3. These demonstrate a good to excellent range of area under the curves (AUCs) with the exception of surface-specific premolars when assessing at the D1 level (lesions restricted to enamel). The sensitivity and specificity values were assessed from a number of studies. For site-specific measurements these were sensitivity 74.8(±11.9) and specificity 87.6(±10), and for surface-specific measurements 63(±2.8) and 79.5(±9.2). The lower efficacy in surface-specific

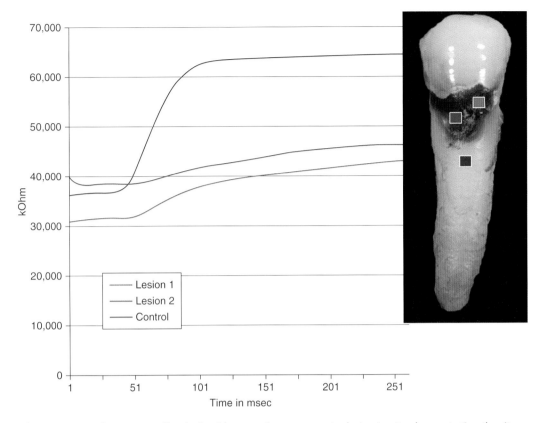

Figure 2-6 A demonstration of an ECM profile obtained from a primary root caries lesion *in vitro* demonstrating the sites assessed.

Table 2-3 ECM ROC areas under the curve

ROC – Area	Diagnostic Threshold	Tooth type	Surface or site specific measurement	Study
0.82	D1	Premolars	Site specific	(Rock and Kidd 1988)
0.80	D1	Molars	Site specific	(Ricketts, Kidd *et al.* 1997)
0.84	D3	Premolars	Site specific	(Rock and Kidd 1988)
0.82	D3	Molars	Site specific	(Verdonschot, Wenzel *et al.* 1993)
0.80	D1	Premolars	Surface specific	(Huysmans, Longbottom *et al.* 1998)
0.67	D1	Premolars	Surface specific	(Huysmans, Longbottom *et al.* 1998)
0.94	D3	Premolars	Surface specific	(Huysmans, Longbottom *et al.* 1998)
0.79	D3	Molars	Surface specific	(Pereira, Huysmans *et al.* 1999)

measurements has led to this area of research being neglected, with the vast majority of publications concentrating on site-specific measurements.

The reproducibility of the device has been assessed in a number of publications and has been rated as good to excellent for both measurement techniques. The intraclass correlation coefficients for site specific were 0.76, and 0.93 for surface specific (Huysmans *et al.* 1998). It is important to note that these high figures relate to the use of the device in a controlled laboratory setting. Further studies *in vitro* are required before the device can be used for monitoring lesions longitudinally. For example, some authors have stated that the limits of agreement

can be as much as ±580KΩ for surface-specific measurements. If the range for an occlusal surface is considered as 100–5,000 KΩ then this could be a substantial source of error (Ekstrand *et al.* 1997).

A clinical trial has been undertaken using the ECM device on root caries, and the successful outcome of this study suggests that dentine may be a more suitable tissue for ECM. The study assessed the effect of 5,000-ppm fluoride dentifrice against 1,100 ppm on 201 subjects with at least one root caries lesion. These were site-specific measurements taken using the airflow function of the ECM unit. After 3 and 6 months, there was statistical difference between the two groups, with the higher fluoride group

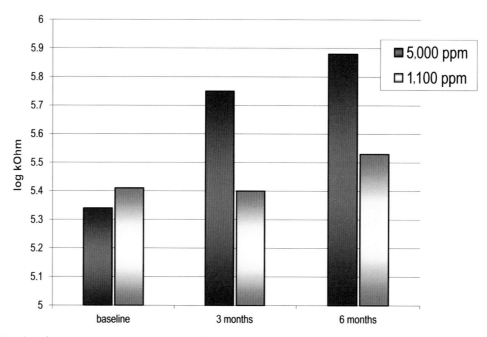

Figure 2-7 ECM values from a root caries study using high and low concentrations of fluoride dentifrices. The increasing ECM values relate to a reduction in porosity and increase in electrical resistance.

showing a better remineralizing capability than the lower fluoride paste users (Baysan *et al.* 2001). See Figure 2-7.

This is good evidence to suggest that ECM is capable of longitudinal monitoring and that clinicians may be able to employ the device to monitor attempts at remineralizing, and thus potentially arresting, root caries lesions in their patients (Baysan *et al.* 2001).

A further application of electronic monitoring of caries is that of Electrical Impedance Spectroscopy (EIS). Unlike ECM which uses a fixed frequency (23 Hz), EIS scans a range of electrical frequencies and provides information on capacitance and impendence among others (Huysmans *et al.* 1996). This process provides the potential for more detailed analysis of the structure of the tooth to be developed, including the presence and extent of caries (Longbottom and Huysmans 2004). A simplified commercial system, CarieScan, has been developed, and this is currently available to the market (www.cariescan.com/) (Longbottom *et al.* 2009). Although there are many published articles describing the technology and theory behind the system, its use and utility in general practice requires further evaluation.

Radiographic techniques

Digital radiographs

Digital radiography has offered the potential to increase the diagnostic yield of dental radiographs, and this has manifested itself in subtraction radiography. A digital radiograph (or a traditional radiograph that has been digitized) is comprised of a number of pixels. Each pixel carries a value between 0 and 255, with 0 being black and 255 being white. The values in between represent shades of gray, and it can be quickly appreciated that a digital radiograph, with a potential of 256 gray levels has significantly lower resolution than a conventional radiograph that contain millions of gray levels. This would suggest that digital radiographs would have a lower diagnostic yield than that of traditional radiographs. Research has confirmed this, with sensitivities and specificities of digital radiographs being significantly lower than those of regular radiographs when assessing small proximal lesions (Verdonschot *et al.* 1992). However, digital radiographs offer the potential of image enhancement by applying a range of algorithms, some of which enhance the white end of the gray scale (such as Rayleigh and hyperbolic logarithmic probability) and others the black end (hyperbolic cube root function). When these enhanced radiographs are assessed, their diagnostic performance is at least as good as conventional radiographs (Verdonschot *et al.* 1999), with reported values of 0.95 (sensitivity) and 0.83 (specificity) for approximal lesions. See Figure 2-8 for an example of this enhancement.

When these findings are considered, one must remember that digital radiographs offer a decrease in radiographic dose and thus offer additional benefits than diagnostic yield. Digital images can also be archived and replicated with ease.

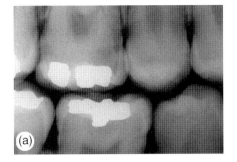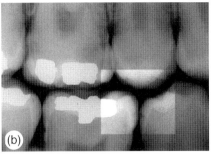

Figure 2-8 Comparison of regular and enhanced digital radiographs: (a) Digital radiograph; (b) Enhance radiograph where the interproximal lesions between first molar and second premolar can be seen more clearly.

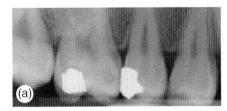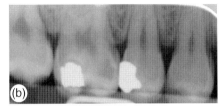

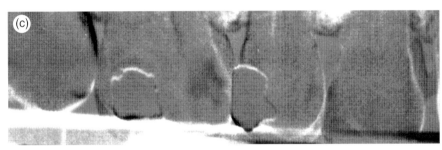

Figure 2-9 Example of a subtraction of two digital bitewing radiographs: (a) Radiograph showing proximal lesion on mesial surface of first molar; (b) Follow-up radiograph taken 12 months later; (c) The areas of difference between the two films are shown as black, that is, in this case the proximal lesion has become more radiolucent and hence has progressed.

Subtraction radiology

As described above, using digital radiographs offers a number of opportunities for image enhancement, processing, and manipulation. One of the most promising technologies in this regard is that of radiographic subtraction, which has been extensively evaluated for both the detection of caries and also the assessment of bone loss in periodontal studies (White *et al.* 1999). The basic premise of subtraction radiology is that two radiographs of the same object can be compared using their pixel values. If the images have been taken using either a geometry stabilizing system (that is, a bitewing holder) or software has been employed to register the images together, then any differences in the pixel values must be due to change in the object (Wenzel *et al.* 1993). The value of the pixels from the first object is subtracted from the second image. If there is no change, the resultant pixel will be scored 0; any value that is not 0 must be attributable to either the onset or progression of demineralization, or regression. Subtraction images therefore emphasise this change and the sensitivity is increased. It is clear from this description that the radiographs must be perfectly aligned, or as close to perfect as possible. Any discrepancies in alignment would result in pixels being incorrectly represented as change (Ellwood *et al.* 1997). Several studies have demonstrated the power of this system, with impressive results for primary and secondary caries. However, uptake of this system has been low, presumably due to the need for well-aligned images. Recent advances in software have enabled two images with moderate alignment to be correctly aligned and then subtracted (Ellwood *et al.* 1997). This may facilitate the introduction of this technology into mainstream practice where such alignment algorithms could be built into practice software currently used for displaying digital radiographs. An example of a subtraction radiograph is shown in Figure 2-9.

Enhanced visual techniques

Fiber Optic Transillumination (FOTI and DiFOTI)

The basis of visual inspection of caries is based upon the phenomenon of light scattering. Sound enamel is comprised of modified hydroxyapatite crystals that are densely packed, producing an almost transparent structure. The color of teeth, for example, is strongly influenced by the underlying dentin shade. When enamel is disrupted, for example in the presence of demineralization, the penetrating photons of light are scattered (that is, they change direction, although do not lose energy), which results in an optical disruption. In normal, visible light, this appears as a 'whiter' area—the so-called white spot (Choksi *et al.* 1994). This appearance is enhanced if the lesion is dried; the water is removed from the porous lesion. Water has a similar refractive index (RI) to enamel, but when it is removed and replaced by air, which has a much lower RI than enamel, the lesion is shown more

clearly. This demonstrates the importance of ensuring the clinical caries examinations are undertaken on clean, *dry* teeth (Cortes *et al.* 2003). See Figure 2-10.

Fiber optic transillumination takes advantage of these optical properties of enamel and enhances them by using a high intensity white light that is presented through a small aperture in the form of a dental handpiece. Light is shone through the tooth, and the scattering effect can be seen as shadows in enamel and dentine, with the device's strength the ability to help discriminate between early enamel and early dentine lesions. See Figure 2-11.

A further benefit of FOTI is that it can be used for the detection of caries on all surfaces and is particularly useful at proximal lesions. The research around FOTI is somewhat polarized, with a recent review finding a mean sensitivity of only 14 and a specificity of 95 when considering occlusal dentine lesions, and 4% and 100% for proximal lesions (Bader *et al.* 2002). This is in contrast to other studies where sensitivity was recorded at 85% and specificity at 99% (Mitropoulos 1985). Many of the differences can be explained by the nature of the ordinal scale used to record the subjective visual assessment and the gold standard used to validate the method. However, one would expect FOTI to be at least as effective as a visual examination.

Recent developments in ordinal scales for visual assessments, such as the ICDAS scoring system (Pitts 2004), may enable a more robust framework for visual exams into which FOTI can be added. One would expect that FOTI would enable discrimination of occlusal lesions to be improved (particularly dentine lesions), as well as detection of proximal lesions (in the absence of radiographs) to be higher (Cortes *et al.* 2003). As a technique, FOTI is an obvious choice for translation into general practice; the equipment is economical, the learning curve

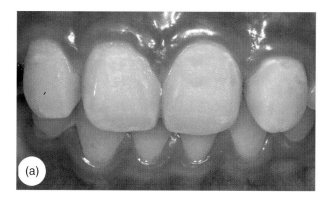

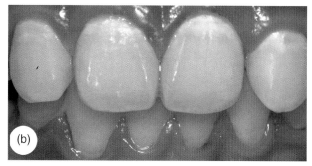

Figure 2-10 Example of early lesions before (a) and after (b) drying.

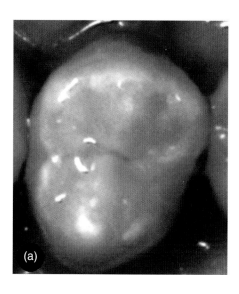

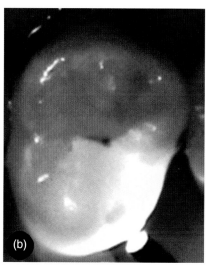

Figure 2-11 Example of FOTI on a tooth: (a) normal clinical vision; (b) with FOTI.

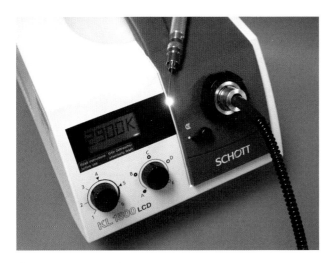

Figure 2-12 FOTI equipment.

is short, and the procedure is not time consuming. Indeed, some work has been undertaken trialling the use of FOTI in practice with encouraging results (Davies *et al.* 2001).

However with the simplicity of the FOTI system comes limitations; the system is subjective rather than objective, there is no continuous data outputted, and it is not possible to record what is seen in the form of an image. Longitudinal monitoring is, therefore, a complex matter, and some degree of training is required in order to be competent at this level of FOTI usage. In order to address some of these concerns, an imaging version of FOTI has been developed—DiFOTI (digital imaging FOIT). This system comprises a high intensity light and gray-scale camera that can be fitted with one of two heads: one for smooth and one for occlusal surfaces. Images are displayed on a computer monitor and can be archived for retrieval at a repeat visit. See Figure 2-12.

However, there is no attempt within the software to quantify the images, and analysis is still undertaken visually by the examiner who makes a subjective call based on the appearance of scattering (Schneiderman *et al.* 1997).

Fluorescent techniques

Visible light fluorescence—QLF

Quantitative light-induced fluorescence (QLF) is a visible light system that offers the opportunity to detect early caries and then longitudinally monitor its progression or regression. Using two forms of fluorescent detection (green and red), it may also be able to determine if a lesion is active or not and predict the likely progression of any given lesion. Fluorescence is a phenomenon by which an object is excited by a particular wavelength of light and the fluorescent (reflected)

light is of a larger wavelength. When the excitation light is in the visible spectrum, the fluorescence will be a different color. In the case of the QLF, the visible light has a wavelength (λ) of 370 nm, which is in the blue region of the spectrum. The resultant auto-fluorescence of human enamel is then detected by filtering out the excitation light using a bandpass filter at λ >540 nm by a small intra-oral camera. This produces an image that is comprised of only green and red channels (the blue having been filtered out), and the predominate color of the enamel is green (de Josselin de Jong *et al.* 1995; Ando *et al.* 1997). Demineralization of enamel results in a reduction of this autofluorescence. This loss can be quantified using proprietary software and has been shown to correlate well with actual mineral loss; r = 0.73–0.86 (van der Veen and de Josselin de Jong 2000).

The source of the autofluorescence is thought to be the enamel dentinal junction (EDJ). The excitation light passes through the transparent enamel and excites fluorophores contained within the EDJ. Studies have shown that when underlying dentine is removed from the enamel, fluorescence is lost, although only a small amount of dentine is required to produce the fluorescence seen (van der Veen and de Josselin de Jong 2000). Decreasing the thickness of enamel results in a higher intensity of fluorescence. The presence of an area of demineralized enamel reduced the fluorescence for two main reasons. The first is that the scattering effect of the lesion results in less excitation light reaching the EDJ in this area, and the second is that any fluorescence from the EDJ is back scattered as it attempts to pass through the lesion.

The QLF equipment is comprised of a light box containing a xenon bulb and a handpiece, similar in appearance to an intra-oral camera. See Figure 2-13.

Light is passed to the handpiece via a liquid light guide, and the handpiece contains the bandpass filter (Angmar-Månsson and ten Bosch 2001). Live images are displayed via a computer, and accompanying software enables patient's details to be entered and individual images of the teeth of interest to be captured and stored. QLF can image all tooth surfaces except interproximally. See Figure 2-14 for an example of QLF images that have been merged to create a montage on the anterior teeth demonstrating resolution of buccal caries over a 1-month period following supervised brushing.

Once an image of a tooth has been captured, the next stage is to analyze any lesions and produce a quantitative assessment of the demineralization status of the tooth. This is undertaken using proprietary software and involves using a patch to define areas of sound enamel around the lesion of interest. Following this the

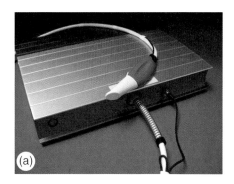

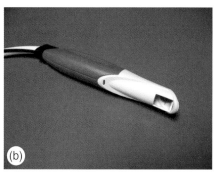

Figure 2-13 QLF Equipment: (a) The QLF unit light box, demonstrating the handpiece and liquid light guide; (b) A close-up of the intra-oral camera featuring a disposable mirror tip that also acts as an ambient light shield.

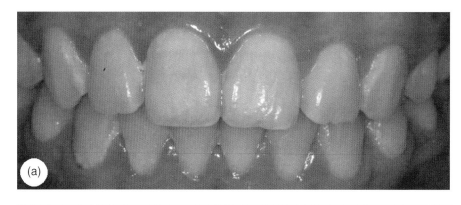

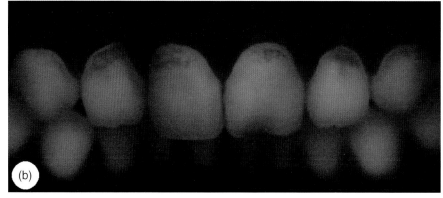

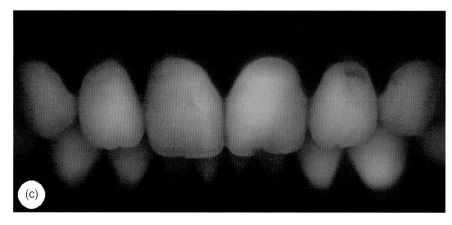

Figure 2-14 Example of QLF images: (a) White light image of early buccal caries affecting the maxillary teeth; (b) QLF image taken at the same time as (a). Note the improved detection of lesions as a result of the increased contrast between sound and demineralized enamel; (c) 6 months after the institution of an oral hygiene program, the lesions have resolved.

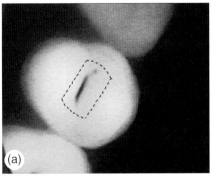
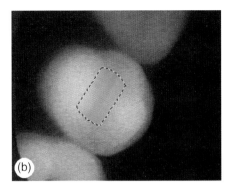
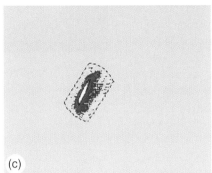

Figure 2-15 An example of lesion analysis using QLF: (a) Lesion on the occlusal surface of a premolar is identified and the analysis patch placed on sound enamel; (b) The reconstruction demonstrates correct patch placement as the surface now looks homogenous; (c) The 'subtracted' lesion is demonstrated in false color indicating the severity of the demineralization; (d) The quantitative output from this analysis at a variety of fluorescent threshold levels.

c:\o14\o14000a.grp
Lesion comment
Extra zoomfactor x,y   1.00, 1.00

Threshold [%]	Delta F [%]	Area [mm²]	Delta Q [mm².%]
-5.0	-16.3	3.3	-53.0
-10.0	-24.1	1.8	-43.3
-15.0	-31.5	1.1	-35.3
-20.0	-37.0	0.8	-30.1
-25.0	-41.3	0.6	-26.1
-30.0	-44.9	0.5	-22.7
-35.0	-47.9	0.4	-19.7
-40.0	-50.7	0.3	-16.5
-45.0	-53.2	0.3	-13.6
-50.0	-55.9	0.2	-9.9

software uses the pixel values of the sound enamel to reconstruct the surface of the tooth and then subtracts those pixels that are considered to be lesions. This is controlled by a threshold of fluorescence loss, and is generally set to 5%. This means that all pixels with a loss of fluorescence greater than 5% of the average sound value will be considered to be part of the lesion. Once the pixels have been assigned "sound" or "lesion," the software then calculates the average fluorescence loss in the lesion, known as %DF, and then the total area of the lesion in mm², a the multiplication of these two variables, results in a third metric output, DQ. See Figure 2-15 for an example of the analysis and the resultant lesion.

When examining lesions longitudinally, the QLF device employs a video repositioning system that enables the precise geometry of the original image to be replicated on subsequent visits.

QLF has been employed to detect a range of lesion types. For occlusal caries, sensitivity has been reported at 0.68 and specificity at 0.70, and this compares well with other systems. Correlations of up to 0.82 have also been reported for QLF metrics and lesion depth. Smooth surfaces, secondary caries, and demineralization adjacent to orthodontic brackets have all been examined. The reliability of both stages of the QLF process, that is, the image capture and the analysis, has been examined and has been shown to be substantial. Intra-class correlation co-efficients have been reported as 0.96 for image capture, with analysis at 0.93 for intra-examiner and 0.92 for inter-examiner comparisons. Again, these compare well to other systems.

The QLF system offers additional benefits beyond those of very early lesion detection and quantification. The images acquired can be stored and transmitted, perhaps for referral purposes, and the images themselves can be used as patient motivators in preventative practice. For clinical research use, the ability to remotely analyze lesions enables increased legitimacy in trials, permitting, for example, a repeat of the analyses to be conducted by a third party. QLF is one of the most promising technologies in the caries detection stable at present, although further research is required to demonstrate its ability to correctly monitor lesion changes over time. There is also a great deal of interest in red fluorescence, and whether or not this can be a predictor of lesion activity, and again, research is currently being undertaken in this area.

Laser fluorescence—DIAGNOdent

The DIAGNOdent (DD) instrument (KaVo, Germany) is another device employing fluorescence to detect the presence of caries. Using a small laser the system produces an excitation wavelength of 655 nm, which produces a red light. This is carried to one of two intra-oral tips: one designed for pits and fissures, and the other for smooth surfaces. The tip both emits the excitation light and collects the resultant fluorescence. Unlike the QLF system, the DD does not produce an image of the tooth; instead it displays a numerical value on two LED displays. The first displays the current reading while the second displays the peak reading for that examination. A small twist of the top of the tip enables the machine to be reset and ready for another site examination, and a calibration device is supplied with the system (Figure 2-16).

There has been some debate over what exactly the DD is measuring; it is not employing the intrinsic changes within the enamel structure in the same way as QLF. This has been demonstrated by the inability of DD to detect artificial lesions in *in vitro* settings. Instead the system is thought to measure the degree of bacterial activity, and this is supported by the fact that the excitation wavelength is suitable for inducing fluorescence from bacterial porphyrins, a by-product of metabolism.

Initial evaluations of the device suggest that it may be a promising tool for clinical use. Correlation with histological depth of lesions was substantial at 0.85, and the sensitivity and specificity for dentinal lesions were 0.75 and 0.96, respectively (Shi *et al.* 2001). Reliability of the device measured by Kappa was 0.88–0.90 for intra-examiner and 0.65–0.73 for inter-examiner (Lussi *et al.* 1999). Further *in vitro* studies have found that the area under the receiver operating characteristic (ROC) was significantly higher for DD (0.96) than that for conventional radiographs (0.66) (Shi *et al.* 2000). However, the device is not without its confounders, and, like many novel caries detection devices, requires teeth to be clean and dry. The presence of stain, calculus, plaque, and, when used in the laboratory, the storage medium, have all be shown to have an adverse effect on the DD readings (Shi *et al.* 2001). Most confounders tend to cause an increase in the DD reading, leading to false positives.

The literature surrounding the DD device was recently assessed in a systematic review (Bader and Shugars 2004). The authors found that, for dentinal caries, the DD device performed well, although there was a great deal of heterogeneity in the studies, and they were all undertaken *in vitro*. The authors stated that these results could not be extrapolated into the clinical setting and then detected a worrying trend for the device to produce more false-positives than traditional diagnostic systems. Their conclusion was therefore that there was insufficient evidence to support the use of the device as a principle means of caries diagnosis in clinical practice (Bader and Shugars 2004). It should be noted that the DD device has not been employed in a clinical trial, so there are no

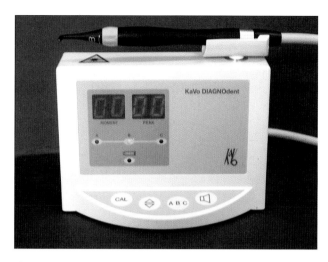

Figure 2-16 The DIAGNOdent device.

data indicating that the system can detect a dose response, for example, to fluoride treatments.

A new DIAGNOdent device, the DIAGNOdent Pen, was launched to market in 2008, and KaVo claim that 45,000 dentists are using the system. Based on the same technology the probe has been adapted to enable readings to be taken inter-proximally. Much of the research on this new device has been undertaken *in vitro*, and there is insufficient evidence available at present to support its use as single tool for detection and monitoring although it may have utility as an adjunct (Aljehani *et al.* 2007; Kuhnisch *et al.* 2007a; Kuhnisch *et al.* 2007b; Farah *et al.* 2008; Huth *et al.* 2008). The popularity of the DD devices may be, in part, due to their pricing. The units are sold below the $2,000 mark, which make them an attractive proposition when compared to other devices.

Photo-thermal Radiometry (PTR)

A new system to the market, the Canary System, is based on the use of combined levels of luminescence and heat released by a tooth that has been excited by a laser. The system is based on the theory that demineralized areas of the tooth will respond to this excitation in different ways than to "sound" areas, and therefore a map of demineralization can be established. A particular benefit of this technology is that the manufacturers claim that the use of pulsed lasers will enable a depth profile of a lesion to be determined (Jeon *et al.* 2004; Jeon *et al.* 2008).

At the time of writing the system was being launched commercially, and the author has not had the opportunity to use or see the system in use. The theory has been well published in both the dental and biomedical optical literature (Jeon *et al.* 2004), but the system's efficacy in general dental practice remains unknown.

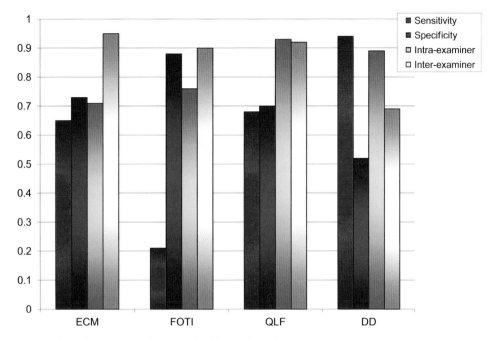

Figure 2-17 A summary of the diagnostic performance (validity and reliability) of a range of novel caries detection systems based on D3 lesions, *in vitro*, on occlusal surfaces. After Pretty 2005.

Other optical techniques

There are a number of other techniques for detecting caries using optical methods. These systems are in their infancy, and many are based solely in laboratories. However, such technologies may prove to be useful in the future. Examples include optical coherence tomography (OCT), and near infra-red imaging (Zakian *et al.* 2009). OCT has been shown to be able to image early enamel caries lesions in extracted teeth (Ngaotheppitak *et al.* 2005) and also on root lesions (Amaechi *et al.* 2004). Like many other novel techniques, it is likely that stain will adversely affect OCT (Hall and Girkin 2004). Work has just begun on using near infra-red, but initial results look promising (Fried *et al.* 2005). One of the advantages of the NIR systems is that they promise the ability to penetrate through stain and hence offer the potential to mitigate this confounding factor that is such an issue in occlusal caries diagnosis. Significant work is involved in developing these systems into clinically and commercially acceptable applications, therefore it could be some time until these new methodologies can be properly assessed in clinical trials.

Ultrasound techniques

The use of ultrasound in caries detection was first suggested over 30 years ago, although developments in this field have been slow. The principle behind the technique is that sound waves can pass through gases, liquids, and solids and through the boundaries between them (Hall and Girkin 2004). Images of tissues can be acquired by collecting the reflected sound waves. In order for sound waves to reach the tooth, they must pass first through a coupling mechanism, and a number of these have been suggested, but those with clinical applications include water and glycerine (Hall and Girkin 2004). A number of studies have been undertaken using ultrasound, with differing levels of success. One study reported that an ultrasound device could discriminate between cavitated and non-cavitated inter-proximal lesions (Matalon *et al.* 2007). A further study found that ultrasonic measurements at 70 approximal sites *in vitro* resulted in a sensitivity of 1.0 and a specificity of 0.92 when compared to a histological gold standard (Ziv *et al.* 1998). Further histological validation has been undertaken by using transverse microradiography and ultrasound (Ng *et al.* 1988). A final *in vivo* study was undertaken using a device described as the Ultrasonic Caries Detector (UCD), which examined 253 approximal sites and claimed a diagnostic improvement over bitewing radiography (Bab *et al.* 1998). Despite these encouraging findings, no further research has been undertaken using the device, and the research has only been published as abstracts.

Conclusion

A range of caries detection systems has been covered in this chapter. A summary of their performance is presented in Figure 2-17.

The pattern of dental caries is changing, with an increasing incidence in occlusal surfaces especially in younger children where prevention has its greatest benefit. This shift has rendered traditional detection systems, particularly bitewing radiographs less useful in the diagnostic protocols of clinicians. High concentration fluoride varnishes have been demonstrated to arrest the progression of early lesions (Weintraub 2003; Weintraub *et al.* 2006), but often traditional methods of detection are too insensitive to permit the most efficacious use of these products. Caries clinical trials involving thousands of subjects over several years employ are no longer commercially viable. For all of these reasons there is a real need for a range of caries detection and quantification systems to augment the clinician's diagnostic pathway.

The evidence supporting each of the systems is currently limited, often by virtue of the *in vitro* nature of the studies or as a result of a failure of standardization of approach to study design making meta-analyses impossible. The Cochrane Oral Health Group is currently undertaking a number of systematic reviews examining the efficiency of dental diagnostic systems, but it is clear that the limited *in vivo* evidence, and range of outcome measures, will require cautious interpretation. However, if we can state with some confidence that the systems do permit earlier detection of enamel lesions, and systems such as QLF and DiFOTI enable images of these lesions to be stored and viewed at a later date, it is worthwhile considering what the purpose may be for supplementing or even replacing well-established dental diagnostic systems. They must offer improved diagnostic efficiency, better patient care pathways, or perhaps comply with legislative changes. There is a paradigm shift occurring in dentistry; we are slowly moving away from a surgical model into one more medically based. The devices described within this chapter, by enabling early detection of caries enable the remineralizing therapies to be correctly prescribed and for their success to be measured. Indeed, it is this ability to longitudinally monitor lesions that have favored devices such as the DIAGNOdent.

The advent of dental auxiliaries who can undertake an increasing number of procedures emphasises the important role that the dentist plays as the leader of the dental team. This leadership role is critically tied to the fact that dental clinicians retain the sole right of diagnosis, and thus the devices and approaches described within the current paper serve only to augment the diagnostic skills of the clinician. Making the *right* decision about the presence or absence of a lesion, its degree of severity, and its likely activity combined with the socio-behavioral aspects of the patient, their risk and modifying factors will continue to rest with the dentist.

References

Agustsdottir, H., Gudmundsdottir, H., Eggertsson, H., et al. (2010) Caries prevalence of permanent teeth: a national survey of children in Iceland using ICDAS. *Community Dentistry and Oral Epidemiology*, 38, 299–309.

Aljehani, A., Yang, L., Shi, X.Q. (2007) In vitro quantification of smooth surface caries with DIAGNOdent and the DIAGNOdent pen. *Acta Odontologica Scandidavica*, 65, 60–63.

al-Khateeb, S., Oliveby, A., de Josselin de Jong, E., et al. (1997) Laser fluorescence quantification of remineralisation in situ of incipient enamel lesions: influence of fluoride supplements. *Caries Research*, 31, 132–140.

Amaechi, B.T. and Higham, S.M. (2001) In vitro remineralisation of eroded enamel lesions by saliva. *Journal Dentistry*, 29, 371–376.

Amaechi, B.T., Podoleanu A.G., Komarov, G., et al. (2004) Quantification of root caries using optical coherence tomography and microradiography: a correlational study. *Oral Health and Preventive Dentistry*, 2, 377–382.

Ando, M., Hall, A.F., Eckert, G.J., et al. (1997) Relative ability of laser fluorescence techniques to quantitate early mineral loss in vitro. *Caries Research*, 31, 125–131.

Angmar-Månsson, B. and ten Bosch, J.J. (2001) Quantitative light-induced fluorescence (QLF): a method for assessment of incipient caries lesions. *Dentomaxillofacial Radiology*, 30, 298–307.

Angmar-Månsson, B.E., al-Khateeb, S., Tranaeus, S. (1998) Caries diagnosis. *Journal of Dental Education*, 62, 771–780.

Bab, I., Ziv, V., Gazit, D., et al. (1998) Diagnosis of approximal caries in adult patients using ultrasonic surface waves (abstract). *Journal of Dental Research*, 77, (Spec Iss A), 255.

Bader, J.D. and Shugars, D.A. (2004) A systematic review of the performance of a laser fluorescence device for detecting caries. *Journal of the American Dental Association*, 135, 1413–1426.

Bader, J.D., Shugars, D.A. Bonito, A.J., et al. (2001) Systematic reviews of selected dental caries diagnostic and management methods. *Journal of Dental Education*, 65, 960–968.

Bader, J.D., Shugars, D.A., Bonito, A.J. (2002) A systematic review of the performance of methods for identifying carious lesions. *Journal of Public Health Dentistry*, 62, 201–213.

Baysan, A., Lynch, E., Ellwood, R., et al. (2001) Reversal of primary root caries using dentifrices containing 5,000 and 1,100 ppm fluoride. *Caries Research*, 35, 41–46.

Braga, M.M., Mendes, F.M., Martignon, S., et al. (2009a) In vitro comparison of Nyvad's system and ICDAS-II with Lesion Activity Assessment for evaluation of severity and activity of occlusal caries lesions in primary teeth. *Caries Research*, 43, 405–412.

Braga, M.M., Oliveira, L.B., Bonini, G.A., et al. (2009b) Feasibility of the International Caries Detection and Assessment System (ICDAS-II) in epidemiological surveys and comparability with standard World Health Organization criteria. *Caries Research*, 43, 245–249.

Choksi, S.K., Brady, J. M., Dang, D.H., et al. (1994) Detecting approximal dental caries with transillumination: a clinical evaluation. *Journal of the American Dental Association*, 125, 1098–1102.

Côrtes, D.F., Ellwood, R.P., Ekstrand, K.R. (2003) An in vitro comparison of a combined FOTI/visual examination of occlusal caries with other caries diagnostic methods and the effect of stain on their diagnostic performance. *Caries Research*, 37, 8–16.

Davies, G.M., Worthington, H.V., Clarkson, J.E. et al. (2001) The use of fibre-optic transillumination in general dental practice. *British Dental Journal*, 191, 145–147.

de Josselin de Jong, E., Sundström, F., Westerling, H., *et al.* (1995) A new method for in vivo quantification of changes in initial enamel caries with laser fluorescence. *Caries Research,* 29, 2–7.

Diniz, M.B., Rodrigues, J.A., Hug, I., *et al.* (2009) Reproducibility and accuracy of the ICDAS-II for occlusal caries detection. *Community Dentistry and Oral Epidemiology,* 37, 399–404.

Ekstrand, K.R., Ricketts, D.N., Kidd, E.A., *et al.* (1997) Reproducibility and accuracy of three methods for assessment of demineralization depth of the occlusal surface: an in vitro examination. *Caries Research,* 31, 224–231.

Ekstrand, K.R., Ricketts, D.N., Kidd, E.A., *et al.* (1998) Detection, diagnosing, monitoring and logical treatment of occlusal caries in relation to lesion activity and severity: an in vivo examination with histological validation. *Caries Research,* 32, 247–254.

Ellwood, R.P., Davies, R.M., Worthington, H.V. (1997) Evaluation of a dental subtraction radiography system. *Journal of Periodontal Research,* 32, 241–248.

Farah, R.A., Drummond, B.K., Swain, M.V., *et al.* (2008) Relationship between laser fluorescence and enamel hypomineralisation. *Journal of Dentistry,* 36, 915–921.

Featherstone, J.D. (2004) The caries balance: the basis for caries management by risk assessment. *Oral Health and Preventive Dentistry,* 2 (Suppl 1), 259–264.

Ferreira Zandoná, A., Santiago, E., Eckert, G., *et al.* (2010) Use of ICDAS combined with quantitative light-induced fluorescence as a caries detection method. *Caries Research,* 44, 317–322.

Fried, D., Featherstone, J.D., Darling, C.L. *et al.* (2005) Early caries imaging and monitoring with near-infrared light. *Dental Clinics of North America,* 49, 771–793, vi.

Hall, A. and Girkin, J.M. (2004) A review of potential new diagnostic modalities for caries lesions. Journal *of Dental Research,* 83 (Spec No C), C89–C94.

Holt, R.D. (2001) Advances in dental public health. *Primary Dental Care,* 8, 99–102.

Huth, K.C., Neuhaus, K.W., Gygax, M., *et al.* (2008) Clinical performance of a new laser fluorescence device for detection of occlusal caries lesions in permanent molars. *Journal of Dentistry,* 36, 1033–1040.

Huysmans, M.C., Longbottom, C., Christie, A.M., *et al.* (2000) Temperature dependence of the electrical resistance of sound and carious teeth. *Journal of Dental Research,* 79, 1464–1468.

Huysmans, M.C., Longbottom C., Hintze, H., *et al.* (1998) Surface-specific electrical occlusal caries diagnosis: reproducibility, correlation with histological lesion depth, and tooth type dependence. *Caries Research,* 32, 330–336.

Huysmans, M.C., Longbottom, C., Pitts, N.B., *et al.* (1996) Impedance spectroscopy of teeth with and without approximal caries lesions—an in vitro study. *Journal of Dental Research,* 75, 1871–1878.

Huysmans, M.C. (2000) Electrical measurements for early caries detection. In: *Early Caries Detection II. Proceedings of the 4th Annual Indiana Conference.* (Ed. G.K. Stookey) Indiana University Press, Indianapolis, Indiana, USA.

Ismail, A.I., Sohn, W., Tellez, M., *et al.* (2007). The International Caries Detection and Assessment System (ICDAS): an integrated system for measuring dental caries. *Community Dentistry and Oral Epidemiology,* 35, 170–178.

Ismail, A.I., Sohn, W., Tellez, M., *et al.* (2008) Risk indicators for dental caries using the International Caries Detection and Assessment System (ICDAS). *Dentistry and Oral Epidemiology,* 36, 55–68.

Jeon, R.J., Han, C., Mandelis, A., *et al.* (2004) Diagnosis of pit and fissure caries using frequency-domain infrared photothermal radiometry and modulated laser luminescence. *Caries Research,* 38, 497–513.

Jeon, R.J., Hellen, A., Matvienko, A., *et al.* (2008) In vitro detection and quantification of enamel and root caries using infrared photothermal radiometry and modulated luminescence. *Journal of Biomedical Optics,* 13, 034025.

Jeon, R.J., Mandelis, A., Sanchez, V., *et al.* (2004) Nonintrusive, non-contacting frequency-domain photothermal radiometry and luminescence depth profilometry of carious and artificial subsurface lesions in human teeth. *Journal of Biomedical Optics,* 9, 804–819.

Kidd, E.A. (1998) The operative management of caries. *Dentistry Update,* 25, 104–108, 110.

Kuhnisch, J., Bücher, K., Henschel, V., *et al.* (2007a) Reproducibility of DIAGNOdent 2095 and DIAGNOdent Pen measurements: results from an in vitro study on occlusal sites. *European Journal of Oral Science,* 115, 206–211.

Kuhnisch, J., Bücher, K., Hickel, R. (2007b) The intra/inter-examiner reproducibility of the new DIAGNOdent Pen on occlusal sites. *Journal of Dentistry,* 35, 509–512.

Longbottom, C., Ekstrand, K., Zero, D. (2009) Novel preventive treatment options. *Monographs in Oral Science,* 21, 156–163.

Longbottom, C. and Huysmans, M.C. (2004) Electrical measurements for use in caries clinical trials. *Journal of Dental Research,* 83 Spec No C, C76–C79.

Lussi, A., Imwinkelried, S., Pitts, N., *et al.* (1999) Performance and reproducibility of a laser fluorescence system for detection of occlusal caries in vitro. *Caries Research,* 33, 261–266.

McIntyre, J.M. (2005) Dental caries: the major cause of tooth damage. In: *Preservation and Restoration of Tooth Structure* (Eds. G.J. Mount and W.R. Hume, 2nd edn. pp. 27. Knowledge Books and Software. Brighton, Queensland AU).

Matalon, S., Feuerstein, O., Caqlderon, S. *et al.* (2007) Detection of cavitated carious lesions in approximal tooth surfaces by ultrasonic caries detector. *Oral Surgery, Oral Pathology, Oral Radiology and Endodontology,* 103, 109–113.

Maupomé, G. and Pretty, I.A. (2004) A closer look at diagnosis in clinical dental practice: part 4. Effectiveness of nonradiographic diagnostic procedures and devices in dental practice. *Journal of the Canadian Dental Association,* 70, 470–474.

Mitropoulos, C.M. (1985) A comparison of fibre-optic transillumination with bitewing radiographs. *British Dental Journal,* 159, 21–23.

Ng, S.Y., Ferguson, M.W., Payne, P.A., *et al.* (1988) Ultrasonic studies of unblemished and artificially demineralized enamel in extracted human teeth: a new method for detecting early caries. *Journal of Dentistry,* 16, 201–209.

Ngaotheppitak, P., Darling, C.L., Fried, D. (2005) Measurement of the severity of natural smooth surface (interproximal) caries lesions with polarization sensitive optical coherence tomography. *Lasers in Surgery and Medicine,* 37, 78–88.

Pitts, N. (2004) "ICDAS"—an international system for caries detection and assessment being developed to facilitate caries epidemiology, research and appropriate clinical management. *Community Dental Health,* 21, 193–198.

Pitts, N.B. (1997) Diagnostic tools and measurements—impact on appropriate care. *Community Dentistry and Oral Epidemiology,* 25, 24–35.

Pitts, N.B. (2001) Clinical diagnosis of dental caries: a European perspective. *Journal of Dental Education,* 65, 972–978.

Pretty, I.A. (2005) A review of the effectiveness of QLF to detect early caries lesions. In: *Early Caries Detection II. Proceedings of the 4th Annual Indiana Conference.* (Ed. G.K. Stookey) Indiana University Press, Indianapolis, Indiana, USA.

Pretty, I.A. and Maupomé, G. (2004a) A closer look at diagnosis in clinical dental practice: part 1. Reliability, validity, specificity and sensitivity of diagnostic procedures. *Journal of the Canadian Dental Association,* 70, 251–255.

Pretty, I.A. and Maupomé, G. (2004b) A closer look at diagnosis in clinical dental practice: part 2. Using predictive values and receiver operating characteristics in assessing diagnostic accuracy. *Journal of the Canadian Dental Association,* 70, 313–316.

Ricketts, D.N., Kidd, E.A. Wilson, R.F. (1997) Electronic diagnosis of occlusal caries *in vitro*: adaptation of the technique for epidemiological purposes. *Community Dentistry and Oral Epidemiology*, 25, 238–341.

Rock, W.P. and Kidd, E.A. (1988) The electronic detection of demineralisation in occlusal fissures. *British Dental Journal,* 164, 243–247.

Schneiderman, A., Elbaum, M., Shultz, T. *et al.* (1997) Assessment of dental caries with Digital Imaging Fiber-Optic TransIllumination (DIFOTI): in vitro study. *Caries Research*, 31, 103–110.

Shi, X.Q., Tranaeus, S., Angmar-Månsson, B. (2001) Validation of DIAGNOdent for quantification of smooth-surface caries: an *in vitro* study. *Acta Odontologica Scandinavica*, 59, 74–78.

Shi, X.Q., Welander, U., Angmar-Månsson, B. (2000) Occlusal caries detection with KaVo DIAGNOdent and radiography: an in vitro comparison. *Caries Research*, 34, 151–158.

van der Veen, M.H. and de Josselin de Jong, E. (2000) Application of quantitative light-induced fluorescence for assessing early caries lesions. *Monographs in Oral Science*, 17, 144–162.

Verdonschot, E.H., Angmar-Månsson, B., ten Bosch, J.J., *et al.* (1999) Developments in caries diagnosis and their relationship to treatment decisions and quality of care. ORCA Saturday Afternoon Symposium 1997. *Caries Research*, 33, 32–40.

Verdonschot, E.H., Kuijpers, J.M., Polder, B.J., *et al.* (1992) Effects of digital grey-scale modification on the diagnosis of small approximal carious lesions. *Journal of Dentistry*, 20, 44–49.

Verdonschot, E.H., Rondel, P., Huysmans, M.C. (1995) Validity of electrical conductance measurements in evaluating the marginal integrity of sealant restorations. *Caries Research*, 29, 100–106.

Verdonschot, E.H., Wenzel, A., Truin, G.L., *et al.* (1993) Performance of electrical resistance measurements adjunct to visual inspection in the early diagnosis of occlusal caries. *Journal of Dentistry*, 21, 332–327.

Verdonschot, E.H. and Angmar-Mansson, B. (2003) Advanced methods of caries diagnosis and quantification. In: *Dental Caries. The disease and its clinical management.* (Eds. O. Fejerskov and E. Kidd) Blackwell Munksgaard, Oxford, England.

Weintraub, J.A. (2003) Fluoride varnish for caries prevention: comparisons with other preventive agents and recommendations for a community-based protocol. *Special Care Dentist*, 23, 180–186.

Weintraub, J.A., Ramos-Gomez, F., Jue, B. *et al.* (2006) Fluoride Varnish Efficacy in Preventing Early Childhood Caries. *Journal of Dental Research,* 85, 172–176.

Wenzel, A., Pitts, N., Verdonschot E.H., *et al.* (1993) Developments in radiographic caries diagnosis. *Journal of Dentistry,* 21, 131–140.

White, S.C., Yoon, D.C., Tedradis S. (1999) Digital radiography in dentistry: what it should do for you. *Journal of the California Dental Association*, 27, 942–952.

Zakian, C., Pretty, I., Ellwood, R. (2009) Near-infrared hyperspectral imaging of teeth for dental caries detection. *Journal of Biomedical Optics*, 14, 064047.

Ziv, V., Gazit, D. Beris D., *et al.* (1998) Correlative ultrasonic histologic and Roentgenographic assessment of approximal caries (Abstract 78). *Caries Research*, 32, 294.

3

Diagnosis of periodontal diseases

Jim Yuan Lai

The periodontium is a group of tissues that are involved with the support of the tooth. The tissues are the gingiva, alveolar mucosa, cementum, periodontal ligament, and alveolar and supporting bone (American Academy of Periodontology 2001). The dynamic relationship between these tissues and the tooth creates an environment that fulfills several functions such as mastication, speech, and aesthetics. However, this interrelationship can lead to the development of periodontal diseases. Part of the tooth is exposed to the external environment while the rest is buried deep within the tissue. Because of this relationship, bacterial colonization may occur on numerous stable surfaces that are close to the tissue.

The healthy periodontium

The purpose of this section is to identify and review key features of a healthy periodontium. The intent is not to provide a comprehensive review of the anatomical and histological components of the periodontium.

The primary functions of the periodontium are attachment and sensation. The dynamic relationship between the tooth and periodontium allows the tooth to remain attached to the jawbone while the tooth is subjected to masticatory forces. Another function of the periodontium is to provide sensory perception of pressure on the tooth.

Alveolar bone and alveolar process

The principle tissues involved with attachment are the gingival fibers and the periodontal ligament fibers that connect to the cementum and to the alveolar bone. The alveolar process is the bone that houses the tooth and is connected to the basal jawbone. The formation of the alveolar process is dependent on the eruption of the tooth. If the tooth does not erupt, the alveolar process is absent. The alveolar process is comprised of the outer cortical plate, the spongiosa, which is trabecular or cancellous bone, and an inner cortical plate that faces the tooth, which is known as the alveolar bone (Figure 3-1). The alveolar bone is identified as the lamina dura radiographically (Figure 3-2). Upon extraction of a tooth, the alveolar bone is lost. The alveolar bone consists of two components, the cribriform plate and bundle bone. The cribriform plate is cortical bone with perforations where blood vessels and nerves travel from the bone marrow spaces to the periodontal ligament. The bundle bone is the inner component of the alveolar bone that faces the tooth and where the principle collagen fiber bundles of the periodontal ligament are embedded (Nanci 2008).

The alveolar crest is formed where the outer cortical bone meets the alveolar bone. For the first three phases of passive eruption, a histologic study of clinically normal human jaws reported the distance from cementoenamel junction to the alveolar crest ranged from 0.04 to 3.36 mm, 0.35 to 5.00 mm, and 0.88 to 3.20 mm (Gargiulo et al. 1961). However, radiographically, it is accepted that there is no evidence of bone loss if the alveolar crest is less than 2 mm from the cementoenamel junction (Hausmann et al. 1991). Radiographic presence of an intact crestal lamina dura is a good indicator of periodontal stability (Figure 3-2). On the other hand, the absence of a crestal lamina dura is not a good predictor of periodontal progression (Rams et al. 1994).

The bone is vascularized with blood vessels housed in the osteons or Haversian system. It also contains undifferentiated progenitor cells that can differentiate into osteoblasts. The bone is constantly undergoing remodeling where there is a delicate balance between bone apposition and resorption.

Comprehensive Preventive Dentistry, First Edition. Edited by Hardy Limeback.
© 2012 John Wiley & Sons, Ltd. Published 2012 by John Wiley & Sons, Ltd.

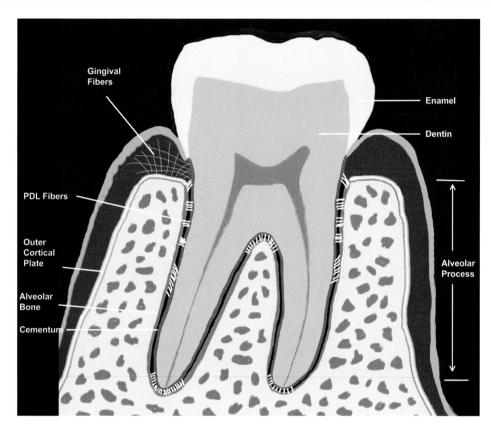

Figure 3-1 Features of the periodontium (alveolar bone [blue], cementum [brown]).

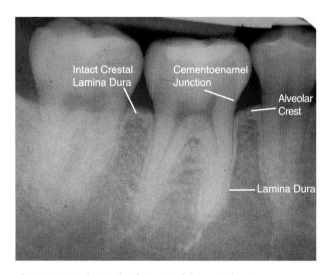

Figure 3-2 Radiographic features of the periodontium.

Periodontal ligament

The periodontal ligament is mainly a fibrous connective tissue to support the tooth, but it also has cellular, neural, and vascular components that allow it to fulfill additional functions of remodeling, nutritive, and sensory. The periodontal ligament supports the tooth by forming a fibrous meshwork attaching the cementum to the alveolar bone. These fibers, which are predominantly type I, III, and XII collagen, originate from both the bone and cementum. On the alveolar bone side, the fibers that are mineralized and embedded in the bundle bone are known as Sharpey's fibers. They are grouped into fiber bundles but start to unravel into smaller fibers as they extend into the periodontal ligament space. Fibers embedded into the cementum are smaller diameter, but they also unravel into smaller fibers and form a tight meshwork with the fibers from the bundle bone, thus forming the periodontal ligament fibers. Based on the anatomic location, there are five groups of principle collagen fiber bundles of the periodontal ligament: (1) alveolar crest fibers, (2) horizontal fibers, (3) oblique fibers, (4) periapical fibers, and (5) interradicular fibers (Figure 3-1) (Nanci 2008).

The width of the periodontal ligament is 0.15 to 0.38 mm. The narrowest portion is around the middle third of the root, and the ligament is the widest at the cervical aspect (Coolidge 1937). The periodontal ligament reacts to occlusal forces and is able to accommodate physiologic forces. There is a thickening of the fiber bundles and the Sharpey's fibers are increased in quantity and size. Consequently, the width of the periodontal ligament is increased. For example, the width of the periodontal ligament in the middle of the alveolus of a premolar in heavy function increases from 0.10 mm to 0.28 mm (Kronfeld 1931).

The width is preserved in the presence of physiologic forces because the periodontal ligament is able to remodel and distribute the forces along the periodontal ligament and alveolar bone. The remodeling capability is due to the presence of cells found in the periodontal ligament. The major cell types are periodontal ligament fibroblasts, undifferentiated ectomesenchymal cells, cementoblasts, cementoclasts, osteoblasts, and osteoclasts. These are the key cells in the breakdown and generation of the cementum, alveolar bone, and the periodontal ligament. The periodontal ligament fibroblast cells are responsible for production of extrinsic collagen fibers and destruction of the fibers by intracellular degradation. In a normal periodontium, there is a significantly high rate of turnover of the ligament. In the presence of inflammation, this balance and the function of the fibroblast can be disturbed, which then can lead to a cumulative loss of collagen. New cementum is produced by the cementoblast. Cementum is not regularly broken down or remodeled whereas the bone is constantly remodeled. There is a balance between bone deposition and resorption. The presence of undifferentiated ectomesenchymal cells in the periodontal ligament is a key source for new cells that are critical to formation of new periodontal ligament since they can differentiate into periodontal ligament fibroblasts, cementoblasts, and osteoblasts (Beersten *et al.* 1997).

Cementum

Cementum is a mineralized connective tissue that covers the root of the tooth. Unlike bone, it is not vascularized. There is some remodeling, but apposition mostly occurs. The cementum is typically thinner at the cervical aspect of the root and becomes thicker apically. The thickness of cementum ranges from 0.05 mm to 0.60 mm. The cementum found at the cervical two-thirds of the tooth is acellular, extrinsic fiber cementum and plays a significant role in supporting the tooth. These extrinsic fibers are produced by periodontal ligament and gingival fibroblasts. The fibers are inserted into the cementum. In the periodontal ligament, they mesh with the fibers from the alveolar bone to form the periodontal ligament fibers while coronal to the alveolar crest, these fibers insert into the connective tissue, periosteum and cementum of other teeth to form the gingival fibers. Cellular, mixed fiber cementum is found at the apical third of the root and in furcations. It has a mixture of intrinsic fibers produced by cementoblasts and extrinsic fibers. Extrinsic fibers are perpendicular to the cementum and are involved with anchorage whereas the intrinsic fibers are orientated parallel to the surface. In this layer, cementocytes are found. Cementocytes are cementoblasts that

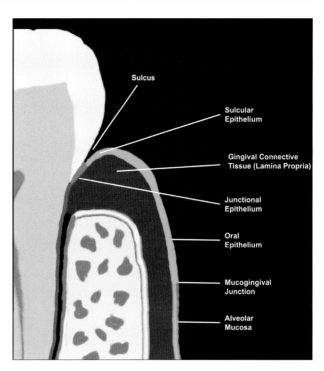

Figure 3-3 Features of the gingiva (junctional epithelium [dark green]).

become surrounded by the cementum. Cementum protects the dentin during tooth movement and wear. The cellular cementum is able to perform repair (Bosshardt and Selvig 1997).

Gingiva

Three types of oral mucosa (masticatory, lining, and specialized mucosa) are found in the oral cavity. The masticatory mucosa that forms a collar around the teeth is defined as the gingiva. The gingiva is attached to the tooth and to the alveolar process. In health, the amount of attached gingiva ranges from 1 mm to 9 mm around the mandibular teeth and on the facial aspect of maxillary teeth. There is great variation in the width, and it is possible to maintain health even in sites with less than 1 mm of attached gingiva (Bowers 1963). The lining mucosa apical to the gingiva is defined as the alveolar mucosa and is loosely bound to the basal aspect of the alveolar process. The gingiva and alveolar mucosa is separated by the mucogingival junction (Figure 3-3).

In a healthy periodontium, the gingiva is typically described to be coral pink and firmly bound whereas the alveolar mucosa is dark-red and movable. In dark-skinned persons, sometimes the gingiva is darker due to melanin pigmentation. On the palatal aspect of maxillary teeth, there is no alveolar mucosa and the palatal gingiva blends with the masticatory mucosa of the palate (Nanci 2008).

The gingiva is comprised of the connective tissue (the lamina propria) and epithelium. The lamina propria contains gingival fibers, ground substance, cells, blood vessels, and nerves. Fifty-five to 60% of the connective tissue is tightly compact fibers bundles that are predominantly collagen. There are also some elastic and oxytalan fibers. Based on their orientation, the collagen fibers are grouped as dentogingival, dentoperiosteal, alveologingival, circular, semicircular, transgingival, intercircular, interpapillary, periosteoginigival, intergingival, and transseptal fibers. These fibers are responsible for supporting the tooth, but they also provide the rigidity and framework of the gingiva. In a healthy periodontium, the gingiva is firm and resilient to frictional forces during mastication. Fibroblast cells are densely populated around these fiber bundles. Other cells present are macrophages, mast cells, neutrophils, and plasma cells, but in health, these cells are in low numbers. During inflammation, the cells dramatically increase in numbers to form dense cell aggregates, which replace the fibers (Schroeder and Listgarten 1997).

The epithelium that lines the lamina propria plays a critical role in protecting the body. It is the first line of defense by providing a physical barrier against bacteria. The epithelium is divided into three parts (Figure 3-3). The oral gingival epithelium is stratified, squamous keratinizing epithelium that extends from the mucogingival junction to the gingival margin. In a healthy periodontium, the gingival margin is typically knife edged and well defined. From the gingival margin to the base of the sulcus, the epithelium that lines the lateral aspect of the gingival sulcus is stratified, squamous non-keratinizing epithelium, known as the oral sulcular epithelium. The base of the sulcus is formed by the coronal aspect of the junctional epithelium. The junctional epithelium is a stratified non-keratinizing epithelium and functions differently from the other two epithelial layers. The oral and sulcular epithelial cells are tightly bound by desmosomes, which provides the gingiva protection from mechanical injury (Nanci 2008).

The junctional epithelial is less resistance to mechanical forces and is more permeable because it is a poorly differentiated tissue with less intercellular junctions. It only has one-third of intercellular junction in comparison to the amount found in the oral and sulcular epithelium. Consequently, there are larger intercellular spaces where fluid and cells can pass through the connective tissue into the sulcus. Invasion of bacteria and its by-products pass through the junctional epithelium more readily. In a healthy gingiva, the junctional epithelium is 15 to 30 cells thick at the coronal aspect and tapers to only 1 to 3 cells thick apically. The entire length of the junctional epithelium provides the seal against the tooth through its two basal laminas. The external basal lamina is attached to the connective tissue, and the internal basal lamina is attached to the tooth. The internal basal lamina attached to the tooth via hemidesmosomes, which provides the epithelial attachment of the gingiva to the tooth (Bosshardt and Lang 2005).

Under experimental condition where the gingiva is completely healthy, there is virtually no gingival sulcus. The coronal aspect of the junctional epithelium is at the level of the gingival margin. Under realistic condition, even for healthy gingiva, there is always a presence of bacteria. As a result, a gingival sulcus is present with elevated level of neutrophils and crevicular fluid (Schroeder 1970). In a healthy periodontium, the histologic sulcus depth has been reported to be from 0 to 2.62 mm (Gargiulo et al. 1961; Wolfram et al. 1974).

In a healthy periodontium, there can be over 200 species in an individual. There is a relatively low bacterial count of 10^3. Seventy-five percent of the bacteria are gram-positive facultative cocci and rods, and 13% are gram-negative rods (Quirynen et al. 2006). Species found in health include *Streptococcus sanguis, Streptococcus mitis, Actinomyces naeslundii, and Actinomyces viscosus* and *Veillonella parvula* (Listgarten 1994). However, red complex bacteria and known periodontal pathogens such as *Porphyromas gingivalis, Tannerella forsythia*, and *Treponema denticola* have been detected in healthy sites (Ximenez-Fyvie et al. 2000).

Because of the constant presence of these bacteria in the healthy periodontium, there continues to be subclinical signs of mild inflammation. Biopsies of clinically healthy gingiva revealed there were predominantly fibroblast cells (57.7%) in the connective tissue, but there was a presence of leukocytes (20.6% neutrophils, 18.4% lymphocytes, and 0.1% plasma cells) (Brecx et al. 1987).

Diagnosis of health

A healthy periodontium is a periodontium that is currently free of any diseases or inflammation and that has not been affected by any irreversible destructive diseases such as periodontitis. Clinical examination of a healthy periodontium should reveal the absence of significant etiologic factors such as plaque, absence of inflammation, and no evidence of clinical attachment loss or periodontal tissue destruction (Figure 3-4).

The instrument used to evaluate the sulcus depth is the periodontal probe. Probing depth is the distance from the gingival margin to the probe tip. Studies have found that the probing depth tends to overestimate the actual sulcus depth. In beagle dogs with healthy gingiva, the probe tip enters into the junctional epithelium and ends, on average, 0.39 mm from the apical termination of junctional epithelium. In beagle dogs with gingivitis, the probe ends

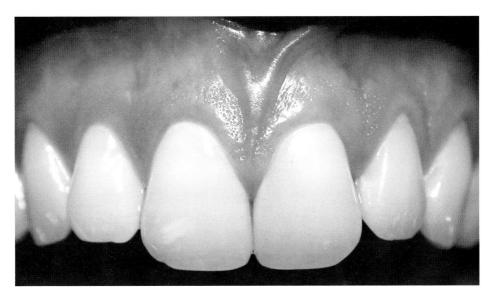

Figure 3-4 Healthy periodontium on maxillary anterior teeth: coral pink, firm gingiva with stippling and knife-edge margins; shallow probing depths; no bleeding on probing, recession, or tooth mobility.

0.10 mm from the apical termination while dogs with periodontitis, the probe passes through the junctional epithelium entirely and ends 0.24 mm into the connective tissue (Armitage *et al.* 1977). In humans, for sites with probing depths less than 4 mm, the probe tip is near (0.01 mm) or slightly beyond (0.02 mm) the apical termination of the junctional epithelium (Magnusson and Listgarten 1980).

In a healthy periodontium, the average sulcus depth is 0.69 mm, and the junctional epithelium is 0.97 mm (Gargiulo *et al.* 1961). Therefore, expected probing depth is close to 2 mm for a healthy status. However, these are averages and there will be variations among individuals.

Healthy status on a reduced periodontium is a clinical situation where the tissue is currently healthy with no signs of inflammation, but there is evidence of past periodontal tissue destruction. This is most frequently found in patients with a past history of periodontitis, but the disease was successfully treated. In other words, the patient regained health and currently is periodontally stable, but there are signs of tissue damage due to past disease (Figures 3-5a and 3-5b).

For sites that have a probing depth more than 4 mm and are inflamed, the probe tip resides in the connective tissue and is 0.29 mm apical to the apical termination of the junctional epithelium during probing. However, one month after daily rinsing with 0.2% chlorhexidine and the teeth are scaled, root planed, and curetted, the probe tip remains in the junctional epithelium and is 0.31 mm coronal to its apical termination during probing (Magnusson and Listgarten 1980).

If the probing depth is deep (greater than 7 mm) and especially in an untreated mouth, there is a likelihood that periodontal pockets and alveolar bone loss exist. However,

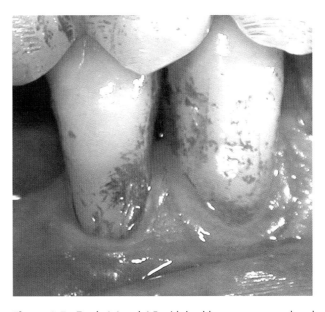

Figure 3-5a Teeth 4.4 and 4.5 with healthy status on a reduced periodontium: coral pink, firm gingiva with knife-edge margins; shallow probing depths; no bleeding on probing or tooth mobility; 2 mm to 3 mm of recession.

moderately deep probing depth (3 to 6 mm) is subject to interpretation. This may be due to pocketing, but it may be also due to the degree of inflammation. A pocket may not exist. Instead the moderately deep probing depth may be due to overestimation of the probe, especially if there is some inflammation (Listgarten 1980).

Furthermore, interpretation of the probing depths can be confounded in sites that have been treated. Periodontitis sites that were treated by periodontal surgery often heal by formation of long junctional epithelium. The length of long junctional epithelium ranged from 1.0 mm to 4.5 mm (Listgarten and Rosenberg 1979). If the long junctional epithelium was 4 mm and there was a slight inflammation, it is possible for the probe tip to pass through the

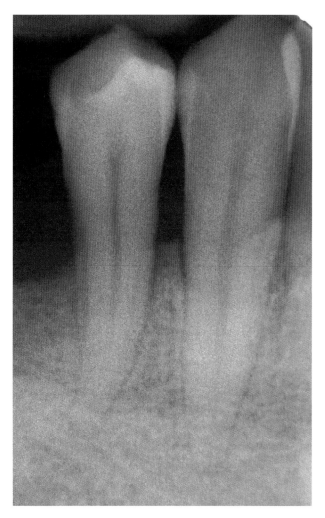

Figure 3-5b Radiograph of Teeth 4.4 and 4.5: presence of horizontal bone loss; alveolar crest is more than 2 mm from the cementoenamel junction.

junctional epithelium to give a probing depth reading of 4 or 5 mm where histologically, there was no significant loss of connective tissue or epithelial attachment. In other words, the sulcus was normal, but the increase in probing depth was due to the degree of inflammation and was not reflective of a true pocket formation (Listgarten 1980).

Tables 3-1 and 3-2 summarize the clinical findings of healthy and healthy on a reduced periodontium. For both healthy and healthy on reduced periodontium, treatment is not necessary. These clinical situations can be maintained through preventive care.

Gingivitis and soft tissue inflammation

Gingivitis is defined as inflammation of the gingiva (American Academy of Periodontology 2001). However, the 1999 International Workshop for the Classification of Periodontal Diseases and Conditions recognized that gingivitis was not a single disease entity. In fact, there are different types of gingival disease, and hence the 1999 Classification defined an entire section to gingival diseases. Common characteristics of all of the gingival diseases include the following:

- signs and symptom being confined to the gingiva
- dental plaque would initiate or exacerbate the lesion
- clinical signs of inflammation
- stable periodontium with no evidence of active loss of attachment
- disease is reversible upon removal of the etiology
- possible role as a precursor to periodontitis (Mariotti 1999)

Examples of gingival diseases include gingivitis associated with dental plaque, puberty-associated gingivitis, pregnancy-associated gingivitis, leukemia-associated gingivitis, drug-influence gingivitis and ascorbic acid-deficiency gingivitis. In this chapter, the focus will only be on plaque-induced gingivitis and plaque-induced gingivitis on a reduced periodontium.

Table 3-1 Clinical features of health

No plaque at gingival margin	
Absence of inflammation	**Absence of periodontal tissue damage**
• Gingival color—coral pink with possible racial pigmentation • Gingival consistency—firm • Gingival margin or contour—knife-edged, positive architecture • Gingival texture—stippling • No bleeding on probing	• Shallow probing depth • No recession • No mobility • No furcation involvement • Radiographic features: No bone loss —Alveolar bone <2 mm from CEJ, intact crestal lamina dura

Table 3-2 Clinical features of healthy on reduced periodontium

No plaque at gingival margin	
Absence of inflammation	Presence of periodontal tissue damage—resolution of previous periodontitis
<ul><li>Gingival color—coral pink with possible racial pigmentation</li><li>Gingival consistency—firm</li><li>Gingival margin or contour—knife-edged, positive architecture</li><li>Gingival texture—stippling</li><li>No bleeding on probing</li></ul>	<ul><li>Shallow to moderate probing depth</li><li>Recession</li><li>Mobility</li><li>Furcation involvement</li><li>Radiographic features: bone loss—Alveolar bone >2 mm from CEJ, intact crestal lamina dura</li></ul>

Epidemiology studies revealed gingivitis is a common disease in both children and adults. In young children, prevalence of gingivitis varied from 9% to 85%, depending on the age and the country of origin (Stamm 1986). Eighty-two percent of adolescents from the United States had gingivitis (Albandar 2002). Various studies reported gingivitis occurring from 75% to 100% of the adult population (Albandar *et al.* 1999).

The primary etiology of gingivitis is plaque. In comparison to health, bacterial count increases from 10^3 to 10^6. About 44% of the bacteria associated with gingivitis are gram-positive facultative cocci and rods, and 40% are gram-negative rods (Quirynen *et al.* 2006). The microbiota shifts toward more gram-negative bacteria, motile rods, and filaments. The bacteria found predominately in gingivitis are *Actinomyces, Streptococcus, Veillonella, Fasobacterium, Treponema* species, and *Prevotella intermedia* (Listgarten 1994). However, the microbiological profile of gingivitis is more similar to the microbiological profile of a healthy periodontium than the profile of periodontitis.

The study by Löe *et al.* (1965) proves that a healthy periodontium developed gingivitis when plaque was allowed to accumulate. Furthermore, this study demonstrated that removal of the plaque led to resolution of the inflammation and return to normal healthy periodontium. Twelve healthy individuals were recruited. They were assessed for the amount of inflammation based on the Gingival Index system and the level of oral hygiene based on the Plaque Index system. The Gingival Index system ranged from 0 to 3 where 0 meant the absence of inflammation, and 3 meant there was severe inflammation with marked redness, hypertrophy, tendency for spontaneous bleeding, and ulceration (Löe and Silness 1963). The Plaque Index system ranged from 0 to 3 where 0 meant no plaque, and 3 had an abundance of plaque within the gingival pocket and/or on the tooth and gingival margin (Silness and Löe 1964).

Then, individuals were instructed not to perform any type of oral hygiene. As the plaque accumulated, the plaque and gingival status were examined at various time intervals. When clinical signs of inflammation appeared, the subjects were then instructed to brush and use wood massage sticks two times per day. The plaque and gingival status were assessed until the gingival and plaque index scores approached 0.

The 12 subjects had an initial mean plaque score of 0.43, which meant they had good oral hygiene with negligible amount of detectable plaque. Upon cessation of oral hygiene, their mean plaque scores increased to 1.67 with large quantities of accumulated soft debris. After reinitiating oral hygiene, the mean plaque score decreased to 0.17.

The gingival condition correlated with the amount of plaque accumulation. The initial mean gingival index was 0.27, which meant virtually no inflammation, and this increased to 1.05 during the period of no oral hygiene. A Gingival Index score of 1 meant mild inflammation with slight change in color and little change in texture. Three subjects developed gingivitis in 10 days; it took 15 to 21 days for the remaining nine subjects to develop gingivitis. The mean gingival index decreased to 0.11 after resuming oral hygiene. The decrease in inflammation took about 5 to 10 days.

This study is useful in educating patients with gingivitis. Some patients may believe that they developed gingivitis because they forgot to brush or floss their teeth the night before. Patients should be educated that the sites with gingivitis have plaque maturing for at least 10 days. Most likely, the plaque has been maturing for at least half a month. In other words, patients need to understand that their oral hygiene routine had been inadequate, and they had been missing those areas for more than half a month. Another point is the patient's expectation in regaining health. The study has demonstrated that after resumption of oral hygiene, it take about 5 to 10 days before there is a lack of inflammation. Patients need to be educated that when they are performing proper oral hygiene such as proper brushing, flossing, or using an interdental brush, the gingiva will continue to be inflamed with bleeding and that these signs will not subside until 5 to 10 days of continuous proper oral hygiene.

The epithelium is the first defense against the bacteria. Page and Schroeder (1976) described the histology changes that occurred when experimental gingivitis developed. Within 2 to 4 days of being exposed to plaque, an initial lesion was formed. The initial lesion was localized to the gingival sulcus with no obvious clinical signs of inflammation. About 5% to 10% of the connective tissue and at the most coronal aspect, the blood vessels dilated, and large numbers of neutrophils migrated from the blood vessels into the junctional epithelium and sulcus. The collagen fibers around these blood vessels were degraded with an increased amount of serum proteins and inflammatory cells. As the inflammation increased, the gingival crevicular fluid flow also increased. The gingival crevicular fluid flowed from the inflamed connective tissue to the gingival sulcus and carried inflammatory cells, enzymes, and cytokines.

The initial lesion then progressed to an early lesion. This usually occurred around 4 to 7 days. A dense lymphoid cell infiltrate dominated by T lymphocytes was formed and occupied about 5% to 15% of the connective tissue. Sixty to 70% of the collagen was lost, and the fibroblasts were altered and increased in size. Proliferation of the basal cells and infiltration of lymphocytes occurred in the junctional epithelium.

Clinical signs of inflammation did not appear until the early lesion became the established lesion. The established lesion was synonymous with gingivitis. It usually took 2 to 3 weeks to develop where there was persistent manifestation of acute inflammation. The lesion only occupied a small portion of the connective tissue and centered near the base of the sulcus. The affected connective tissue predominantly contained B lymphocytes and plasma cells. Immunoglobulins were detected in both the connective tissue and junctional epithelium. There was continued loss of collagen. The junctional epithelium proliferated into the connective tissue. The desmosomal junctions were ruptured, and spaces between the epithelial cells were increased. This distention was due to the migration of the inflammatory cells and fluid exudates that passed through the junctional epithelium. The established lesions were either transient or persistent. If untreated, most established lesions did not progress. A small proportion of the established lesions progressed to periodontitis, but it was uncertain when and what will trigger gingivitis to become periodontitis.

Diagnosis of gingivitis

Gingivitis is inflammation that is superimposed on a normal periodontium. Clinical examination should reveal gingival inflammation but with no evidence of clinical attachment loss or periodontal tissue destruction (Figures 3-6a and 3.6b). However, moderately deep probing depths may arise due to the formation of pseudopockets or gingival pockets. There is no loss of attachment, but due to the inflammation, the gingival margin migrates coronally. As a result, there is an increase in probing depth. Also, depending on the severity of the inflammation, the probe tip may pass through the junctional epithelium and rest on the coronal portion of the connective tissue attachment (Magnusson and Listgarten 1980).

The concept of gingivitis on a reduced periodontium was introduced at the 1999 International Workshop for the Classification of Periodontal Diseases and Conditions (Mariotti 1999). The following describes the clinical situation where gingivitis on a reduced periodontium may develop. First, the patient has periodontitis and experiences irreversible clinical attachment and bone loss. Then, after periodontal therapy, the inflammation is resolved, and periodontal health is established. In other words, the periodontal status is healthy on a reduced periodontium. Then, if oral hygiene is not maintained and plaque eventually accumulates, gingival inflammation will develop within 15 to 20 days. Often this gingival inflammation is transient or reversible. In such cases, the clinical diagnosis is gingivitis on a reduced periodontium. The understanding is the inflammation is caused by the bacteria, but there is no active periodontitis and no evidence of progressive attachment loss. Table 3-3 and Table 3-4 summarize the clinical findings of gingivitis and gingivitis on a reduced periodontium.

Treatment of both gingivitis and gingivitis on a reduced periodontium is to remove the primary etiology. Proper oral hygiene care and removal of plaque and calculus are effective in elimination of the inflammation and in returning the periodontium to healthy or healthy on a reduced periodontium status. The disease is reversible, and there is no evidence of further periodontal tissue destruction.

Periodontitis and its progression

Periodontitis is defined as inflammation of the supporting tissues of the teeth (American Academy of Periodontology 2001). The inflammation results in clinical attachment loss where there is progressive destruction of the alveolar bone, periodontal ligament, and the gingival connective tissue attachment. Bacteria

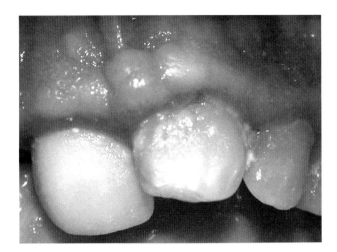

Figure 3-6a Teeth 1.1, 2.1, 2.2 with gingivitis: erythematous gingival margin with rolled border; presence of plaque on the teeth; shallow probing depths with bleeding on probing; no recession or tooth mobility.

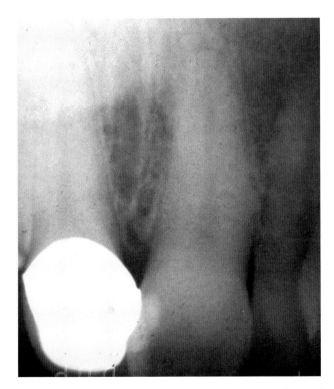

Figure 3-6b Radiograph of Teeth 1.1, 2.1, 2.2: no evidence of bone loss; alveolar crest is less than 2 mm from the cementoenamel junction.

are needed to initiate this disease, but most of the destruction is the result of the host inflammatory response. The ultimate endpoint of periodontitis is tooth loss due to the inadequate support. There are different clinical forms of periodontitis. The most common form is chronic periodontitis. Other forms of periodontitis include aggressive periodontitis, periodontitis as a manifestation of systemic diseases, necrotizing ulcerative periodontitis, and periodontitis associated with endodontic lesion. In this section, the discussion will only focus on chronic periodontitis (Armitage 1999).

Chronic periodontitis is most prevalent in adults but can occur at a younger age. Epidemiological studies have reported the prevalence of periodontitis in the United States to be from 4.2% to 87.4% (Cobb *et al.* 2009). The wide range is due to the lack of consensus on how periodontitis is measured. Albander (2011) reported, based on the NHANES III studies (1988–1994), the prevalence of periodontitis among the American population age 30 and older are 30.5% for mild periodontitis, 13.3% for moderate periodontitis, and 4.3% for advanced periodontitis. In other words, 48.2% of the American adult population has some form of periodontitis.

The primary etiology of chronic periodontitis is bacteria. Periodontitis is unlike other infectious diseases. Many infectious diseases involve the invasion of an exogenous bacterium that eventually overwhelms the body's defense. Periodontitis is caused by a mixed infection involving a diverse group of bacteria. These bacteria are found in biofilms that result in complex interactions between the various bacteria and its environment. *Porphyromonas gingivalis, Tannerella forsythia*, and *Aggregatibacter actinomycetemcomitans* are bacteria that cause periodontitis. Numerous other bacteria are also associated with periodontitis such as *Campylobacter rectus, Eubacterium nodatum, Prevotella intermedia, Prevotella nigrescens, Parvimonas micra*, and *Treponema denticola* (Genco *et al.* 1996). In comparison to both healthy and gingivitis patients, there is a significant shift toward gram-negative anaerobic bacteria in periodontitis patients with about 10% to 13% of the bacteria being gram-positive facultative cocci and rods, and 74% are gram-negative rods (Quirynen *et al.* 2006). Because these bacteria exist in biofilms, there tend to be coaggregation. Six closely associated groups of bacteria species were identified, and many of the putative periodontal pathogens were found to be in the orange and red complexes (Socransky *et al.* 1998). Based on DNA probe count, supragingival plaque from healthy patients contains 0.5% red complex bacteria and 13.8% orange complex bacteria; subgingival plaque contains 2.3% red complex bacteria and 22.5% orange complex bacteria. From periodontitis patients, the supragingival plaque contains 2.8% red complex bacteria and 17.5% orange complex bacteria; subgingival plaque contains 7.0% red complex bacteria and 27.6% orange complex bacteria (Ximenez-Fyvie *et al.* 2000).

Initiation of periodontitis by these periodontal pathogens will be dependent on the specific host

Table 3-3 Clinical features of gingivitis

Presence of plaque at gingival margin	
Presence of inflammation	Absence of periodontal tissue damage
• Gingival color—erythematous	• Shallow to moderate probing depth—possible formation of pseudopockets
• Gingival consistency—edematous, friable, or fibrotic	• No recession
• Gingival margin or contour—rolled, enlarge	• No mobility
• Gingival texture—shiny, smooth, loss of stippling	• No furcation involvement
• Bleeding on probing	• Radiographic features: No bone loss—Alveolar bone <2 mm from CEJ, intact crestal lamina dura
Reversible with plaque removal	

Table 3-4 Clinical features of gingivitis on a reduced periodontium

Presence of plaque at gingival margin	
Presence of inflammation	Presence of periodontal tissue damage—resolution of previous periodontitis
• Gingival color—erythematous	• Shallow to moderate probing depth—possible formation of pseudopockets
• Gingival consistency—edematous, friable, or fibrotic	• Recession
• Gingival margin or contour—rolled, enlarge	• Mobility
• Gingival texture—shiny, smooth, loss of stippling	• Furcation involvement
• Bleeding on probing	• Radiographic features: bone loss—Alveolar bone >2 mm from CEJ
Reversible with plaque removal	

immunoinflammatory response. For individuals who are not susceptible to periodontitis, the oral biofilm in the gingival sulcus will be prevented from advancing further by the host defense mechanism. As a result there will be no formation of periodontal pockets.

Individuals who are susceptible to periodontitis have a different host response. Environmental, acquired, and genetic risk factors such as tobacco smoking, systemic diseases, stress, compromised host defense, and increasing age play a role in determining the susceptibility of the host to periodontitis (Page 1998). The biofilm in the sulcus leads to an inflammatory reaction of the connective tissue. The blood vessels become permeable to neutrophils. The neutrophils travel to the sulcus with their primary purpose of destroying the bacteria. However, during this process, the neutrophils are releasing high levels of matrix metalloproteinases, which results in destruction of the collagen fibers. Consequently, there is a dense inflammatory infiltrate that builds up in the area where collagen destruction has occurred. The junctional epithelium starts to detach from the tooth surface when neutrophils occupy more than 60% of the junctional

epithelium (Carranza and Camargo 2006). This detachment leads to periodontal pocket formation. The periodontal pocket is defined as "a pathologic fissure between a tooth and the crevicular epithelium. It is an abnormal apical extension of the gingival crevice caused by migration of the junctional epithelium along the root as the periodontal ligament is detached by a disease process" (American Academy of Periodontology 2001).

The junctional epithelium transforms into pocket epithelium and become thin and ulcerated. This allows greater access of bacterial virulence factors such as lipopolysaccharides and antigens into the connective tissue. As more collagen fibers are degraded, the pocket epithelium migrates apically. The inflammatory infiltrate is composed mostly of neutrophils, T and B lymphocytes, plasma cells, and macrophages. In the presence of virulence factors, numerous host cells such as monocytes, macrophages, lymphocytes, and fibroblasts produce high levels of pro-inflammatory cytokines. The production of these pro-inflammatory cytokines such as interleukin-1β, tumor necrosis factor-α, interleukin-6, and prostagladin E_2 leads to further destruction of collagen, components of the gingival connective tissue, and the periodontal ligament (Page 1998). Furthermore, these cytokines upset the delicate balance between bone formation and resorption. In the presence of cytokines such as interleukin-1, -6, -11, tumor necrosis factor-α, bradykinin, and kallidin, osteoblasts increase expression of RANKL (receptor activator of nuclear factor-kappa B ligand) on their cell surface. RANKL binds to RANK (receptor activator of nuclear factor-kappa B), which is found on osteoclast precursor cells. This binding leads to osteoclast activation and bone resorption (Cochran 2008).

This lesion is described as the advance lesion and is synonymous with periodontitis. In summary, features of the advanced lesion include the following:

- extension of the lesion into alveolar bone and periodontal ligament
- significant bone loss
- continued loss of collagen subjacent to the pocket epithelium with fibrosis at distant sites
- presence of cytopathically altered plasma cells
- formation of periodontal pockets
- conversion of the bone marrow distant from the lesion into fibrous connective tissue (Page and Schroeder 1976)

Chronic periodontitis is characterized by short periods of activity and long periods of quiescence. During those short burst of exacerbation, there is destruction of the periodontium. The intensity of each episode varies. During the quiescent phase, tissue repair occurs. During this phase, there is reduced inflammatory response with little or no loss of attachment. However, over time, the amount of destruction is greater than the amount of repair, which consequently leads to cumulative loss of attachment (Listgarten 1986). Furthermore, the time of onset and extent of destruction varies from site to site. There is no consistent pattern in terms of how many teeth are involved. Some sites do not exhibit activity whereas other sites may have one or several bursts of activity (Haffajee and Sokransky 1986). The typical convention in the cumulative destruction of chronic periodontitis is considered to be slow where the amount of attachment loss was averaged to be from 0.04 mm to 1.04 mm per year (Fleming 1999). This average tends to mask what is occurring at site-specific levels. A group of patients with periodontitis who did not receive any periodontal therapy were monitored for a period of 6 years (Lindhe *et al.* 1983). Majority of the sites had less than 2 mm of attachment loss, and progression of disease occurred infrequently. However, 1.6% to 3.9% of the sites had more than 2 mm of attachment loss over a 3-year time interval, while 11.6% of sites had more than 2 mm of attachment loss based on a 6-year time interval.

Diagnosis of periodontitis

A site with chronic periodontitis demonstrates signs of inflammation superimposed on sites with a reduced periodontium (Figures 3-7a, 3.7b, and 3.7c). The signs of inflammation are similar to gingivitis such as gingival erythema, edema, and bleeding on probing. These signs are superimposed on sites that exhibit formation of periodontal pockets, alveolar bone and periodontal ligament loss, clinical attachment loss, and tooth mobility. The amount of subgingival plaque and calculus often correlate with the amount of destruction that has occurred.

Number of risk factors and indicators are known to modify the severity of the disease. Demonstrated by longitudinal studies, risk factors are variables that are associated with increased risk of developing periodontitis whereas risk indicators are variables that are identified by cross-sectional studies. Tobacco use and uncontrolled glycemic levels for diabetics are the two strongest risk factors for periodontitis. Individuals with these risk factors are likely to have more periodontal destructions. Other risk factors and indicators include immunosuppression, psychological stress, poor access to dental care, lower socioeconomic status, increase in age, and ethnicity. Table 3-5 summarizes the clinical findings of chronic periodontitis.

If untreated, the ultimate outcome of periodontitis is tooth loss. Treatment of periodontitis involves elimination of the etiology by reducing the bacterial burden, control of the risk factors, and modulation of the host response. Current treatment is often successful in

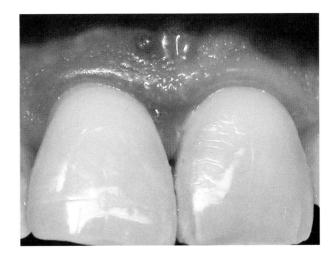

Figure 3-7a Periodontitis on tooth 1.1: erythematous gingiva with enlarged mesial papilla; presence of fistula with deep probing depth and bleeding on probing; slight mobility.

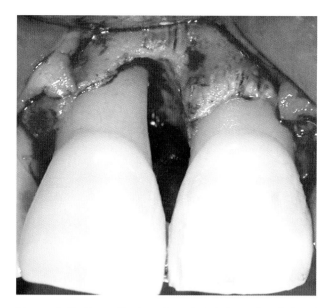

Figure 3-7b Flap reflection of tooth 1.1: loss of periodontal ligament and bone on the mesial aspect.

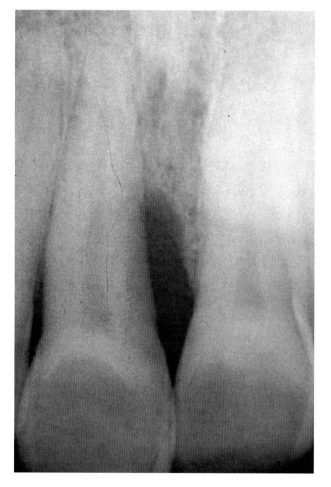

Figure 3-7c Radiograph of tooth 1.1: evidence of bone loss on the mesial aspect; alveolar crest is more than 2 mm from the cementoenamel junction.

elimination of the disease, but there is irreversible destruction of the periodontium. Periodontal maintenance therapy is a critical component to monitor for any recurrence of the disease.

Dental calculus

Dental calculus is a secondary contributing factor to periodontitis. It is formed when the plaque is calcified. As a result, it is a hard mineralized substance that is formed around teeth and dental prostheses. Calculus does not induce the inflammatory response. A study on rhesus monkeys demonstrated that junctional epithelium is able to attach onto the calculus surface if plaque formation was inhibited by daily application of 2% chlorhexidine gluconate (Listgarten and Ellegaard 1973). In other words, the calculus did not trigger any destructive inflammatory response. Instead, if plaque formation was inhibited, healing by repair still occurred despite the presence of the calculus. However, calculus usually exists with a soft loose layer of microorganisms covering its surface (Friskopp and Hammarström 1980). Plaque accumulation is easier on the porous and roughen surface of the calculus, which will eventually lead to a host immunoinflammatory response.

Supragingival or salivary calculus is found coronal to the gingival margin; subgingival or seruminal calculus is formed apical to the gingival margin (American Academy of Periodontology 2001).

The National Survey of Oral Health in US Schoolchildren by the National Institute of Dental Research (1986–1987) revealed supragingival calculus was observed in 33.7% of children and subgingival calculus in 22.8% of children (Bhat 1991). The 1998 United Kingdom Adult Dental Health survey found 73% of adults had calculus (Morris 2001). Sixty-one percent of adults between ages 16 and 24 years had calculus. This prevalence grew to 83% in adults who were age 65 and over.

Calculus formation varies among individuals. Typically, the rate of calculus formation occurs more rapidly in the first 2 to 3 weeks. Mineralization has been observed within 3 days of plaque formation. Calculus formation plateaus off around week 4 (Conroy and Sturzenberger 1968). Age, gender, ethnicity, diet, oral hygiene, bacterial composition, access to professional cleaning, prescribed medications, and mental or physical handicaps are some of the variables that can affect the amount of calculus formation (White 1997). Tobacco smoking has a strong impact on subgingival calculus formation. The mean subgingival calculus load for smokers was much higher (3.4 affected sites per person or a mean proportion of 6.2%) in comparison to former smokers (1.2 affected sites per person or 2.4%) and

Table 3-5 Clinical features of chronic periodontitis

Presence of subgingival plaque and calculus	
Presence of inflammation	Presence of periodontal tissue damage
• Gingival color—erythematous • Gingival consistency—edematous, friable, or fibrotic • Gingival margin or contour—rolled, enlarge • Gingival texture—shiny, smooth, loss of stippling • Bleeding on probing	• Moderate to deep probing depth—periodontal pockets • Recession • Mobility • Furcation involvement • Radiographic features: bone loss—Alveolar bone >2 mm from CEJ
Presence of periodontal risk factors and indicators	

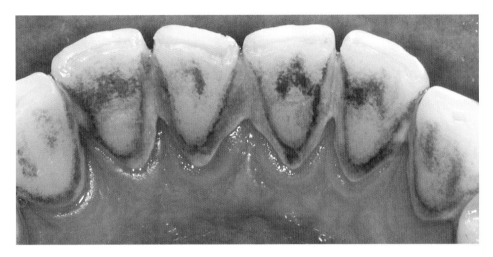

Figure 3-8 Supragingival calculus on the lingual aspect of mandibular incisors.

non-smokers (0.6 affected sites per person or 1.1%) (Bergstrom 2005).

Supragingival calculus is typically a yellow to whitish mass (Figure 3-8). The composition of supragingival calculus is primarily inorganic (75.97% $Ca_3(PO_4)_2$, 3.77% $Mg_3(PO_4)_2$, 3.17% $CaCO_3$). The primary source of the calcium and phosphate is from the saliva. It is frequently found on the buccal aspects of maxillary first molars and on the lingual aspect of mandibular incisors (Corbett and Dawes 1998). These teeth are close to the salivary ducts. The Stensen's duct delivers saliva from the parotid salivary gland and exit adjacent to the maxillary first molar; the Wharton's duct and Bartholin's duct deliver saliva from the submaxillary and sublingual glands to the anterior floor of the mouth (Alexander 1971).

Two-thirds of the inorganic components are in crystalline form (58% hydroxyapatite, 21% magnesium whitlockite, 12% octacalcium phosphate, 9% brushite) (Hinrichs 2006). The organic component is comprised of 8.34% protein, 2.71% fat, and 6.04% water (Glock 1938). There is a mixture of protein-polysaccharide complexes, desquamated epithelial cells, and leukocytes.

Subgingival calculus is dark brown or greenish-black and strongly adheres to the root surface (Figure 3-9). It has similar composition to supragingival calculus but is generally harder than supragingival calculus. The supragingival calculus average mineral content is 36% by volume in comparison to 58% by volume of subgingival calculus (Friskopp and Isacsson 1984).

The mineral component of subgingival calculus is derived from inflammatory and serum exudates in the gingival crevice. The dark color may be due to the iron heme pigments associated with the bleeding of the inflamed gingiva (Wirthlin 2004).

The accumulation of subgingival calculus is less site specific than supragingival calculus. Subgingival calculus is found on mesial and distal surfaces of the lower anterior teeth and on the lingual aspect of mandibular molars (Alexander 1971).

There are numerous theories on how calculus is formed. Two common theories are either mineral precipitation occurs when there is a rise in degree of saturation of calcium and phosphate ions or seeding agents induce foci of calcification. Certain bacteria also have the ability to calcify. They include *S. Sanguis*,

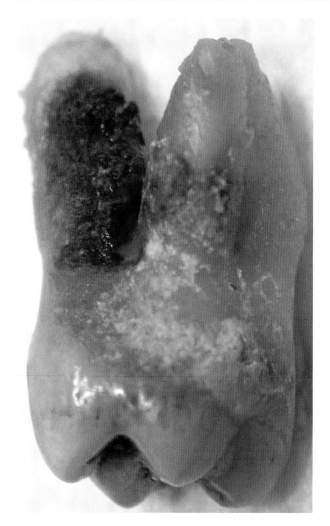

Figure 3-9 Extracted tooth with subgingival calculus on its roots.

S. Salivarius, Bacterionema matruchotii, A. naeslundii, A. viscosus, S. aureus, E. corrodens, Veillonella alcalescens, P. gingivalis, and *Eubacterium saburreum* (Sidaway 1978).

Although calculus is not the primary etiology of periodontitis, removal of the calculus, especially subgingival calculus, is an important goal in terms of periodontal therapy because there is a propensity for plaque to accumulate on its surfaces.

New technologies in detecting periodontal disease progression

The ultimate goal in periodontal therapy is tooth retention. This can be achieved by prevention and early detection of periodontitis. If one can detect when there is active destruction, appropriate intervention to arrest the disease can occur in a timely manner. Periodontitis is a disease that cycles between periods of active destruction and quiescence. Determining when the disease is in its destructive phase is a challenge due to the limitation of the current diagnostic tools.

The ideal diagnostic test should be both highly sensitive and highly specific. Sensitivity is the ability to detect subjects who have the disease; specificity is the ability to correctly identify the subjects who do not have the disease. In other words, the intent is to minimize the number of false positive and negative test results (Listgarten 1986).

The current methods in detecting disease progression are based on subjective evaluation of the combined presence of inflammation and evidence of periodontal destruction. If one solely relies on residual probing depth, a 6-mm residual probing depth has only 37% diagnostic predictability for future attachment loss. The diagnostic predictability improves to 62% if there is a site with 6-mm residual probing depth and bleeds on probing more than 75% of the time over a span of 42 months (Claffey 1990). However, 62% predictability is still a poor percentage.

Current diagnostic technology is largely subjective and relies on experience of the clinician. The concern is that there may be significant amounts of undetected and untreated periodontitis. As a result, appropriate therapy may be occurring too late.

Research in improving diagnostic capability has been focused on identifying biomarkers found during periodontal disease activity. These include assessing for the presence or absence of periodontal pathogens and quantifying markers for inflammation, host immunoinflammatory response, and host tissue destruction. One of the continuing challenges with using these biomarkers is due to the complexity of periodontitis. Currently, there are no universally accepted biomarkers that are specific for periodontitis (Chapple 2009).

Since the discovery of pathogens that are specifically associated with periodontitis, the use of microbiological testing has been used to determine presence or absence of these bacteria. The techniques used range from bacterial culturing, use of immunological assays (for example, enzyme-linked immunosorbent assay, indirect immunofluorescent microscopy assays) and molecular biology techniques (that is, checkerboard DNA-DNA hybridization technology, qualitative and quantitative polymerase chain reaction). These techniques identify the type and amount of periodontal pathogens that exist in the subgingival plaque samples. Culturing determines the antibiotic susceptibility of the pathogens (Sanz *et al.* 2004).

In order for microbial diagnosis to be of value, the results of the microbiological testing should affect the diagnosis and the treatment planning (Listgarten and Loomer 2003). This has not been the case. Microbiological testing is not used on a routine basis for diagnosis. The mere presence of these periodontal pathogens is not adequate to determine disease activity. Periodontal pathogens are found in healthy individuals (Ximenez-Fyvie et al. 2000). The absence of pathogens is a better predictor of periodontal health as opposed to using the presence of pathogens to predict periodontal disease (Wennstrom et al. 1987; Dahlen and Rosling 1998). Furthermore, microbiological testing is unable to differentiate between patients with aggressive and chronic periodontitis (Mombelli et al. 2002). Similarly, microbiological testing on refractory periodontitis patients revealed practically insignificant levels of periodontal pathogens, and yet these patients continue to have significant amount of destruction and attachment loss (Bhide et al. 2006).

With a better understanding that the periodontal pathogens initiate the disease while the host immunoinflammatory response leads to destruction of the periodontal tissue, the research is starting to focus more on the correlation of disease activity with biomarkers of inflammation, host immunoinflammatory response, and host tissue destruction. Examples of these biomarkers include interleukin-1β and -2, tumor necrosis factor-α, interferon-γ (Gorska et al. 2003), matrix metalloproteinase-8 (Mancini 1999), β-glucuronidase (Lamster et al. 1994), alkaline phosphatase (Chapple 1999), and elastase (Eley et al. 1996). These biomarkers can be collected from subgingival plaque, gingival crevicular fluid, saliva, tissue biopsy, and serum (Chapple 1997).

General use of these biomarkers for diagnosis of periodontitis has not been adopted in clinical practice due to a number of reasons. Collection of subgingival plaque and gingival crevicular fluid require selection of sites within the mouth. It is uncertain how many sites would accurately reflect the disease activity. The techniques used to collect the samples are also considered to be time consuming, labor intensive, and complex.

Numerous diagnostic tests have been produced for the market. PerioScan or the BANA test was able to detect the trypsin-like activity of Treponema denticola, Porphyromonas gingivalis, and Tanneralla forsythia. However, the test had a sensitivity of 85% and specificity of 53% for the presence of the periodontal pathogens (Loesche et al. 1990). PerioGard detected the presence of aspartate aminotransferase (AST). AST is an intracellular cytoplasmic enzyme that is released upon cell death. AST levels in gingival crevicular fluid increase during periodontal tissue destruction. PerioGard had 100% sensitivity but only 42% specificity in detecting disease-active sites (Persson et al. 1990). The Periodontal Susceptibility Test detects the presence of two interleukin genes (allele 2 at IL1A + 889 and IL1B + 3953 loci). If patients have both alleles, they were defined to be genotype positive and assumed to be at higher risk

(odds ratio of 18.9) of developing periodontitis. However, in smokers, this specific genotype was not associated with periodontitis (Kornman et al. 1997). Subsequent clinical studies have failed to demonstrate PerioGard as a definitive diagnostic test (Greenstein and Hart 2002). In other words, the current diagnostics kits on the market have performed relatively poorly. One of the reason is the diagnostic kits have focused on a single biomarker.

Proteonomics and genomics are the study of proteins and genes on a large scale. The use of multiple biomarkers can increase the sensitivity and specificity of diagnostic tests. High salivary levels of matrix metalloproteinase-8 or interleukin-1β increase the risk of higher probing depths, clinical attachment loss, and bleeding on probing with an odds ratio of 11 to 15.4. The combined elevated levels of matrix metalloproteinase-8 and interleukin-1β increased the risk of periodontal disease by 45 times (Miller et al. 2006). Another study evaluated if the salivary levels of interleukin-1β is 43.9 pg/ml and levels of matrix metalloproteinase-8 is 264.4 ng/ml, individually, for interleukin-1β, sensitivity is 66%, specificity is 98.3%, positive predictive value is 91.7%, and negative predictive value is 91.2%. For matrix metalloproteinase-8, sensitivity is 40%, specificity is 98.3%, positive predictive value is 90%, and negative predictive value is 85.5% for diagnosis of periodontitis. If both levels are evaluated together, the positive predictive value increases to 96%, and the negative predictive value is 82% (Miller et al. 2010).

For a diagnostic test to be useful and practical from a clinical viewpoint, the test needs to be quantitative, highly sensitive and specific, reproducible, rapid and simple to perform, noninvasive, versatile in terms of sample handling, storage, and transport, amenable to chairside use, economical, and dependent upon simple and robust instrumentation (Chapple 2009).

One of the promising technologies in identifying disease progression is the use of proteomics, genomics, biosensors, and nanotechnology. These technologies have the potential to provide an accurate, portable, and easy-to-use diagnostic platform where the sampling methods are easy, noninvasive, economical, and allow clinicians to identify definitive protein and genetic markers associated with periodontitis (Wong 2006).

The National Institute of Dental and Craniofacial Research funded the development of microfluidics and microelectromechanical (MEMS) systems. These LAB-ON-A-CHIP (LOC) assay systems will provide the capability to analyze fluids and biomarkers. LOC systems allow complex assays to be performed with short analysis time and small samples and reagent volumes (Christodoulides et al. 2007).

Although biomarkers are in higher quantity in the serum and gingival crevicular fluid, the focus is on the use of saliva as the source. Saliva has the advantage of being easily accessible and less labor intensive in its collection. Furthermore, the technologies of these systems are more sensitive to make up the shortfall of biomarkers being in lower amounts in the saliva. As a whole mouth analysis, a disadvantage of using saliva is the lack of site-specific information (Wong 2006).

A variety of researchers are developing and have developed LOC prototypes to measure proteins, DNA, mRNA, bacteria, electrolytes, and small molecules in saliva. These prototypes are handheld, automated sensors that allow for rapid detection of multiple proteins (Zhang *et al.* 2009).

The Integrated Microfluidic Platform for Oral Diagnostics (IMPOD) was developed to measure a variety of putative periodontal disease biomarkers (tumor necrosis factor-α, interleukin-6, matrix metalloproteinase-8) from saliva (Herr 2007a). The IMPOD analyzed 20 μl of saliva in less than 10 minutes for the level of matrix metalloproteinase-8. There was significant correlation between the measured matrix metalloproteinase-8 concentration in saliva with periodontal pocket depth (r = 0.884), clinical attachment loss of >3 mm (r = 0.8223), and degree of radiographic bone loss (r = 0.548) (Herr *et al.* 2007b).

Another LOC system, the LabNow analyzer and Nano-Biochip, evaluated levels of C-reactive protein, matrix metalloproteinase-8 and interleukin-1β. This system was able to determine that the salivary levels of interleukin-1β and matrix metalloproteinase-8 were 2.6 times and 2.0 times higher, respectively, for periodontitis patients than for healthy patients (Christodoulides *et al.* 2007).

These LOC systems are still prototypes. More research is required, and studies need to validate whether these systems are accurate enough to be used as diagnostic tools.

In summary, the ongoing challenge of the clinician is to differentiate between the non-destructive forms of periodontal diseases (gingivitis) from the destructive forms (periodontitis). Periodontitis is a complex disease with a dynamic relationship between the biofilm and the host immunoinflammatory response.

Traditional diagnostic methods in the future will be enhanced by using biomarkers of inflammation, host immunoinflammatory response, and host tissue destruction. Advances in the knowledge of proteomics, genomics, biosensors, and nanotechnology will aid in development of point-of-care diagnostic tools. The value of these point-of-care diagnostic tools can enhance the diagnostic ability of the clinician by providing an accurate, portable, and easy-to-use diagnostic platform where the sampling methods are easy, noninvasive, and economical.

References

Albandar, J.M. (2002) Periodontal diseases in North America. *Periodontology 2000*, 29, 31–69.

Albandar, J.M. (2011) Underestimation of Periodontitis in NHANES surveys. *Journal of Periodontology*, 82, 337–341.

Albandar, J.M., Brunelle, J.A., Kingman, A. (1999) Destructive periodontal disease in adults 30 years of age and older in the United States. *Journal of Periodontology*, 70, 13–29.

Alexander, A.G. (1971) A study of distribution of supra-and subgingival calculus, bacterial plaque, and gingival inflammation in the mouths of 400 individuals. *Journal of Periodontology*, 42, 21–28.

American Academy of Periodontology (2001) *Glossary of Periodontal Terms 4th edn*. Chicago, Illinois.

Armitage, G.C. (1999) Development of a classification system for periodontal diseases and conditions. *Annals of Periodontology*, 4, 1–6.

Armitage, G.C. (2010) Comparison of the microbiological features of chronic and aggressive periodontitis. Development of a classification system for periodontal diseases and conditions. *Periodontology 2000*, 53, 70–88.

Armitage, G.C., Svanberg, G.K., Löe, H. (1977) Microscopic evaluation of clinical measurements of connective tissue attachment levels. *Journal of Clinical Periodontology*, 14, 173–190.

Beertsen, W., McCulloch, C.A.G., Sodek, J. (1997) The periodontal ligament: a unique, multifunctional connective tissue. *Periodontology 2000*, 13, 20–40.

Bergstrom, J. (2005) Tobacco smoking and subgingival dental calculus. *Journal of Clinical Periodontology*, 32, 81–88.

Bhat, M. (1991) Periodontal health of 14–17-year-old US schoolchildren. *Journal of Public Health Dentistry*, 51, 5–11.

Bhide, V.M., Tenenbaum, H.C., Goldberg, M.B. (2006) Characterization of patients presenting for treatment to a university refractory periodontal diseases unit: three case reports. *Journal of Periodontology*, 77, 316–322.

Bosshardt, D.D. and Lang, N.P. (2005) The junctional epithelium: from health to disease. *Journal of Dental Research*, 84, 9–20.

Bosshardt, D.D. and Selvig, K.A. (1997) Dental cementum: the dynamic tissue covering of the root. *Periodontology 2000*, 13, 41–75.

Bowers, G.M. (1963) A study of the width of attached gingiva. *Journal of Periodontology*, 34, 201–209.

Brecx, M.C., Gautschi, M., Gehr, P., *et al.* (1987) Variability of histologic criteria in clinically healthy human gingiva. *Journal of Periodontal Research*, 22, 468–472.

Carranza, F.A. and Camargo, P.M. (2006) The periodontal pocket. In: *Carranza's Clinical Periodontology*, (Eds. M.G. Newman, H.H. Takei, P.R. Klokkevold), 10th edn., pp. 434–451. Saunders, St. Louis.

Chapple, I.L.C. (1997) Periodontal disease diagnosis: current status and future developments. *Journal of Dentistry*, 25, 3–15.

Chapple, I.L.C. (2009) Periodontal diagnosis and treatment—where does the future lie? *Periodontology 2000*, 51, 9–24.

Chapple, I.L.C., Garner, I., Saxby, M.S. *et al.* (1999) Prediction and diagnosis of attachment loss by enhanced chemiluminescent assay of crevicular fluid alkaline phosphastase levels. *Journal of Clinical Periodontology*, 26, 190–198.

Christodoulides, N., Floriano, P.N., Miller, C.S., *et al.* (2007) Lab-on-a-chip methods for point-of-care measurements of salivary biomarkers of periodontitis. *Annals of the New York Academy of Sciences*, 1098, 411–428.

Claffy, N., Nylund, K., Kiger, R., *et al.* (1990) Diagnostic predictability of scores of plaque, bleeding, suppuration and probing depth for probing attachment loss. 3-1/2 years of observation following initial periodontal therapy. *Journal of Clinical Periodontology*, 17, 108–114.

Cobb, C.M., Williams, K.B., Gerkovitch, M.M. (2009) Is the prevalence of periodontitis in the USA in decline? *Periodontology 2000*, 50, 13–24.

Cochran, D.L. (2008) Inflammation and bone loss in periodontal disease. *Journal of Periodontology*, 79, 1569–1576.

Conroy, C.W. and Sturzenberger, O.P. (1968) The rate of calculus formation in adults. *Journal of Periodontology*, 39, 142–144.

Coolidge, E.D. (1937) The thickness of the human periodontal membrane. *Journal of the American Dental Association*, 24, 1260–1270.

Corbett, T.L. and Dawes, C. (1998). A comparison of the site-specificity of supragingival and subgingival calculus deposition. *Journal of Periodontology*, 69, 1–8.

Dahlen, G. and Rosling, B. (1998) Identification of bacterial markers by culture technique in evaluation of periodontal therapy. *International Dental Journal*, 48, 104–110.

Eley, B.M. and Cox, S.W. (1996) A 2-year longitudinal study of elastase in human gingival crevicular fluid and periodontal attachment loss. *Journal of Clinical Periodontology*, 23, 681–692.

Fleming, T.F. (1999) Periodontitis. *Annals of Periodontology*, 4, 32–37.

Friskopp, J. and Hammarström, L. (1980) A comparative, scanning electron microscopic study of supragingival and subgingival calculus. *Journal of Periodontology*, 51, 553–562.

Friskopp, J. and Isacsson, G. (1984) A quantitative microradiographic study of mineral content of supragingival and subgingival dental calculus. *Scandinavian Journal of Dental Research*, 92, 25–32.

Gargiulo, A.W., Wentz, F.M., Orban, B. (1961) Dimensions and Relations of the Dentogingival Junction in Humans. *Journal of Periodontology*, 32, 261–267.

Genco, R., Kornman, K., Williams, R., *et al.* (1996) Consensus report periodontal diseases: pathogenesis and microbial factors. *Annals of Periodontology*, 1, 926–932.

Glock, G. and Murray, M. (1938) Chemical investigation of salivary calculus. *Journal of Dental Research*, 17, 257–264.

Gorska, R., Gregorek, H., Kowalski, J., *et al.* (2003) Relationship between clinical parameters and cytokine profiles in inflamed gingival tissue and serum samples from patients with chronic periodontitis. *Journal of Clinical Periodontology*, 30, 1046–1052.

Greenstein, G. and Hart, T.C. (2002) Clinical utility of a genetic susceptibility test for severe chronic periodontitis: a critical evaluation. *Journal of American Dental Association*, 133, 452–459.

Haffajee, A.D. and Socransky S.S. (1986) Attachment level changes in destructive periodontal diseases. *Journal of Clinical Periodontology*, 13, 461–472.

Hausmann, E., Allen, K., Clerehugh, V. (1991) What alveolar crest level on a bite-wing radiograph represents bone loss? *Journal of Periodontology*, 62, 570–572.

Herr, A.E., Hatch, A.V., Giannobile, W.V. *et al.* (2007a) Integrated microfluidic platform for oral diagnostics. *Annals of the New York Academy of Sciences*, 1098, 362–374.

Herr, A.E., Hatch, A.V., Throckmorton, D.J. *et al.* (2007b) Microfluidic immunoassays as rapid saliva-based clinical diagnostics. *Proceedings of the National Academy of Sciences of the United States of America*, 104, 5268–5273.

Hinrichs, J.E. (2006) The role of dental calculus and other predisposing factors. In: *Carranza's Clinical Periodontology*, (Eds. M.G. Newman, H.H. Takei, P.R. Klokkevold), 10th edn. pp. 170–192. Saunders, St. Louis.

Kornman, K.S., Crane, A., Wang, H.Y., *et al.* (1997) The interleukin-1 genotype as a severity factor in adult periodontal disease. *Journal of Clinical Periodontology*, 24, 72–77.

Kronfeld, R. (1931) Histologic study of the influence of function on the human periodontal membrane. *Journal of the American Dental Association*, 18, 1242–1274.

Lamster, I.B., Holmes, L.G., Grass, K.B.W. *et al.* (1994) The relationship of β-glucuronidase activity in crevicular fluid to clinical parameters of periodontal disease. Findings from a multicenter study. *Journal of Clinical Periodontology*, 21, 118–127.

Lindhe, J., Haffajee, A.D., Socransky, S.S. (1983) Progression of periodontal disease in adult subjects in the absence of periodontal therapy. *Journal of Clinical Periodontology*, 10, 433–442.

Listgarten, M.A. (1980) Periodontal probing: what does it mean? *Journal of Clinical Periodontology*, 7, 165–176.

Listgarten, M.A. (1986) A perspective on periodontal diagnosis. *Journal of Clinical Periodontology*, 13, 175–181.

Listgarten, M.A. (1994) The structure of dental plaque. *Periodontology 2000*, 5, 52–65.

Listgarten, M.A. (1998) A perspective on periodontal diagnosis. *Journal of Clinical Periodontology*, 13, 175–181.

Listgarten, M.A. and Ellegaard, B. (1973) Electron microscopic evidence of a cellular attachment between junctional epithelium and dental calculus. *Journal of Periodontal Research*, 8, 143–150.

Listgarten, M.A. and Loomer, P.M. (2003) Microbial identification in the management of periodontal diseases. A systemic review. *Annals of Periodontology*, 8, 182–192.

Listgarten, M.A. and Rosenberg, M. (1979) Histological study of repair following new attachment procedures in human periodontal lesions. *Journal of Periodontology*, 50, 333–344.

Löe, H. and Silness, J. (1963) Periodontal disease in pregnancy. I. Prevalence and severity. *Acta Odontologica Scandinavica*, 21, 533–551.

Löe, H., Theilade, E., Jensen, S.B. (1965) Experimental gingivitis in man. *Journal of Periodontology*, 36, 177–183.

Loesche, W.J., Bretz, W.A., Kerschensteiner, D., *et al.* (1990) Development of a diagnostic test for anaerobic periodontal infections based on plaque hydrolysis of benzoyl-DL-arginine-naphthylamide *Journal of Clinical Microbiology*, 28, 1551–1559.

Magnusson, I. and Listgarten, M.A. (1980) Histological evaluation of probing depth following periodontal treatment. *Journal of Clinical Periodontology*, 7, 26–31.

Mancini, S., Romanelli, R., Laschinger, C.A., *et al.* (1999) Assessment of a novel screening test for neutrophils collagenase activity in the diagnosis of periodontal diseases. *Journal of Periodontology*, 70, 1292–1302.

Mariotti, A. (1999) Dental plaque-induced gingival diseases. *Annals of Periodontology*, 4, 7–17.

Miller, C.S., Foley, J.D., Bailey, A.L., *et al.* (2010) Current developments in salivary diagnostics. *Biomarkers in Medicine*, 4, 171–189.

Miller, C.S., King, C.P., Langub, C., *et al.* (2006) Salivary biomarkers of existing periodontal disease. A cross-sectional study. *Journal of American Dental Association*, 137, 322–329.

Mombelli, A., Casagni, F., Madianos, P.N. (2002) Can presence or absence of periodontal pathogens distinguish between subjects with chronic and aggressive periodontitis? A systematic review. *Journal of Clinical Periodontology*, 29, 10–21.

Morris, A.J., Steele, J., White, D.A. (2001) The oral cleanliness and periodontal health of UK adults in 1998. *British Dental Journal*, 191, 186–192.

Nanci, A. (2008) *Ten Cate's Oral Histology: Development, Structure and Function*, 7th edn., Mosby, Inc. St. Louis, Missouri.

Page, R.C. (1998) The pathobiology of periodontal diseases may affect systemic diseases: inversion of a paradigm. *Annals of Periodontology*, 3, 108–120.

Page, R.C. and Schroeder, H.E. (1976) Pathogenesis of inflammatory periodontal disease: A summary of current work. *Laboratory Investigation*, 34, 235–249.

Persson, G. R., DeRouen, T. A., Page, R.C. (1990) Relationship between gingival crevicular fluid levels of aspartate aminotransferase and active tissue destruction in treated chronic periodontitis patients. *Journal of Periodontal Research*, 25, 81–87.

Quirynen, M., Teughels, W., Kinder Haake, S., *et al.* (2006) Microbiology of periodontal disease. In: *Carranza's Clinical Periodontology* (Eds. M.G. Newman, H.H. Takei, P.R. Klokkevold) 10th edn. pp. 134–169. Saunders, St. Louis.

Rams, T.E., Listgarten, M.A., Slots, J. (1994) Utility of radiographic crestal lamina dura for predicting periodontitis disease activity. *Journal of Clinical Periodontology*, 21, 571–576.

Sanz, M., Lau, L., Herrera, D., *et al.* (2004) Methods of detection of *Actinobacillus actinomycetemcomitans, Porphyromonas gingivalis* and *Tannerella forsythensis* in periodontal microbiology, with special emphasis on advanced molecular techniques: a review. *Journal of Clinical Periodontology*, 31, 1037–1047.

Schroeder, H.E. (1970) Quantitative parameters of early human gingival inflammation. *Archives of Oral Biology*, 15, 383–400.

Schroeder, H.E. and Listgarten, M.A. (1997) The gingival tissues: the architecture of periodontal protection. *Periodontology 2000*, 13, 91–120.

Sidaway, D.A. (1978) A microbiological study of dental calculus. II. The in vitro calcification of microorganisms from dental calculus. *Journal of Periodontal Research*, 13, 360–366.

Silness, J. and Löe, H. (1964) Periodontal disease in pregnancy. II. Correlation between oral hygiene and periodontal condition. *Acta Odontologica Scandinavica*, 22, 121–135.

Socransky, S.S., Haffajee, A.D., Cugini, M.A., *et al.* (1998) Microbial complexes in subgingival plaque. *Journal of Clinical Periodontology*, 25, 134–144.

Stamm, J.W. (1986) Epidemiology of gingivitis. *Journal of Clinical Periodontology*, 13, 360–366.

Wennstrom, J.L, Dahlen, G., Svensson, J., *et al.* (1987) *Actinobacillus actinomycetemcomitans, Bacteroides gingivalis* and *Bacteroides intermedius*: Predictors of attachment loss? *Oral Microbiology and Immunology*, 2, 158–163.

White, D.J. (1997) Dental calculus: recent insights into occurrence, formation, prevention, removal and oral health effects of supragingival and subgingival deposits. *European Journal of Oral Sciences*, 105, 508–522.

Wirthline, M.R. and Armitage, G.C. (2004) Dental plaque and calculus: microbial biofilms and periodontal diseases. In: *Periodontics: Medicine, Surgery, and Implants.* (Eds. L.F. Rose, B.L. Mealey, R.J. Genco, R.J., D.W. Cohen) pp. 99–116. Mosby, St. Louis.

Wolfram, K., Egelberg, J., Hornbucle, C., *et al.* (1974) Effect of tooth cleaning procedures on gingival sulcus depth. *Journal of Periodontal Research*, 9, 44–49.

Wong, D. (2006) Salivary diagnostics powered by nanotechnologies, proteomics and genomics. *Journal of American Dental Association*, 137, 284–286.

Ximenez-Fyvie, L.A., Haffajee, A.D., Socransky, S.S. (2000) Comparison of the microbiota of supra- and subgingival plaque in subjects in health and Periodontitis. *Journal of Clinical Periodontology*, 27, 648–657.

Zhang, L., Henson, B.S, Camargo, P.M., *et al.* (2009) The clinical value of salivary biomarkers for periodontal disease. *Periodontology 2000*, 51, 25–37.

4

Oral cancer

Grace Bradley and Iona Leong

Introduction

Oral cancer refers to malignant tumors of the oral soft and hard tissues, hence the term encompasses many types of malignant tumors including squamous cell carcinoma, sarcoma of soft tissues and bone, and lymphoma and melanoma that affect the oral cavity. However, more than 90% of malignant oral tumors are squamous cell carcinomas arising from the mucosal epithelium (Neville *et al.* 2009), and this chapter will focus on the prevention of oral squamous cell carcinomas.

Oral cancer can arise from any mucosal site to invade and destroy adjacent normal tissues. It is associated with significant morbidity and mortality because of the importance of oral tissues in chewing, swallowing, speaking, and facial appearance. Furthermore, the carcinoma can metastasize to regional lymph nodes of the neck and distant sites such as lungs, liver, and bone and cause death by disseminated tumor growth and invasion of vital structures (Johnson *et al.* 2005).

The overall 5-year disease-free survival rate of patients with oral cancer has remained at 50% to 60% for several decades (Neville *et al.* 2009), despite advances in techniques of surgical resection and reconstruction and radiation therapy. The prognosis correlates with the stage, or clinical extent, of malignant disease. Localized lesions of oral cancer with no evidence of metastasis are associated with a 5-year survival of greater than 80%. In contrast, advanced oral cancer with distant metastasis has a 5-year survival of about 30% (Jemal *et al.* 2010).

Prevention and early detection are the key approaches to reduce the incidence, morbidity, and mortality of oral cancer. Successful prevention requires an understanding of the epidemiology and risk factors of oral cancer; early detection is based on diagnosis and management of precursor lesions, an understanding of the varied appearance of early stage oral cancer and effective use of biopsy for definitive diagnosis of cancer. The cornerstone of prevention and early detection of oral cancer is regular examination of the oral mucosa by health care professionals with clinical experience in the mode of presentation of oral cancer. During the last 2 decades, advances have been made in understanding the molecular biology of oral cancer, with translation of this knowledge into molecular techniques of cancer prevention and detection (Lingen 2010b; Molinolo *et al.* 2009; Pitiyage *et al.* 2009). These should be validated as adjunctive tools to extend the capability of clinical examination and biopsy of suspicious lesions to control oral cancer.

Among all health care professionals, dentists and dental hygienists have the best opportunity to perform regular, thorough examination of the oral mucosa and to educate patients on risk factors for oral cancer. Sustained efforts to prevent oral cancer must be an integral part of any comprehensive oral health care program.

Epidemiology of oral cancer

Epidemiologic studies have shown the burden of oral cancer as a malignant disease with a wide geographic distribution. There are large variations in the occurrence of oral cancer among different countries and some notable trends in the disease over the past few decades.

The occurrence of disease in a population can be expressed in terms of incidence and prevalence. Incidence is the number of new cases arising in a given period in a

Comprehensive Preventive Dentistry, First Edition. Edited by Hardy Limeback.
© 2012 John Wiley & Sons, Ltd. Published 2012 by John Wiley & Sons, Ltd.

specified population and is usually expressed as the number of cases per year or as a rate per 100,000 persons per year. The prevalence of a particular disease can be defined as the number of persons in a defined population who have been diagnosed with that disease, and who are still alive at a given point in time. Most epidemiologic studies have reported on the incidence of oral cancer, as well as the mortality rate.

Incidence

Oral cancer is the sixth most common cancer in the world today, with an annual estimated incidence of 263,000 (Ferlay *et al*. 2010b). Although oral cancer is

Table 4-1 Lip and oral cavity cancer incidence and mortality rates in more developed and less developed countries

	Incidence number of new cases		Mortality number of deaths	
	Males	Females	Males	Females
Less developed regions	107,739	64,133	61,231	35,734
More developed regions	65,757	28,391	21,878	8,811

Incidence: Population weighted average of the country rates applied to the 2008 area population.
Mortality: Population weighted average of the country rates applied to the 2008 area population.
Source: Ferlay *et al*. (2010b)

uncommon in developed countries, it is a significant and growing problem in other parts of the world (Table 4-1). The highest incidence rates are found in developing countries in South and Southeast Asia, Latin America, and Eastern Europe. In India, Sri Lanka, and Pakistan oral cancer is one of the most common cancers in males, accounting for up to 30% of all new cases of cancer (Table 4-2), whereas in the United States oral cancer accounts for less than 3% of all cancers in males (ACS 2010; Ferlay *et al*. 2010b). The highest age-standardized incidence rates for tongue and mouth cancer in males and females in the world is in Pakistan (Ferlay *et al*. 2010a). Other countries with high incidence rates include Brazil, France, Hungary, Slovakia, Slovenia, Uruguay, Puerto Rico, Papua New Guinea, and Melanesia. Regional variations in the incidence of oral cancer are largely due to differences in exposure to major risk factors such as tobacco and alcohol. The rates in Southeast Asia and certain African countries are directly related to risk behaviors such as chewing tobacco (for example, betel nut chewing, use of qat), in addition to smoking and alcohol consumption.

Age and sex

Oral cancer is more common in men than in women, reflecting the greater exposure of men to risk factors such as tobacco, alcohol, and in the case of lip cancer, sunlight (Table 4-1 and Table 4-2). The risk of developing oral cancer increases with age. Most cases of oral

Table 4-2 Age-standardized incidence rates and number of new cases for cancer of the lip and oral cavity (excluding pharyngeal cancer) in select countries for 2008

Country	Men			Women		
	Rank*	New cases	ASR	Rank*	New cases	ASR
Hungary	5	1,141	16.5	15	348	3.6
Sri Lanka	1	1,701	16.5	8	589	5.0
Pakistan	2	6,803	11.0	3	4,895	8.6
India	2	45,445	9.8	4	24,375	5.2
France	10	3,815	8.1	14	2,026	3.4
Brazil	6	6,474	7.6		2,508	2.3
United States	10	15,817	7.3		7,355	2.8
Canada	12	1,378	5.3		909	3.1
United Kingdom	14	2,293	4.9		1,415	2.4
World	10	170,496	5.3		95,524	2.5

*Rank of oral cancer among 15 most frequent cancers
ASR: Age-standardized rate is the number of new cases per 100,000 persons per year adjusted to the standard age structure. Standardization is necessary when comparing several populations because age has a powerful influence on the risk of cancer.
Source: Ferlay *et al*. (2010b)

cancer occur in people over the age of 50 years, but approximately 6% occur in people under the age of 45 years (Macfarlane *et al.* 1987; Shiboski *et al.* 2005).

Anatomic sites

In the European Union and the United States, the tongue accounts for 40–50% of oral cancers and is the most common anatomic site for oral cancer. Among Asian populations, carcinoma of the buccal mucosa is more common due to betel quid/tobacco chewing habits.

Survival

Survival from a specific cancer can be expressed as the proportion of people diagnosed with that cancer who are still alive 5 years after the diagnosis. For most countries the 5-year survival rate for oral cancer is approximately 50% (Warnakulasuriya 2009b). The oral cancer survival rate is affected by the extent or stage of the disease at the time of diagnosis and whether treatment is available. For example, the relative 5-year survival rate for localized oral cancer is 83%, compared with 32% for cancer with metastases to distant sites. This is also discussed on p. 73 and summarized in Table 4-8. Worldwide variations in 5-year survival rates from oral cancer may be the result of earlier detection and improved treatment in developed countries compared with developing countries (Table 4-3).

Table 4-3 Age-standardized mortality rates and numbers of deaths due to cancer of the lips and oral cavity (excluding cancer of the pharynx) in select countries for 2008

Country	Number of cases men	ASR men	Number of cases women	ASR women
Sri Lanka	1,180	11.5	405	3.4
Hungary	621	8.6	151	1.5
India	31,102	6.8	16,551	3.6
Pakistan	2,996	5.2	2,167	4.1
Brazil	2,780	3.3	920	0.8
France	1,088	2.2	412	0.6
United Kingdom	775	1.5	452	0.6
Canada	354	1.3	226	0.6
United States	2,435	1.1	1,411	0.4
World	83,109	2.6	44,545	1.2

ASR—Age-standardized rate is the number of deaths per 100,000 persons per year adjusted to a standard age structure.
Standardization is necessary when comparing several populations because age has a powerful influence on the risk of cancer.
Source: Ferlay *et al.* (2010b)

Even within a country, significant variations in stage at time of diagnosis and survival rates occur. The overall 5-year relative survival rate for oral cancer in the US in 2010 was estimated to be 61%. For example, the 5-year survival rate in Caucasians is 63% compared with 43% in African Americans, although 36% of Caucasians are diagnosed with early stage disease compared with 22% of African Americans.

Mortality

Mortality is the number of deaths occurring in a given period in a specified population and can be expressed as number of deaths per year or as a rate per 100,000 persons per year. The age-standardized global death rate from oral cancer is estimated at 2.6 per 100,000 men and 1.2 per 100,000 women (Ferlay *et al.* 2010b). The majority of deaths due to oral cancer occur in the less developed countries, with the greatest burden seen in India (Tables 4-1 and 4-3). Declining oral cancer death rates in Western Europe since the late 1980s stand in contrast to the increasing mortality rates seen in Central Europe and Eastern Europe, especially in Hungary, Slovakia, Slovenia, and the Russian Federation (La Vecchia *et al.* 2004). Regional variations in the mortality rates due to oral cancer are largely due to differences in exposure to major risk factors such as tobacco and alcohol consumption, availability and quality of treatment, completeness of reporting, and age structure of the population.

Trends

Trends in oral cancer incidence are not uniform in the world. For example, there is an increasing trend in oral cavity and tongue cancer incidence in men and women in North and Eastern Europe, Asia, China, and India. Declining rates are seen in men in France and Italy; however, rates for oral and tongue cancer are increasing in women in France, Germany, the UK, and Japan. In South America the rates are stable for men and increasing for women.

The incidence of cancer of the oral cavity and pharynx in the United States has been declining in men since 1975 and in women since 1980, although recent studies have shown that the incidence is increasing for those cancers related to human papillomavirus (HPV) infection (ACS 2010).

Changes in alcohol and tobacco consumption may modify trends in oral cancer incidence and mortality. Death rates in the United States from oral cavity and pharynx cancer have decreased by more than 2% per year since 1980 in men and since 1990 in women (ACS

Table 4-4 Trends in 5-year relative survival rates in US

Cancer type	1975–77	1984–86	1999–2005
All sites	50%	54%	68%*
Oral cavity and pharynx	53%	55%	63%*

*The difference in rates between 1975–1977 and 1999–2005 is statistically significant (p<0.05).
Survival rates are adjusted for normal life expectancy and are based on cases diagnosed in the SEER 9 areas from 1975–1977, 1984–1986, 1999–2005, and followed through 2006.
Source: American Cancer Society, Cancer Facts and Figures 2010.

2010) and is probably related to changes in tobacco and alcohol consumption (Table 4-4).

Conclusion

The high incidence of oral cancer in many countries with limited health care resources emphasizes the importance of a preventive approach to control this disease. The geographic pattern and trend over time indicate the importance of lifestyle and habits in the development of oral cancer. Large-scale, multicenter studies have allowed the evaluation of a number of lifestyle- and habit-related risk factors, which should help to direct ongoing efforts at primary prevention.

Risk factors

Risk factors are habits, aspects of lifestyle and chronic health problems that increase the likelihood of developing a disease. For oral cancer, the firmly established risk factors are tobacco use, excessive alcohol consumption, and betel quid/areca nut chewing, while sun exposure is the major risk factor for cancer of the vermilion border of lip. Other potential risk factors have been proposed, including infection by HPV, marijuana smoking, chronic periodontal disease, and low intake of fruit and vegetables, but the evidence for these associations is not as strong (Table 4-5).

Investigations into the risk factors for oral cancer have been helpful in understanding the global epidemiologic patterns of this disease, and allow the identification of individuals who are at high risk for oral cancer. Primary prevention of oral cancer is largely based on controlling or eliminating tobacco and alcohol consumption. However, the mechanisms by which the known risk factors contribute to the multistep process of oral cancer development are not well understood. Oral cancer can develop in individuals with no known risk factors, and it is important that diagnosis is not delayed or missed in patients who do not fit the high-risk profile.

Table 4-5 Risk factors for oral cancer

Strong associations
Tobacco smoking
Smokeless tobacco
Alcohol consumption
Betel quid and areca nut chewing
Sun exposure (cancer of the lip)

Weak associations
Human Papillomavirus infection (strong association with oropharyngeal cancer)
Marijuana smoking
Chronic periodontal disease
Low intake of fruit and vegetable

The risk factors listed in Table 4-5 represent our understanding of the extrinsic or environmental factors in cancer development.

Recent studies have examined genetic susceptibility to account for variations in the response to carcinogenic factors, such as metabolism of carcinogens (both activation and inactivation), capacity for DNA repair, and also immunologic response to viral infection. Elucidation of host factors such as deficient DNA repair may also help in understanding the development of oral cancer in the absence of known risk factors.

Tobacco and alcohol use

Large-scale epidemiologic studies have indicated that approximately 75% of head and neck cancers, which include cancer of the oral cavity, oropharynx, hypopharynx, and larynx, are attributable to cigarette smoking and alcohol drinking (Hashibe et al. 2007; Marron et al. 2010). All forms of tobacco use, including cigarette, cigar, and pipe smoking and various types of smokeless tobacco, are associated with an increased risk of oral cancer, although the most extensive epidemiologic data concern cigarette smoking because of its high prevalence. Cigarette smokers have a higher risk of developing head and neck cancer than never-smokers (odds ratio = 2 for all levels of smoking combined) in the absence of alcohol consumption. There is a dose-response effect, in that the risk of cancer is proportional to the number of cigarettes smoked per day, the duration of smoking and pack-years of cigarette use. (Smoking one pack per day for 1 year will give the cumulative measure of 1 pack-year.) The odds ratio for head and neck cancer rises above 4 in people who have more than 30 pack-years of cumulative exposure (Blot et al. 1988, Hashibe et al. 2007). When the head and neck subsites are considered separately, the risk of laryngeal cancer is most strongly associated with cigarette smoking, followed by oral and pharyngeal cancer. Cigarette smoking is thought to cause diffuse alterations throughout the mucosa of the upper aerodigestive tract that predispose to cancer, described as 'field cancerization.' Patients who continue to smoke after treatment of oral cancer have an increased risk of developing a second primary cancer within the upper aerodigestive tract.

Alcohol has not been found to be a strong risk factor in the absence of tobacco use. Heavy drinkers who consume three or more drinks per day have twice the risk of head and neck cancer, in the absence of tobacco use. (One drink is 12 ounces of beer, 5 ounces of wine, or 1 ounce of liquor or aperitif.) The effect is greatest for pharyngeal cancer and less for oral cancer (Hashibe et al. 2007). However, there is a synergistic effect (greater than expected joint effect) when smoking is combined with alcohol drinking. In a large epidemiologic study of head and neck cancer, tobacco users who were nondrinkers have a twofold risk of cancer, alcohol drinkers who did not use tobacco do not show a significantly increased risk of cancer, but tobacco users who were drinkers have 5 times the risk of cancer. For oral cancer, the greatest risk is seen among smokers who also consume three or more drinks per day, where the risk is 10- to 15-fold compared to nonsmokers who were also nondrinkers (Hashibe et al. 2009).

The effect of tobacco use and alcohol drinking on the incidence of head and neck cancer is illustrated by the population attributable risk (PAR), which represents the reduction in incidence of the disease that would be observed if the population were entirely unexposed to these risk factors alone or in combination (Figure 4-1). Approximately 72% of head and neck cancer can be attributed to tobacco use or alcohol drinking, singly or in combination. The PAR for tobacco and/or alcohol is lower for oral cancer (64%) than pharyngeal and laryngeal cancer (72% and 88%, respectively). For all head and neck sites taken together, the PAR for tobacco and/or alcohol is lower for women (58%) than men (75%) and very much lower for the under-45 age group (44%) compared to those over 45 (77%) (Hashibe et al. 2009). The PAR values show the importance of controlling tobacco and alcohol use in prevention of head and neck cancer, but they also demonstrate that a significant fraction of head and neck cancer cannot be attributed to these two major risk factors. This is especially notable for oral cancer compared to pharyngeal and laryngeal cancer, for young patients under 45, and female patients. For the never smoker-never drinkers who develop oral cancer, there is a need to investigate other risk factors such as human papillomavirus, marijuana use, involuntary or second-hand smoke, and dietary factors (Dahlstrom et al. 2008) so that preventive measures can be instituted.

Cessation of tobacco smoking or alcohol drinking has been reported to reduce the risk of head and neck cancer, but it takes years before the cancer risk returns to the level of never smoker-never drinkers (Marron et al. 2010). Oral cancer risk is reduced among individuals who stopped smoking 1 to 4 years ago and continues to decrease with increasing time since cessation (Figure 4-2). The risk returns to the level of never smokers 20 years after quitting. The prolonged effect of tobacco smoking suggests that the cellular and molecular changes produced by tobacco carcinogens are only corrected after many generations of epithelial proliferation.

In accordance with the synergistic effect of tobacco use and alcohol drinking, the reduction in cancer risk after smoking cessation is seen among current and former alcohol drinkers but is less consistent among never-drinkers. Cessation of alcohol drinking is beneficial in reducing oral cancer risk, especially after 10 or more years (Figure 4-2). Among individuals who smoke and drink alcohol, the data suggest that quitting both habits is slightly better in cancer risk reduction compared to quitting smoking only (Marron et al. 2010). Overall, the data emphasize that the best approach to oral cancer prevention is to avoid tobacco use in the first place and to stop smoking in those who have taken up the habit.

Betel quid and areca nut chewing

Areca nut chewing is a widespread habit in many parts of Asia, particularly India, Sri Lanka, Taiwan, the southern part of China, Papua New Guinea, and among immigrants from these areas to Western countries. Areca nut is consumed for social and religious reasons. It produces a sense of euphoria and heightened alertness, and it is addictive. The most common form of areca nut chewing is the betel quid, which consists of areca nut, slaked lime, and spices, with or without tobacco, wrapped in a betel leaf. The betel quid is typically placed in the labial or buccal vestibule and either slowly chewed or left to rest on the mucosa for hours. In many communities, children and teenagers are encouraged to take up the habit, often with sweetened products to appeal to them. It is not uncommon for areca nut chewers to have a history of 5 or 6 decades of chewing (Auluck et al. 2009).

Areca nut and betel quid chewing, with or without tobacco, is associated with oral cancer. Numerous studies done in geographic regions with high prevalence of these habits have shown an increased risk of oral cancer among chewers. Betel quid chewing is in fact the predominant risk factor for oral cancer in many parts of South Asia and Southeast Asia (IARC 2004; Secretan et al. 2009). The cancer usually develops in the area of oral mucosa chronically exposed to the areca nut or betel quid, and is frequently preceded by leukoplakia and erythroplakia

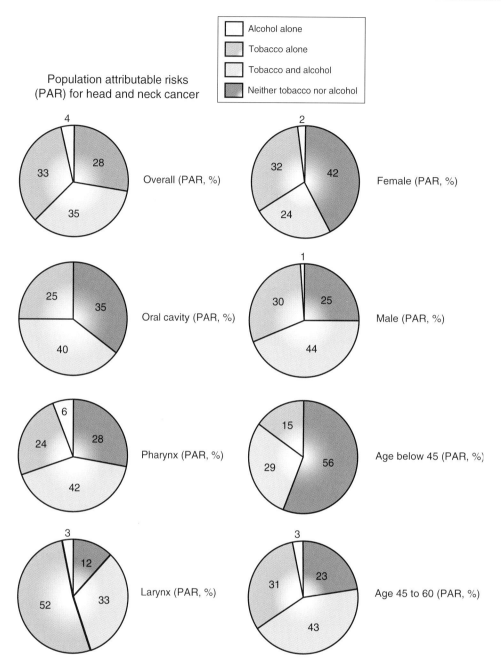

Figure 4-1 Population attributable risks for head and neck cancer, overall, and by site, sex and age group, showing the proportion of cancer cases that may be attributed to tobacco and/or alcohol.

(white and red patches) or by oral submucous fibrosis. The latter is an irreversible condition specifically associated with areca nut chewing and is characterized by blanching and stiffening of the labial and buccal mucosa and soft palate, resulting in inability to open and obliteration of the labial and buccal vestibules. Chewing betel quid with tobacco is associated with 6 to 9 times the risk of oral cancer compared to non-chewers. The increase in cancer risk is smaller for betel quid chewing without tobacco, but this varies among studies, possibly due to

differences in the constituents of the chewed material. A dose-response relationship has been demonstrated, with increasing risk of cancer associated with increased duration of the habit and larger number of betel quids chewed per day (IARC 2004; Thomas *et al.* 2007).

In view of the well-documented association between betel quid chewing and oral cancer, it is important for health professionals to be aware of the oral manifestations of betel quid chewing, to inquire about this group of habits, and counsel patients accordingly.

Reduction of risk of oral cancer upon cessation of tobacco smoking or alcohol drinking

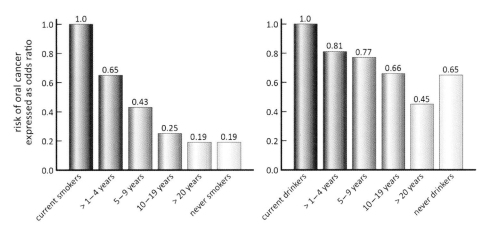

Figure 4-2 Graphs of relative risk of oral cancer showing the gradual decrease in risk over 20 years following cessation of tobacco or alcohol use.

Human papillomavirus

Human papillomavirus (HPV) is a causative factor for carcinoma of the uterine cervix. At least 90% of cervical carcinomas contain the DNA of high risk HPV (types 16 and 18), and infection with this virus is now thought to be necessary for the development of cervical carcinomas. Extensive studies of HPV in head and neck carcinomas have indicated that HPV infection is not necessary for the development of carcinomas across all head and neck sites. However, carcinoma of the oropharynx, particularly the tonsils and base of tongue, is strongly associated with HPV type 16, with up to 60% of carcinomas in this subsite found to contain HPV DNA in high copy number and in transcriptionally active form. Carcinomas of other head and neck sites, including oral cavity, are less likely to contain HPV, with reported detection rates of around 4% for oral carcinomas (Gillison and Lowy 2004; Adelstein *et al.* 2009).

HPV-associated head and neck cancer has a distinct risk factor profile from non HPV-associated cancer. Certain sexual practices, such as oral-genital contact and high number of sexual partners, are associated with increased risk of HPV-positive oropharyngeal cancer, suggesting that oral-genital contact is the predominant route of infection of the oral and pharyngeal mucosa (Gillison *et al.* 2008; Heck *et al.* 2010). Use of marijuana is also a risk factor for HPV-positive carcinoma but not for HPV-negative carcinoma, and the magnitude of the risk is proportional to cumulative joint-years of marijuana smoking (Gillison *et al.* 2008). Conversely, smoking and alcohol drinking are strong risk factors for HPV-negative cancer but not for HPV-positive cancer.

Seropositivity to HPV 16 capsid protein L1 was found to be associated with carcinoma of the oropharynx and oral cavity. However, the presence of antibodies to HPV reflects infection in all susceptible mucosal sites including the upper aerodigestive tract and anogenital mucosa. Conversely, not all individuals exposed to HPV seroconvert or continue to be seropositive over time (Herrero *et al.* 2003). These considerations may complicate the use of serologic tests for HPV infection as a risk marker for oral and oropharyngeal cancer.

The presence of HPV in exfoliated oral mucosal cells was not associated with cancer of the oral cavity or oropharynx (Herrero *et al.* 2003). To date, there are no cohort studies that demonstrate an association between detection of HPV in exfoliated oral cells and risk of head and neck carcinoma. Thus, the usefulness of HPV testing to indicate risk of oral and oropharyngeal cancer has not been established (Gillison and Lowy 2004; Lingen 2010a).

The demonstration of an association between oropharyngeal carcinoma and high risk HPV has implications for the prevention of these cancers by vaccination. Currently, two HPV vaccines that are effective in preventing infection are available, with one vaccine targeting both low and high risk types to prevent genital warts and cervical carcinomas and the other vaccine targeting only the high risk types. Several countries, including Australia, the UK, and Canada have instituted publicly funded vaccination programs for girls prior to sexual activity and exposure to HPV. The effect of mass vaccination programs for young people of both sexes on the incidence of oral and pharyngeal cancer will require large-scale cohort studies (Adelstein *et al.* 2009).

Other risk factors for oral cancer

Several potential risk factors have been considered for oral cancer, although their role has not been firmly established, either in conjunction with tobacco and alcohol use, or as independent factors that may contribute to oral cancer in non-smokers who are also non-drinkers.

Marijuana smoking produces carcinogens similar to tobacco smoking (for example, nitrosamines and polycyclic aromatic hydrocarbons), even though the cannabinoids themselves have not been shown to be carcinogenic. Worldwide, marijuana is the most common illegal drug, and is used by an estimated 4% of the world population in the 15- to 64-age group (Berthiller *et al.* 2009). According to a 2007 report by the United Nations, the prevalence of marijuana use is highest in Micronesia and Papua New Guinea (29%), Ghana (21.5%), Zambia (17.7%), Canada (16.8%), Australia and New Zealand (13.4%), and the US (12.6%). Small-scale studies have reported an association between marijuana smoking and upper aerodigestive tract cancer, but this has not been confirmed in other studies (Warnakulasuriya 2009a). A large epidemiologic study did not find an association between marijuana smoking and head and neck cancer either overall, or among never users of tobacco and never drinkers (Berthiller *et al.* 2009). There is evidence to suggest an association with oropharyngeal cancer, specifically with HPV 16-positive squamous cell carcinoma. The majority of these carcinomas are found in the palatine tonsils and the base of the tongue, which form part of the Waldeyer's ring of lymphoid tissue, and it has been suggested that cannabinoids might contribute to HPV-associated carcinogenesis through modulation of immune function. Tobacco smoking and alcohol consumption are both prevalent among marijuana users, so the role of marijuana may be confounded by the strong combined effect of tobacco and alcohol. Analysis of the association between marijuana use and head and neck cancer is further complicated by variation in the frequency and duration of the habit and the potency/formulation of the consumed product as joints, pipes, or others. At this time, it is not possible to exclude marijuana smoking as a risk factor for oral cancer, and further studies that control for smoking and alcohol consumption are warranted.

Reducing the risk of oral cancer

Diet

The role of low vegetable and fruit intake has been examined as a risk factor for several cancer types, including colorectal, stomach, esophageal, oral, and oropharyngeal cancer (Danaei *et al.* 2005). Other studies have looked at the protective effect of high consumption of vegetables and fruit against cancer development. Many different constituents of plants may help to prevent cancer, including carotenoids, flavonoids, ascorbate, folate, and fiber, and they may act in combination to affect different steps in cancer development. There is no uniform system to measure vegetable and fruit intake, and no single definition of a unit of intake. Some studies use broad categories (such as, all vegetables and fruit) while others consider categories that may be botanical or culinary. Dietary habits are affected by smoking, which is a strong risk factor for oral and oropharyngeal cancer, so it is important to control for the effect of smoking in studies of diet and oral cancer. Several studies have shown a decreased risk of head and neck cancer in individuals with high intake of vegetables and fruit compared to those with low intake with a relative risk of about 0.7 (AICR 2009; Freedman *et al.* 2008). Other studies did not show a significant effect. Overall, the current evidence indicates that non-starchy vegetables and fruits probably protect against cancer of the mouth, pharynx, and larynx (AICR 2009).

Improved oral hygiene

Poor oral health and chronic periodontal disease have been reported as risk factors for head and neck cancer. The underlying mechanism(s) for this association is not clear. Bacterial enzymes in dental plaque may activate carcinogens in tobacco or dietary constituents and thus increase the risk of cancer. Chronic inflammation leads to tissue damage, which stimulates attempts at regeneration and repair, and this may contribute to cancer development. Two hospital-based, case-control studies conducted in Eastern Europe and Latin America showed that poor oral hygiene, as assessed by a trained interviewer, was associated with increased risk of cancer of the oral cavity, pharynx, and larynx. A significant association was found for current smokers and drinkers but not for non-smokers, former smokers, or non-drinkers. Number of missing teeth was not associated with cancer at these sites (Guha *et al.* 2007). A case-control study that was based on a single cancer center in the US demonstrated an association between risk of head and neck cancer and alveolar bone loss measured in panoramic radiographs. The association was strongest among former smokers, followed by non-smokers and current smokers, and was found among both users and non-users of alcohol. Number of missing teeth did not show a significant association with head and neck cancer (Tezal *et al.* 2009).

Further investigations of oral hygiene and chronic periodontitis as risk factors for head and neck cancer are warranted, and may increase our understanding of the role of microorganisms in mucosal cancer. On the other hand, it is well established that prevention and treatment of periodontal disease are important for optimal oral health and function, and these recent studies that suggest a cancer risk from poor oral hygiene and periodontal disease provide an additional rationale for maintenance of good oral hygiene.

Genetic predisposition/molecular epidemiology

Although tobacco use and alcohol drinking are major risk factors for oral cancer, not all smokers and drinkers develop cancer in their lifetime. This suggests that there is variation in susceptibility to carcinogens from tobacco and alcohol (Hashibe et al. 2003; Wang et al. 2010). Cigarette smoke contains DNA damaging agents (mutagens) such as benzo(a)pyrene, which can form DNA adducts that interfere with gene transcription and DNA replication. Many carcinogens require biochemical activation by cytochrome enzymes (for example, CYP1A1) and are metabolized to biologically inactive forms by detoxifying enzymes, notably glutathione-S transferases (GST-M,T,P). Cells with damaged DNA may repair the damage by multi-enzyme pathways such as the nucleotide excision repair pathway. Recent studies have investigated the association between genetic polymorphisms of these enzymes and development of head and neck cancer. Lack of functional GST-M or GST-T is associated with a modest increase in risk (less than twofold) of head and neck cancer, probably due to reduced ability to detoxify tobacco carcinogens (Hashibe et al. 2003). Polymorphism (variations of gene sequence that can be detected within a population) of several DNA repair genes are also reported to be associated with a moderate increase in head and neck cancer risk, probably due to decreased DNA repair capacity (Huang et al. 2005; An et al. 2007). Reports of genetic polymorphisms as cancer risk factors are often inconsistent and difficult to interpret, because of the large number of genetic variants, the varying prevalence of each variant in different geographic locations, and the relatively small effect on risk that is conferred by an individual variant. Future studies will likely focus on combinations of genetic polymorphisms and their interaction with different levels of tobacco and alcohol exposure. At present, there is no reliable genetic test of susceptibility or resistance to tobacco carcinogens. Avoidance of tobacco and alcohol is the most effective way to prevent oral cancer.

Premalignant or potentially malignant oral lesions

Oral cancer develops through a multi-step process, in which premalignant, or potentially malignant, epithelial lesions can be recognized. These premalignant lesions are often clinically detectable as white or red patches, called leukoplakia and erythroplakia, respectively. Considerable efforts have been made over the past 30 to 40 years to define leukoplakia and erythroplakia, in order to separate them from other oral white and red patches that are inflammatory, reactive, or infectious in nature and are not associated with cancer development (Warnakulasuriya et al. 2007). Longitudinal studies have shown that oral premalignant lesions may have different outcomes that are generally difficult to predict. A minority of these lesions progress to an invasive malignant lesion, while others remain unchanged for years, decrease in size, or become larger and more irregular in shape and texture. Long-term follow-up studies of leukoplakia in Europe and North America have shown that between 1% and 18% of these lesions developed into carcinoma, over a period that varied from a few months after initial diagnosis of leukoplakia to more than 10 years (Napier and Speight 2008). Accurate diagnosis of leukoplakia and erythroplakia, assessment of the risk of progression to cancer, and optimal management of these lesions form an approach to the secondary prevention of oral cancer.

A widely used definition of leukoplakia is 'a predominantly white lesion of the oral mucosa that cannot be characterized as any other definable disease' (Axell et al. 1996). Recently, this definition has been amended to state that 'the term leukoplakia should be used to recognize white plaques of questionable risk having excluded known diseases or disorders that carry no increased risk for cancer' (Warnakulasuriya et al. 2007). It is clear that the diagnosis of leukoplakia is one of exclusion, and requires that other causes of oral white lesions have been excluded (Table 4-6).

Erythroplakia is the red counterpart of leukoplakia and is defined as a red patch that cannot be characterized as any other definable disease. This is again a diagnosis of exclusion and requires that red patches of inflammatory or infectious nature have been ruled out (Table 4-6). Following a provisional diagnosis of leukoplakia or erythroplakia that is based on history and clinical examination, biopsy is required to confirm that the white or red patch is not due to other diseases, and to examine for the presence and severity of epithelial dysplasia (Warnakulasuriya et al. 2007).

Leukoplakia is a fairly common oral lesion, and the overall prevalence rate based on studies worldwide is estimated to be between 1% and 5%. The reported prevalence rate varies among different studies, because of differences in the populations being studied and the diagnostic criteria used for leukoplakia (Napier and Speight 2008). A subset of leukoplakia has a red component and is called erythroleukoplakia, although predominantly red lesions or erythroplakia are rare. It is important to recognize

Table 4-6 Causes of white and red patches that should be excluded to make the diagnoses of leukoplakia and erythroplakia, respectively. Modified from Warnakulasuriya *et al.* (2007)

White patches

---

frictional keratosis
keratosis from habitual cheek biting
leukoedema
acute pseudomembranous candidiasis
chemical injury
lichen planus (plaque type)
lichenoid reaction, such as to amalgam
white sponge nevus
hairy leukoplakia

Red patches

---

traumatic lesion (frictional irritation or thermal burn)
non-specific gingivitis
atrophic candidiasis
erythematous lichen planus
hypersensitivity reaction

---

erythroplakia despite its rarity because of a much stronger association with carcinoma (Neville and Day 2002).

Leukoplakia is seen over a wide age range but is much more common in middle-aged and older persons, and is more prevalent among males. Studies in Asia, Europe, and North America have shown that the occurrence of leukoplakia corresponds closely with tobacco use, including various forms of smoking and smokeless tobacco. The anatomic distribution of these lesions varies among studies in different geographic locations, and again there is a relationship with pattern of tobacco use. Lesions are commonly found on the buccal mucosa and commissures, gingiva, and tongue, followed by the palate and floor of the mouth. Despite the close association between leukoplakia and tobacco use, a significant number of leukoplakias occur in persons who have never smoked and are considered idiopathic (Napier and Speight 2008).

The clinical appearance of leukoplakia ranges from thin, flat, greyish-white patches to thick, opaque-white patches with a rough or fissured surface. Some lesions have papillary surface projections and are called verrucous or verruciform leukoplakia. Lesions that are mixed red and white often have a granular or nodular surface and are called erythroleukoplakia, speckled, or nodular leukoplakia. Erythroplakia appears as a smooth red patch that may be sharply demarcated or have vague borders. The extent and number of lesions also vary from a single, small, well-defined lesion to large lesions with indistinct borders covering several square centimeters (Figure 4-3). An uncommon form of leukoplakia, called proliferative verrucous leukoplakia, is characterized by multifocal lesions, which progress from flat white patches to thick, verrucous lesions that occupy a large part of the oral mucosa (Axell *et al.* 1996; Neville and Day 2002).

Assessment of the risk of progression to carcinoma is based on clinical and histologic features (Table 4-7).

The risk is higher in persons over age 50 and in females. Lesions in the floor of the mouth and lateral-ventral tongue are more likely to progress than those in the buccal mucosa and commissures.

Although the majority of leukoplakias are associated with tobacco use, the idiopathic lesions in non-tobacco users are more likely to become malignant. This seemingly paradoxical observation should not diminish the importance of tobacco in oral cancer development, but it may indicate that idiopathic leukoplakias result from less reversible alterations of the epithelium. Larger size and non-homogenous appearance of the lesion have been reported to be associated with increased risk of carcinoma (Napier and Speight 2008). In a recent study, lesions that were mixed white and red (erythroleukoplakia) and those that were larger than $200\,mm^2$ showed an increased risk of progression to cancer (Holmstrup *et al.* 2006). Erythroplakia carries a higher risk of malignancy than even erythroleukoplakia, and a significant proportion of these lesions actually are early lesions of squamous carcinoma (Mashberg and Samit 1995).

Histologic assessment of the presence and severity of epithelial dysplasia helps to predict the risk of malignant transformation. Lesions graded as moderate or severe dysplasia or carcinoma in situ are more likely to progress to cancer, but those with mild dysplasia may also develop into cancer, apparently without progressing through increasing grades of dysplasia before the onset of invasion into underlying structures (Bradley *et al.* 2010; Warnakulasuriya *et al.* 2008). Despite numerous studies of premalignant lesions, there is no consensus on an accurate predictor of cancer risk (Napier and Speight 2008).

Removal of the premalignant lesion, by scalpel excision, laser excision or ablation or by cryotherapy is the major approach to treatment. For each patient, the assessment of risk of cancer based on clinical and histologic examination is weighed against the feasibility and morbidity from excision of the lesion, which is influenced by the location and extent of the lesion and the medical status of the patient. Excision of the clinically detectable mucosal lesion may be followed by recurrence. This may be due to the inability to clinically delineate the abnormal area of epithelium that has undergone neoplastic transformation. A recent review of the management of oral premalignant lesions pointed out a lack of controlled clinical trials to demonstrate that removal of these lesions can reliably prevent recurrence or

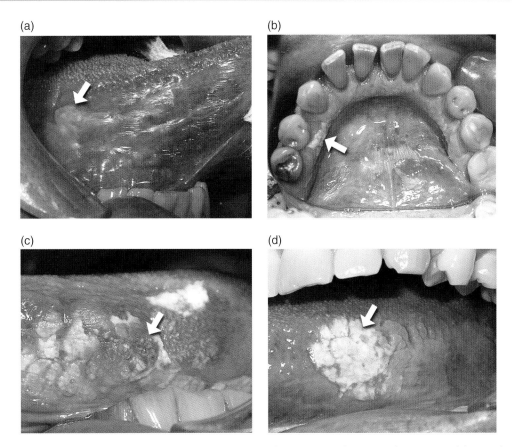

Figure 4-3 (a) Asymptomatic white patch of the right lateral-ventral tongue in a heavy smoker. Incisional biopsy (*arrow*) showed hyperkeratosis with mild dysplasia. (b) Asymptomatic, extensive white patch of the floor of mouth and mandibular mucosa in a former heavy smoker. Incisional biopsy (*arrow*) showed verrucous hyperplasia. After biopsy, the mucosa healed to a similar, white verrucous appearance. (c) Tender, red and white lesion (*arrow*) that developed within a longstanding, rough white patch of the left lateral tongue; biopsy showed squamous cell carcinoma. (d) Asymptomatic white patch of the left lateral tongue in a non-smoker; incisional biopsy of the thick, rough area (*arrow*) showed hyperkeratosis with moderate dysplasia; excision was recommended but patient was lost to follow up until an ulcer developed in this area 7 months later, biopsy showed squamous cell carcinoma.

Table 4-7 Clinical and histologic features of oral premalignant lesions that have been reported to be associated with increased risk of cancer development

Clinical features
age over 50
female
location in floor of mouth, lateral-ventral tongue
idiopathic
large size, for example, area greater than 200 mm²
presence of red component—erythroleukoplakia and erythroplakia

Histologic features
moderate or severe dysplasia
carcinoma *in situ*

development of carcinoma (Lodi and Porter 2008). Medical therapy or chemoprevention has been tested as treatment of leukoplakia. Most of these studies employed local or systemic retinoids or beta-carotene, or local antineoplastic agents such as bleomycin. Although some of these studies reported improvement of the lesions, the systemic agents produced significant side effects, and there were frequent recurrences when treatment was stopped. There is no convincing evidence that chemoprevention approaches are effective in preventing malignant transformation (Lodi and Porter 2008).

Despite the difficulty with prediction of malignant change and the inability to reliably eliminate lesions that were deemed to be high risk, the diagnosis and treatment of oral premalignant lesions have provided an opportunity to intervene in the carcinogenic process. It is now understood that the presence of an oral premalignant lesion signifies an increased risk of cancer in the oral cavity and elsewhere in the upper aerodigestive tract, and long-term monitoring of the patient is needed. Clinical surveillance supported by biopsy where indicated, coupled with patient education, will enable early diagnosis of cancer that develops in these patients. (See the next section.)

Early diagnosis of oral cancer

Early stage oral cancer disrupts the normal structure of the oral mucosa, resulting in the clinical appearance of a red, or red and white patch that may be associated with a shallow ulcer (Mashberg and Samit 1995; Neville and Day 2002). Oral cancer at this stage is asymptomatic or mildly sensitive and is often dismissed as a traumatic or infective lesion, but biopsy will show invasion of malignant squamous epithelium into underlying connective tissue (Figure 4-4 a, b, c, d, e). Early lesions of oral cancer are treated with surgical removal that results in minimal functional and

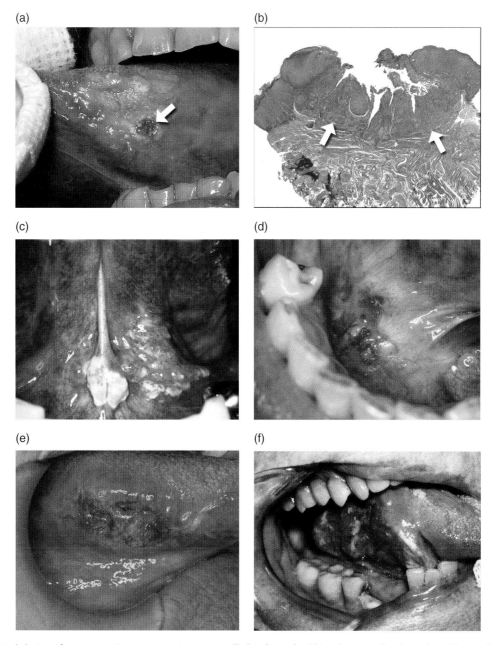

(a)

(b)

(c)

(d)

(e)

(f)

Figure 4-4 (a) Early lesion of tongue carcinoma presenting as a small ulcer (*arrow*) within a longstanding irregular white patch. (b) Low power view of the biopsy of the lesion shown in (a), showing squamous cell carcinoma that has invaded into the lamina propria of the mucosa and the superficial aspect of the tongue musculature (*arrows*). (c) Carcinoma of the anterior floor of mouth presenting as irregular, slightly raised white patches associated with a poorly demarcated area of erythema. (d) Carcinoma of the right anterior floor of mouth, seen as a granular red patch with a white border. (e) Carcinoma of the right lateral tongue. (f) Advanced carcinoma of the tongue presenting as a raised, ulcerated mass. The lesion had invaded deep into the tongue muscle and across the midline, and also involved the adjacent floor of mouth.

Table 4-8 Distribution of stage at diagnosis and 5-year relative survival rates for patients with cancer of the oral cavity and pharynx in the United States 1999 to 2005. Data from Jemal *et al.* (2010)

Stage at Diagnosis	Stage Distribution (%)	5-year Relative Survival (%)
Localized (confined to primary site)	34	83
Regional (metastasis to lymph nodes of the neck)	46	54
Distant (metastasis to distant sites)	14	32

cosmetic deficit, and the prognosis for disease-free survival is good.

Failure to detect and treat oral cancer at the early stage will lead to progressive destruction of mucosa, submucosa, skeletal muscle, minor and major salivary glands and bone, as well as metastasis to lymph nodes of the neck and distant sites such as lungs and liver (Figure 4-4 f). The prognosis worsens with spread of the disease to regional lymph nodes and to distant sites. Data from the Surveillance, Epidemiology and End Results (SEER) program of the US National Cancer Institute for 1999 to 2005 showed 5-year relative survival rates of patients with oral and pharyngeal cancer to vary from 83% for localized disease, to 54% for disease with regional spread, to 32% for disease with distant metastases (Table 4-8). (Relative survival rates are used by SEER to measure survival of cancer patients in comparison to the general population to estimate the effect of cancer.)

Unfortunately, the majority of oral and pharyngeal cancers are diagnosed at a late stage, when regional or distant spread has already occurred (Table 4-8). Treatment of late stage oral cancer entails severe, long-term side effects, risk of recurrence, and is associated with a high mortality rate.

Improvement in early diagnosis and treatment of oral cancer can be achieved by education of the public on the early signs of oral cancer, coupled with regular examination of oral tissues by knowledgeable health professionals. Increased public awareness should help to reduce the delay from first symptom to examination by a dentist or physician (Peacock *et al.* 2008). However, early lesions of oral cancer are often asymptomatic and discovered during routine oral examination or an office visit for unrelated reasons (Figure 4-5). A study of patients newly diagnosed with oral and pharyngeal cancer showed that patients who had a regular primary care dentist, and those who received an oral cancer examination at their last dental visit were significantly more likely to have early stage disease compared to patients who did not have this level of oral health care (Watson *et al.* 2009).

Another study with a smaller sample of patients recently diagnosed with oral and oropharyngeal squamous cancer demonstrated that detection of an asymptomatic malignant lesion during a routine office visit was associated with a significantly smaller lesion and earlier clinical stage of disease. Detection of oral cancer during a non-symptom-driven examination was more likely to occur in a dental office than a physician's office (Holmes *et al.* 2003).

A well-equipped dental office provides the optimal setting for a thorough examination of the oral tissues, with particular attention to the 'high-risk' areas for oral cancer, which are the posterior-lateral and ventral tongue, the floor of the mouth, the soft palate, and tonsillar pillars (Mashberg and Samit 1995; Neville and Day 2002). The evaluation of asymptomatic and symptomatic oral lesions must be based on a comprehensive knowledge of variations of normal anatomy and benign and malignant lesions. The majority of oral lesions that are encountered in a dental office are reactive or inflammatory lesions due to dental infection or various forms of irritation, but any unexplained, persistent mucosal lesion should be investigated, regardless of whether the patient belongs to a high risk group for oral cancer. A lesion suspicious for cancer should be subjected to incisional biopsy of adequate depth. The diagnosis of mucosal carcinoma is made by demonstration of invasion of malignant epithelial cells into underlying tissues. Non-invasive procedures such as cytologic testing cannot provide a definitive diagnosis and should not be used as an alternative to biopsy (Neville and Day 2002; Lingen *et al.* 2008). When the biopsy diagnosis is oral squamous carcinoma, the clinician is responsible for informing and counseling the patient and referring the patient for cancer treatment.

The pathway from examination of a patient to the initiation of treatment typically involves several health care professionals and may be delayed at various points, as a result of inadequate clinical evaluation of a suspicious lesion, improper biopsy technique or interpretation, inappropriate referral, and lack of accessible cancer treatment (Figure 4-5). The relative importance of these barriers varies among different geographical and socio-economical settings. Better understanding of factors that cause delay in diagnosis and correction of these problems will eventually reduce the morbidity and mortality of oral cancer (Gomez *et al.* 2010).

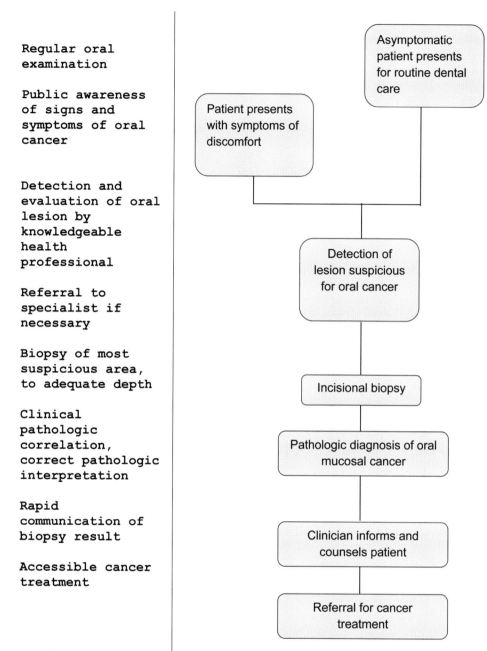

Regular oral
examination

Public awareness
of signs and
symptoms of oral
cancer

Detection and
evaluation of oral
lesion by
knowledgeable
health
professional

Referral to
specialist if
necessary

Biopsy of most
suspicious area,
to adequate depth

Clinical
pathologic
correlation,
correct pathologic
interpretation

Rapid
communication of
biopsy result

Accessible cancer
treatment

Asymptomatic patient presents for routine dental care

Patient presents with symptoms of discomfort

Detection of lesion suspicious for oral cancer

Incisional biopsy

Pathologic diagnosis of oral mucosal cancer

Clinician informs and counsels patient

Referral for cancer treatment

Figure 4-5 Pathway to diagnosis and treatment of oral cancer and factors that favor early diagnosis and treatment.

Screening for oral cancer

Introduction

Screening is a means of detecting disease early in asymptomatic individuals. The aim of screening is to reduce mortality and morbidity from the disease, either by preventing progression of the disease or by facilitating simpler and more effective treatment of the disease early in its natural history (Hakama and Auvinen 2008). Screening tests are usually not diagnostic of cancer, but instead indicate that a cancer may be present. Definitive diagnosis of cancer requires surgical biopsy and pathologic confirmation.

Cancer screening may be offered to a population opportunistically or as part of an organized program (Miles *et al.* 2004). Organized screening is distinguished from opportunistic screening primarily on the basis of how invitations to screening are extended. In organized screening programs, which are also known as mass screening programs, the target group is invited to participate specifically for the purpose of detecting potentially malignant lesions. In opportunistic screening, also known as spontaneous or unorganized screening, individuals are invited to be screened during health care visits for reasons unrelated to cancer. Opportunistic screening in the dental setting occurs when oral cancer screening is incorporated into the comprehensive hard and soft tissue oral examination (Miles *et al.* 2004).

Organized screening programs require considerable organization and planning. These programs are centrally coordinated, and offer a standardized system of care, with implemented guidelines on who is to be screened and how any abnormalities detected by screening should be followed and treated. The overall quality of the program (quality assurance) is assessed by targets such as population uptake rates, cancer detection rates, and false-positive and false-negative rates (Miles *et al.* 2004).

Opportunistic screening depends on individuals to request screening or on their health care providers to recommend screening. Guidelines for opportunistic screening are not as structured, and quality assurance may be more variable. Opportunistic screening may not target those groups at high risk of cancer, and those who do receive screening may be screened either too frequently or too infrequently (Miles *et al.* 2004).

The accuracy or ability of a screening test to discriminate disease is described by four indices: sensitivity, specificity, positive predictive value, and negative predictive value. The sensitivity of a screening test indicates the extent to which early disease is identified and is the proportion of persons who have a positive test among those with the disease. Sensitivity is a basic measure of the success of screening, indicating the yield. Specificity describes the proportion of individuals who do not have the disease and who have a negative screening test result. Specificity is a measure of the ability of the test to correctly identify that the disease is not present. Poor specificity results in high financial costs and adverse effects as a result of false-positive tests (Hakama and Auvinen 2008).

A false positive is an erroneously positive screening result. A false-positive screening test can result in unnecessary anxiety and possible costly and invasive medical intervention. A false negative is an erroneously negative screening result. A false-negative screening test provides undue reassurance and may result in delayed diagnosis and worse outcome due to treatment delay (Hakama and Auvinen 2008).

Predictive values describe the performance of the test from the point of view of the person screened. Positive predictive value refers to the proportion of people in a specified population with positive test results who have the disease. Negative predictive value refers to the proportion of people in a specified population with negative test results who are disease free (Hakama and Auvinen 2008).

Screening resulting in early cancer detection may not produce an improved outcome (reduced mortality rate) for all cancer types. A screening test should only be applied to a cancer that can be effectively treated or where intervention will prevent progression of the cancer. Screening may reveal borderline abnormalities that would not progress even if untreated. One of the adverse effects of screening is overdiagnosis, where detection of indolent disease and its unnecessary treatment result in unnecessary anxiety and morbidity. Because of the financial, social, and psychological costs associated with screening, the benefits of screening should outweigh the costs before a screening program is implemented. A good screening test is simple, safe, and acceptable to the public, detects disease early in its natural history, and discriminates between innocuous lesions and lesions likely to progress. Cancer screening programs should be undertaken only if the prevalence of the cancer is high enough to justify the costs and efforts of screening, and adequate resources and facilities are available for the diagnosis and treatment of the disease (Hakama and Auvinen 2008).

Oral cancer screening

Oral cancer is a disease for which screening is potentially beneficial. The oral cavity is easily accessible for routine visual examination. Early detection is feasible because many oral cancers are preceded by clinically visible precursor lesions, and surgical treatment of early oral cancer is very effective. How effective is screening for oral cancer in reducing mortality rates due to oral cancer? A randomized, controlled screening trial with cancer-specific mortality applied to an appropriate target population provides the strongest support for a screening intervention. Investigations of the effectiveness of oral cancer screening have been limited by study design flaws, including small sample numbers, lack of appropriate controls, sample selection bias, and absence of histopathological confirmation. In some studies the sample populations were groups at high risk of developing oral cancer and not representative of the general population at whom screening is typically targeted (Kujan *et al.* 2006; Lingen *et al.* 2008; Patton *et al.* 2008; Fedele 2009; Brocklehurst *et al.* 2010; Rethman *et al.* 2010). Oral cancer screening methods are discussed in the sections below (Table 4-9).

Screening by visual and tactile examination

The standard method for oral cancer screening is a conventional visual and tactile examination of the oral soft tissues using normal incandescent light (Kujan *et al.* 2006; Lingen *et al.* 2008; Patton *et al.* 2008; Rethman *et al.* 2010; Brocklehurst *et al.* 2010). Although oral cancer screening may potentially reduce mortality rates, a

Table 4-9 Oral cancer screening methods

Standard screening method

Visual and tactile examination under conventional lighting

Diagnostic adjuncts

Oral cytology
Toluidine blue
Light-based detection systems
- Chemiluminescence (for example, ViziLite)
- Narrow-emission tissue fluorescence (VELscope)
Biomarkers, salivary diagnostic tests

---

randomized controlled trial of a large organized screening program did not show a statistically significant decrease in oral cancer mortality rate in the general population who were deemed to be at low risk of oral cancer. However, the same mass screening program did result in earlier intervention and a statistically significant reduction in mortality in a population at high risk of oral cancer characterized by tobacco and alcohol use (Sankaranarayanan *et al*. 2005; Subramanian *et al*. 2009; Brocklehurst *et al*. 2010).

Adjunctive screening aids

Some cancers arise from clinically normal mucosa, and some clinically visible precursor lesions do not progress to cancer. Adjunctive screening aids have been marketed to enhance visual examination, to detect precancerous lesions in clinically normal oral mucosa, and to assess the biologic potential of mucosal lesions. Adjunctive screening aids do not replace conventional visual and tactile examination of the oral soft tissues and are not diagnostic tests. Diagnosis of oral cancer and its precursor lesions requires histopathologic examination of biopsy samples. Adjunctive screening methods include light-based devices, transepithelial cytology, and toluidine blue staining (Lingen *et al*. 2008; Patton *et al*. 2008; Fedele 2009; Rethman *et al*. 2010).

Light-based devices

Commercially available light-based devices are auxiliary aids to visual examination and are designed to assist in lesion detection. Normal and abnormal mucosal tissues show different absorbance and reflectance profiles when exposed to various forms of energy or light. Light-based devices consist of light sources that provide blue (400–460 nm) or white illumination. Some tests based on chemiluminescence and tissue reflectance require application of 1% acetic acid to mucosa, which causes abnormal squamous epithelium to show as a distinctly white (acetowhite) area when it is exposed to the light (for example, MicroluxDL, Orascoptic DK, and ViziLite Plus). Devices based on autofluorescence reveal patterns of absorbance and reflectance of naturally occurring fluorophores in the oral soft tissues exposed to excitation wavelengths. Abnormal tissue exhibits decreased levels of autofluorescence, appearing dark compared with the normal tissue, which emits a green autofluorescence when viewed through a filter (VELscope). The device may potentially assist in the determination of surgical margins and selection of the optimal biopsy site in large or multifocal lesions (Lingen *et al*. 2008; Patton *et al*. 2008; Rethman *et al*. 2010).

Light-based devices enhance lesions already visible to the clinician and cannot replace standard visual examination. False positive results may result from the detection of inflammatory, pigmented, and other noncancerous lesions. The utility of light-based devices in the general dental setting is questionable, because the devices do not allow discrimination of innocuous lesions from biologically aggressive ones. Currently there is insufficient evidence that devices based on tissue reflectance and autofluorescence improve the detection of potentially malignant lesions beyond that of a conventional visual and tactile examination (Lingen *et al*. 2008; Patton *et al*. 2008; Rethman *et al*. 2010).

Transepithelial cytology

Atypical cells that may indicate malignancy are identified in transepithelial samples by computer-assisted analysis and interpretation by a pathologist (OralCDx BrushTest, OralCDx Laboratories, Suffern, NY). Confirmatory biopsy is recommended when atypical cells, abnormal cells of uncertain significance, dysplastic, or cancerous cells are reported, because the test does not provide a final diagnosis. Transepithelial cytology is intended for the evaluation of lesions deemed to be at low risk for malignancy. The test is an unnecessary extra procedure for lesions clinically suspicious for cancer, as such lesions require surgical biopsy for diagnosis irrespective of the cytology results. Atypical findings are frequently obtained when this test is performed on inflammatory or reactive lesions. False positive results may lead to unwarranted patient anxiety, referral for further evaluation, and possible unnecessary biopsies. Transepithelial cytology is potentially useful in specific situations where biopsy may be difficult to perform, such as for the assessment of patients with multiple oral lesions but no history of oral cancer, for screening medically complex patients who cannot safely tolerate a surgical procedure, or for patients with access to care restraints (Lingen *et al*. 2008; Patton *et al*. 2008; Rethman *et al*. 2010).

Toluidine blue staining

Toluidine blue, also known as tolonium chloride, is a metachromatic dye that preferentially binds to tissues undergoing rapid cell division and to sites of DNA damage. High numbers of false positive stains occur as toluidine blue will stain inflammatory and regenerative lesions in addition to dysplastic and cancerous tissues, making it less useful in primary care settings and in the general population. Investigations of toluidine blue staining as an adjunct to clinical examination indicate that it is best used by experienced clinicians in high-risk individuals such as those with a history of oral cancer or older patients who are heavy consumers of tobacco and alcohol (Lingen *et al.* 2008; Patton *et al.* 2008; Rethman *et al.* 2010).

Biomarkers and salivary diagnostics

A biomarker or molecular marker is a biological molecule found in blood, other body fluids, or tissues that can be objectively measured and evaluated as an indicator of normal biological processes, pathologic processes, or responses to a therapeutic intervention. Biomarkers may be DNA, RNA, and/or proteins and thus may be detected by methods used in genomics, transcriptomics, and proteomics (Schaaij-Visser *et al.* 2010).

The histological finding of dysplasia in tissue samples is used to assess the likelihood of transformation of a lesion to cancer. Dysplasia is not a completely reliable indicator of the malignant potential of a lesion. Not all dysplastic lesions progress to cancer, while some non-dysplastic lesions show molecular markers of premalignancy and progress to cancer. Biomarker assessment may potentially predict the biologic behavior of a precancerous lesion. It is likely that not one biomarker, but a panel of biomarkers, will be required to be clinically useful. Because tests for biomarkers may be based on blood and other body fluids such as saliva, non-invasive screening tests can potentially be developed. Currently there are no established biomarker panel sets for oral precancer and cancer that have a sufficient degree of specificity and sensitivity to indicate the prognosis of a given lesion. The effectiveness of biomarker assays as oral cancer screening tools have yet to be assessed in randomized controlled studies (Lingen 2010b).

Human papillomavirus tests

Although high-risk types of the human papillomavirus (HPV) may be an etiologic factor in cancers of the tonsil, the base of the tongue, and the oropharynx, HPV does not appear to play a significant role in the pathogenesis of cancers of the oral cavity proper. Furthermore, the presence of HPV in a saliva test does not necessarily establish a patient as being at higher risk for developing cancer because the natural history of oral HPV infection is not fully understood. Therefore, tests to detect HPV, such as recently introduced saliva-based HPV tests, have limited value in the screening for oral cancer (Lingen 2010a).

Conclusions

Despite insufficient scientific evidence to show that oral cancer screening results in decreased mortality from oral cancer, routine screening for oral cancer should be an integral component of dental examinations. Screening by visual and tactile examination may result in early detection of potentially malignant lesions and oral cancer. Commercial screening adjunctive aids add to the costs of screening and have not been found to significantly improve the detection of potentially malignant lesions over conventional visual and tactile examination. Moreover screening adjuncts cannot discriminate between lesions that are potentially malignant and that are of little clinical significance.

Oral cancer screening is not a diagnostic procedure in itself and can produce false positive and false negative results. Clinicians must therefore be aware of the limitations of the particular screening method used, be able to interpret the results of the screening test, and correlate the screening results with the clinical findings. Tissue biopsy remains the gold standard for diagnosing an oral premalignant lesion or oral cancer. Further education and training of primary health care providers to promote a systematic and rigorous approach to early detection of oral cancer and an understanding of the natural history of oral cancer are essential for the success of a screening program. To improve the outcome of oral cancer through screening in the primary care setting, further research in the development, implementation, and evaluation of screening methods is required.

Role of the dental team

Periodic encounters with dentists, either for acute care or for checkups, offer the opportunity for health counseling, cancer screening, and case finding. Oral cancer can be prevented by educating and counseling patients about the risk factors for oral cancer and by promoting cessation of tobacco and alcohol use in patients. The evaluation of cancer risk involves assessment of the type, quantity, frequency, and duration of consumption of these products. High-risk patients can be taught to recognize possible warning signs of cancer and be encouraged to take prompt action leading to early diagnosis.

Many dentists routinely perform opportunistic screening for oral cancer during regular dental visits.

The standard screening method for oral cancer is a simple, non-invasive procedure that involves a visual and tactile inspection of the oral mucosa with adequate lighting, gauze, and gloves (Rethman *et al.* 2010). Most oral cancers and their precursor lesions are detectable at the time of a comprehensive oral examination. Although adjunctive screening tools may be considered, the use of these adjunctive aids requires appropriate training and experience (Rethman *et al.* 2010). Adjunctive screening tools include exfoliative cytology, toluidine blue staining, and direct fluorescence visualization (Lingen *et al.* 2008; Patton *et al.* 2008; Rethman *et al.* 2010). The vast majority of oral cancers occur in older individuals who are heavy consumers of tobacco and alcohol use. Nevertheless, clinicians should be aware that oral cancer can occur in younger patients without known risk factors, validating opportunistic screening in the setting of primary dental care (BC Oral Cancer Prevention Program 2008).

Any lesions identified by screening require further action. Innocuous and reactive lesions detected by oral cancer screening contribute to false positive results (Rethman *et al.* 2010). Possible causes of lesions thought to be reactive in nature should be eliminated. Confirmatory biopsy may be considered for lesions that are found to persist at follow up 1 to 2 weeks after removal of all etiologic factors and for lesions that raise clinical suspicion for malignancy (Rethman *et al.* 2010). The risk of performing an unnecessary biopsy of a lesion of unknown clinical significance can be reduced by obtaining a second opinion from a clinician with advanced training and experience in oral mucosal diagnosis (Rethman *et al.* 2010).

Appropriate management of biopsy-proven dysplasia includes assessment of risk of malignant transformation and selection of appropriate therapy, such as long-term monitoring and/or surgical therapy. The diagnosis of invasive oral cancer by biopsy (case finding) should be followed by prompt referral to an appropriate cancer treatment center.

Dental treatment for the oral cancer patient includes comprehensive evaluation and preparation of the patient prior to cancer therapy, provision of dental care during cancer treatment, and dental management of the patient after completion of cancer therapy. Radiation therapy to the head and neck region and chemotherapy may be associated with oral complications such as xerostomia, mucositis, caries, dysphagia, infection, and osteonecrosis. Some side effects are transient, disappearing shortly after completion of cancer treatment, while others may be permanent. Oral hygiene measures, patient education, and preventive treatment, such as fluoride therapy and removal of potential sources of infection, should be provided before, during, and after cancer therapy to avoid the need for invasive dental treatments and to prevent osteonecrosis. After cancer therapy is completed, the dentist plays a continuing role in surveillance for tumor recurrence or for development of second primary tumors. The dental team should continue to counsel patients to avoid risk factors to prevent the development of a second malignancy.

References

ACS. (2010) American Cancer Society. Cancer Facts & Figures. Atlanta.

Adelstein, D.J., Ridge, J.A., Gillison, M.L., *et al.* (2009) Head and neck squamous cell cancer and the human papillomavirus: summary of a National Cancer Institute State of the Science Meeting, November 9–10, 2008, Washington, D.C. *Head and Neck,* 31, 1393–1422.

AICR. (2009) Food, nutrition, physical activity and the prevention of cancer: a global perspective; the second report of the World Cancer Research Fund and American Institute for Cancer Research available online at http://www.dietandcancerreport.org/?p=ER.

An, J., Liu, Z., Hu, Z., *et al.* (2007) Potentially functional single nucleotide polymorphisms in the core nucleotide excision repair genes and risk of squamous cell carcinoma of the head and neck. *Cancer Epidemiology Biomarkers and Prevention,* 16, 1633–1638.

Auluck, A., Hislop, G., Poh, C., *et al.* (2009) Areca nut and betel quid chewing among South Asian immigrants to Western countries and its implications for oral cancer screening. *Rural and Remote Health,* 9, 1118.

Axell, T., Pindborg, J.J., Smith, C.J., *et al.* (1996) Oral white lesions with special reference to precancerous and tobacco- related lesions: conclusions of an international symposium held in Uppsala, Sweden, May 18–21 1994. International Collaborative Group on Oral White Lesions. *Journal of Oral Pathology and Medicine,* 25, 49–54.

BC Oral Cancer Prevention Program. (2008) Clinical Practice Guidelines. Guideline for the early detection of oral cancer in British Columbia. College of Dental Surgeons of British Columbia.

Berthiller, J., Lee, Y.C., Boffetta, P., *et al.* (2009) Marijuana smoking and the risk of head and neck cancer: pooled analysis in the INHANCE consortium. *Cancer Epidemiology Biomarkers and Prevention,* 18, 1544–1551.

Blot, W.J., McLaughlin, J.K., Winn, D.M., *et al.* (1988) Smoking and drinking in relation to oral and pharyngeal cancer. *Cancer Research,* 48, 3282–3287.

Bradley, G., Odell, E.W., Raphael, S., *et al.* (2010) Abnormal DNA content in oral epithelial dysplasia is associated with increased risk of progression to carcinoma. *British Journal of Cancer,* 103, 1432–1442.

Brocklehurst, P., Kujan, O., Glenny, A.M., *et al.* (2010) Screening programmes for the early detection and prevention of oral cancer. *Cochrane Database Systematic Reviews,* CD004150.

Dahlstrom, K.R., Little, J.A., Zafereo, M.E., *et al.* (2008) Squamous cell carcinoma of the head and neck in never smoker-never drinkers: a descriptive epidemiologic study. *Head and Neck,* 30, 75–84.

Danaei, G., Vander Hoorn, S., Lopez, A.D., *et al.* (2005) Causes of cancer in the world: comparative risk assessment of nine behavioural and environmental risk factors. *Lancet,* 366, 1784–1793.

Fedele, S. (2009) Diagnostic aids in the screening of oral cancer. *Head and Neck Oncology,* 1, 5.

Ferlay, J., Parkin, D.M., Curado, M.P., *et al.* (2010a) Cancer Incidence in Five Continents, Volumes I to IX: IARC CancerBase No.9 available onine at http://ci5.iarc.fr.

Ferlay, J., Shin, H.R., Bray, F., *et al.* (2010b) GLOBOCAN 2008 v1.2, Cancer Incidence and Mortality Worldwide: IARC CancerBase No. 10 [Online]. Lyon, France: International Agency for Research on Cancer. Available at: http://globocan.iarc.fr, accessed on 24/03/2011.

Freedman, N.D., Park, Y., Subar, A.F., *et al.* (2008) Fruit and vegetable intake and head and neck cancer risk in a large United States prospective cohort study. *International Journal of Cancer,* 122, 2330–2336.

Gillison, M.L., D'Souza, G., Westra, W., *et al.* (2008) Distinct risk factor profiles for human papillomavirus type 16-positive and human papillomavirus type 16-negative head and neck cancers. *Journal of the National Cancer Institute,* 100, 407–420.

Gillison, M.L. and Lowy, D.R. (2004) A causal role for human papillomavirus in head and neck cancer. *Lancet,* 363, 1488–1489.

Gomez, I., Warnakulasuriya, S., Varela-Centelles, P.I., *et al.* (2010) Is early diagnosis of oral cancer a feasible objective? Who is to blame for diagnostic delay? *Oral Diseases,* 16, 333–342.

Guha, N., Boffetta, P., Wunsch Filho, V., *et al.* (2007) Oral health and risk of squamous cell carcinoma of the head and neck and esophagus: results of two multicentric case-control studies. *American Journal of Epidemiology,* 166, 1159–1173.

Hakama, M. and Auvinen, A. (2008) Cancer screening. *International Encyclopedia of Public Health,* 464–480.

Hashibe, M., Brennan, P., Benhamou, S.V., *et al.* (2007) Alcohol drinking in never users of tobacco, cigarette smoking in never drinkers, and the risk of head and neck cancer: pooled analysis in the International Head and Neck Cancer Epidemiology Consortium. *Journal of the National Cancer Institute,* 99, 777–789.

Hashibe, M., Brennan, P., Chuang, S.C., *et al.* (2009) Interaction between tobacco and alcohol use and the risk of head and neck cancer: pooled analysis in the International Head and Neck Cancer Epidemiology Consortium. *Cancer Epidemiology, Biomarkers and Prevention,* 18, 541–550.

Hashibe, M., Brennan, P., Strange, R.C., *et al.* (2003) Meta- and pooled analyses of GSTM1, GSTT1, GSTP1, and CYP1A1 genotypes and risk of head and neck cancer. *Cancer Epidemiology, Biomarkers and Prevention,* 12, 1509–1517.

Heck, J.E., Berthiller, J., Vaccarella, S., *et al.* (2010) Sexual behaviours and the risk of head and neck cancers: a pooled analysis in the International Head and Neck Cancer Epidemiology (INHANCE) consortium. *International Journal of Epidemiology,* 39, 166–181.

Herrero, R., Castellsague, X., Pawlita, M., *et al.* (2003) Human papillomavirus and oral cancer: the International Agency for Research on Cancer multicenter study. *Journal of the National Cancer Institute,* 95, 1772–1783.

Holmes, J.D., Dierks, E.J., Homer, L.D. *et al.* (2003) Is detection of oral and oropharyngeal squamous cancer by a dental health care provider associated with a lower stage at diagnosis? *Journal of Oral Maxillofacial Surgery,* 61, 285–291.

Holmstrup, P., Vedtofte, P., Reibel, J., *et al.* (2006) Long-term treatment outcome of oral premalignant lesions. *Oral Oncology,* 42, 461–474.

Huang, W.Y., Olshan, A.F., Schwartz, S.M., *et al.* (2005) Selected genetic polymorphisms in MGMT, XRCC1, XPD, and XRCC3 and risk of head and neck cancer: a pooled analysis. Cancer *Epidemiology, Biomarkers and Prevention,* 14, 1747–1753.

IARC. (2004) Betel-quid and areca-nut chewing and some areca-nut derived nitrosamines. *IARC Monographs in Evaluating Carcinogenic Risks in Humans,* 85, 1–334.

Jemal, A., Siegel, R., Xu, J., *et al.* (2010) Cancer statistics, 2010. *CA: A Cancer Journal for Clinicians,* 60, 277–300.

Johnson, N., Franceschi, S., Ferlay, J., et al. (2005) Squamous cell carcinoma. In: *Pathology and Genetics of Head and Neck Tumours* (Eds. L. Barnes, J.W. Eveson, P. Reichart, and D. Sidransky), pp. 168–175. IARC Press, Lyon.

Kujan, O., Glenny, A.M., Oliver, R.J., *et al.* (2006) Screening programmes for the early detection and prevention of oral cancer. *Cochrane Database Systematic Reviews,* 3, CD004150.

La Vecchia, C., Lucchini, F., Negri, E., *et al.* (2004) Trends in oral cancer mortality in Europe. *Oral Oncology,* 40, 433–439.

Lingen, M.W. (2010a) Can saliva-based HPV tests establish cancer risk and guide patient management? *Oral Surgery, Oral Medicine, Oral Pathology, Oral Radiology and Endodontics,* 110, 273–274.

Lingen, M.W. (2010b) Screening for oral premalignancy and cancer: what platform and which biomarkers? *Cancer Prevention Research (Phila),* 3, 1056–1059.

Lingen, M.W., Kalmar, J.R., Karrison, T., *et al.* (2008) Critical evaluation of diagnostic aids for the detection of oral cancer. *Oral Oncology,* 44, 10–22.

Lodi, G. and Porter, S. (2008) Management of potentially malignant disorders: evidence and critique. *Journal of Oral Pathology and Medicine,* 37, 63–69.

Macfarlane, G.J., Boyle, P., Scully, C. (1987) Rising mortality from cancer of the tongue in young Scottish males. *Lancet,* 2, 912.

Marron, M., Boffetta, P., Zhang, Z.F. *et al.* (2010) Cessation of alcohol drinking, tobacco smoking and the reversal of head and neck cancer risk. *International Journal of Epidemiology,* 39, 182–196.

Mashberg, A. and Samit, A. (1995) Early diagnosis of asymptomatic oral and oropharyngeal squamous cancers. *CA: A Cancer Journal for Clinicians,* 45, 328–351.

Miles, A., Cockburn, J., Smith, R.A. *et al.* (2004) A perspective from countries using organized screening programs. *Cancer,* 101, 1201–1213.

Molinolo, A.A., Amornphimoltham, P., Squarize, C.H., *et al.* (2009) Dysregulated molecular networks in head and neck carcinogenesis. *Oral Oncology,* 45, 324–334.

Napier, S.S. and Speight, P.M. (2008) Natural history of potentially malignant oral lesions and conditions: an overview of the literature. *Journal of Oral Pathology and Medicine,* 37, 1–10.

Neville, B., Damm, D., Allen, C., *et al.* (2009) In: *Oral and Maxillofacial Pathology,* 3rd edition, pp. 409–421. Saunders Elsevier, St. Louis, Missouri.

Neville, B.W. and Day, T.A. (2002) Oral cancer and precancerous lesions. *CA: A Cancer Journal for Clinicians,* 52, 195–215.

Patton, L.L., Epstein, J.B., Kerr, A.R. (2008) Adjunctive techniques for oral cancer examination and lesion diagnosis: a systematic review of the literature. *Journal of the American Dental Association,* 139, 896–905.

Peacock, Z.S., Pogrel, M.A., Schmidt, B.L. (2008) Exploring the reasons for delay in treatment of oral cancer. *Journal of the American Dental Association,* 139, 1346–1352.

Pitiyage, G., Tilakaratne, W.M., Tavassoli, M., *et al.* (2009) Molecular markers in oral epithelial dysplasia: review. *Journal of Oral Pathology and Medicine,* 38, 737–752.

Rethman, M.P., Carpenter, W., Cohen, E.E., *et al.* (2010) Evidence-based clinical recommendations regarding screening for oral squamous cell carcinomas. *Journal of the American Dental Association,* 141, 509–520.

Sankaranarayanan, R., Ramadas, K., Thomas, G., *et al.* (2005) Effect of screening on oral cancer mortality in Kerala, India: a cluster-randomised controlled trial. *Lancet,* 365, 1927–1933.

Schaaij-Visser, T.B.M., Brakenhoff, R.H., Leemans, C.R., *et al.* (2010) Protein biomarker discovery for head and neck cancer. *Journal of Proteomics,* 73, 1790–1803.

Secretan, B., Straif, K., Baan, R., *et al.* (2009) A review of human carcinogens—Part E: tobacco, areca nut, alcohol, coal smoke, and salted fish. *Lancet Oncology,* 10, 1033–1034.

Shiboski, C.H., Schmidt, B.L., Jordan, R.C. (2005) Tongue and tonsil carcinoma: increasing trends in the U.S. population ages 20–44 years. *Cancer,* 103, 1843–1849.

Subramanian, S., Sankaranarayanan, R., Bapat, B., *et al.* (2009) Cost-effectiveness of oral cancer screening: results from a cluster randomized controlled trial in India. *Bulletin of the World Health Organization,* 87, 200–206.

Tezal, M., Sullivan, M.A., Hyland, A., *et al.* (2009) Chronic periodontitis and the incidence of head and neck squamous cell carcinoma. *Cancer Epidemiology, Biomarkers and Prevention,* 18, 2406–2412.

Thomas, S.J., Bain, C.J., Battistutta, D., *et al.* (2007) Betel quid not containing tobacco and oral cancer: a report on a case-control study in Papua New Guinea and a meta-analysis of current evidence. *International Journal of Cancer,* 120, 1318–1323.

Wang, L.E., Hu, Z., Sturgis, E.M., *et al.* (2010) Reduced DNA repair capacity for removing tobacco carcinogen-induced DNA adducts contributes to risk of head and neck cancer but not tumor characteristics. *Clinical Cancer Research,* 16, 764–774.

Warnakulasuriya, S. (2009a) Causes of oral cancer—an appraisal of controversies. *British Dental Journal,* 207, 471–475.

Warnakulasuriya, S. (2009b) Global epidemiology of oral and oropharyngeal cancer. *Oral Oncology,* 45, 309–316.

Warnakulasuriya, S., Johnson, N.W., van der Waal, I. (2007) Nomenclature and classification of potentially malignant disorders of the oral mucosa. *Journal of Oral Pathology and Medicine,* 36, 575–580.

Warnakulasuriya, S., Reibel, J., Bouquot, J. (2008) Oral epithelial dysplasia classification systems: predictive value, utility, weaknesses and scope for improvement. *Journal of Oral Pathology and Medicine,* 37, 127–133.

Watson, J.M., Logan, H.L., Tomar, S.L., *et al.* (2009) Factors associated with early-stage diagnosis of oral and pharyngeal cancer. *Community Dentistry and Oral Epidemiology,* 37, 333–341.

5

Evidence-based dentistry

Amir Azarpazhooh, David Locker, and Prakeshkumar S. Shah

Introduction

The concept of evidence-based health care exists as far back as the origin of medicine. Long before the first known documentation of the so-called randomized controlled trial of citrus solution to treat scurvy on the British Navy, practitioners have adopted the principle of utilizing the available information from their past knowledge, practice, and wisdom to provide the best possible care for their patient. This is the fundamental basis of evidence-based health care. This concept was formalized in the 1970s by Guyatt, which resulted in proliferation of information and misinformation regarding evidence-based medicine. It is ignorantly conceived by many that randomized controlled trial is the other name of evidence-based medicine. The concept has evolved in the last 4 decades, and formal acknowledgement of all types of evidence and involvement of all subspecialties of health care provision has been embraced. The concept is well summarized in the following definition: "Evidence based health care takes place when decisions that affect the care of patients are taken with due weight accorded to all valid, relevant information" (Hicks 2011).

The impetus here is accorded to "decisions that affect the care of patients," "due weight," "all," "valid," and "information." A topic with different levels of information (unbiased versus biased) is considered after appropriate assignment of relative importance to the type of information, and importantly all of the available information is captured in the proper manner and its validity is assessed in applying this to the decisions we make for improvements in the care we deliver for the patient in front of us. In dentistry, since the 1990s, there has been an increasing interest in evidence-based concepts internationally and from a wide variety of dental groups with the ultimate goal of improving patient care. For example, the American Dental Association "supports the concept of evidence-based dentistry developed through systematic examination of the best available scientific data, and will use this information to help shape the Association's Research Agenda" (American Dental Association 2008). The evidence-based education and practice must promote understanding of both basic and applied science, the management of uncertainty, and the development of new knowledge. Consequently, the evidence-based dental practices would update and change in the clinical procedures based on the new knowledge (Pitts 2004).

To understand the concepts of evidence-based dentistry, it is important to understand the basis of epidemiology, the nature of a given research question, and the best study designs that would provide the evidence to such a question. Therefore, in this chapter, we will cover the following topics:

1. Epidemiology and the sequence of epidemiological reasoning
2. Study designs in clinical research (descriptive, analytical, interventional) and their analytical framework
3. Research syntheses and their value in evidence-based dentistry
4. The importance of knowledge of these topics for any practitioner for the critical appraisal of research, for which the general guidelines are discussed at the end of the chapter

Comprehensive Preventive Dentistry, First Edition. Edited by Hardy Limeback.
© 2012 John Wiley & Sons, Ltd. Published 2012 by John Wiley & Sons, Ltd.

Epidemiology

Epidemiology is the study of the frequency, distribution, and determinants of health conditions or events (including disease) in human populations and the application of such study to control diseases and other health problems (U.S. Department of Health and Human Services 2006). With the origins in the study of epidemics (the sudden increase in the rate of occurrence of a disease), epidemiology is considered as the core scientific discipline of public and population health practice and has an important role in clinical practice. Oral epidemiology is that branch of the discipline that studies oral health and disease through its central concern with **causation** and the relationships among various **exposures** or **interventions** and their **outcomes.** Clinical epidemiology follows the same logical and quantitative concepts and methods of epidemiology to clinical delivery of care (diagnostic, prognostic, therapeutic, and preventive) to individual patients. All health professionals need to be familiar with epidemiology, its principles and procedures, for the following reasons:

1. It provides for a comprehensive understanding of health and disease in individuals and populations, and the forces and factors that influence them. This is consistent with the mission of the health care system and health care professionals, which is to eliminate disease from and improve the health of individuals and populations.
2. It provides for an understanding of the scientific methods used to produce the knowledge base on which health care practice is founded.
3. Epidemiological principles are beginning to play an important role in clinical decisions for individual patients.

In determining the cause of disease, epidemiology proceeds in the following way, hence, the sequence of epidemiological reasoning:

1. *Observation:* An initial observation of the distribution of a disease in a population leads to the **suspicion** that a given factor influences the occurrence of disease. Such observation can be initiated from clinical practice based on clinicians' observations of their patients, from data that governments routinely collect, from laboratory research, from examination of disease patterns (that is, comparison of people with a disease to determine what characteristics they have in common, or comparisons of people with and without a disease to determine in what ways they differ), or from theoretical speculation from existing knowledge of disease prevention and causation models. For example, in the 1920s and 1930s, it was observed that the rate of lung cancer was increasing as the consumption of cigarettes in the general population increased.
2. *Formulation of specific hypotheses:* The suspicions concerning influence of a particular factor on disease occurrence is stated as a formal **hypothesis,** a tentative plausible theory and a supposition that links the onset of disease with some factor in a form that will allow it to be tested and refuted (U.S. Department of Health and Human Services 2006). Obviously, not all hypotheses are worth pursuing. They have to have some degree of plausibility (either through biological pathways or through epidemiological data showing that high rates of disease exist in populations where the factor of interest is also common) before time and resources are invested in testing them.
3. *Conduct study and assess validity of association:* A plausible hypothesis is tested by means of an epidemiological study. For this purpose, study population is assembled from individuals with disease or outcome of interest, and an appropriate comparison group and data are collected and analyzed to determine if the observed association really exists and if it is a valid statistical associations between factors and disease occurrence exist or there are alternative explanations for the association (such as chance, bias, confounding to be discussed below).
4. *Make a judgement on causation:* An association exists if two variables appear to be related by a mathematical relationship; with a change of one appears to be related to the change in the other in the opposite direction (that is, negative or inverse relationship) or in the parallel direction (such as positive or direct relationship). However, association alone does not necessarily mean a cause and effect relationship. All available evidence has to be considered to make a casual inference. Once cause and effect has been established, we can proceed to prevention by modifying the factor in question. (The difference will be discussed in more details below.)

Study designs in epidemiologic studies and their analytical framework

Study design is the way in which health status and risk factor data are to be measured and collected and a hypothesis is tested. The design of a study is very important because:

1. It determines broadly who and what is to be studied.
2. A badly designed study can lead to erroneous results or it may not answer the question presented.

3. It determines the methods used to analyze the data.
4. It is considered with a view of how the data will later be analyzed.
5. It can rarely be changed once the study has begun (Levin 2005).

Main types of epidemiological studies

There are four main types of epidemiological studies: descriptive studies; analytical studies; interventional studies; and research synthesis. These main types are briefly described as follows.

Descriptive studies

Descriptive studies include activities related to characterizing the distribution of diseases within a population. It is the aspect of epidemiology concerned with organizing and summarizing data regarding the persons affected (for example, the characteristics of those who became ill such as demographics, sex, age, ethnicity, marital status, occupation, socioeconomic status, lifestyle, etc.), time (such as, when they become ill), and place (for instance, where they might have been exposed to the cause of illness) (U.S. Department of Health and Human Services 2006). Descriptive studies are often the first tentative approach to a new disease, health status of communities, or area of inquiry (Grimes and Schulz 2002c) and are useful for documenting the health of populations, monitoring trends and planning for public health resources, and formulating hypotheses or showing that there is an association between a given disease and a specific factor that may be related to onset. They are relatively easy to conduct, less expensive, and may provide important information to formulate further research hypothesis. However, they are "concerned with and designed only to describe the existing distribution of variables, without regard to causal or other hypotheses" (Last 1988). There are two major groups in descriptive studies: (1) Those that deal with individuals, such as (a) case report, (b) case-series report, (c) cross-sectional studies, and (d) surveillance; and (2) those that relate to populations, such as ecological or correlational studies. The brief summary of these studies and some dental examples follow.

Descriptive studies: case report

A case report is the most basic, yet one of the most common, types of descriptive studies. It is the least publishable unit in the medical/dental literature and consists of a detailed profile and report of a health problem by the observant clinician in one single patient, that is, the case. The report usually describes the diagnosis, manifestations, clinical course, and clinical outcome of that case.

A single case report is anecdotal and thus provides little empirical evidence to the clinician. Such observation may prompt further investigations with more rigorous study designs (Grimes and Schulz 2002c). As an example, Torabinejad and Turman (2011) reported on the use of platelet-rich plasma for pulp regeneration in an 11-year-old boy whose maxillary second premolar tooth had developed pulpal necrosis and symptomatic apical periodontitis after the traumatic avulsion and replantation.

Case reports document unusual occurrences that may be interesting anomalies or may represent the first clue of the emergence of a new disease or risk to health. For example, in 1961 a case report was published of a young woman with pulmonary embolism (Jordan 1961). This disease is usually seen in older women. The woman concerned had just started taking oral contraceptives. This was the first indication of that oral contraceptives increased the risk of blood clotting disorders, and this was subsequently confirmed by larger population-based studies.

Descriptive studies: case series

A case series is a report of description of individual cases that appear to have what may be a new disease or side effect of treatment. Again, the report describes the diagnosis, manifestations, clinical course, and clinical outcome of a condition. No control group is involved in case series. As an example, Block (2011) illustrated a technique for immediate placement of implants into 35 consecutive molar extraction sites. A case series provides weak empirical evidence and at best can be considered as a source of hypotheses for investigation by stronger study designs. That said, case report and case series are the most common study type in the clinical literature. Case series, like case reports, may give rise to useful hypotheses but cannot establish that an association does exist between a risk factor and a disease. Case series can also constitute the case group for a case-control study, a relatively stronger design that can explore the hunches about causes of disease. Whereas a report of a single unusual case might not trigger further investigation, a case-series of several unusual cases (in excess of what might be expected) adds to the concern. A convenient feature of case-series reports is that they can constitute the case group for a case-control study, which can then explore hunches about causes of disease. Although a single case may document an interesting oddity, it may not trigger further investigation. In contrast, a case-series of several unusual cases adds to the concern and provides the basis for a useful hypothesis about a disease (Grimes and Schulz 2002c). Sometimes, the appearance of several similar cases in a short period heralds an epidemic. For example, in the period October 1980 to May 1981, five young men, all active homosexuals, were treated for biopsy-confirmed *Pneumocystis carinii* pneumonia at three different hospitals in Los Angeles, California. One case may have been an anomaly, but five cases suggested the emergence of a new disease. This was the first published report of what, a year later, became known as acquired immunodeficiency syndrome (AIDS). Because all of these men were homosexual and the cluster was identified on the basis of sexual contact, it was suggested that various forms of sexual behaviors were related to the risk of disease and the infectious agents were sexually transmitted among homosexually active males (Centers for Disease Control and Prevention 1982).

Descriptive studies: cross-sectional surveys

A cross-sectional survey (also known as a frequency survey or a prevalence study) is a study at one point of time, in which a sample of persons from a population are enrolled and their exposures and health outcomes are measured simultaneously (US Department of Health and Human Services 2006). Measurement of the prevalence of a given disease (usually expressed as a percentage or proportion or number of cases per unit population) and the severity of that disease (usually expressed as a mean value derived from an appropriate scale or index) requires a cross-sectional survey. This is a survey undertaken at one point in time and provides a snapshot of the health of the population at that time. As an example, Statistics Canada collected data for the Canadian Health Measures Survey (CHMS) from about 6,000 people in 15 communities randomly selected across Canada between March 2007 and February 2009. The sample represents 97% of the Canadian population aged 6 to 79 years old. The study collected data on the health of Canadians by means of direct physical measurements such as blood pressure, height, weight, and physical fitness. As part of the CHMS, a clinical oral health examination and questionnaire was also performed. The study provided the important information on epidemiology of oral diseases in Canada. For example, we now know that 57% of 6 to 11 year olds and 59% of 12 to 19 year olds have or have had a cavity. Six percent of adult Canadians no longer have any natural teeth, and 21% of adults with teeth have, or have had, moderate or severe periodontal diseases (Health Canada 2010).

Cross-sectional studies are relatively inexpensive, take up little time to conduct, can assess many outcomes and risk indicators at the same time, and are useful for public health planning to develop targeting strategies, understanding disease etiology and for generation of hypotheses (Levin 2006). Typically, a random sample of the population of interest is drawn and the number of cases of a given disease occurring in the sample is determined by clinical examination or questionnaire. Therefore, cross-sectional surveys can estimate prevalence of outcome of interest. At the same time information is collected, again by examination or questionnaire, on various attributes and characteristics that may be related to the disease under study. However, cross-sectional studies do not tell us the direction of that association (that is, the temporal relation) as they lack any information on timing of exposure and outcome relationships. It is not possible to determine from this kind of study whether the putative risk factor preceded the onset of disease, and the situation may provide differing results if another time frame had been chosen.

Another type of survey that measures prevalence is the repeated cross-sectional survey. As the name implies, these surveys are cross-sectional studies, but they are repeated at regular and specified intervals in the same population. There is no attempt to survey the same individuals. This survey looks at a different group of people at each point in time and gives information about how the prevalence of disease is changing over time. For example, in the UK, the national cross-sectional surveys of 5-year-old children (the British Association for the Study of Community Dentistry Survey) are examined annually. This study provides information on prevalence and trends in oral disease for this age group. As mentioned above, such information is important for the public health planning.

Descriptive studies: surveillance

Surveillance studies are ongoing systematic collection, analysis, and interpretation of health data that are essential to the planning, implementation, and evaluation of public health practice, closely integrated with the timely dissemination of these data to those who need to know (Centers for Disease Control 1986). Surveillance can be thought of as watchfulness over a community (Grimes and Schulz 2002c). The best example of the impact of such studies is the eradication of smallpox. Following global vaccination campaigns to cover at least 80% of the population, rigorous disease surveillance was implemented to detect outbreaks and target them with focused containment measures. Through the surveillance studies, whenever the "index" cases with smallpox were identified, all close contacts of the index case and all close contacts of those people were vaccinated. This method effectively isolated the index case. With only human-to-human transmission and no animal reservoir for the disease, the chain of transmission was broken and the virus died out and the disease was eradicated in 1980, leading to an extraordinary public-health achievement (Fenner *et al.* 1988). Thus, surveillance studies are important from population-health perspectives.

Descriptive studies: ecologic studies

Ecologic studies have populations or groups as the unit of analysis. The ecological studies can therefore measure prevalence and incidence of disease, particularly when disease is rare and can monitor population health so that public health strategies may be developed and directed. In ecological studies, aggregated secondary data on risk factors and disease prevalence from different population groups is compared to identify associations. Such design can study the relationship between population-level exposure to risk factors and disease and may be useful for suggesting hypotheses but cannot be used to test them. Also, because these studies are performed at the population level, associations between two variables at the group level (or ecological level) may differ from associations between analogous variables measured at the individual level (that is, ecological fallacy) (Schwartz 1994). Therefore, the presence of a correlation in an ecologic study does not mean that an association will be found when studies of individuals are undertaken. Conversely, the absence of a correlation in an ecologic study does not mean that the factor in question is not related to the onset of disease in an individual.

Analytical studies

Descriptive studies are useful for formulating hypotheses or showing that there is an association between a given disease and a specific factor that may be related to onset. However, none of the designs enable us to determine cause-and-effect relationships. Analytic study designs allow us to test hypotheses concerning causal relationships. They are concerned with why and how a health problem occurs. In analytic epidemiology, comparison groups are used to provide baseline or expected values. In this way, the associations between exposures and outcomes can be quantified, and hypotheses about the cause of the problem can be tested (US Department of Health and Human Services 2006). Consequently, the strength of analytical designs stems from the following facts:

1. They compare people with and without a disease or with and without exposure to a potential risk factor.
2. They are able to establish whether the risk factor preceded the onset of the disease or not.
3. They give a quantitative estimate of the strength of association between a risk factor and disease.
4. They can take account of factors other than the one we are interested in which may influence disease onset.

In analytical studies, groups are compared to identify and quantify associations, test hypotheses, and identify causes. Two common types are cohort studies and case-control studies (US Department of Health and Human

Services 2006). Before discussing these two designs, to avoid any uncertainty in terminology, we shall start by defining some keywords/concepts used in clinical epidemiology. *Risk* is the probability that people who are exposed to certain "risk factors" will subsequently develop a particular disease, injury, or other health condition within a specified time or age span, more often than similar people who are not exposed (Flethcer 2005; US Department of Health and Human Services 2006). *Risk Factor* is "...an environmental [e.g., infectious agents, drugs, and toxins], behavioral [e.g., smoking, excessive alcohol drinking], or biologic factor [or inherited factors such as specific genes] confirmed by temporal sequence, usually in longitudinal studies, which if present directly increases the probability of a disease occurring, and if absent or removed reduces the probability. Risk factors are part of the causal chain, or expose the host to the causal chain. Once disease occurs, removal of a risk factor may not result in a cure." (Beck 1998).

Analytical studies: cohort studies

Cohort by definition applies to a well-defined group of people who have something in common (such as a common experience or exposure) when they are first assembled and who are then followed up for a period of time to see what happens to them (US Department of Health and Human Services 2006). Cohort studies proceed in a logical sequence: from exposure to outcome (Grimes and Schulz 2002d). The observation is carried forward over time to see which of the participants experience the outcome (hence also called longitudinal studies or prospective studies). The observation period should be a meaningful period of time based on the natural history of the disease in question. At the end of the study, the comparison in the rates of the outcome events in the exposed and unexposed groups is performed to examine how potential risk factors relate to subsequent outcome events. If the exposed group develops a higher incidence of the outcome than the unexposed, then the exposure is associated with an increased risk of the outcome (Grimes and Schulz 2002d). In particular, the association between exposure and disease can be measured using the following measures of effect according to Fletcher (2005):

- **Absolute Risk** or the number of new cases of disease arising during a given period of time in a defined population that is initially free of the condition, hence incidence of disease in exposed and non-exposed.
- **Attributable Risk** indicates the additional risk (incidence) of disease following exposure, over and above that experienced by people who are not exposed.
- **Relative Risk** (RR) indicates how many times exposed population are more likely to get the disease relative to

non-exposed population (that is, the incidence of disease in exposed population divided by that of the non-exposed population). This is the most commonly reported result in studies of risk and is useful for expressing the strength of a causal relationship.

Cohort studies can be done by going ahead in time from the present (prospective cohort study) (Figure 5-1) or, alternatively, by going back in time to comprise the cohorts and following them up to the present (retrospective cohort study) (Figure 5-2). In the latter case, the investigator might use existing medical records and go back in time several years to identify those exposed and not exposed to the factor in question. He would then track them forward through records to note the outcome

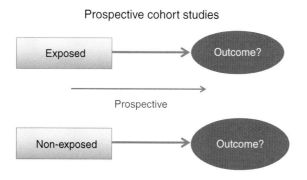

Prospective cohort studies

Is outcome more prevalent among exposed than unexposed?

Figure 5-1 Prospective cohort studies. The overall design of a cohort study: the exposed and non-exposed groups to a particular factor of interest are followed up for a meaningful period of time to evaluate whether the outcome of interest is more prevalent among exposed than non-exposed group.

Retrospective cohort studies

Is outcome more prevalent among exposed than unexposed?

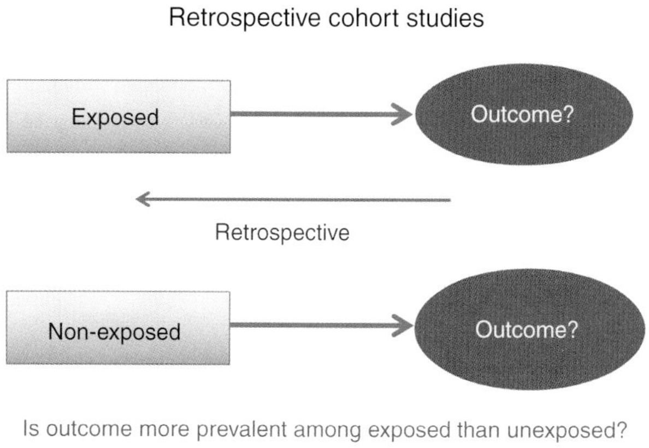

Figure 5-2 Retrospective cohort studies. The overall design of a cohort study: the exposed and non-exposed groups to a particular factor of interest are followed up for a meaningful period of time to evaluate whether the outcome of interest is more prevalent among exposed than non-exposed group.

of interest. Again, the study moves from exposure to outcome, although the data collection occurred after the fact. The apparent advantage of historical cohort studies is that the information is available immediately, although the quality of such information depends on the quality of recorded information (Grimes and Schulz 2002b).

As an example, a prospective cohort study that will be ongoing in Australia aims to explore the interactions between risk and protective factors in the development of early childhood caries, in particular the effects of infant feeding practices. Mothers living in disadvantaged areas in Southwestern Sydney will be invited to join the study soon after the birth of their child at the time of the first home visit by Child and Family Health Nurses and data on feeding practices (for example, initiation and duration of breastfeeding, introduction of solid food, intake of cariogenic and non-cariogenic foods) and dental health behaviors (for example, fluoride exposure, oral hygiene practices) will be gathered using a telephone interview when the children are 4, 8, and 12 months old, and thereafter at six monthly intervals until the child is aged 5 years. Children will have a dental and anthropometric examination at 2 and 5 years of age, and the main outcome measures will be oral health quality of life, caries prevalence, and caries incidence.

Cohort studies can establish the temporal dimension, whereby exposure is seen to occur before outcome giving some indication of causality. Since the healthy population at the inception is followed over time, such studies can be used to study more than one outcome (disease) and to measure the change in exposure and outcome over time. They are also useful for the study of rare exposures. However, cohort studies are inefficient for diseases that are relatively rare because very large numbers need to be followed for long periods of time until a rare incident is established. They also are expensive because of resources necessary to study many people over time, and their results are not available for a long time. There is also a risk of loss to follow-up; over time, participants may leave the study for any reason resulting in incomplete data that can misrepresent the true state of risk factor if the reason for drop out is related to outcome. There is also a potential for selection bias. That is, a difference in incidence of the outcome of interest between those who participated and those who did not would give biased results (Grimes and Schulz 2002b; Fletcher 2005).

Analytical studies: case control studies

A case-control study is an observational study that enrolls one group of persons with a certain disease, chronic condition, or type of injury (case patients) and a group of persons without the health problem (control subjects) and compares differences in exposures, behaviors, and other characteristics to identify and quantify associations, test hypotheses, and identify causes (US Department of Health and Human Services 2006). Therefore, the case-control studies work backwards. They start with an outcome and look for exposures that might have caused the outcome (Grimes and Schulz 2002d). As an example, Leung *et al.* (2011) compared the periodontal status of 36 dentate Hong Kong Chinese patients with systemic sclerosis who were age- and sex-matched to systemically healthy controls who attended a dental hospital.

The design of a case-control study is simple. From the members of the same base population, a group of cases (people with the disease) and controls (people without the disease) are selected. These cases and controls would meet the same criteria for inclusion in the study and are matched with a set of characteristics not related to the exposure under study. In other words, controls should be similar to cases in all important respects except the cases do not have the outcome in question. Using chart reviews, interviews, or other means, information on prior exposure to the factor of interest is obtained for both cases and controls to examine how potential risk factors in the past history relate to the current status of disease. If the prevalence of the exposure is higher among cases than among controls, then the exposure is associated with an increased risk of the outcome (Grimes and Schulz 2002d). In particular, the association between exposure to the potential risk factor in the past and disease in the current time can be measured using odds ratio (OR), that is, the odds that a case is exposed divided by the odds that a control is exposed (Figure 5-3).

Case-control studies are commonly used for initial, inexpensive, and quick evaluation of risk factors and are particularly suited to the study of rare diseases or diseases with long latency periods such as cardiovascular disease and cancer. These studies often require less time, effort, and money than would cohort studies (Grimes and Schulz 2002d). However, difficulties remain in overcoming potential bias and confounding. For example, successful selection of both cases and controls who are representative of their respective populations is often difficult. Moreover, the collected information on exposure to the factor relies on subjects' recall or health records; both can be inaccurate. For example, there may be a better recollection of exposures among the cases than among the controls (recall bias), a persistent difficulty in studies that rely on memory (Grimes and Schulz 2002b; Grimes and Schulz 2002d; Schulz and Grimes 2002a). They are also inefficient in studying rare risk factors, since the possibility of encountering with them in the past is slim for both cases and controls.

Experimental or interventional studies

So far we understand that descriptive studies enable us to develop plausible hypotheses about risk factors, and analytical studies allow us to test those hypotheses. The next step is to produce evidence that allow us to ascertain whether or not various therapeutic or preventive interventions improve a patient's clinical condition, reduce the frequency of disease in populations, or improve population health. Such evidence can be generated through experimental or interventional studies. In experimental and intervention studies, the investigator intervenes and then observes the outcomes of that intervention. Clearly, for ethical reasons, these interventions must be ones that are believed to do more good than harm. Consequently, experimental and interventional studies are limited to the assessment of new ways of preventing or treating disease. These studies are usually referred to under the general name of clinical trials, which can be *prophylactic*, that test interventions to PREVENT disease (vaccination, dietary change) or *therapeutic*, that test interventions to TREAT disease or reduce disability (a new drug; implants versus dentures).

When a new preventive or therapeutic treatment or procedure is developed, there is often a degree of doubt concerning its benefits. When penicillin was introduced, death rates from pneumococcal pneumonia fell from around 95% to 15%. This was such a dramatic change that clinical trials were neither necessary nor ethical. Mere observation of the difference was sufficient to confirm the benefits of antibiotic therapy. More often however, new interventions produce small to moderate benefits, around 10 to 20% improvement compared to conventional treatments. In these cases, observational studies, because of their limitations, cannot establish with any degree of certainty that a new treatment is

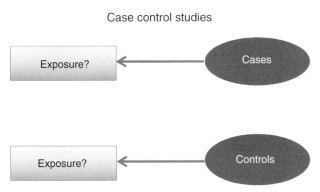

Case control studies

Is exposure more prevalent among cases than controls?

Figure 5-3 Case control studies. The overall design of a case-control study: People with the disease (cases) and without the disease (controls) are being compared to examine how potential risk factors in the past history relate to the present status of disease.

Randomized clinical trials

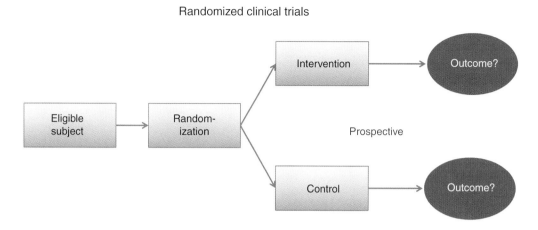

Is outcome more prevalent among intervention group than control group?

Figure 5-4 Randomized clinical trials. The overall design of a randomized clinical trial: The eligible subjects are randomly assigned to an intervention group to receive the new intervention or to a control group to receive a placebo, existing intervention, or nothing. They will then be followed over a meaningful period of time to evaluate whether the outcome of interest is more prevalent among intervention than the control group.

beneficial, and clinical trials must be undertaken to confirm that benefit.

A typical intervention study is a randomized controlled trial.

Description of a randomized controlled trial

When we talk about clinical trials we generally mean a randomized controlled clinical trial or RCT. This is a prospective, experimental study that involves primary data generated in the clinical environment. This design approximates the controlled experiment of basic science and resembles the cohort study in several respects, with the important exception of randomization of participants to exposures (Grimes and Schulz 2002d). Randomized trial is the strongest evidence of the clinical efficacy of preventive and therapeutic procedures in the clinical setting. However, it should also be noted that RCTs are expensive (both time and money) and may have high drop out (for example, undesirable side effects for an intervention, or little incentive for participants). A randomized trial has the following basic design (Figure 5-4):

1. Assemble group of individuals at risk (prophylactic) or who have the disease (therapeutic)
2. Randomly allocate to EXPERIMENTAL and CONTROL groups
3. Give experimental group the new intervention
4. Give control group a placebo or an existing intervention (or in some cases, nothing)
5. Follow over time and measure OUTCOMES in both groups
6. Assess if differences are statistically and clinically significant

The way in which good and poor outcomes are assessed will vary according to the type of intervention being assessed. For example, the following trial compared the effect of a drug "captopril" (angiotensin-converting enzyme inhibitor used for the treatment of hypertension) with a placebo on death rates among patients with myocardial infarction (heart attack) (Table 5-1).

In this case, the relative risk can be calculated as: RR=71.9/76.9=0.94. Since the RR is less than 1, it indicates the protective effect of the drug.

However, a clinical trial to compare the quality of life outcomes of implant therapy and dentures for edentulous patients would look at changes in scores on a measure of oral health-related quality of life. Here the patients in each group would be assessed prior to therapy and 6 months after therapy and the amount of change in each group compared. For example in the following RCT (Awad *et al.* 2000), 54 patients received implant supported dentures and 48 received conventional dentures. The oral health related quality of life scale (the Oral Health Impact Profile) was administered prior to and following therapy. In this case the columns of the table refer to pre- and post-treatment scores. Note high scores mean poorer quality of functional and psychosocial well being (Table 5-2).

These data indicate that implant-supported dentures bring about a greater improvement in quality of life than conventional dentures among this group of patients.

Within the domain of randomized controlled trial several other subtypes have been used by investigators. These include the following:

- Quasi-randomized clinical trial: Cost, ethical issues, and logistical problems may prevent the use of the

Table 5-1 Relative risk example

			Outcome		
			Deaths	Survivors	Death rate per 1,000
Randomization	↗	Captopril	2,088	26,940	71.9
	↘	Placebo	2,231	26,791	76.9

Table 5-2 Quality of life outcomes example

			Outcome		
			Mean score Pre-treatment	Mean score Post-treatment	% Change
Randomization	↗	Implant	100	66	34
	↘	Conventional	99	89	10

RCT in many settings. Here, non-randomized trial design is often used. These differ from the RCT in that allocation of patients to experimental and control groups is not based on random allocation but is based on a predictable variable such as date of birth (odd or even), day of admission (odd or even), ward A versus ward B or hospital number (odd or even), etc. (Grimes and Schulz 2002d). The study groups may differ from one another and bias can be introduced whether to enroll patient or not in the study depending upon known allocation. Thus, in these types of study design there are many threats to internal validity. A dental example is a study on flare-up rate related to root canal treatment of asymptomatic nonvital maxillary central incisor teeth performed in one and two appointments. Patients were assigned *consecutively* to either one- or two-visit treatment (Al-Negrish and Habahbeh 2006).

- Split mouth trial: These trials take advantage of the fact that the mouth has two halves so that two treatments can be given simultaneously to the same individual. In each individual in the trial, the treatments are assigned to a randomly selected side of the mouth. The obvious advantage of such design is each subject will serve as his/her own control, which can remove a lot of inter-individual variability from the estimates of the treatment effect and increase statistical efficiency. Also on average fewer patients are needed. However, the statistical analysis of split-mouth designs is, in general, more complicated than the analysis of a classical whole-mouth study (Lesaffre *et al.* 2007; Lesaffre *et al.* 2009) This type of trial has been typically used to evaluate different types of dental sealant in terms of retention rates and caries preventive potential. For

example, Lygidakis and Oulis (1999) selected 112 subjects of 7–8 years of age who had four newly erupted first molar teeth. In each subject, one side of the mouth was randomly selected to receive a conventional sealant and the other a fluoride-containing sealant. The children were followed for 4 years to compare percentages of teeth in which the sealants were still in place and the percentage of teeth that had decayed.

- Crossover randomized trial: In a crossover trial, individuals serve as their own control. However, in this case all subjects receive the treatments to be compared, but the treatments are applied sequentially. The participants are randomly allocated to one of two treatment groups, and, after a sufficient treatment period and often a washout period, are switched to the other treatment for the same period. Preferably the order in which the treatments are given should be random. For example, Tang *et al.* (1997) gave 10 patients a four-implant long-bar overdenture and 6 patients a two-implant hybrid prosthesis. After a 2-month adaptation period, patients' ratings of stability and comfort and tests of chewing function were undertaken. The treatments were then switched and the assessments repeated after another 2-month adaptation period. The two types of implant-supported denture were then compared. The advantage of this design is that you would need only half the number of subjects for the study; however, the disadvantage is that the "leftover" or "residual" treatment effect of first intervention may have an influence on the second treatment, and there would be some dependency in assessment when data are collected in the same subject. Analyses of such studies require special adjustments.

- Cluster randomized trial: In cluster RCT, the intervention involves an entire community rather than individual patients, and there may be as few as two units of observation. The design of a community trial is as follows:
  - ○ Select two communities as similar as possible in size, composition, and other characteristics.
  - ○ Select one at random to be the experimental community and another as a control community.
  - ○ Assess disease rates in each community to confirm that they are similar.
  - ○ Implement the intervention in the experimental community.
  - ○ After a suitable length of time, compare disease rates in the two communities.

As an example, in 1965, Brown and Poplove (1965) compared rates of dental caries between the Canadian towns of Brantford and Sarnia. Brantford, Ontario had the fluoride content of its water supply brought up from negligible levels to 1.0 to 1.2 parts per million. The effect on caries rates was assessed by comparing Brantford with Sarnia, the non-fluoridated control community. After 15 years, the mean number of decayed, missing, and filled permanent teeth (DMFT) of 12- to 14-year olds in Brantford was 3.23, 57% less than the mean of 7.46 observed in Sarnia. The advantage of cluster-randomized trials is the ability to conduct studies in situations where it is ethically or practically impossible to randomize patients in two groups within each setting due to spill-over effect. The disadvantage of cluster RCT is that results are not generalizable at individual patient level.

Irrespective of the design of RCT, several issues need to be carefully considered in either design or interpretation of results of RCT.

1. Randomization

   The hallmark of RCT is assignment of participants to exposures purely by chance. The assignment of patients to experimental or control treatment should be randomized, that is by methods such as tossing a coin, which ensure the equal chance of allocation. This is the most important aspect of an RCT and ensures that patients had equal chance of receiving either experimental or control intervention. The purpose is to end up in two groups that have similar characteristics in terms of all known and unknown factors, which may influence the outcome. Moreover, anything short of proper randomization courts selection and confounding biases (Schulz and Grimes 2002c). In other words, proper implementation of a randomization has three major advantages:

   1) it ensures that the allocation bias and confounding are minimized

   2) it ensures the internal validity of the study, that is, the outcome observed was the result of the intervention and the intervention alone

   3) it facilitates the statistical analysis

2. Subject selection

   Unlike the observational study, RCTs depend upon patients volunteering to take part and pass through a screening process (Grimes and Schulz 2002d). Moreover, RCTs are usually undertaken on highly selected groups of patients to make it easier to distinguish the "signal" (treatment effect) from the "noise" (bias and chance). Most have quite stringent entry criteria that determine who is and is not eligible to participate in a trial. Whereas the internal validity of a proper RCT is high (that is, it measures what it sets out to measure), it might not have external validity (Grimes and Schulz 2002d). External validity (also called generalizability or applicability) is the extent to which the results of a study can be generalized to other circumstances (Campbell 1957). For example, the Physicians' Health Study was a large RCT undertaken to determine if low doses of aspirin would reduce total cardiovascular mortality (Grimes and Schulz 2002d). Participants were 22,071 male physicians aged 40 to 84 years. Males of that age were chosen because high rates of cardiovascular disease in that population meant that sufficient endpoints for analysis (deaths from heart disease) would accumulate fairly quickly. Moreover, physicians are easy to follow over time and are more likely to comply with the requirements of the clinical trial, thus enhancing internal validity. However, can the results of the trial be generalized to all males? They may apply to all men aged 40 years and over, but do they apply to women?

3. Intervention

   It is important to consider an intervention that sufficiently differs from alternative managements, with a reasonable expectation that the outcome will be affected. Similarly, it is important to consider an intervention that is likely to be implemented in usual clinical practice, not a complex intervention that is beyond the real-world treatment plans (that is, effectiveness versus efficacy).

4. Placebo

   Most contemporary trials compare a new therapy with an existing therapy. In particular, if the usual existing care is already known to be effective, then a more effective (or economical) outcome should be expected for a new therapy. If the control group is not given an alternative therapy then they are given a placebo intervention that is indistinguishable from the active treatment. Examples of placebo in drug trial are sugar pills or saline injections that match the physical appearance, color, taste, or smell of the test medicine but that does not have a specific, known mechanism of action. In this way, the placebo effect can be controlled, that is, the benefits obtained from a drug or intervention are over and above its therapeutic effect.

5. Measurement of Outcomes–Blinding

If the measurement of outcomes involves clinical judgments or patient reports then these may be biased if the clinician or patient knows which group they are in. This is controlled by blinding (also known as masking), which refers to keeping trial participants, investigators (usually health care providers), or assessors (those collecting outcome data) unaware of an assigned intervention (Schulz and Grimes 2002b). Blinding is an important safeguard against bias, particularly when assessing subjective outcomes (Wood *et al.* 2008). In a single blind trial, the subjects do not know to which group they have been allocated; in a double blind trial, neither patients nor physicians know; and in a triple blind trial, patients, physicians, nor the person analyzing the data know which patients are experimental and which are controls. The groups are usually designated as A and B, and one person not involved in the trial has the key that identifies experimental and control patients.

6. Measurement of outcomes–All relevant clinical outcomes

All relevant outcomes must be measured to get a complete clinical picture of the efficacy of an intervention. For example, two drugs may be equally effective at controlling a disease, but one may have significant quality of life effects such as nausea, insomnia, and/or irritability. Consequently, we should always consider whether or not all relevant clinical, economic, and patient-based outcomes have been considered. For example, in a study of comparing the caries-preventive effect of sodium fluoride varnish and acidulated phosphate fluoride (APF) gel, Seppa *et al.*(1995) randomly allocated 245 children aged 12–13 years with high past caries experience into varnish/gel groups. The participants received semi-annual applications of either fluoride varnish or APF gel for 3 years, and the examination/radiographs were taken at baseline and follow-up. Although the mean total decayed, missing, filled permanent tooth surfaces (DMFS) increments of the varnish and gel groups were comparable, fluoride varnish was superior to fluoride gel with respect to treatment time/costs, patient acceptability, and short-term side effects/discomfort (such as nausea, vomiting, burning).

7. Statistical Versus Clinical Significance

An RCT may indicate that there is a statistically significant difference in the outcomes of two inter-

ventions. However, is the difference also of clinical significance? For example, a new drug may result in a statistically significant reduction in blood pressure when compared to an existing drug, but is this reduction likely to reduce the patient's risk of a heart attack to any significant degree? Similarly, implant therapy may result in a statistically significant improvement in scores on a quality of life measure when compared to denture therapy, but is this difference meaningful to the patient? Any benefit in improved health outcomes must be statistically significant, but specifically, it should be clinically significant, that is, it should be beyond or equal to the smallest difference that clinicians and patients feel improves oral health or wellness. If there is no benefit at the threshold of both clinical and statistical health improvement, then the procedure should not be used for that purpose.

8. Ethical Issues

For ethical reasons, a clinical trial should usually only be undertaken when there is reason to believe that the new treatment approach is beneficial (for example, based on prior knowledge) but sufficient doubt remains about the extent of that benefit or safety. For example, if there is no doubt that a new treatment is better than an old treatment, it is unethical to withhold it from patients for the purposes of a clinical trial. Many, and sometimes complex, ethical issues are involved in clinical trials. Prior to the conduct of an RCT, its methods and procedures must be carefully scrutinized by an ethics committee to ensure that it is justified.

9. Efficacy Versus Effectiveness

When we are satisfied with the above-mentioned issues, in order to consider the results of RCTs of new dental treatment/product, we should consider two concepts: **efficacy** and **effectiveness**. RCTs establish **efficacy,** the benefit of the intervention to a defined group of patients treated under ideal conditions. Subjects in RCTs are a highly selected group, and the trial is usually performed by clinical experts in centers of excellence, usually university-based dental schools. **Effectiveness** refers to the benefit of the intervention in the real world (that is, to the typical patient treated under ordinary conditions by the average practitioner). In such case, the true practice effectiveness is usually less than the efficacy measured in an RCT because the diagnostic accuracy in identifying the suitable patients that benefit from the therapy, and the quality and quantity of practitioners' and patients' compliance to the treatment protocol would affect the achieved outcome. Consequently, studies are also needed of the outcomes of new therapies when used in the average clinical practice to confirm that the benefits obtained in clinical trials accrue to all patients.

Research synthesis

It has been well known now that a busy general practitioner in the community needs to read at least 17 to 20 articles every day to keep him/her self apprised of the latest evidence on the topics of interest in his/her daily clinical practice. This might well be true, albeit the number may be low, for a dental practitioner. Thus, reliance on a summative synthesis has gained vast popularity in recent days. There are two main types of synthesis articles.

1. Informal or narrative review: These reviews are conducted by experts in the field, most commonly without an explicit question or search methods. Based on their knowledge, these individuals, mostly when appraising a relevant research paper published in the same issue of the journal, will provide an expert commentary on the subject highlighting a smaller question based on their expertise. They are mostly opinion-based, limited in scope, and do not contain critical assessment of quality of the included studies. At times though, these are the only types of syntheses you may encounter for the clinical situation at hand; however, care is warranted in the interpretation of such results. An example of this would be the recent article on internal root resorption that reviewed the prevalence, etiology, pathogenesis, histological manifestations, differential diagnosis with cone beam computed tomography, and treatment perspectives (Patel *et al.* 2010).

2. Formal or systematic review (with or without meta-analysis): On the other hand, a systematic review consists of "a review of a clearly formulated question that uses systematic and explicit methods to identify, select, and critically appraise relevant research, and to collect and analyze data from the studies that are included in the review" (Higgins 2006). Prior to conducting a systematic review, authors develop a specific and pertinent research question and method to conduct a particular review. It is decided *a priori* what search methods will be used, how the identified literature will be selected and critically appraised, what data will be collected, and how data will be analyzed, summarized, and reported. A systematic review may or may not include a meta-analysis. Meta-analysis is a statistical technique of combining available data from various studies that are relatively homogeneous and deriving a summary estimate. In the hierarchy of evidence-based health care, a well-conducted systematic review with meta-analysis is considered the highest possible

evidence. Cochrane Collaboration, an independent entity heavily involved in the production of several systematic reviews in various fields including dental care, produces high quality systematic reviews of various health care interventions and constantly updates these reviews with new information on a regular basis. Some view this as a "cookbook" approach to the provision of recommendations on health care; however, well-conducted reviews have now formed the basis for sound practice parameters and guidelines. Systematic reviews at times stop at providing recommendations, and professional organizations or a similar body will take into consideration all evidence including performing their own systematic reviews and coming up with guidelines for practice. An example of well-conducted systematic reviews (which would encourage the clinician to implement the practice in dental care) would be a series of publications by Cochrane Oral Health Group that evaluate the effectiveness and safety of four topical fluoride treatments (toothpastes, gels, varnishes, and mouth rinses) in preventing caries in children and adolescents (Marinho *et al.* 2003a; Marinho *et al.* 2003b; Marinho *et al.* 2003c; Marinho *et al.* 2004a; Marinho *et al.* 2004b). More examples of other well-conducted systematic reviews can be found in the Oral Health Group of the Cochrane library.

When we know various types of study design, the most important question comes to mind. Busy dental practitioners who have somewhat limited knowledge and skill will ask themselves a question: How can I make sense of all this? How would I be able to differentiate a good quality article from not-so good quality of care? In the following section, we describe a generic approach to critical appraisal of any article. The purpose of this section is not to be "critical and shed all articles" because fault finding is easy. The purpose is to find the good qualities within this article and highlight its weak points and think how the latter could be overcome.

Critical appraisal of research: general guidelines

When one reads an article on a certain topic, he/she should be able to differentiate a good manuscript from a not-so-helpful manuscript. At the same time, it must be kept in mind that there is not a single paper that does not have one or another fallacy. The purpose of critically reviewing an article is to determine whether the biases inherent in the current study are severe enough that it not only creates doubts about external validity but also doubts internal validity of the study. This process is an art that can be learned only by practicing it often. When critically appraising an article, no matter what type of article it is, three important concepts need to be kept in mind: validity, reliability, and applicability.

- **Validity** of an article is assessed by asking questions like the following: (a) Did the study address a clearly focused research question?, (b) Did the investigator perform the right type of study for question?, (c) What is the quality of the study?, and (d) If there are confounders, did the investigator address them?
- **Reliability** is assessed by the confidence one can place in the findings of the study. The investigators must report confidence margins around their estimate or there should be sufficient information from the study available to calculate the confidence limits.
- Finally **applicability** of the results is ascertained by asking the following questions: (a) Can the results be applied to the population that I see in my dental clinic or hospital unit?, (b) Did the investigators considered all of the important outcomes?, and (c) Should policy or practice change as a result of the evidence contained in this study?

There are several tools available for critical appraisal of different types of study and one of the constellations of such toolkits is available at the Centre for Evidence-based Medicine (2011).

Finally, when readers have completed reading an article, often readers would ask these questions: What is the strength of this evidence? Are the findings strong enough to develop recommendations for care?

In the next section, the hierarchy of study designs and relative strengths of various types of studies in generating or contributing to evidence pool is discussed.

Levels of evidence

In 1979, the Canadian Task Force on the Periodic Health Examination published for the first time a guideline that characterized the level of evidence underlying health care recommendations and the strength of recommendations (Canadian Task Force on the Periodic Health Examination 1979). This system includes a hierarchy of evidence as the highest (Level I) being a properly randomized controlled trial to the lowest (Level III) being opinions of respected authorities, based on clinical experience, descriptive studies, or reports of expert committees. This system also includes a bidirectional classification of its recommendations for specific clinical preventive actions (Grades A–E, and I with Grade A showing good evidence to recommend for the clinical preventive action to Grade E showing good evidence to recommend against the clinical preventive action, and Grade I showing insufficient evidence, in quantity and/or quality, to make a recommendation) (Table 5-3).

Since then several other organizations have proposed criteria to classify clinical practice guidelines. For example, the US Preventive Services Task Force (USPSTF) followed the same research design rating as the Canadian Task Force on Preventive Health Care but assigns one of five letter grades to each of its recommendations (A, B, C, D, or I). The recent revision of the USPSTF grade definitions (May 2007) is shown in Tables 5-4 and 5-5 (US Preventive Services Task Force 2008).

Concept of cause and effect in epidemiological studies

The final section of this chapter is devoted to the idea that when a researcher reports on higher risk of certain exposure in patients who had disease compared to those without disease, how can we conclude that there is a cause and effect relationship between exposure and outcome? In clinical medicine and dentistry, risk factor is mainly used to predict the occurrence of disease. However, it should be appreciated that just because a risk factor may predict the disease, it does not necessarily mean that the risk factors cause the disease (Fletcher and Fletcher 2005). For example, analytic epidemiological studies tell us if there is an association between a given factor (for example, smoking) and a disease (such as, periodontal disease). However, the presence of even a strong risk factor in an individual does not necessarily mean that an individual will get the disease. Simply because an association exists does not necessarily mean there is a cause and effect relationship between the factor and the disease, and this must be taken into account. Sir Bradford Hill suggested criteria for understanding cause and effect relationships. These criteria follow (Hill 1965):

1. Strength of the association: How strong is the effect, measured as relative risk or odds ratio? The stronger the association between the factor and the disease, the more likely a cause and effect relationship exists. An odds ratio or relative risk of 3–5 would be considered quite strong, but 1–2 would be considered weak. Odds ratios and relative risks linking periodontal disease and heart disease range from 1.5 to 2.7, which can be considered to be weak to moderate.
2. Consistency of association with other studies: Has the effect been seen by others? If studies with different designs, conducted by different investigators in different places using different populations all show the same result, this points to a cause and effect relationship. For example, results of studies done around the world have consistently shown an association between smoking and periodontal disease.

Table 5-3 This system includes a hierarchy of evidence as the highest (Level I) being properly randomized controlled trial to the lowest (Level III) being opinions of respected authorities, based on clinical experience, descriptive studies or reports of expert committees. This system also includes recommendations grades (A–E, I) for specific clinical preventive actions: Grade A showing good evidence to recommend the clinical preventive action) to Grade E showing good evidence to recommend against the clinical preventive action, and Grade I showing insufficient evidence (in quantity and/or quality) to make a recommendation

Recommendations Grades for Specific Clinical Preventive Actions

A	The CTF concludes that there is **good** evidence to recommend the clinical preventive action.
B	The CTF concludes that there is **fair** evidence to recommend the clinical preventive action.
C	The CTF concludes that the existing evidence is **conflicting** and does not allow making a recommendation for or against use of the clinical preventive action, however other factors may influence decision-making.
D	The CTF concludes that there is **fair** evidence to recommend against the clinical preventive action.
E	The CTF concludes that there is **good** evidence to recommend against the clinical preventive action.
I	The CTF concludes that there is **insufficient** evidence (in quantity and/or quality) to make a recommendation, however other factors may influence decision-making.

The CTF recognizes that in many cases patient-specific factors need to be considered and discussed, such as the value the patient places on the clinical preventive action; its possible positive and negative outcomes; and the context and/or personal circumstances of the patient (medical and other). In certain circumstances where the evidence is complex, conflicting, or insufficient, a more detailed discussion may be required.

Levels of Evidence—Research Design Rating

I	Evidence from randomized controlled trial(s)
II-1	Evidence from controlled trial(s) without randomization
II-2	Evidence from cohort or case-control analytic studies, preferably from more than one center or research group
II-3	Evidence from comparisons between times or places with or without the intervention; dramatic results in uncontrolled experiments could be included here
III	Opinions of respected authorities, based on clinical experience; descriptive studies or reports of expert committees

Source: Canadian Task Force on Preventive Health Care (Canadian Task Force on Preventive Health Care 1997)

Table 5-4 The table summarizes the US Preventive Service Task Force (USPSTF) definitions of the grades that can be assigned to recommendations about a service and the suggested implications in practice associated with each grade. The USPSTF assigns a certainty level based on the nature of the overall evidence available to assess the net benefit of a preventive service. The USPSTF defines certainty as "likelihood that the USPSTF assessment of the net benefit of a preventive service is correct." The net benefit is defined as benefit minus harm of the preventive service as implemented in a general, primary care population

Grade	Definition	Suggestions for Practice
A	The USPSTF recommends the service. There is high certainty that the net benefit is substantial.	Offer or provide this service.
B	The USPSTF recommends the service. There is high certainty that the net benefit is moderate or there is moderate certainty that the net benefit is moderate to substantial.	Offer or provide this service.
C	The USPSTF recommends against routinely providing the service. There may be considerations that support providing the service in an individual patient. There is at least moderate certainty that the net benefit is small.	Offer or provide this service only if other considerations support the offering or providing the service in an individual patient.
D	The USPSTF recommends against the service. There is moderate or high certainty that the service has no net benefit or that the harms outweigh the benefits.	Discourage the use of this service.
I Statement	The USPSTF concludes that the current evidence is insufficient to assess the balance of benefits and harms of the service. Evidence is lacking, of poor quality, or conflicting, and the balance of benefits and harms cannot be determined.	Read the clinical considerations section of USPSTF Recommendation Statement. If the service is offered, patients should understand the uncertainty about the balance of benefits and harms.

Table 5-5 Levels of certainty regarding net benefit

Level of Certainty	Description
High	The available evidence usually includes consistent results from well-designed, well-conducted studies in representative primary care populations. These studies assess the effects of the preventive service on health outcomes. This conclusion is therefore unlikely to be strongly affected by the results of future studies.
Moderate	The available evidence is sufficient to determine the effects of the preventive service on health outcomes, but confidence in the estimate is constrained by such factors as: ● The number, size, or quality of individual studies. ● Inconsistency of findings across individual studies. ● Limited generalizability of findings to routine primary care practice. ● Lack of coherence in the chain of evidence. As more information becomes available, the magnitude or direction of the observed effect could change, and this change may be large enough to alter the conclusion.
Low	The available evidence is insufficient to assess effects on health outcomes. Evidence is insufficient because of: ● The limited number or size of studies. ● Important flaws in study design or methods. ● Inconsistency of findings across individual studies. ● Gaps in the chain of evidence. ● Findings not generalizable to routine primary care practice. ● Lack of information on important health outcomes. ● More information may allow estimation of effects on health outcomes.

Source: US Preventive Services Task Force (2008)

3. Specificity of association: Does exposure lead only to outcome? If an association is highly specific, this provides support for causality. This may be the case for acute infectious diseases (poliomyelitis and tetanus) and for genetic diseases; however, since many exposures such as cigarette smoking lead to numerous outcomes, lack of specificity does not argue against causation (Grimes and Schulz 2002a; Fletcher and Fletcher 2005).

4. Temporal Sequence: Did the study clearly demonstrate that the exposure preceded the onset of the disease? This is a fundamental self-evident principle that the causes should precede effects. The use of a cohort study design provides the best evidence with respect to the temporal sequence of cause and effect.

5. Biological gradient (dose-response relation): Does the risk of disease increase with increasing exposure to the factor under investigation? If this is the case, then it strengthens the argument for a cause and effect relationship. However, it should be noted that the absence of a dose-response relationship is relatively weak evidence against causation because of the role of the confounders and the fact that not all causal associations exhibit a dose-response relationship (Fletcher and Fletcher 2005).

6. Biologic plausibility: Does the association make sense? If we can identify possible biological mechanisms whereby the factor causes the disease, then our conclu-

sion of a cause and effect relationship is strengthened. In the case of smoking and periodontal disease, we know that smoking affects the physiology of the oral cavity and has a direct effect on the gingival tissues. Plausible biological pathways for linking periodontal disease and heart disease have also been described. However, the biological plausibility depends on the state of medical knowledge and the lack of it may indicate the limitations of medical knowledge, rather than the lack of a causal association (Grimes and Schulz 2002a; Fletcher and Fletcher 2005).

7. Coherence: Does the evidence fit with what is known regarding the natural history and biology of the outcome? Coherence between epidemiological and laboratory findings increases the likelihood of an effect. However, Hill noted that "…lack of such [laboratory] evidence cannot nullify the epidemiological effect on associations" (Hill 1965).

8. Reversibility: If a factor is causally related to a disease then the reduction in exposure is followed by lower rates of disease. Again it should be noted that the reversible associations are strong, but not infallible, evidence of a causal relationship (due to the role of confounders) (Fletcher and Fletcher 2005).

9. Reasoning by analogy: Is the observed association supported by similar associations? In other words, does the total body of evidence support a judgment of cause and effect?

Table 5-6 Association example

		New periodontal disease in 1992		
		Yes	No	Total
1989	Smokers	100	200	300
	Non-smokers	60	540	600

Let's consider these questions using smoking and periodontal disease as an example. In the hypothetical study of smoking and periodontal disease, we considered in a previous lecture, 900 people (300 smokers and 600 non-smokers) were observed over a 3-year period. From Table 5-6, 33% of smokers had additional loss of periodontal attachment compared to 10% of non-smokers so that the relative risk of new disease among smokers compared to non-smokers is 3.3.

Does the observed association between smoking and periodontal disease document a real relationship or is it due to chance, bias, or confounding?

- Chance: This refers to a statistical issue. It refers to the random error that is inherent in all observations. Epidemiologists (like all scientists) work with samples or small groups drawn from the population of interest. We infer what is happening within that population based on the experience of the sample we study. Consequently, there is always the possibility that an observed association could have arisen by chance. We evaluate this by applying appropriate statistical tests to the data, to examine whether an effect (difference) is present or is not by using statistical tests to examine the hypothesis (the "null hypothesis") that there is no difference. With respect to the example above, these tests tell us how likely it is that the differences between smokers and non-smokers we observed would have occurred by chance if there is no relationship between smoking and periodontal disease in the population from which the study subjects were drawn. This is defined as the probability that a result as extreme as the one we obtained could have occurred by chance alone if there is truly no relationship between the exposure (smoking) and the disease (periodontal disease) in the population we are studying. Usual notation for this test is p value. If a p value is less than 0.05, we refer to the result as statistically significant (that is, unlikely to be purely be chance). If the p value is greater than 0.05, we cannot rule out chance as an explanation of the observed association, and the result is not statistically signifi-

cant. In addition to p values, one needs to look at the confidence that can be placed in the reported findings; this is usually reported as 95% confidence interval (CI). This means that if this experiment is repeated 100 times, the value of the estimate will fall within these limits in 95 of such experiments. It is important to interpret results carefully and, if required, with the help of a statistician.

- Bias: Unlike the conventional meaning of bias—that is, prejudice—bias in research denotes a systematic error (such as the result of any processes or effect at any stage of a study [design, execution, application of generated information]) that causes observations to differ systematically from truth. Bias undermines the internal validity of research (Grimes and Schulz 2002a). Bias cannot be corrected for at the analysis; it can only be reduced by proper study design and implementation and not by increasing sample size (which only increases precision and reduces the impact of chance). Observational study designs are inherently more susceptible to bias than are experimental study designs. However, many randomized controlled trials (Schulz et al. 1995; Moher et al. 1998) have built-in bias. We evaluate this by looking very closely at how the study was conducted to identify possible sources of bias. In an RCT, bias can occur if patients are not properly randomized to experimental and control groups or if clinical examiners are not blind to the subject's status when evaluating outcomes.

- Confounding: Confounding is a mixing or blurring of effects. It refers to the probability that an observed association between two variables is explained by a third variable. This variable is called confounder. Confounder is causally related to outcome but is also associated with exposure. An example is the apparent relationship between having gray hair and death:

Gray hair → Death

is in fact explained by a third variable, age.

$$Age \nearrow \text{Gray hair}$$
$$\searrow \text{Death}$$

If we control for age, then the observed association between gray hair and death will disappear. Thus, age is a confounder in this relationship. Confounding can then be controlled for at the analysis stage, provided that confounding was anticipated and the requisite information was gathered. In this way, we can examine if the association we are interested in still appears or if its strength has been modified. If we fail to collect this data, then we cannot assess the potential role of confounding.

Conclusions

Clinical practice used to be based on clinical experience and clinical opinion. Although these are still relevant, decisions regarding a patient's health problems and how to treat them are increasingly based on scientific evidence. It is important that one understands various types of study design and develops ability to critically appraise the scientific literature. In turn, the ability to distinguish good from poor science leads to evidence-based care.

Acknowledgement

The idea of a chapter in evidence-based dentistry started between Amir Azarpazhooh and David Locker in 2008 when compiling a manual for teaching evidence-based dentistry to students in the Faculty of Dentistry, University of Toronto. David Locker passed away in April 2010. Much of this material stems from our several years of teaching in the Faculty of Dentistry, and Faculty of Medicine, University of Toronto, Toronto, Canada.

References

Allen, P.F., McMillan, A.S., Walshaw, D. (1999) Patient expectations of oral implant-retained prostheses in a UK dental hospital. *British Dental Journal,* 186, 80–84.

Al-Negrish, A.R. and Habahbeh, R. (2006) Flare up rate related to root canal treatment of asymptomatic pulpally necrotic central incisor teeth in patients attending a military hospital. *Journal of Dentistry,* 34, 635–640.

American Dental Association. (2008) *Policy on Evidence-Based Dentistry.* Chicago, IL.

Awad, M.A., Locker, D., Korner-Bitensky, N., *et al.* (2000) Measuring the effect of intra-oral implant rehabilitation on health-related quality of life in a randomized controlled clinical trial. *Journal of Dental Research,* 79, 1659–1663.

Beck, J.D. (1998) Risk revisited. *Community Dentistry and Oral Epidemiology,* 26, 220–225.

Block, M.S. (2011) Placement of implants into fresh molar sites: results of 35 cases. *Journal of Maxillofacial & Oral Surgery,* 69, 170–174.

Brown, H.K. and Poplove, M. (1965) The Brantford-Sarnia-Stratford fluoridation caries study: final survey, 1963. *Canadian journal of public health. Revue canadienne de santé publique,* 56, 319–324.

Campbell, D.T. (1957) Factors relevant to the validity of experiments in social settings. *Psychological bulletin,* 54, 297–312.

Canadian Task Force on the Periodic Health Examination. (1979) The periodic health examination. *Canadian Medical Association Journal,* 121, 1193–1254.

Canadian Task Force on Preventive Health Care. (1997) *Canadian Task Force Methodology, Levels of Evidence—Research Design Rating* [Online]. Ottawa, Canada: Health Canada. Available at http://www.ctfphc.org.

Centers for Disease Control. (1986) Comprehensive plan for epidemiologic surveillance. Atlanta, GA: Centers for Disease Control.

Centers for Disease Control and Prevention. (1982) A Cluster of Kaposi's Sarcoma and Pneumocystis carinii Pneumonia among Homosexual Male Residents of Los Angeles and range Counties, California. *Morbidity and Mortality Weekly Report,* 31, 305–307.

Centre for Evidence-based Medicine. (2011) Tools for each step of the EBM process. [online] Available at http://www.cebm.net/index.aspx?o=1023.

Fenner, F., Henderson, D., Arita, I., *et al.* (1988) *Smallpox and its eradication,* Geneva, World Health Organization.

Fletcher, R.W. and Fletcher, S.W. (2005) *Clinical Epidemiology: The Essentials,* Lippincott Williams & Wilkins, Baltimore MD, USA.

Grimes, D.A. and Schulz, K.F. (2002a) Bias and causal associations in observational research. *Lancet,* 359, 248–252.

Grimes, D.A. and Schulz, K.F. (2002b) Cohort studies: marching towards outcomes. *Lancet,* 359, 341–345.

Grimes, D.A. and Schulz, K.F. (2002c) Descriptive studies: what they can and cannot do. *Lancet,* 359, 145–149.

Grimes, D.A. and Schulz, K.F. (2002d) An overview of clinical research: the lay of the land. *Lancet,* 359, 57–61.

Health Canada. (2010) *Oral Health Statistics 2007–2009.* [online] available at http://www.hc-sc.gc.ca/hl-vs/pubs/oral-bucco/fact-fiche-oral-bucco-stat-eng.php. Ottawa.

Hicks, N. (2011) Evidence based thinking about health care. [online] available at http://www.medicine.ox.ac.uk/bandolier/band39/b39-9.html.

Higgins, J. and Green, S. (2006) *Cochrane Handbook for Systematic Reviews of Interventions. The Cochrane Library, Issue 4.* John Wiley & Sons, Ltd., Chichester, UK.

Hill, A.B. (1965) The Environment and Disease: Association or Causation? *Proceedings of the Royal Society of Medicine,* 58, 295–300.

Jordan, W. (1961) Pulmonary embolism. *Lancet,* ii, 1146–1147.

Last, J.M. (1988) *A dictionary of epidemiology,* Oxford University Press, New York, NY.

Lesaffre, E., Garcia Zattera, M.J., Redmond, C., *et al.* (2007) Reported methodological quality of split-mouth studies. *Journal of Clinical Periodontology,* 34, 756–761.

Lesaffre, E., Philstrom, B., Needleman, I., *et al.* (2009) The design and analysis of split-mouth studies: what statisticians and clinicians should know. *Statistics in Medicine,* 28, 3470–3482.

Leung, W.K., Chu, C.H., Mok, M.Y., *et al.* (2011) Periodontal Status of Adults With Systemic Sclerosis: Case-Control Study. *Journal of periodontology* (August).

Levin, K.A. (2005) Study design I. *Evidence-based Dentistry,* 6, 78–79.

Levin, K.A. (2006) Study design III: Cross-sectional studies. *Evidence-based dentistry,* 7, 24–25.

Lygidakis, N.A. and Oulis, K.I. (1999) A comparison of Fluroshield with Delton fissure sealant: four year results. *Pediatric Dentistry,* 21, 429–431.

Marinho, V.C., Higgins, J.P., Logan, S., *et al.* (2003a) Fluoride mouthrinses for preventing dental caries in children and adolescents. *The Cochrane Database of Systematic Reviews [electronic resource],* CD002284.

Marinho, V.C., Higgins, J.P., Logan, S., *et al.* (2003b) Topical fluoride (toothpastes, mouthrinses, gels or varnishes) for preventing dental caries in children and adolescents. *The Cochrane Database of Systematic Reviews [electronic resource],* CD002782.

Marinho, V.C., Higgins, J.P., Sheiham, A., *et al.* (2003c) Fluoride toothpastes for preventing dental caries in children and adolescents. *The Cochrane Database of Systematic Reviews [electronic resource],* CD002278.

Marinho, V.C., Higgins, J.P., Sheiham, A., *et al.* (2004a). Combinations of topical fluoride (toothpastes, mouthrinses, gels, varnishes) versus single topical fluoride for preventing dental caries in children and adolescents. *The Cochrane Database of Systematic Reviews [electronic resource],* CD002781.

Marinho, V.C., Higgins, J.P., Sheiham, A., *et al.* (2004b) One topical fluoride (toothpastes, or mouthrinses, or gels, or varnishes) versus another for preventing dental caries in children and adolescents. *The Cochrane Database of Systematic Reviews [electronic resource]*, CD002780.

Moher, D., Pham, B., Jones, A., *et al.* (1998) Does quality of reports of randomised trials affect estimates of intervention efficacy reported in meta-analyses? *Lancet*, 352, 609–613.

Patel, S., Ricucci, D., Durak, C., *et al.* (2010) Internal root resorption: a review. *Journal of Endodontics*, 36, 1107–1121.

Pitts, N. (2004) Understanding the jigsaw of evidence-based dentistry. 2. Dissemination of research results. *Evidence-Based Dentistry*, 5, 33–35.

Schulz, K.F., Chalmers, I., Hayes, R.J., *et al.* (1995) Empirical evidence of bias. Dimensions of methodological quality associated with estimates of treatment effects in controlled trials. *Journal of the American Medical Association*, 273, 408–412.

Schulz, K.F. and Grimes, D.A. (2002a) Case-control studies: research in reverse. *Lancet*, 359, 431–434.

Schulz, K.F. and Grimes, D.A. (2002b) Blinding in randomised trials: hiding who got what. *Lancet*, 359, 696–700.

Schulz, K.F. and Grimes, D.A. (2002c) Generation of allocation sequences in randomised trials: chance, not choice. *Lancet*, 359, 515–519.

Schwartz, S. (1994) The fallacy of the ecological fallacy: the potential misuse of a concept and the consequences. *American Journal of Public Health*, 84, 819–824.

Seppa, L., Leppanen, T., and Hausen, H. (1995) Fluoride varnish versus acidulated phosphate fluoride gel: a 3-year clinical trial. *Caries Research*, 29, 327–330.

Tang, L., Lund, J.P., Tache, R., *et al.* (1997) A within-subject comparison of mandibular long-bar and hybrid implant-supported prostheses: psychometric evaluation and patient preference. *Journal of Dental Research*, 76, 1675–1683.

Torabinejad, M. and Turman, M. (2011) Revitalization of tooth with necrotic pulp and open apex by using platelet-rich plasma: a case report. *Journal of Endodontics*, 37, 265–268.

U.S. Department of Health and Human Services, Office of Workforce and Career Development, Career Development Division. (2006) *Principles of Epidemiology in Public Health Practice*, Public Health Foundation, Atlanta, GA.

U.S. Preventive Services Task Force. (2008) *Grade Definitions*. [online] available at http://www.uspreventiveservicestaskforce.org/uspstf/grades.htm [Online].

Wood, L., Egger, M., Gluud, L.L., *et al.* (2008) Empirical evidence of bias in treatment effect estimates in controlled trials with different interventions and outcomes: meta-epidemiological study. *British Medical Journal*, 336, 601–605.

6

The role of diet in the prevention of dental diseases

Paula Moynihan

Introduction

Despite an increased awareness of the importance of oral health and advances made in the use of fluoride as a preventive measure, the prevalence of dental caries remains unacceptably high in many industrialized countries. Levels of dental caries have increased in some developing countries where the intake of sugars has increased due to nutrition transition toward a more 'westernized diet.' There is strong evidence from epidemiological studies for an association between the amount and frequency of free sugars intake and dental caries. Studies of human populations show that diets that are rich in complex carbohydrates from starchy staple foods and diets that are high in fresh fruit are associated with low levels of dental caries. The important role that fluoride plays in the prevention of dental caries is indisputable, however exposure to fluoride through drinking water and increased used of fluoride-containing dentifrice has not eliminated dental caries, and furthermore many countries do not have access to fluoridated water and/or dental hygiene products.

Current global guidelines on the intake of free sugars recommend that the intake of free sugars should not exceed 10% of energy intake because when consumption of free sugars is 15–20 kg/person per year (which equates to 6–10% energy intake), the level of dental caries observed is low. Available evidence on the association between frequency of consumption of sugars and dental caries suggests that when the frequency of consumption of sugar-containing foods is limited to less that four times per day caries development is low.

Dental diseases in which diet plays an etiological role include enamel developmental defects, dental caries, tooth wear, and periodontal disease. The main cause of tooth loss is dental caries, and in adults the main cause of tooth loss is periodontal disease. The main focus of this chapter is diet and dental caries, but other conditions relevant to diet will be considered in brief.

The impact of dental diseases on well being

Dental disease is associated with a low mortality, but nonetheless dental disease impacts self esteem, social integration into society, and the ability to speak and eat. Oral disease is associated with impaired social functioning in both children and adults (Chen *et al.* 1997) and causes considerable pain and anxiety (Kelly *et al.* 2000) especially in societies with limited access to treatment. Surveys in many countries including Thailand, China, and Madagascar (Petersen *et al.* 1991; Minguan *et al.* 2000) have shown a high percentage of children who report dental pain and suffer tooth extractions.

Dental caries and periodontal disease result in tooth loss, which reduces enjoyment of eating and the confidence to socialize and in some vulnerable groups such as the very old, is associated with increased risk of under nutrition (Lamy *et al.* 1999; *Dion et al.* 2007; *De marchi et al.* 2008). The edentulous have been shown to have a diet that is lower in fruits, vegetables, and fiber and higher in saturated fat compared with the dentate, though a causal relationship has not been established. Nonetheless, the edentulous are a group that would potentially benefit from dietary advice.

Comprehensive Preventive Dentistry, First Edition. Edited by Hardy Limeback.
© 2012 John Wiley & Sons, Ltd. Published 2012 by John Wiley & Sons, Ltd.

The systemic effect of nutrition on the teeth

Nutritional status affects the teeth during the pre-eruptive stage. Deficiencies of vitamin D, vitamin A, and protein energy malnutrition (PEM) have been associated with enamel hypoplasia, a condition in which the mineralization process is disrupted and manifests as pits and fissures and larger areas deficient in enamel on the enamel surface that become stained on eruption. Teeth with hypoplasia of enamel are more susceptible to dental caries (Rugg-Gunn 1993).

Nutrient deficiencies including protein deficiency and vitamin A deficiency are associated with salivary gland atrophy. This will result in reduced saliva flow and may impact on the buffering capacity of saliva, which will reduce the ability of saliva to neutralize plaque acids. Protein deficiency and deficiencies of micronutrients, such as some vitamins, zinc, and iron, can influence the amount and composition of saliva reducing the protective effects of saliva in the mouth (Navia 1996). Malnutrition may therefore increase the susceptibility to dental caries when sugars are available in the diet. In developing countries where malnutrition exists, the level of dental caries observed is higher than expected for the level of sugar exposure (based on observations from developed countries). However, in the absence of dietary sugars, malnutrition is not associated with dental caries.

Periodontal disease

For many years texts have claimed that, with the exception of vitamin C deficiency-related scurvy, nutrition shows little association with periodontal disease. The main overriding factor in the etiology of periodontal disease is the presence of plaque, and prevention measures focus on oral hygiene. In recognition of the etiological role of plaque, early research focused on the impact of diet on plaque volume and showed that a high sucrose intake is associated with increased plaque volume due to the production of extracellular glucans. Human intervention studies have shown higher plaque volumes and increased gingivitis with high sucrose diets compared with low sucrose diets (Scheinen *et al.* 1976; Sidi and Ashley 1984). However, the maximum reduction in sugar in the diet that is practical would not prevent the development of gingivitis (Gaengler *et al.* 1986).

Advice on diet and nutrition are not routinely part of the management or prevention of periodontal disease. However, with an increased understanding of the disease at the cellular level coupled with improved means of assessing nutritional status, emerging evidence suggests a significant role of diet in the etiology of periodontitis

and strong associations between systemic inflammatory diet-related conditions and periodontal disease.

Periodontal disease progresses more rapidly in undernourished populations and the important role of nutrition in immune function is the probable explanation of this observation (Enwonwu 1995).

Analysis of data from the National Health and Nutrition Examination Survey (NHANES) III in the USA has shown an inverse relationship between intake of calcium and periodontitis in adults. The risk of periodontitis in women increased by 27% and 54% when the intake of calcium fell below 800 mg and 499 mg per day, respectively (Nishida *et al.* 2000). Requirements for folate are high in tissues that have a high cellular turnover rate, such as the gingival epithelium, and an independent association between low blood folate status and risk of periodontitis has recently been reported (Yu *et al.* 2007). The important roles of vitamin C in the tissues of the periodontium are well established, and recent studies support an association between low serum vitamin C status and periodontitis. This reflects vitamin C's important role in collagen formation and the structural integrity of the periodontal ligament, blood vessel walls, and its role in the formation of the alveolar bone matrix. However, vitamin C is also important for optimum immune function and is a powerful antioxidant. Dietary antioxidants are thought to play an important role in protecting the gingival from oxidative damage from free radicals. Several studies show that antioxidant status is compromised in periodontitis, and data from NHANES III have shown an inverse relationship between serum total antioxidant capacity and periodontitis (Chapple *et al.* 2007). Fruits, vegetables, and whole grain foods are the major sources of antioxidants in the diet and may offer protection against periodontal inflammation. However, the impact of dietary modification to improve antioxidant status on the progression of periodontitis remains to be determined. Diet plays a key role in the etiology of obesity and of diabetes, and both of these conditions are associated with increased risk of periodontitis. Therefore, lifestyle interventions to address being overweight and obesity may also positively impact periodontal health.

The intraoral effect of diet on the teeth

Teeth are most susceptible to dental caries soon after they erupt; therefore, the peak ages for dental caries are 2–5 years for the deciduous dentition and early adolescence for the permanent dentition. In developed countries, there is a trend for older adults now to retain their teeth for longer, however, periodontal recession may lead to exposure of the root surfaces and being relatively less mineralized than the tooth crowns, roots are susceptible to root caries.

Dietary sugars and dental caries

Sugars are undoubtedly the most important dietary factor in the development of dental caries. In this chapter the term 'sugars' refers to all mono- and disaccharides; the term 'sugar' only refers to sucrose; the term 'free sugars' refers to all mono- and disaccharides added to foods by the manufacturer, cook, or consumer, plus sugars naturally present in honey, fruit juices, and syrups; and the term 'fermentable carbohydrate' refers to free sugars, glucose polymers, fermentable oligosaccharides, and highly refined starches.

Population studies

Sugar intake and levels of dental caries can be compared country by country. Sreebny (1982) correlated the dental caries experience of primary dentition (dmft) of 5- and 6-year-old children and the permanent dentition (DMFT) of 12-year-old children with sugar supplies data of 23 and 47 countries, respectively. A correlation of borderline significance (+0.31) was observed for deciduous dentition, and a strong positive and highly significant correlation was found for the permanent dentition (+0.72, p<0.0005). For the 21 countries where sugars availability was less than 50 g/day, the associated DMFT was below 3, thus showing that low sugar availability is associated with low levels of caries. For seven countries with very high sugar availability (43.8 kg per person per year, that is 120 g/day), the DMFT was greater than 5. The data showed that 52% of the variation in caries levels could be explained by the per capita availability of sugar.

Woodward and Walker (1994) matched per capita sugar availability data with mean DMFT values for 12-year-old children using data from 90 countries. Overall there was a trend for DMFT to increase with increasing sugar availability, with sugar availability accounting for 28% of variation in dental caries levels, a substantial amount considering the crudeness of the analysis (that is, different examiners and accuracy of sugar supply data regarding actual consumption by 12-year-olds; the fact that dental data are not necessarily based on representative samples; and the level of confounding factors, such as fluoride exposure and frequency of sugar intake). For industrialized countries the correlation was not significant. This is probably due to the fact that in industrialized countries where people are exposed to high levels of sugars, changing sugars by a few kilograms per year does not affect the caries attack (Nadanovsky 1994). It has also been suggested that the relationship between sugars consumption and dental caries is sigmoid in nature; at very high intakes the graph flattens. Therefore, those countries with high intakes that fall on the flattened part of the curve, the relationship between per capita sugar availability and levels of dental caries is not apparent (Sheiham 2001).

The data from the analysis of Woodward and Walker (1994) show that 23 of the 26 countries with sugars availability below 50 g/d had a mean DMFT for 12-year-old children of below 3, whereas only half of the countries with sugar availability above this level had achieved DMFT >3.

Ruxton *et al.* (1999) devised a simple scatter plot based on data from the papers by Sreebny (1982) and Woodwood and Walker (1994) of changes in sugars supply against changes in mean DMFT at age 12 years in 67 countries. DMFT had dropped in 18 countries that had declines in sugar supply. In 25 countries DMFT had declined despite increases in sugar supply. In three countries sugar declined and DMFT increased. In 18 countries caries levels increased and sugar supply increased. Overall the relationship between sugar and dental caries levels was supported by 36 countries and not supported by 28.

The weaker association between sugar availability and dental caries in developed countries is in part accounted for by the fact that many sugars other than sucrose are contributing to total sugars intake in modern society. In the USA there is widespread use of high fructose corn syrup, and in other industrialized countries the use of glucose polymers and fruit juice concentrates is common.

There are a number of population studies that have shown a marked change in the incidence and or prevalence of dental caries following a reduction in sugars consumption. Good examples of this are provided by studies that measured both sugars availability and levels of dental caries before, during, and after World War II during which the intake of sugars was restricted due to food shortages.

Schulerud (1950) examined oral health data from Norwegian studies of children, aged 3 to 12 years before, during, and following World War II. The data showed a reduction in the proportion of decayed teeth during the war of approximately 50% for 6- and 7-year-old children. Norwegian National Survey data show that during World War II, the intake of sucrose was in the region of 28 g per person day (10.4 kg per person per year).

The data reported by Toverud (1957) show that changes in the intake of sugar before, during, and following World War II in Scandinavia were mirrored by changes in caries prevalence and the annual incidence of dental caries. This study reported that in Norway sugar availability fell to only 36–42 g/day (approximately 7.5–9% total energy), and annual caries incidence more than halved. Similar reductions in dental caries were found for Denmark and Finland, but for all countries, dental caries increased markedly again following the sharp rise in sugar in post-war diets. Similarly, a series of reports based on Japanese data (Takahashi 1961; Takeuchi 1962) show a close correlation (r = +0.7−+0.8) between annual caries incidence in the first permanent molars and annual sugar availability before, during, and after World War II. In these studies it was noted that when annual sugar consumption was less that 10 kg/year, which is equivalent to 40 g/day, caries incidence was very low.

The studies relating to the World War II sugar restrictions were conducted before widespread use of fluoride, so one must question whether sugars reduction would have such an impact if the protection offered by fluoride were available. However, Weaver (1950) observed a reduction in dental caries between 1943 and 1949 in areas of North England with both optimum and low water-fluoride concentrations with caries levels in the fluoridated area decreasing by approximately 50% following a reduction in sugars intake. This suggests that maximum caries prevention is achieved when populations are exposed to fluoride in addition to restricting intake of sugars.

Evidence for an association between dental caries and sugars intake is also provided by observational studies of dental caries levels in populations before and after an increase in sugar consumption. Populations that move from a traditional diet consistently low in sugar to a more 'westernized diet' containing increased amounts of sugars experience a marked increase in the prevalence of dental caries. Examples of this trend include the Alaskan Inuit (Bang and Kristoffersen 1972), many African populations (MacGregor 1963; Emslie 1966; Sheiham 1967; Olsson 1979), and inhabitants of the Island of Tristan da Cunha (Fisher 1968). More recently Jamel et al. (2004) reported on the impact of the UN sanctions in Iraq on sugars availability and levels of dental caries in children in Iraq. The UN sanctions in Iraq had a marked impact on sugar intake with per capita sugar availability falling from 50 kg to 12 kg per person per year. In a repeat dental survey of Iraqi children before and following the UN sanctions, the average DMFT of 6- to 7-year-old children fell from 4.8 to 2.3; in 11- to 12-year-old children, DMFT fell from 4.2 to 1.6; and in the 14- to 15-year-old age group, DMFT fell from 5.3 to 1.9. Before the sanctions, 34.2% of 6- to 7-year-old children, 31.9% of 11- to 12-year-old children, and 28.1% of 14- to 15-year-old children were caries free whereas following the sugar restriction 56.8%, 52%, and 48.9% were caries free, respectively.

Groups of people with habitually high consumption of sugars have relatively high levels of caries compared with the population average. Examples include children requiring long-term sugared medicines (before sugar-free formulations were widely available) and confectionery industry workers (Anaise 1978; Roberts 1979; Katayama et al. 1979; Masalin et al. 1990). On the other hand, a lower than average caries experience has been reported in population groups that habitually consume little sugars. Examples include children living in institutions that adhered to strict dietary regimens, and children with Hereditary Fructose Intolerance who have to consume a sucrose- and fructose-free diet.

Hopewood House (Harris 1963) in Australia was a home for children aged up to 12 years who were examined in repeated dental and dietary surveys between 1947 and 1962. The diet of the children was closely supervised and contained minimal sugar up to the age of 12. After the age of 12 children moved out of the home although they maintained links with the home. Up to the age of 12, as many as 46% of the children were caries free compared with 1% in state schools. However, after the children left the home, the rate of caries was similar to that of the children in state schools.

Newbrun et al. (1980) conducted a case-control study in adults with hereditary fructose intolerance (HFI) in which the level of dental caries was compared between participants with HFI who followed a low-sucrose diet and controls on a normal sucrose-containing diet. Mean daily sugar intake was 48.2 g/day in control subjects and 2.5 g/day in HFI participants. Mean DMFT was 14.3 in controls compared with 2.1 in those with HFI. Mean DMFS was 36.1 in controls and 3.3 in those with HFI.

A weakness of the data from observations of populations is that changes in intake of sugars are often associated with changes in the intake of other carbohydrates such as refined flour, and some argue therefore that changes in levels of dental caries cannot be solely attributed to increases in sugars intake. However, in HFI, intake of starchy carbohydrate is not limited yet caries remains low, thus indicating that the main contributor to development of caries is indeed dietary sugars.

Human intervention studies

Dietary intervention studies that measure the impact on caries development of modifying the intake of dietary sugars are rare probably due to the difficulty in prescribing a diet for the long period of time required to measure a change in caries development (usually at least 18 months). Two oft-quoted intervention studies are the Vipeholm Study (Gustafsson et al. 1954), which was conducted in a hospital for patients with mental impairments shortly after World War II, and the Turku Sugar Studies (Sheinin et al. 1976), conducted in Finland in the early 1970s. Both studies were conducted on highly selected groups of people before the widespread use of fluoride and would not be possible to repeat today due to more stringent ethical codes of practice. Nonetheless the findings are still relevant today.

The Vipeholm study investigated the effect of consuming sugary foods of varying stickiness and at different frequencies on the caries increment. It was found that sugars, even when consumed in large amounts, had little effect on caries increment if consumed up to a maximum of four times a day at mealtimes only. However, increased frequency of consumption of sugar between meals was associated with a marked increase in dental caries. It was also found that the increase in dental caries activity disappears on withdrawal of sugars. The study demonstrates the important effect of frequency of sugars consumption and the significance of mealtime consumption (that is, consumption when salivary flow rate is increased and buffering capacity is therefore increased).

The Turku Study evaluated the effect of almost total substitution of sucrose in the normal Finnish diet with either fructose or xylitol on caries development. Three groups of participants (n = 125 in total) aged 12–53 years, with the majority in their twenties, consumed a diet containing either sucrose, fructose, or the non-sugar sweetener xylitol for a period of 25 months. Dental caries increment was measured at 6-month periods. Foods were specially manufactured for the fructose and xylitol groups. Subjects were asked to avoid sweet fruits such as dried fruits, as sugars in these foods could not be substituted. An 85% reduction in dental caries was observed in the xylitol group (who had removed sugar from their diet) compared with the sucrose group, indicating that almost total removal of sugars from the diet resulted in a markedly lower development of caries.

In a more recent dietary study by Rodrigues et al. (1999), the development of dental caries was compared between nursery school children, initially aged 3 years, who were attending nursery schools that had introduced guidelines on reducing added sugars intake, with children attending nurseries that had not adopted the sugars guidelines. The children attending nurseries that had adopted dietary guidelines consumed less than 10% energy intake as added sugars (22.9 g per day: approximately 33 g equates to 10% energy for this age group). The children attending nurseries that had not adopted the guidelines consumed on average 53 g/day. Children with an intake of sugars >10% energy intake had three times the risk of dental caries.

Observational studies of sugars and dental caries

Many studies exist where the intake of sugars has been compared with the level of dental caries at one point in time (that is, a cross-sectional design). However, dental caries develops over time, and therefore simultaneous measurements of dental caries levels and sugars intake may not provide a true reflection of the role of diet in the development of caries. It is the diet several years earlier that is responsible for current caries levels. Cross-sectional studies therefore provide much weaker evidence for the role of diet in the development of dental caries; data from studies of this design should be interpreted with caution. In a recent systematic analysis of published data on the association between amount of sugars intake and dental caries, it was found that of the 22 studies of cross-sectional design identified, 13 studies found a significant association between sugars and caries, and 8 studies did not (Moynihan and Kelly, 2012). In a recent study, Masson et al. (2010) investigated the strength of the association between sugars intake and treatment for dental decay in Scottish children aged 3–17 years. Intake of free sugars increased the risk of having had treatment for decay: adjusted OR 1.84 for the highest tertile of NMES intake (>20% EI) versus the lowest tertile (<14.8%).

It has been suggested that the reasons why many older studies failed to show a relationship between sugars intake and development of dental caries is because many of these were of poor methodological design (for example, cross sectional), used unsuitable dietary methodologies, and were underpowered (Marthaler 1990). Correlations between individuals' sugars consumption and dental caries increments may be weak due to the limited range of sugars intake in the study population, that is, variation in sugars intake within populations is too low to show an effect on caries occurrence. If all people within a population are exposed to the disease risk factor, the relationship between the risk factor and the disease will not be apparent (Rose 1993). There is more between country variation in intake of sugars, which is why a stronger association between sugar availability and dental caries levels is found from analysis of worldwide data.

For the study of diet and dental caries, a longitudinal design in which sugars consumption is related to dental caries increment is more appropriate and therefore provides stronger evidence. Because this design requires repeated oral examinations, it is a more costly and time consuming and is therefore relatively rare. However, the large majority of studies relating amount of sugars intake to caries increment have reported a significant positive association. Seven out of eight longitudinal studies were identified (Moynihan and Kelly, 2012).

In a study of Argentinean children (Battellino et al. 1997), 1-year caries incidence was significantly correlated with intake of sucrose (r=0.4). MacKeown et al. (2000) in a cohort study of South African children initially aged

1 year found that change in dmfs and prevalence of dental caries between the ages of 1 and 5 years was not significantly associated with added sugars intake at age 1 year. In a larger cross-sectional analysis of dmft and caries prevalence at age 5, a significant relationship between dental caries and added sugars intake was reported.

Karjalainen *et al.* (2001) showed that the sucrose intake of Finnish children that developed dental caries between the ages of 3 and 6 years was significantly higher than children that remained caries free. The mean sucrose intake of those that developed caries at age 6 was 33.4 g/day (10.7% of energy intake) compared with 26.5 g (8.8% energy intake). Thus, those that remained caries free consumed <10% energy intake as sugars.

Ruottinen *et al.* (2004) compared DMFT at age 10 years between the top and bottom 5% of sugars consumers from birth. The mean sucrose intake of the high sucrose consumers was 48.4 g/day, and for the low sucrose consumers it was 22.5 g/day. The sugar consumption of the high group exceeded 10% of energy intake after 13 months of age. In the low sugar group, intake of sugar did not exceed 7% of energy intake at any age. The mean DMFT at age 10 was 1.4 in the high group compared with 0.5 in the low group.

In study of more than 400 children aged 11–12 years old from England (Rugg-Gunn *et al.* 1984), a low but highly significant, correlation between caries increment over 2 years and amount of total sugars in the diet was observed. The 31 children who consumed the most dietary sugars (131 g/day) developed 56% more caries than the 31 children with the lowest sugars consumption (<78g/day). The study was conducted in a low fluoride area, but fluoride toothpaste was used and the relationship between sugars and dental caries remained after controlling for brushing habits.

Stecksen-Blicks and Gustaffson (1986) investigated the relationship between intake of dietary sugar and caries increment over 1 year in Swedish children aged 8 and 13 years. Children who developed fewer carious surfaces over the study period had a significantly lower intake of dietary sugars (52.4 g) compared with those who developed three or more carious lesions (76.9g). Though the level of fluoride in water was low, it is likely that most children would have used fluoride toothpaste.

The Michigan Study (Burt *et al.* 1988; Burt and Szpuner 1994) was carried out in the USA between 1982 and 1985 in a non-fluoridated area and investigated the relationship between total sugars intake and dental caries increment over 3 years in children initially aged 10–15 years. This study also found a weak but significant relationship between the amount of dietary sugars and dental caries increment. Children who consumed a higher proportion of their total dietary energy as sugars

had a higher caries increment for approximal caries, though there was no significant association between sugars intake and pit and fissure caries. However, intake of sugars was generally high for all subjects in this study with only 20 out of 499 children consuming less than 75 g/day, and the average intake of the lowest quartile of consumption being 109 g/day or 23.4% of energy intake. Burt and Szpunar (1994) recognized that, in the Michigan Study, the reason for the low relative risk of caries development in the high sugars consumers was that small variances were found both for caries increment and intake of sugars.

A number of studies have investigated the association between consumption of sugars-rich foods (as opposed to total amount of sugars intake) and caries development. In a group of Swedish children, Sundin *et al.* (1992) found a strong correlation between caries increment and the consumption of sweets. The relationship was strongest for those with poor compared with good oral hygiene. Lachapelle-Harvey and Sevigny (1985) compared the diets of 11-year-old Canadian children with caries development over a 20-month period. Consumption of chocolate or sugared chewing gum in-between meals and consumption of iced cakes at meal times were associated with caries development. Grindefjord *et al.* (1996) observed a significant relationship between frequent consumption of sugary foods and drinks and caries increment in a cohort of young Swedish children between the ages of 1 and 3.5 years.

Which is more important—frequency of sugars consumption or the amount of sugars consumed?

In the past there has been some debate as to whether it is the total amount of sugars consumed or the frequency with which they are consumed that is more strongly related to the development of dental caries. The evidence discussed so far clearly shows an association between total amount of sugars consumed and dental caries. However, the two variables are highly correlated so that when the frequency of consumption increases so does the total amount consumed (World Health Organization 1990). Likewise a reduction in frequency in intake of sugars should result in a reduction in the total amount of sugars consumed.

The findings of animal experiments have added to the understanding of the importance of frequency of intake. As in animal studies, the frequency of consumption of sugars can be altered while keeping the amount constant. Such studies showed that dental caries experience increases with the increasing frequency of intake of sugars when the amount of sugars eaten remains the same (Konig *et al.* 1968). It has also been shown in animal studies that fewer dental caries develop when the time between meals is increased (Firestone *et al.* 1984). Animal studies have also been used to investigate the relationship between amount of sugars consumed and the development of dental caries. Mikx *et al.* (1975) found a significant relationship between the sugar concentration of the diet fed to rats and the development of dental caries. Hefti and Schmid (1979) found that dental caries severity increased with increasing sugars concentrations up to 40%.

Human epidemiological studies have also indicated that the frequency of sugars intake is associated with development of dental caries (Holbrook *et al.* 1989; Holbrook *et al.* 1995). The aforementioned Vipeholm study (Gustafsson *et al.* 1954) showed that caries development was low when sugars were consumed up to 4 times a day at mealtimes. The studies of Holbrook *et al.* (1989; 1995) of children in Iceland also suggest that the safe threshold for frequency of consumption of sugars is 4 times a day: children with a frequency of sugars intake of 4 or more per day or more than 3 snacks per day had significantly increased caries scores. For children that developed ≥3 carious lesions, the mean frequency of sugar intake was 5.1 times per day compared with 2.1 times a day for children who developed ≤3 carious lesions. Data from a longitudinal study of preschool children in the UK showed that development of caries was higher in children who consumed more than 4 sweetened snacks or drinks per day compared with children who consumed 1 of these items a day or less (Holt *et al.* 1982).

The findings of human epidemiological studies therefore suggest that sugars intake should be limited to no more than 4 intakes per day. Many more studies have investigated the relationship between the frequency of sugars intake than have investigated the relationship between amount of sugars intake and caries; this is primarily because assessing frequency of intake is relatively straightforward through the use of a food frequency questionnaire. However, to accurately assess the total amount (weight) of sugars consumed, a prospective method of dietary analysis such as a food diary is required as is the use of food compositional tables to derive the absolute amount of sugars in all foods consumed. Fewer studies have undertaken this more comprehensive approach to dietary assessment, however, unless both variables have been measured in the same population, the relative importance of frequency and amount cannot be judged.

Several human epidemiological studies show amount of sugars intake to be more important that frequency (Rugg-Gunn *et al.* 1984; Burt *et al.* 1988; Szpuner *et al.* 1995). Kleemola-Kujala and Räsänen (1982) found that dental caries increased with increasing amount of sugars consumption only when oral hygiene was poor. Jamel *et al.* (1996), in a study of young adults in Iraq, found that the number of cups of tea consumed and the amount of sugar added to tea were positively related to the level of dental caries, thus indicating that both the frequency and the amount of sugar intake are associated with caries development. Evidence shows a strong correlation between the amount and frequency of sugars consumption. In an analysis of dietary data from more than 400 11–12 year-old children in the north of England, Rugg-Gunn *et al.* (1984) found a strong and highly significant correlation between frequency of intake of sugars-rich foods and total weight consumed. Likewise, Cleaton-Jones *et al.* (1984) reported significant associations between frequency and amount of sugar intake in a number of South African ethnic groups. In the aforementioned study of Rodrigues *et al.* (1999), a direct relationship between frequency and amount of sugar consumption was found in nursery school children in Brazil. Those with a frequency of sugars intake of 4–5 times per day were 6 times more likely to develop high caries levels over 1 year compared with children with the lowest frequency of sugars intake. A significant association between the frequency and amount of sugared drink consumption has also been reported for American children (Ismail *et al.* 1984). It was found that both increased frequency and amount of sugared drinks consumption were associated with higher caries risk. Those who consumed three sugared drinks per day had more than twice the risk of developing dental caries than those that consumed sugared drinks no more than 1 per day. Overall, the evidence shows that both the amount of sugars consumed and the frequency with which sugars are consumed are related to the development of dental caries. The evidence shows that these two variables are highly associated and so efforts to control one impact on the other. At a population level it is important to set a goal in terms of amount of sugars because this will drive health promotion and provide a standard against which the diet of populations and the outcomes of health promotion initiatives may be judged. However, at the level of the individual, when providing chairside advice, it is much easier to set goals in terms of frequency because it is more straightforward for the patient to conceptualize.

Does the cariogenicity of different types of sugar differ?

Nowadays diets contain many different sugars including sucrose, glucose, lactose, fructose, glucose syrups, high fructose corn syrups, and other carbohydrates including synthetic oligosaccharides and highly processed starches that are fermentable in the mouth. The oral bacteria can metabolise mono- and disaccharides to produce acid, and salivary amylase can break down other refined starches to glucose and maltose, which can subsequently be metabolized to produce acids. All mono- and disaccharides are cariogenic, and some evidence suggests that sucrose in particular is cariogenic. Sucrose is the substrate for extracellular glucan synthesis, and clinical studies show that glucan formation increases the porosity of plaque, which permits deeper penetration of dietary sugars and increased acid production adjacent to the tooth surface (Zero 2004). Evidence also shows that lactose is less cariogenic compared with other mono and disaccharides (Jenkins and Ferguson 1966). However, the aforementioned Turku study (Scheinin *et al.* 1976) showed no difference in caries development between subjects on diets sweetened with sucrose compared with fructose. Substituting one mono- or disaccharide for another is unlikely to have a marked effect on dental caries levels.

There is less information available on the relative cariogenicity of other fermentable carbohydrates. Invert sugar when substituted for sucrose has been shown to cause approximately 20% fewer caries to develop (Frostell *et al.* 1991). Glucose polymers (maltodextrins and glucose syrups) are increasing being used in diets, and therefore, it is important to consider the cariogenic potential of these carbohydrates. Glucose polymers comprise a mixture of short-chain saccharides and alpha-limit dextrins. The limited available data from animal studies, plaque pH studies, and studies *in vitro* indicate glucose polymers are cariogenic. The use of synthetic non-digestible oligosaccharides (prebiotics) is also increasing. Plaque pH studies and experiments *in vitro* suggest that isomaltooligosaccharides and glucooligosaccharides are not as cariogenic as sugars such as sucrose (Roberts *et al.* 1980; Koga *et al.* 1988; Ooshima *et al.* 1998), but fructooligosaccharides, which are more widely available in foods, are as cariogenic as sucrose (Hartmink *et al.* 1995).

Does reducing sugars intake remain important when a population is exposed to fluoride?

Systemically ingested fluoride can become incorporated into the developing teeth up to the age of around 6 years, increasing the resistance of the teeth, once erupted, to acid attack. However, the main action of fluoride is a lifelong topical protection at the enamel surface after eruption. Fluoride makes the teeth more resistant to acid-induced demineralization and promotes remineralization following a plaque acid challenge. In the oral cavity, fluoride replaces the hydroxyl groups in hydroxyapatite to form fluoroapatite, which is more resistant to demineralization. Remineralization of enamel in the presence of fluoride results in the porous lesion being remineralized with fluoroapatite rather than hydroxylapatite. The reader is referred to the chapter on fluoride in this book for an in-depth analysis of how fluoride protects teeth from a cariogenic diet.

More than 800 controlled trials of the effect of fluoride on dental caries have been conducted and show that fluoride is the most effective preventive agent against caries (Murray 1986). Exposure to fluoride largely accounts for the decline in dental caries that has been observed in developed countries over the past 4 decades. Fluoride reduces dental caries in children by up to 40%; however, it does not eliminate dental caries nor eradicate the cause of caries—the high and frequent consumption of sugars (Moynihan and Petersen 2004).

Earlier studies of the association between intake of dietary sugars and dental caries were conducted before there was widespread use of fluoride. More recent studies of the relationship between sugars and dental caries are confounded by the presence of fluoride but show that a relationship between sugars intake and caries still exists in the presence of fluoride. In many studies of the relationship between intake of dietary sugars and dental caries levels in children, the relationships between sugars intake and development of dental caries remains after controlling for oral hygiene and fluoride exposure (Holt *et al.* 1991; Beighton *et al.* 1996). The aforementioned study of Weaver (1950) indicated that adequate exposure to fluoride did not totally override the effect of sugars in the diet. Marthaler (1990) reviewed the changes in the prevalence of dental caries and concluded that, even when preventive measures such as use of fluoride are employed, a relationship between sugars intake and caries still exists and that sugars continue to be the main threat to dental health despite progress made using fluorides. It is likely that, in industrialized countries where there is adequate exposure to fluoride, a further reduction in the prevalence and severity of dental caries will not be achieved without a reduction in free sugars intake.

A comprehensive review of the literature, which included 36 studies that met quality-related inclusion criteria (Burt and Pai 2001), addressed this question: "In the modern age of extensive fluoride exposure, do individuals with a high level of sugars intake, experience greater caries severity relative to those with a lower level of intake?" No paper failed to find a relationship between sugars intake and caries. The conclusions of the systematic review follow: (1) where there is good exposure to fluoride, sugars consumption is a moderate risk factor for caries in most people; (2) sugars consumption is likely to be a more powerful indicator for risk of caries in persons who do not have regular exposure to fluoride; and (3) with widespread use of fluoride, sugars consumption still has a role to play in the prevention of caries, but this role is not as strong as it is without exposure to fluoride.

It should be noted that although exposure to fluoride will go a long way to protect against the detrimental impact of sugars on dental health, it will not protect against the potential wider health implications of a high sugars intake. An energy dense diet that is high in fats and/or sugars, and a high intake of sugared drinks have also been associated with being overweight and obesity (WHO 2003; James and Kerr 2005; Francis et al. 2009).

Does starch cause dental caries?

Starch is a complex polymer of glucose that is heterogeneous in nature and is present in an array of foods both desirable and less desirable in terms of health. Starch varies in botanical origin. It may be highly refined or consumed in its natural state. It is sometimes consumed raw for example in fruits and vegetables but is predominantly consumed in a cooked form. All of these factors should be considered when assessing the potential cariogenicity of starch-containing foods. Current dietary guidelines promote the increased consumption of starchy staple foods, for example bread, cereals, rice, and potatoes. It is recommended that 50–70% of energy intake should be provided by starch-rich carbohydrates. It is important therefore to consider the impact of consumption of starches on dental health.

Oral bacteria cannot metabolize starch to acids, therefore, in order to contribute to the caries process, cooked and processed starches have to be hydrolyzed to glucose, maltose, or maltotriose by salivary amylase in order to be metabolized to acid.

Plaque pH studies measure the change in pH in the dental plaque on consuming a food or drink. Some plaque pH studies use an indwelling plaque electrode, which has the tendency to give an all or nothing response to any carbohydrate. The indwelling electrode technique is therefore not appropriate for discriminating the acidogenic potential between carbohydrates (Edgar 1985). Studies using this method have shown starch-containing foods (for example, white bread) can depress plaque pH below 5.5. Plaque pH studies may also employ the 'harvesting method' where plaque is removed from all areas of the mouth and pH is subsequently measured. This method is more able to discriminate between the acidogenic potential of different carbohydrates. Studies using the harvesting method have shown that starch-

containing foods are less acidogenic compared with sucrose or sucrose-rich foods. Foods high in starch have been shown to produce as much acid as high-sucrose products (Lingström et al. 2000). Pollard et al. (1995) showed that breakfast cereals, bread, rice, and pasta reduced plaque pH but not below critical pH and significantly less so than sucrose. However, plaque pH studies measure acidogenic potential of a food (that is, acid production on ingestion which is used as a proxy for caries development). A weakness of this type of study is that it takes no account of the caries protective factors found in some starch-containing food, or account for the effect of foods on stimulation of salivary flow.

Animal studies have enabled the effect on caries of defined types, frequencies, and amounts of carbohydrates to be studied. In a review of evidence for the role of starch in caries development from animal studies it was concluded that raw starch is of low cariogenicity, cooked starch may cause dental caries but only about half the amount caused by sucrose, and mixtures of starch and sucrose are more cariogenic than starch alone, and the level of caries that develops is related to the sucrose concentration in the mix (Rugg-Gunn 1993). Caution needs to be applied when extrapolating the results of animal studies to humans due to differences in tooth morphology, plaque bacterial ecology, salivary flow and composition, and the form in which the diet is provided (usually powdered form in animal experiments).

Populations that consume a high-starch diet low in sugars have low caries experience compared with populations who consume diets relatively low in starch but high in sugars. In the Hopewood House study (Harris et al. 1963), the intake of unrefined starchy staple foods was high and children had low levels of caries. In the Turku study (Scheinin et al. 1976), intake of starch was not limited yet low caries occurred in the group that did not consume sugars. In Hereditary Fructose Intolerance diets, sucrose cannot be consumed yet glucose and therefore starch may be consumed freely. People with HFI have low caries despite consuming plenty starchy foods (Newbrun et al. 1980).

During World War II, dental caries declined due to the limited sugars availability. During the same period the intake of starch increased in many countries including England, Norway, and Japan. Furthermore, when diet and caries levels are compared at a country level no relationship is seen between per capita availability of cereals such as wheat once sugars intake is controlled for. Yet the relationship between sugars availability and levels of dental caries remains when cereal availability is controlled for suggesting starchy cereals do not play a significant role in the development of caries (Rugg-Gunn

1993). Longitudinal observations studies have also shown that those who develop few caries have significantly higher intakes of starch compared with those who develop high levels of caries (Ruottinen *et al.* 2004; Larsson *et al.* 1992). Less refined starchy staple foods (for example, whole grain foods) have properties that protect the teeth from decay and may require more mastication thereby promoting increased secretion of saliva, increasing plaque-acid buffering capacity.

Overall the evidence shows that staple starchy foods such as rice, potatoes, and bread are of low cariogenicity. Highly refined and heat-treated starch can cause dental caries but less so than sugars. Foods containing cooked starch and substantial amounts of sucrose appear to be as cariogenic as similar quantities of sucrose. In industrialized countries, the number of processed starchy foods has increased, and many of these foods are also high in fats and/or free sugars and salt (such as corn snacks, sweetened breakfast cereals, cakes, and biscuits [cookies]). It is not the intake of these types of starchy foods but the increased intake of starchy staple foods (for example bread, potatoes, and whole grain foods) that is being encouraged by nutritionists and other health professionals.

Does fruit cause dental caries?

There is little evidence to show that fruit consumption is an important factor in the development of dental caries when consumed as part of the mixed human diet. Some plaque pH studies have found fruit to be acidogenic (though less so than sucrose) (Ludwig and Bibby 1957; Hussein *et al.* 1996), and in the study of Pollard (1995), although fruit consumption depressed plaque pH it did not fall below the critical pH in any of the participants. Fruits also contain factors that protect against dental decay including many polyphenolic compounds, and plaque pH studies do not account for this nor the fact of the stimulating effect that fruit consumption has on salivary flow.

Animal studies have shown that fruit causes caries, but in these studies fruit consumption was at high frequencies (for example, 17 times a day) (Imfeld *et al.* 1991; Stephan 1966), but nonetheless, the caries caused by fruit consumption was significantly less than that caused by sucrose. Epidemiological studies of human populations have shown that fruit is of low cariogenicity. In a study of Finnish children aged 5, 9, and 13 years, no differences in vitamin C intake (as an index of fruit consumption) were found between children with high compared with low caries (Kleemola-Kujala and Rasanen 1979). Studies of longitudinal design (Clancy *et al.* 1977; Rugg-Gunn *et al.* 1984) have reported a negative association between fruit

consumption and caries development. One study that did find an association between consumption of fruit and levels of dental caries was that of Grobler and Blignaut (1989) in which the dental caries experience of workers on apple and grape farms was found to be higher than that of workers on grain farms. The level of fruit consumption by the fruit farm workers averaged eight apples per day or three bunches of grapes per day. The high DMFT levels were largely due to missing teeth, the cause of which was unknown.

Theoretically dried fruit may potentially be more cariogenic since the drying process breaks down the cellular structure of the fruit, releasing free sugars. Dried fruits tend to have a longer oral clearance. However research has shown that dried fruits contain many factors that protect against decay in addition to being a good source of dietary fiber and micronutrients making them a valuable contribution to fruit intake. When limiting intake of sugars, it is preferable to focus on sources of sugars that provide little other nourishment.

Based on current evidence it can be concluded that increasing consumption of fresh fruit in order to replace free sugars in the diet is likely to decrease the level of dental caries in a population.

Classification of sugars for dental health and general health purposes

For dental health purposes, it is important to distinguish between sugars naturally present in fruits, vegetables, cereal, grains, and milk as these foods are not associated with dental caries. Current dietary guidelines promote the increased consumption of fruits, vegetables, starchy staple foods, and milk makes an important contribution to calcium intake. In view of this the sugars associated with dental caries were classified by WHO as 'free sugars' and defined as 'all added sugars (by manufacturer, cook or consumer) and sugars present in fruit juices, honey and syrups' (WHO 2003).

Strategies to prevent dental caries: modification of free sugars consumption

A summary of the research informing safe levels of intake for free sugars is given in Table 6-1.

Newbrun and Sheiham have postulated that the relationship between dental caries and level of sugar is sigmoid in nature (Newbrun 1982; Sheiham 1983). When the level of sugar intake is below 10 kg/person/year, which is equivalent to less than 30 g/day, the level of dental caries is very low. When intake of sugars rises above 15 kg/person/year (about 40 g/day), dental caries increases and intensifies with increasing sugars intake. At high levels of sugar intake in the region of

Table 6-1 Summary of the evidence for a low level of sugars intake

Author year	Population	Sugars levels and dental caries
Ruottinen et al. 2004	Finnish children aged 10 years	The top 5% of sugars consumers consumed >10% energy as sugars after 13 months of age. Mean dmft/DMFT was 3.9. The bottom 5% sugar consumers did not consume >7% of energy intake as sugars. The mean dmft/DMFT (mixed dentition) was 1.9.
Jamel et al. 2004	Iraqi children aged 6–7, 11–12, and 14–15 years	At a sugars intake of 12 kg per year, the mean DMFT values were below 2.0.
Karjalainen et al. 2001	Finnish children aged 3–6 years	The mean sucrose intake of those that developed caries at age 6 was 33.4 g per day (10.7% of energy intake) compared with 26.5 g per day (8.8% energy intake).
MacKeown et al. 2000	South African children initially aged 1 year	Prevalence of dental caries increased from 1.5% at age 1 (when sugars intake equated to 17 g per day or ~6% E) to 62.2% at age 5 years when sugars intake was in excess of 10% E (48g/d = approximately 14% E).
Rodrigues et al. 1999	Pre-school children aged 3 years in Brazil	When sugars intake was >12.3 kg per person per year, caries in the deciduous dentition was 29% more likely.
Miyazaki and Morimoto 1996	Data from Japan 1945–1987	When sugars intake was <15 kg per person per year, DMFT was <3.0. Caries levels increased as sugar intake increased until a peak was reached at 29 kg per year in 1973. Thereafter, sugars intake decreased and so did caries. A correlation of +0.9 was observed.
Woodwood and Walker 1994	12-year-old children from different countries using data from WHO and FAO	When sugars intake was <10 kg per person per year, 78% of countries had a DMFT of <2.0. 30% of countries with a sugars intake of >10 kg per year had a DMFT of <2.0.
Steyn et al. 1987	South African children	For all ethnic groups studied, sucrose intake was above 50 g per day and DMFT was above 3.0.
Sheiham 1983	Children aged 12 years from different countries using data from WHO	When sugars intake is <10 kg per person per year, caries is low. When sugars intake is <15 kg per year, caries is low if there is exposure to fluoride.
Sreebny 1982	Children aged 12 years from different countries using data from WHO	When sugars intake was <18.25 kg per person per year, DMFT was <3.0.
Scheinin et al. 1976	Turku study of Finnish adults	56% fewer caries when sucrose was removed from diet.
Martinsson 1972	Swedish children aged 14 years	Boys with the highest caries consumed on average 14.8% E as sugars compared with 9.6% in those with low caries. Girls with the highest caries levels consumed 15.4% E as sugars compared with 10.6% E in the girls with low levels of caries.
Buttner 1971	Data from 18 countries in 1959	When intake of sugars was <20 kg per person per year, dental caries was very low.
Takeuchi 1962	Children in Japan	At a sugars intake of <10 kg per person per year, dental caries were seldom found in the first two post eruptive years in the first permanent molars. At a sugars intake of >15 kg per person per year, caries occurred in the first post eruptive year and caries intensified.
Takahashi 1961	Children in Japan	Annual caries increment was positively related to sugars when annual sugars intake ranged from 0.2–15 kg per person per year.
Toverud 1957		In Norway during World War II when sugar availability fell to only 36–42 g/day (~7.5–9 % E) annual caries incidence more than halved.
Schulerud 1950	Children aged 6 and 7 years	During World War II there was a 50% reduction in dental caries for 6- and 7-year-old children. Intake of sucrose was in the region of 28 g per day (10.4 kg per person per year).
Knowles 1946	3–7 year old children in Jersey during WWII	When sugars intake was <10 kg per person per year, over 50% of children were caries free.

35 kg/person/year (about 96 g/person/day), a saturation level is reached so that a further increase in sugar intake beyond this level does not increase caries to any appreciable extent. Some of the studies summarized in Table 6-1 were conducted on populations that were not exposed to fluoride. Exposure to fluoride may increase the level of safe intake for sugars. Sheiham (1983) postulated that where fluoride in drinking water is at 0.7–1 ppm, or where more than 90% of toothpastes available are fluoridated, the sugars caries relationship shifts and increases the safe level of sugars consumption from 10 kg/person/year to 15 kg/person/year.

What are the current recommendations for levels of sugars intake in different countries?

It is important that goals for sugars intake are set at the population level because a wealth of evidence shows that when free sugars intake by a population is low, dental caries levels are low. A population goal based on amount of free sugars intake also enables the dental health risks of populations to be assessed and health promotion goals monitored. In 1990 the WHO was the first organization to set a numerical cap on sugars intake recommending that free sugars should contribute no more than 10% to energy intake (WHO 1990). Numerous countries have set recommendations for levels of free sugars (also referred to as 'added,' 'purified,' 'non-milk extrinsic,' or refined') intake, which are summarized in Table 6-2.

In a worldwide review of national recommendations for levels of sugars intake, Freire *et al.* (1994) reported that 23 countries had set goals for sugars consumption.

Following the 2002 WHO consultation on Diet, Nutrition and the Prevention of Chronic Disease, the conclusions and recommendations relating to the prevention of dental diseases were published (WHO 2003) and are summarized below.

It was concluded that the level of dental caries is low in countries where the consumption of free sugars is below 15–20 kg/person/year. This is equivalent to a daily intake of 40–55 g, and the values equate to approximately 6–10% of energy intake.

It was therefore recommended that countries that currently have low consumption of free sugars (<15–20 kg/person/year) do not increase consumption levels and that countries with levels of consumption above this amount formulate country-specific and community-specific goals for reducing the amount of consumption of free sugars, aiming toward the recommended maximum of 10% of energy intake.

Furthermore, it was recommended that the frequency of consumption of foods and/or drinks containing free sugars should be limited to a maximum of four times per day.

With respect to the important preventive role of fluoride, it was recommended that there should be adequate exposure to fluoride using appropriate vehicles such as water and milk and availability of affordable toothpastes, especially in countries that are currently undergoing nutrition transition (and adopting a more westernized diet).

The WHO report also highlighted that governments needed to be aware of the potential financial consequence of failing to prevent dental diseases, especially to governments of countries that currently have low levels of disease but that are undergoing nutrition transition.

The importance of regular monitoring of the prevalence and severity of dental diseases in different age groups and different countries as well as the collation of information on levels on sugars intake using appropriate and standardized methods was highlighted.

Table 6-2 Policies and recommendations on levels of free sugars intake by a number of countries and the World Health Organization

Year	Organization	Recommendation for threshold of free sugars intake as a percent of energy intake
1986	Netherlands, Ministry of Health	0–10%
1987	Australia, Department of Health	≤12%
1987	Finland, Board of Nutrition	≤10%
1989	Poland, National Institute	<10%
1990	World Health Organization	≤10%
1991	United Kingdom, Department of Health	≤10%
1996	Nordic Nutrition Recommendations	≤10%
1997	Sweden	≤10%
2003	World Health Organization	≤10%

The report also recommended that all health professionals including the dental profession should received adequate training in nutrition and that nutrition health professions receive information on dental health issues during training. This is essential if advice for dental health is to be consistent with advice for general health. With respect to training and education, it was also recognized that school children should received education about diet and oral health.

In this regard, the reader may find the following guide to snack foods useful (Table 6-3).

What research is required to advance knowledge in the field of nutrition and oral health?

More information is required on the intake of free sugars and the dietary sources of sugars by different populations and age groups, especially in countries undergoing economic growth and nutrition transition. There is also a need for more research into the optimum levels of fluoride ingestion for different ages, climates, and nutritional status. However, the role of sugars in the etiology of

Table 6-3 Snack guide for dental health

Snack category (examples, list not exhaustive)	"Traffic Light" guide and comments
Low in sugars and in line with healthier eating advice	
Vegetable snacks	– low calorie, good source of vitamins and fiber
Bread sticks	– low calorie, less cariogenic
Yogurt, natural/artificially sweetened	– low calorie, good source of calcium, probiotic source
Sandwiches with savory fillings	– choose lower fat choices, such as lean meat, fish salad
Unsweetened breakfast cereals	– good source of energy, mineral, vitamins, and fiber
Milk	– choose lower fat varieties[a], good source of calcium
Lower fat cheeses	– good source of calcium
Water	– stimulates saliva, replaces sweet drinks
Tea and coffee without added sugar	– tea has fluoride
Low in sugars but not as healthy	
Salted nuts	– high in salt
Plain potato chips	– high in salt and added fat
Full fat cheeses	– good source of calcium, protein, and fat soluble vitamins but high in saturated fat and sodium so eat in moderation
Sugar free confectionery	– may be high in fat and calories
Sugar free soft drinks, soda pop, cordials	– can cause acid erosion of teeth, low in nutrients
Plain popcorn	– may be high in salt and fat if buttered
Potentially cariogenic but otherwise in line with healthier eating advice	
Fruit juice including natural unsweetened	– a good source of vitamin C but is high in free sugars and may cause acid erosion so drink no more than one glass a day
Dried fruits	– contain free sugars but a very good source of fiber and micronutrients – eat as part of a meal rather than a snack
Fruit smoothies	– high in free sugars but a good source of calcium if made with milk and also contribute to fruit intake
Sweetened milk drinks	– a good source of calcium and protein but high in free sugars
Cariogenic and less healthy options	
All sugared and chocolate confectionery	– high in fat and or free sugars
Flavored potato chips and corn snacks	– high in fat, salt and free sugars
Cakes, biscuits, cookies, donuts	– high in fat, free sugars, processed starch
Sugared soft drinks, soda pop, cordials	– erosive, high in free sugar, low nutrition value
Pepperoni sticks and beef jerky	– sugars often added, high in saturated fat and salt
Fruit leathers	– high in free sugars
Ice cream	– high in saturated fat and free sugars
Jam	– high in free sugars
Sugared popcorn	– high in sugars and processed starch

[a] reduced fat milks are unsuitable for children under 2 years

dental caries is indisputable, and there is a need for future research to focus on dietary intervention strategies at the national, community, and individual level to find pragmatic and affordable means of reducing sugars intake while increasing the intake of fruits, vegetables, and starchy staple foods in line with dietary advice for general health.

References

Anaise, J.Z. (1978) Prevalence of dental caries among workers in the sweets industry in Israel. *Community Dentistry and Oral Epidemiology*, 8, 142–145.

Bang, G. and Kristoffersen, T. (1972) Dental caries and diet in an Alaskan Eskimo population. *Scandinavian Journal of Dental Research*, 80, 440–444.

Battellino, L.J., Cornejo, L.S., Dorronsoro de Cattoni, S.T., *et al.* (1997). [Oral health status evaluation of pre-school children: longitudinal epidemiologic study (1993–1994), Cordoba, Argentina]. *Revista de Saude Publica*, 31, 272–281.

Beighton, D., Adamson, A., Rugg-Gunn, A. (1996) Associations between dietary intake, dental caries experience and salivary bacterial levels in 12-year-old English schoolchildren. *Archives of Oral Biology*, 41, 271–280.

Burt, B. and Pai, S. (2001) Sugar consumption and caries risk: a systematic review. *Journal of Dental Education*, 65, 1017–1023.

Burt, B. and Szpunar, S.M. (1994) The Michigan Study: relationship between sugars intake and dental caries over 3 years. *International Dental Journal*, 44, 230–240.

Burt, B.A., Eklund, S.A., Morgan, K.J., *et al.* (1988) The effects of sugars intake and frequency of ingestion on dental caries increment in a 3-year longitudinal study. *Journal of Dental Research*, 67, 1422–9.

Büttner, M. (1971) *Zuckeraufnahme und Karies.* [Sugar intake and caries.] In: *Grundfragen der Ernährungswissenschaft* (Ed. H.D. Cremer), pp. 175–191, Rombach, Freiburg im Breisgau, Germany. [Cited by Marthaler, T. M. (1979) Health and Sugar Substitutes. In: *Proceedings of ERGOB Conference on Sugar Substitutes* (Ed. B. Guggenheim) pp. 27–34, Karger, Basel, Switzerland].

Chapple, I.L.C., Milward, M.R., Dietrich, T. (2007) The prevalence of inflammatory periodontitis is negatively associated with serum antioxidant concentrations. *The Journal of Nutrition*, 137, 657–664.

Chen, M., Andersen, R.M., Barmes, D.E., *et al.* (1997) *Comparing Oral Health Systems. A Second International Collaborative Study.* Geneva: World Health Organization.

Clancy, K.L., Bibby, B.G., Goldberg, H.J.V., *et al.* (1977) Snack food intake of adolescents and caries development. *Journal of Dental Research*, 56, 568–573.

Cleaton-Jones, P., Richardson, B.D., Winter, G.B. *et al.* (1984) Dental caries and sucrose intake in five South African pre-school groups. *Community Dentistry and Oral Epidemiology*, 12, 381–385.

De Marchi, R.J., Hugo, F.N., Hilgert, J.B., *et al.* (2008) Association between oral health status and *nutritional* status in south Brazilian independent-living older people. *Nutrition*, 24, 546–553.

Dion, N., Cotart, J-L., Rabilloud, M. (2007) Correction of nutrition test errors for more accurate quantification of the link between dental health and malnutrition. *Nutrition*, 23, 301–307.

Edgar, W.M. (1985) Prediction of the cariogenicity of various foods. *International Dental Journal*, 35, 190–194.

Emslie, D.R. (1966) A dental health survey in the Republic of Sudan. *British Dental Journal*, 120, 167–178.

Enwonwu, C.O. (1995) Interface of malnutrition and periodontal diseases. *American Journal of Clinical Nutrition* 61 (Suppl.), 430S–436S.

Firestone, A.R., Imfeld, T., Muhlemann, H.R. (1984) Effect of the length and number of intervals between meals on caries in rats. *Caries Research*, 18, 128–133.

Fisher, F.J. (1968) A field study of dental caries, periodontal disease and enamel defects in Tristan da Cunha. *British Dental Journal*, 125, 447–453.

Francis, D.K., Van den Broeck, J., Younger, N., *et al.* (2009) Fast food and sweetened beverage consumption: association with overweight and high waist circumference in adolescents. *Public Health Nutrition*, 12, 1106–1114.

Frostell, G., Birkhed, D., Edwardsson, S., *et al.* (1991) Effect of partial substitution of invert sugar from sucrose in combination with duraphat treatment on caries development in pre-school children: the Malmo Study. *Caries Research*, 25, 304–310.

Gaengler, P., Pfister, W., Sproessig, M., et al. (1986) The effects of carbohydrate-reduced diet on development of gingivitis. *Clinical Preventive Dentistry*, 8, 17–23.

Grindefjord, M., Dahllof, G., Nilsson, B. *et al.* (1996) Stepwise prediction of dental caries in children up to 3.5 years of age. *Caries Research*, 30, 256–266.

Grobler, S.R. and Blignaut, J.B. (1989) The effect of a high consumption of apples or grapes on dental caries and periodontal disease in humans. *Clinical Preventive Dentistry*, 11, 8–12.

Gustafsson, B.E., Quensel, C.E., Lanke, L.S., *et al.* (1954) The Vipeholm dental caries study. The effect of different levels of carbohydrate intake on caries activity in 436 individuals observed for 5 years. *Acta Odontologica Scandinavica*, 11, 232–364.

Harris, R. (1963) Biology of the children of Hopewood House, Bowral, Australia, 4. Observations on dental caries experience extending over 5 years (1957–61). *Journal of Dental Research*, 42, 1387–1399.

Hartmink, R., Quataert, M.C., van Leare, K.M., *et al.* (1995) Degradation and fermentation of fructooligosaccharides by oral streptococci. *Journal of Applied Bacteriology*, 79, 551–557.

Hefti, A. and Schmid, R. (1979) Effect on caries incidence in rats of increasing dietary sucrose levels. *Caries Research*, 13, 298–300.

Holbrook, W.P., Arnadóttir, I.B., Takazoe, I., *et al.* (1995) Longitudinal study of caries, cariogenic bacteria and diet in children just before and after starting school. *European Journal of Oral Sciences*, 103, 42–45.

Holbrook, W.P., Kristinsson, M.J., Gunnarsdottir, S. (1989) Caries prevalence, *streptococcus mutans* and sugar intake among 4-year-old urban children in Iceland. *Community Dentistry and Oral Epidemiology*, 17, 292–295.

Holt, R.D. (1991) Foods and drinks at four daily time intervals in a group of young children. *British Dental Journal*, 170, 137–143.

Holt, R.D., Joels, D., Winter, G.B. (1982) Caries in preschool children; the Camden study. *British Dental Journal*, 153, 107–109.

Hussein, I., Pollard, M.A., Curzon, M.E.J. (1996) A comparison of the effects of some extrinsic and intrinsic sugars on dental plaque pH. *International Journal of Paediatric Dentistry*, 6, 81–86.

Imfeld, T.N., Schmid, R., Lutz, F., *et al.* (1991) Cariogenicity of Milchschnitte (Ferrero-GmbH) and apple in programme-fed rats. *Caries Research*, 25, 352–358.

Ismail, A.I., Burt, B.A., Eklund, S.A. (1984) The cariogenicity of soft drinks in the United States. *Journal of the American Dental Association*, 109, 241–245.

Jamel, H.A., Sheiham, A., Watt, R.G., *et al.* (1996) Sweet preference, consumption of sweet tea and dental caries: studies in urban and rural Iraqi populations. *International Dental Journal*, 47, 213–217.

Jamel, H., Plasschaert, A., Sheiham, A., *et al.* (2004). Dental caries experience and availability of sugars in Iraqi children before and after the United Nations sanctions. *International Dental Journal,* 54, 21–25.

James, J. and Kerr, D. (2005) Preventing childhood obesity by reducing soft drinks. *International Journal of Obesity,* 29 (suppl 2), S54–S57.

Jenkins, G.N. and Ferguson, D.B. (1966) Milk and dental caries. *British Dental Journal,* 120, 472–477.

Karjalainen, S., Soderling, E., Sewon, L., *et al.* (2001). A prospective study on sucrose consumption, visible plaque and caries in children from 3 to 6 years of age. *Community Dentistry and Oral Epidemiology,* 29, 136–142.

Katayama, T., Nagagawa, N., Honda, O., *et al.* (1979) Incidence and distribution of Strep mutans in plaque from confectionery workers. *Journal of Dental Research,* 58 (Special issue), 2251.

Kelly, M., Steele, J., Nuttall, N., *et al.* (2000) Adult Dental Health Survey. In: *Oral Health in the United Kingdom 1998.* The Stationery Office, London, UK.

Kleemola-Kujala, E. and Räsänen, L. (1982) Relationship of oral hygiene and sugar consumption to risk of caries in children. *Community Dentistry and Oral Epidemiology,* 10, 224–233.

Kleemola-Kujala, E. and Räsänen L. (1979) Dietary pattern of Finnish children with low and high caries experience. *Community Dentistry and Oral Epidemiology,* 7, 199–205.

Knowles, E.M. (1946) The effects of enemy occupation on the dental condition of children in the Channel Islands. *Monthly Bulletin of the Ministry of Health and the Public Health Laboratory Service,* 1946, 161–172.

Koga, T., Horikoshi, T., Fujiwarra, T., *et al.* (1988) Effects of panose on glucan synthesis and cellular adherence Streptococcus mutans. *Microbiology and Immunology,* 32, 25–31.

Konig, K.P., Schmid, P., Schmid, R. (1968) An apparatus for frequency controlled feeding of small rodents and its use in dental caries experiments. *Archives of Oral Biology,* 13, 13–26.

Lachapelle-Harvey, D. and Sevigny, J. (1985) Multiple regression analysis of dental status and related food behaviour of French Canadian adolescents. *Community Dentistry and Oral Epidemiology,* 13, 226–229.

Lamy, M., Mojon, P., Kalykakis, G., *et al.* (1999) Oral status and nutrition in the institutionalized elderly. *Journal of Dentistry,* 27, 443–448.

Larsson, B., Johansson, I., Ericson, T. (1992) Prevalence of caries in adolescents in relation to diet. *Community Dentistry and Oral Epidemiology,* 20, 133–137.

Lingström, P., van Houte, J., Kashket, S. (2000) Food starches and dental caries. *Critical Reviews in Oral Biology and Medicine,* 11, 366–380.

Ludwig, T.G. and Bibby, B.G. (1957) Acid production from different carbohydrate foods in plaque and saliva. *Journal of Dental Research,* 36, 56–60.

MacGregor, A.B. (1963) Increasing caries incidence and changing diet in Ghana. *International Dental Journal,* 13, 516–522.

MacKeown, J.M., Cleaton-Jones, P.E., Edwards, A.W. (2000) Energy and macronutrient intake in relation to dental caries incidence in urban black South African preschool children in 1991 and 1995: the Birth-to-Ten study. *Public Health Nutrition,* 3, 313–319.

Marthaler, T. (1990) Changes in the prevalence of dental caries: how much can be attributed to changes in diet? *Caries Research,* 24, 3–15.

Martinsson, T. (1972) Socio-economic investigation of school children with high and low caries frequency. 3. A dietary study based on information given by the children. *Odontologisk Revy,* 23, 93–113.

Masalin, K., Murtamaa, H., Meurman, J.H. (1990) Oral health of workers in the modern Finnish confectionery industry. *Community Dentistry and Oral Epidemiology,* 18, 126–130.

Masson, L.F., Blackburn, A., Sheehy, C., *et al.* (2010) Sugar intake and dental decay: results from a national survey of children in Scotland. *British Journal of Nutrition,* 104, 1555–1564.

Mikx, F.H.M., Hoevel, J.Svd., Plasschaert, A.J.M., *et al.* (1975) Effect of *Actinomyces viscosus* on the establishment and symbiosis of *Streptococcus mutans* and *Streptococcus sanguis* on SPF rats on different sucrose diets. *Caries Research,* 9, 1–20.

Minquan, D., Petersen, P.E., Fan, M.W., *et al.* (2000) Oral health services in PR China as evaluated by dentist and patients. *International Dental Journal,* 50, 175–183.

Miyazaki, H. and Morimoto, M. (1996) Changes in caries prevalence in Japan. *European Journal of Oral Sciences,* 104, 452–458.

Moynihan, P.J. and Kelly, A.A.M. (2012) A systematic review of the evidence for a relationship between the amount of sugars consumption and dental caries in humans. Report compiled for WHO.

Moynihan, P.J. and Petersen, P. E. (2004) Diet, nutrition and dental diseases (Background paper for the Joint WHO/FAO Expert Consultation on diet, nutrition and the prevention of chronic diseases. Geneva 28 Jan–1 Feb 2002). *Public Health Nutrition,* 7, 201–226.

Murray, J.J. (1986) *Appropriate Use of Fluorides for Human Health.* World Health Organization, Geneva, Switzerland.

Nadanovsky, P. (1994) Letter. *British Dental Journal,* 177, 280.

Navia, J.M. (1996) Nutrition and dental caries: ten findings to be remembered. *International Dental Journal,* 46 (Suppl. 1), 381–387.

Newbrun, E. (1982) Sucrose in the dynamics of the carious process. *International Dental Journal,* 32, 13–23.

Newbrun, E., Hoover, C., Mettraux, G., *et al.* (1980) Comparison of dietary habits and dental health of subjects with hereditary fructose intolerance and control subjects. *Journal of the American Dental Association,* 101, 619–626.

Nishida, M., Grossi, S.G., Dunford, R.G., *et al.* (2000) Calcium and the risk for periodontal disease. *Journal of Periodontology,* 71, 1057–1066.

Olsson, B. (1979) Dental health situation in privileged children in Addis Ababa Ethiopia. *Community Dentistry and Oral Epidemiology,* 7, 37–41.

Ooshima, T., Fujiwarra, T., Taki, T., *et al.* (1998) The caries inhibitory effects of GOS-sugar in vitro and in rat experiments. *Microbiology and Immunology,* 32, 1093–1105.

Petersen, P.E. (1983) Dental health among workers at a Danish chocolate factory. *Community Dentistry and Oral Epidemiology,* 11, 337–341.

Petersen, P.E., Poulsen, V.J., Ramahaleo, J.J., *et al.* (1991) Dental caries and dental health behaviour situation among 6- and 12-year old urban schoolchildren in Madagascar. *African Dental Journal,* 5, 1–7.

Pollard, M.A. (1995) Potential cariogenicity of starches and fruits as assessed by the plaque sampling method and intraoral cariogenicity test. *Caries Research,* 29, 68–74.

Roberts, I.F. and Roberts, G.J. (1979) Relation between medicines sweetened with sucrose and dental disease. *British Medical Journal,* 2, 14–16.

Roberts, P.G. and Hayes, M.L. (1980) Effects of 20-deoxy-D-glucose and other sugar analogues on acid production from sugars by human dental plaque bacteria. *Scandinavian Journal of Dental Research,* 88, 201–209.

Rodriguez, C.S., Watt, R.G., Sheiham, A. (1999) The effects of dietary guidelines on sugar intake and dental caries in 3-year-olds attending nurseries. *Health Promotion International,* 14, 329–335.

Rose, G. (1993) *The Strategy of Preventive Medicine.* Oxford University Press, Oxford UK.

Rugg-Gunn, A.J. (1993) *Nutrition and Dental Health.* Oxford Medical Publications, Oxford UK.

Rugg-Gunn, A.J., Hackett, A.F., Appleton, D.R., *et al.* (1984) Relationship between dietary habits and caries increment assessed over two years in 405 English adolescent schoolchildren. *Archives of Oral Biology*, 29, 983–992.

Ruottinen, S., Karjalainen, S., Pienihakkinen, K., *et al.* (2004) Sucrose intake since infancy and dental health in 10-year-old children. *Caries Research,* 38, 142–148.

Ruxton, C.H.S., Garceau, F.J.S., Cottrell, R.C. (1999) Guidelines for sugar consumption in Europe. Is a qualitative approach justified? *European Journal of Clinical Nutrition*, 53, 503–513.

Scheinin, A., Makinen, K.K., Ylitalo, K. (1976) Turku sugar studies V. Final report on the effect of sucrose, fructose and xylitol diets on the caries incidence in man. *Acta Odontologica Scandinavica*, 34, 179–198.

Schulerud, A. (1950) Dental Caries and Nutrition During Wartime in Norway. *Fabritius and Sonners Trykkeri,* Oslo, Norway.

Sheiham, A. (1967) The prevalence of dental caries in Nigerian populations. *British Dental Journal*, 123, 144–148.

Sheiham, A. (1983) Sugars and dental caries. *Lancet*, 1, 282–284.

Sheiham, A. (2001) Dietary effects on dental diseases. *Public Health Nutrition*, 4, 569–591.

Sidi, A.D. and Ashley, P.F. (1994) Influence of frequent sugar intake on experimental gingivitis. *Journal of Periodontology*, 55, 419–423.

Sreebny, L.M. (1982) Sugar availability, sugar consumption and dental caries. *Community Dentistry and Oral Epidemiology*, 10, 1–7.

Stecksen-Blicks, C. and Gustafsson, L. (1986) Impact of oral hygiene and use of fluorides on caries increment in children during one year. *Community Dentistry and Oral Epidemiology,* 14, 185–189.

Stephan, R.M. (1996) Effects of different types of foods on dental health in experimental animals. *Journal of Dental Research,* 45, 1551–1561.

Steyn, N.P., Albertse, E.C., van Wyk Kotze, T.J., *et al.* (1987) Sucrose consumption and dental caries in twelve-year-old children of all ethnic groups residing in Cape Town. *Journal of the Dental Association of South Africa*, 42, 43–49.

Sundin, B., Granath, L., Birkhed, D. (1992) Variation of posterior approximal caries incidence with consumption of sweets with regard to other caries-related factors in 15–18-year olds. *Community Dentistry and Oral Epidemiology*, 20, 76–80.

Szpunar, S.M., Eklund, S.A., Burt, B.A. (1995) Sugar consumption and caries risk in schoolchildren with low caries experience. *Community Dentistry and Oral Epidemiology*, 23, 142–146.

Takahashi, K. (1961) Statistical study on caries incidence in the first molar in relation to the amount of sugar consumption. *Bulletin of the Tokyo Dental College*, 2, 44–57.

Takeuchi, M. (1962) On the epidemiological principles in dental caries attack. *Bulletin of the Tokyo Dental College*, 3, 96–111.

Toverud, G. (1957) The influence of war and post-war conditions on the teeth of Norwegian schoolchildren. *Millbank Memorial Fund Quarterly,* 25, 373–459.

Weaver, R. (1950) Fluorine and war-time diet. *British Dental Journal*, 88, 231–239.

Woodward, M. and Walker, A.R.P. (1994) Sugar and dental caries: The evidence from 90 countries. *British Dental Journal*, 176, 297–302.

World Health Organization. (1990) *Diet, Nutrition and the Prevention of Chronic Diseases. Technical Report Series No 797,* World Health Organization, Geneva.

World Health Organization. (2003) *Diet, Nutrition and the Prevention of Chronic Diseases.* Technical Report Series 916. FAO/WHO, Geneva.

Yu, Y–H., Kuo, H–K., Lai, Y-L. (2007) The association between serum folate levels and periodontal disease in older adults: data from the National Health and Nutrition Examination Survey 2001/02. *Journal of the American Geriatrics Society,* 55, 108–113.

Zero, D. (2004) Sugars—The Arch Criminal? *Caries Research*, 38, 277–285.

7

Probiotics and dental caries risk

Eva Söderling

Introduction

The Food and Agriculture Organization (FAO)/World Health Organization (WHO) have defined probiotics as "live micro-organisms, which when administered in adequate amounts, confer a health benefit to the host." They should preferably be of human origin and be able to temporarily colonize the gastrointestinal tract and survive in it. They must also be non-pathogenic and non-toxic. Existing evidence suggests that probiotic health effects are strain specific.

Probiotics are used in the prevention and treatment of infectious diseases and allergies. (For review, see Hatakka and Saxelin 2008.) In some countries probiotics are recommended for infants because of their long-term enhancement of the immune responses of children. Combinations of probiotics, like *Bifidobacterium lactis* BB-12, and *Lactobacillus rhamnosus* GG, appear to be most effective in this respect (Rautava *et al.* 2009). Figure 7-1 summarizes the potential mechanisms by which probiotic bacteria may exert their antagonism against pathogenic organisms. Probiotics are mainly ingested orally, and the gastrointestinal tract is thus the primary target organ for probiotic microorganisms. However, when ingested in the form of, for example, tablets, chewing gums, cheese, and milk, the oral cavity is exposed to the probiotics. With the worldwide increase in the use of probiotics, their effects on oral health have become a hot topic.

The probiotic species most often investigated and widely used in foods are lactobacilli and bifidobacteria. This chapter focuses mainly on these genera even though other microorganisms are also used as probiotics.

Caries-related mechanisms of probiotic activity

In the gut the probiotic bacteria enhance the immune responses of the host (Figure 7-1) It can be hypothesized that systemic effects of probiotics could also influence oral health. Total SIgA levels in saliva were, however, not affected by the use of probiotics as shown by Paineau *et al.* (2008).

Lactobacilli and bifidobacteria are both acidogenic and aciduric. Some lactobacilli and bifidobacteria, including *L. rhamnosus* GG and *B. lactis* BB-12, do not ferment sucrose (Haukioja *et al.* 2008). Considering dental caries, sucrose fermentation is an important virulence factor of probiotics that is seldom discussed in the literature. The low pH generated by most probiotics is also crucial for their antimicrobial actions. Several studies have demonstrated that probiotic lactobacilli may inhibit caries-associated microorganisms via antimicrobial substances active at a low pH. The growth inhibition of *S. mutans in vitro* has been attributed to the generation of a low pH either via organic acid production and/or production of bacteriocins or metabolites active at a low pH (Simark-Mattsson *et al.*, 2009).

The adhesion capacity and persistence on the oral mucosa and teeth is an important property of probiotics from an oral health point of view. *In vitro* studies have demonstrated that probiotic lactobacilli show varying degrees of adhesion to saliva-coated hydroxyapatite surfaces, *L. rhamnosus* strains adhering better than *L. reuteri* strains (Haukioja *et al.* 2006). However, interactions between oral microorganisms and probiotics influence adhesion. Probiotics may modify the protein composition

Comprehensive Preventive Dentistry, First Edition. Edited by Hardy Limeback.
© 2012 John Wiley & Sons, Ltd. Published 2012 by John Wiley & Sons, Ltd.

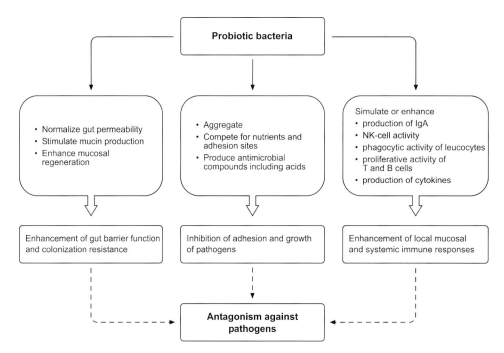

Figure 7-1 Potential mechanisms by which probiotic bacteria may exert their antagonistic effects against pathogenic organisms. Modified from Hatakka and Saxelin (2008), with permission from Bentham Science Publishers Ltd.

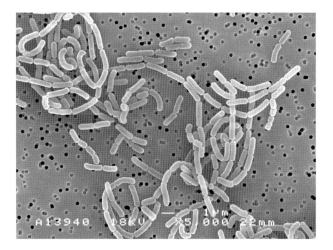

Figure 7-2 Scanning electron micrograph of *Lactobacillus rhamnosus* GG. By courtesy of Valio Ltd, Helsinki, Finland.

of the pellicle and specifically prevent adhesion of other bacteria. Haukioja *et al.* (2006) showed that *Fusobacterium nucleatum*-coating of hydroxyapatite modified the binding of probiotics *in vitro*. So far, only a few studies have addressed the *in vivo* binding of probiotics to the oral cavity. *L. rhamnosus* GG and *L. reuteri* ATCC 55730 have shown rather rapid oral clearance in adults (Yli-Knuuttila *et al.* 2006; Caglar *et al.* 2009). Recently, the persistence of *L. rhamnosus* GG and LC705, *Propionibacterium freudenreichii* and *B. lactis* BB-12 administered as capsules, yoghurt, or cheese was compared. *L. rhamnosus* GG was the only probiotic strain regularly recovered in saliva

samples during and after the 2-week intervention (Saxelin *et al.* 2010). Within ten days *L. rhamnosus* GG was, however, eliminated from the saliva of approximately 80% of the subjects (Saxelin *et al.* 2010). Interestingly, some probiotic lactobacilli have inhibited biofilm formation of mutans streptococci (MS) (Comelli *et al.* 2002; Söderling *et al.* 2010). For a scanning electron micrograph of *L. rhamnosus* GG, see Figure 7-2.

A phenomenon closely related to adhesion is co-aggregation between probiotic bacteria and caries-associated strains. Some lactobacilli were demonstrated to co-aggregate with MS (Twetman *et al.* 2009a). Recently *L. paracasei* DSMZ16671 selectively co-aggregated *S. mutans* and also reduced caries occurrence in rats inoculated with *S. mutans* (Lang *et al.* 2010; Tanzer *et al.* 2010).

Probiotics and counts of *mutans streptococci*

Most clinical studies on probiotics and oral health have focused on measuring changes in counts of MS. (For review, see Stamatova and Meurman 2009a) In adults, even high counts of MS in the plaque/saliva do not necessarily mean an increased caries risk. However, decreasing MS without affecting the "normal flora" should improve the microbiological composition of the plaque and make it less virulent. The majority of studies dealing with probiotics and counts of MS have been performed with *L. reuteri* SD2112 (ATCC 55730). This probiotic, sometimes combined with *L. reuteri* PTA 5289, has been administered in short-term clinical studies in adults via straws, tablets, medical devices, milk, and chewing gums, all studies resulting in a decrease of MS counts (Caglar *et al.* 2007, Stamatova and Meurman 2009a). Also some bifidobacteria have been associated in clinical studies with decreases in MS counts (Stamatova and Meurman 2009a). *L. rhamnosus* GG was, however, associated with minor changes (Näse *et al.* 2001; Ahola *et al.* 2002) and *L. rhamnosus* LB21 with no changes (Stecksen-Blicks *et al.* 2009) in MS counts. Some of the above studies have included determination of oral counts of lactobacilli in addition to MS; however, no data on long-term consumption of probiotics on the composition of the oral microbiota have been published.

In some countries probiotics are recommended for infants. Thus, a major concern is the effect the administration may have on the colonization of erupting teeth and the future dental health of the child. The only clinical trial so far on the effects of probiotics on oral colonization in infants indicates that early administration of *B. lactis* BB-12 (twice a day, daily dose log 10 CFU, mean administration time 15 months) had no effect on the microbiota of the erupting teeth or the mucosa, including *S. mutans*, in the children monitored at the ages of 8 months and 2 years (Taipale *et al.* 2012).

Probiotics and caries occurrence

Probiotics, mostly lactobacilli or bifidobacteria, are aciduric and acidogenic microorganisms. Such bacteria are usually connected with caries occurrence, not its prevention. So far the few studies on probiotics and caries occurrence suggest that probiotics could rather promote dental health than be a hazard to it. In a Finnish study, 594 children ages 1 to 6 years old attending a day-care center, received *L. rhamnosus* GG-containing milk for 7 months. The milk use reduced the caries risk significantly in the 3- to 4-year-old children (Näse *et al.* 2001). In a recent Swedish study, 248 preschool children ages 1 to 5 years -old received either a control milk or a test milk supplemented with both fluoride and *L. rhamnosus* LB21 for 21 months (Stecksen-Blicks *et al.* 2009). Caries occurrence decreased significantly in the test group, but as the authors themselves state, it is difficult to establish the role of the probiotic organism in that study.

Other than caries-related effects of probiotics on oral health

Probiotics have also been studied for their effects on periodontal diseases and oral yeast infections (Stamatova and Meurman 2009b). Interesting results have been obtained by using a mixture of *S. sanguinis*, *S. salivarius* and *S. mitis* in guiding periodontal pocket recolonization in an animal model. However, bacterial replacement

does not meet the traditional criteria of probiotic therapy. As discussed above, the combination of two *L. reuteri* strains (ATCC 55730 and PTA 5289; available as tablets with the trade name RELADENT® in Europe and GUM® PerioBalance® in the USA) was connected with a reduction in the counts of MS (Caglar *et al.* 2007). With this strain combination Twetman *et al.* (2009b) showed in a 2-week intervention study a decrease in bleeding on probing and pro-inflammatory cytokines of the crevicular fluid. In a different 2-week study with 59 patients *L. reuteri* was suggested to decrease gum bleeding and gingivitis (Krasse *et al.* 2006), but the strains used in the study were not defined. *L. salivarius* WB21-containing tablets (trade name WAKAMATE D®) were used in three clinical studies lasting 4–8 weeks. According to these studies, the use of the probiotic tablet may have beneficial effects on periodontal health, but the results should be verified with higher numbers of subjects. A combination of *S. oralis* strain KJ3sm, *S. uberis* KJ2sm, and *S. rattus* JH 145 is used in probiotic products like mouthwashes and mints with the trade name ProBiora3™. So far, the health claims connected with these products are backed up by one 4-week mouthwash pilot study suggesting that the mouthwash reduced *S. mutans* and *Porphyromonas gingivalis* counts.

The effects of a probiotic cheese containing *a.o.* *L. rhamnosus* GG and *L. rhamnosus* LC705 on the prevalence of oral *Candida* were studied in 192 elderly subjects in a high-quality RCT trial. The probiotic intervention lasted 16 weeks and resulted in a significant reduction of high yeast counts (Hatakka *et al.* 2007). This result can be applicable for example in homes for elderly.

Conclusions

The actions of probiotic bacteria in the gastrointestinal tract are well known. So far, it is not known whether probiotics could, for example, modulate the immune response in the mouth as has been suggested to take place in the gut. New probiotics are emerging, and several research groups have identified resident lactobacilli in the oral microbiota of healthy subjects as potential probiotics. Probiotics could also be genetically modified to improve their beneficial properties. With such probiotics, safety issues are the main obstacles. The probiotics must undergo massive safety evaluations before they are accepted for use, for example, in probiotic products targeted to children. Such probiotics may have their main applications in products that are not ingested, like mouthwashes used to prevent periodontal diseases or halitosis.

Optimally, "old" probiotics with proven benefits for general health could be used to benefit dental health. Combinations of probiotics appear to be more effective in benefiting general health than single probiotics; this may be the case also in promoting oral health. The existing *in vitro* studies and short-term clinical studies help in understanding the mechanisms of action of probiotics. Long-term, randomized, and controlled clinical trials are, however, needed to demonstrate beneficial effects of probiotics on oral health. The administration of the probiotics should not at least be a hazard to dental health. As for the vehicles of administration, dairy products containing no carbohydrate sweeteners, tablets, and chewing gums could be optimal probiotic vehicles.

References

Ahola, A.J., Yli-Knuuttila, H., Suomalainen, T., *et al.* (2002) Short-term consumption of probiotic-containing cheese and its effect on dental caries risk factors. *Archive of Oral Biology*, 47, 799–804.

Caglar, E., Kavaloglu, S.C., Kuscu, O.O., *et al.* (2007) Effect of chewing gums containing xylitol or probiotic bacteria on salivary MS and lactobacilli. *Clinical Oral Investigation*, 11, 425–429.

Caglar, E., Topcuoglu, N., Cildir, S.K., *et al.* (2009) Oral colonization by *Lactobacillus reuteri* ATCC 55730 after exposure to probiotics. *International Journal of Paediatric Dentistry*, 19, 377–381.

Comelli, E.M., Guggenheim, B., Stingele, F., *et al.* (2002) Selection of dairy bacterial strains as probiotics for oral health. *European Journal of Oral Science*, 110, 218–224.

Hatakka, K., Ahola, A.J., Yli-knuuttila, H., *et al.* (2007) Probiotics reduce the prevalence of oral *Candida* in the elderly – a randomized, controlled trial. *Journal of Dental Research*, 86, 125–130.

Hatakka, K. and Saxelin, M. (2008) Probiotics in intestinal and non-intestinal infectious diseases—clinical evidence. *Current Pharmaceutical Design*, 14, 1351–1367.

Haukioja, A., Söderling, E., Tenovuo, J. (2008) Acid production from sugars and sugar alcohols by probiotic lactobacilli and bifidobacteria in vitro. *Caries Research*, 42, 449–453.

Haukioja, A., Yli-Knuuttila, H., Loimaranta, V. *et al.* (2006) Oral adhesion and survival of probiotic and other lactobacilli and bifidobacteria in vitro. *Oral Microbiology and Immunology*, 21, 326–332.

Lang, C., Böttner, M., Holz, C., *et al.* (2009) Specific lactobacillus/mutans streptococcus co-aggregation. *Journal of Dental Research*, 89, 175–179.

Näse, L., Hatakka, K., Savilahti, E., *et al.* (2001) Effect of long-term consumption of a probiotic bacterium, *Lactobacillus rhamnosus* GG, in milk on dental caries and caries risk in children. *Caries Research*, 35, 412–420.

Paineau, D., Carcano, D., Leyer, G., *et al.* (2008) Effects of seven potential probiotic strains on specific immune responses in healthy adults: a double-blind, randomized, controlled trial. *FEMS Immunology and Medical Microbiology*, 53, 107–113.

Rautava, S., Salminen, S., Isolauri, E. (2009) Specific probiotics in reducing the risk of acute infections in infancy—a randomised, double-blind, placebo-controlled study. *British Journal of Nutrition*, 101, 1722–1726.

Simark-Mattsson, C., Jonsson, R., Emilson, C.G., *et al.* (2009) Final pH affects the interference capacity of naturally occurring oral *Lactobacillus* strains against mutans streptococci. *Archive of Oral Biology*, 54, 602–607.

Stamatova, I. and Meurman, J.H. (2009a) Probiotics: health benefits in the mouth. *American Journal of Dentistry*, 22, 329–338.

Stamatova, I. and Meurman, J.H. (2009b) Probiotics and periodontal disease. *Periodontology*, 51, 141–151.

Stecksén-Blicks, C., Sjöström, I., Twetman, S. (2009) Effect of long-term consumption of milk supplemented with probiotic lactobacilli and fluoride on dental caries and general health in preschool children: a cluster-randomized study. *Caries Research*, 43, 374–381.

Söderling, E.M., Marttinen, A.M., Haukioja, A.L. (2010) Probiotic Lactobacilli Interfere with *Streptococcus mutans* biofilm formation in vitro. *Current Microbiology*, Sep 11. (Epub ahead of print).

Taipale, T., Pienihäkkinen, K., Salminen, S. *et al.* (2012) Bifidobacteriumanimalis subsp. lactis BB-12 Administration in early childhood: a randomized clinical trial of effects on oral colonization by mutans streptococci and the probiotic. *Caries Research*, 46, 69–77.

Tanzer, J.M., Thompson, A., Lang, C., *et al.* (2010) Caries inhibition by and safety of *Lactobacillus paracasei* DSMZ16671. *Journal of Dental Research*, 89, 921–926.

Twetman, L., Larsen, U., Fiehn, N.E., *et al.* (2009a) Coaggregation between probiotic bacteria and caries-associated strains: an in vitro study. *Acta Odontologica Scandinavica*, 27, 1–5.

Twetman, S., Derawi, B., Keller, *et al.* (2009b) Short-term effect of chewing gums containing probiotic *Lactobacillus reuteri* on the levels of inflammatory mediators in gingival crevicular fluid. *Acta Odontologica Scandinavica*, 67, 19–24.

Yli-Knuuttila, H., Snäll, J., Kari, K., *et al.* (2006) Colonization of *Lactobacillus rhamnosus* GG in the oral cavity. *Oral Microbiology and Immunology*, 21, 129–131.

8

Mechanical plaque removal

Shirley Gutkowski

Introduction: why remove oral biofilm?

It may seem obvious to the readers of this book why biofilm management is important. It may be so innate that describing the reasons to fellow health care practitioners may be difficult; hence, this section of the chapter is here to support your efforts in collaborating with other health care providers. The nature of biofilm is such that it allows for pathogens from many species to cohabitate and proliferate. The film grows from the anchoring of non-pathogenic species within a short period of time, and the bacterium congregate and start building a defense mechanism called slime. As it matures all types of microbes from bacteria, virus, fungus, amoebae, and nematodes are invited in. Left unchecked and undisturbed, these biofilm can mature into a biomass harboring untold numbers of bacteria and concentrations of opportunistic pathogens that can alter the health of those who are vulnerable to them.

Vulnerable people include those who are sick or infirm, or those who depend on others for their Activities of Daily Living (ADL). In these groups the idea of *oral biofilm reduction* is significant. For good reason the caregivers are very reluctant to provide oral care in the form of traditional mechanical removal of the oral biofilm. They are fearful of being bitten or spat on. The caregivers often have to spend valuable time coaxing people to open their mouths. The caregivers are unprepared to provide oral care to a non-willing participant considering they are not quite willing to provide this type of care in the first place. Caregivers are much more comfortable cleaning the perineal area than the teeth/mouth.

Residents in long-term care can be very sincere in their assertion that the oral care was already provided, although it may not have been. Residents are very much like willful children; their lust for life may be whittled down to the joy of aggravating another person, or their autonomy may have been stripped to where deciding whether or not they want someone to clean their teeth is all they have left. Most decisions are made for them. The problems related to assisted living and oral care in long-term care homes are dealt with in detail in Chapter 20.

Alternatives to traditional biofilm removal are quite effective in controlling harmful bacteria. Dietary adjustments (Chapter 6); functional foods (Yamanaka *et al.* 2004), probiotics (Chapter 7); xylitol (Chapter 9); chlorhexidine mouth rinses (Chapter 10); and fluorides (Chapter 16) are all part of a comprehensive approach when good oral hygiene is not possible. Focusing on biofilm management instead of just its mechanical removal will create a better outcome and decrease stress in the caregiver who may be trying to remove biofilm every day and failing to keep the growth to a minimum. Oral biofilm management is important because these people, those who cannot provide ADL for themselves, are at risk for pneumonia (Limeback 1998; Scannapieco *et al.* 2003), inability to control blood glucose (Grossi *et al.* 1997; O'Connell *et al.* 2008; Makiura *et al.* 2008), fetid halitosis, infections of the mouth/head (Mylonas *et al.* 2007), pain associated with broken teeth, nutritional imbalance (Mojon *et al.* 1999; Chai *et al.* 2006; De Marchi *et al.* 2008), lethargy, depression (Dumitrescu and Kawamura 2010), hunger, isolation, and impending early death (Kokubo *et al.* 2008) due to any or all of the above.

Comprehensive Preventive Dentistry, First Edition. Edited by Hardy Limeback.
© 2012 John Wiley & Sons, Ltd. Published 2012 by John Wiley & Sons, Ltd.

The dental health care provider can be cognizant of these hurdles and provide alternatives and modifications to traditional brushing and flossing for the dependent adult cohort (Nishiyama et al. 2010; Adachi et al. 2007). When teaching oral care to caregivers, dental care providers should have input. For the most part, education in tooth brushing is taught by nurses to nurses or nursing assistants. Very rarely are dental hygienists asked to prepare and deliver the didactic and or practical lectures for these students. Textbooks are also managed by nurses and perpetuate information that may no longer be accurate. The oral care section should be included in the section on wound care, not cosmetics (Glassman and Subar 2010).

In hospital cases, oral infection control is increasingly becoming a key component in protocols (Buehlmann et al. 2008). Starting in acute situations such as ventilator or tube fed patients, increasing awareness of biofilm management is evident (Berry and Davidson 2006; Powers et al. 2007). Chlorhexidine is playing a confusing roll. Some studies find patients' risk for respiratory infections less (Tantipong et al. 2008) and some find the same risk (Panchabhai et al. 2009; Pobo et al. 2009). The missing component may be a dental hygienist specializing in this type of care. A dental hygienist is uniquely trained in management of oral biofilm and could play a vital role in this practice setting.

The next issue discussed is the less acute condition of those undergoing elective surgery. Oral disinfection is helpful to reduce the respiratory pathogens counts before intubation (Ogata et al. 2004). Children with high risk for Early Childhood Caries (ECC) are at increased risk for acute or chronic otitis media (Alaki et al. 2008). So the care of both infections should be addressed equally and at the same time (Danhauer et al. 2010).

In the USA nurses are applying fluoride varnish to children's teeth to avoid dental decay. The fluoride varnish does not alter the children's biofilm. Once again those uniquely qualified to manage the biofilm, educate parents, and treat the effects of the biofilm infections are left out of the loop. Dental hygienists often train the nurses in fluoride varnish application and never get a chance to provide anticipatory guidance in oral care, tooth eruption, jaw growth, airway and tongue thrust, pacifier use/abuse, and a host of other orocentric effects.

The third tier of hospital cases affected by oral pathogens affects those who have a cross over with other diseases where dental disease becomes an opportunistic infection. Examples are overt cardiac patients, oncology, endocrine (diabetes), respiratory, obstetrics, gynecology, geriatric, and rheumatology (Sjögren's).

Candida infections can kill and are seldom addressed as such. Candida is listed as an opportunistic infection,

and it often has its beginnings in the oral cavity. This fungus can travel and join a biofilm in many distant locations. Incidence of Candida in those with and without oral care shows that professional oral care can decrease this problem and allow patients to recover without succumbing to this type of infection. Falls and debilitating illness or treatments such as chemotherapy of radiation for cancer treatment set up a situation where oral biofilm harboring these opportunistic microbes can and does contribute to the downfall of these susceptible people.

The unchecked presence of oral biofilm is the beginning of a cascade of oral and systemic events. As the biofilm grows the interior of the film houses anaerobic microbes that are slowly multiplying. The perimeter is populated by more active microbes. The films' architecture mushrooms as the complexity of the film increases; channels develop to bring in food and take away waste. The film harbors pathogens that enter into the film and contribute to the society. On occasion different inhabitants of the film escape or are, in effect, asked to leave using quorum sensing.

Inhabitants leave the biofilm as planktonic bacteria. When leaving en mass the term *planktonic shower* describes the event. In the event that this "shower" is within the closed system of the human body, symptoms and manifestations of disease occur.

In the case of periodontal disease, a number of planktonic bacteria enter into the soft tissue wall of the periodontal pocket where they continue to break down tissue. Two separate biofilms grow on both walls of the pocket. The oxygen level is very low in the film and within the tight quarters of the pocket. Anaerobes take hold and the entire body focuses on ridding the body of the invaders. Due to the nature of the biofilm, the body's defenses are useless against the invaders. DNA shifting occurs to protect them even further. Antibiotics are ineffective because the dormant bacteria at the heart of the film are unaffected by the antibiotics targeting rapidly multiplying DNA. When the danger has passed, they reanimate and build another biofilm, or join one already in progress. They grow quietly and then symptoms start to accumulate once more. This occurrence is very evident in a child suffering ear infections. Antibiotics may help, but the child often suffers again and again. The biofilm is never really destroyed. The survivors are altered, and a new antibiotic must be used.

In the modern world oral biofilm removal is often part of the discussion of sweet breath and white teeth. The motivation to brush is immaterial. Whatever it takes is what it should take. The upshot of the infection to the dental team is the loss of the tooth. Collagenase, protease, and other enzymes produced by the body and volatile sulfur compounds (VSC) from the bacteria break down the periodontal fibers as well as inhibit osteoblast proliferation and apoptosis (Zhang *et al.* 2010). Each of these outcomes acts as a negative loop affording stretching room for yet another or larger biofilm. The VSC also contribute to the soft tissue wall porosity allowing not only the white blood cells into the pocket but oral pathogens, from the planktonic showers, into the blood stream to join a biofilm in the vasculature. This also manifests more obviously to bleeding on probing. This gaseous waste product of protein breakdown also affects the fibroblast DNA. These specialized connective tissue cells secrete proteins and molecular collagen that form the extracellular matrix of connective tissue. Collagenase induced by cytokines during an immune response stimulate fibroblasts and osteoblasts and cause indirect tissue damage breaking down collagen in the skin as well as the periodontal fibers.

Currently those outside of dentistry hesitate to incorporate oral health care providers into their protocols; however, the science is screaming out to them. Oral health care should be provided by those who have a firm grasp on how, why, what, and when.

The term 'plaque removal' has taken dentistry and dental hygiene down a garden path. Our utopia is based on teaching people a technical skill that relies heavily on their relationship with oral health, their dexterity, and their level of medical/dental IQ, not to mention their motivation, their level of distractedness, and their life commitments that divert their needs or best intentions.

As a profession clinical dentistry has taken little time to incorporate anything short of mechanical removal of perceived pathogens from the oral surfaces. Little effort is placed on the patients' or clients' uniqueness. The patient's/client's physicality, physiology, or the biology of the oral inhabitants is very rarely taken into consideration. Clinicians resort to badgering, head shaking, and finger wagging in an effort to get people to use a brush and floss as a panacea for all dental illnesses from halitosis to dental decay to oral cancer.

A more accurate term for clinicians to grasp onto is 'biofilm management' as the reference for decreasing pathogens in the oral cavity. Biofilm management can be achieved mechanically by all oral health care providers and by most non-dental professionals. However, we are now fortunate to live in a time when we have much more at our disposal than just brushing and flossing. By using the more accurate term, biofilm management, we are freeing ourselves from the tyranny of the toothbrush and the limitations of dental floss, which is not to say it's time to retire them. This chapter will delve deeply into the mechanical means of biofilm management for the clinician and the non-clinician patient/client to reduce biofilm to a healthy level.

Consumers purchase what they think we would like them to have or use. They will also repurchase what we give them in the dental office, whether it works for them or not. They will also try to follow directions for a very short time then lapse into autopilot brushing mindlessly. Regardless of the style or design of the brush, bristles, handle, color, or material, the bristle end of the brush must touch the teeth and move. Toothbrush designers try to create toothbrushes that take operator error out of the equation; however, each person has a unique error that can be addressed.

Aside from the traditional stick toothbrush, many other designs are on the market, and each fills a niche. There is no 'one-size-fits-all' toothbrush. People need a different tool for mechanical biofilm management as they go through life stages from birth to adulthood, from health to debilitating physical or mental illness.

The toothbrush

Design

The toothbrush has been around for centuries (as a stick brush; see below). The modern toothbrush has not evolved much from that idea. There are three parts to the brush:

- The head
- The neck (shank)
- The handle

All three components have undergone modifications over time. The handle has built-in properties to assist users in brushing their teeth. Currently the Bass technique has garnered favor as a technique for massaging the soft tissue and removing the most debris from the hard tissue (Poyato-Ferrera *et al.* 2003). This Bass technique was modified to incorporate the sulcular space, a distance of up to 3 millimeters; however, the bristle tip has limited access.

Bristles or filaments

The actual brush is made of a cluster of nylon filaments fastened together and attached to the brush head with a fastener resembling a staple. Over the centuries the bristles have evolved from animal hair (boar or horse) to man-made nylon or polyester materials.

Modern bristles

Bristles are almost exclusively made of nylon in North America. They are routinely between five to eight thousandths of an inch in diameter. The smaller the diameter, the more flexibility it has. Small diameter filaments are used in soft bristles, and even smaller diameter filaments are used in the sensitive designation for the bristles. The filament diameter is not the only determining factor of brush stiffness, sometimes called hardness of the brush. The length of the filament and the angle of the tuft to the handle determine the stiffness sensation as well.

Imagine the bristle tuft inserted into the handle perpendicularly. As the user moves the brush back and forth from the front of the mouth to the back (anterior to posterior), the bristles move freely in either direction. If the tuft is inserted with the smaller angle toward the head of the brush and the larger angle toward the neck of the brush, the bristles will feel stiffer moving posteriorly as compared to moving anteriorly.

Placing the bristles in rows alternating anterior-leaning and posterior-leaning gives the impression of better-cleaning, stiffer bristles to the user. Patients, it seems, like the feeling of a stiffer-bristled toothbrush, which is why industry is inventive in tufting angles. See Figure 8-1.

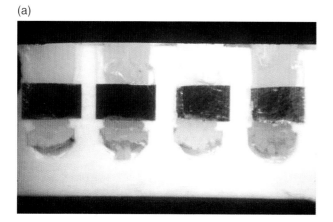

Figure 8-1 Toothbrush with angled insertion of bristles.

Too stiff a brush will harm the soft tissue (Zimmer and Oztürk 2011). Soft bristle brushes are recommended, in general, for that reason. There are new brushes with silicone bristles. A PubMed search on this type of bristle did not reveal any research on this kind of addition. This would be a good topic for a class research project.

Of course this is not for everyone. It's amazing how many people have different views of what works for them. Just the idea of using a new brush, a new brush design, or even a new color may increase the user's time with the brush. Time, of course, is still the most important aspect of using any brush.

Figure 8-2 shows how the majority of bristles are anchored to the brush. Upon close inspection the space left by the staple is visible. A grouping of filaments is called a tuft. If the required number of filaments per tuft is 30, for instance, 15 filaments are used and folded in half by a staple that is forced into the plastic of the brush head. This staple holds the bristles in place creating a tuft of bristles. In most brushes, the tuft is perpendicular to the head, and the filament ends are polished, called end rounding. The end rounding of the bristle tufts protects the soft tissue from abrasion, and is an important part of the manufacturing process (Carvalho *et al.* 2007).

Very inexpensive brushes often have poorly fastened tufts. They also do not have consistent end rounding of the filaments. The lack of attention to these two manufacturing processes makes the brushing experience less than satisfactory because the bristles are likely to abrade the gingiva and/or to fall out. Very inexpensive toothbrushes also use handle material that bends easily with the pressure necessary to brush the teeth.

(a)

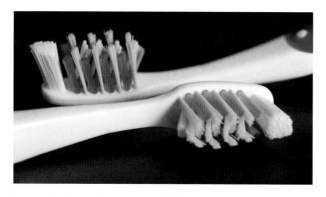

(b)

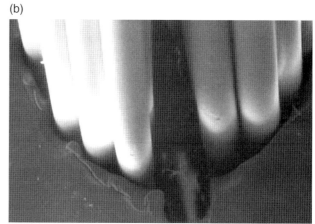

Figure 8-2 Tuft anchoring. Toothbrush filaments are anchored in three ways. This figure shows staple-set tufting. (a) shows a longitudinal section of the toothbrush head. The bundles are not fixed tightly enough to the synthetic material. This creates gaps and holes, which form part of the outer surface. The gaps are made visible by the scanning electron microscope (b). From Wetzel *et al.* (2005). © 2005 American Dental Association. All rights reserved. Reprinted by permission.

(a)

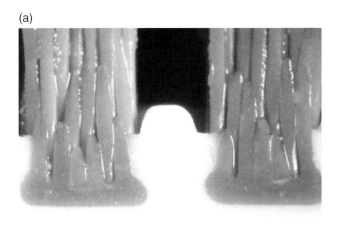

(b)

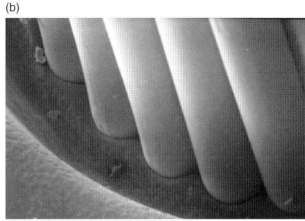

Figure 8-3 In-mold tufting. The photographs show that the bases of the bundles are joined closely to the head of the toothbrush (a). Only a few gaps are visible; however, they do not reach the outer surface. The scanning electron microscope analysis revealed tight anchoring (b). From Wetzel *et al.* (2005). © 2005 American Dental Association. All rights reserved. Reprinted by permission.

(a)

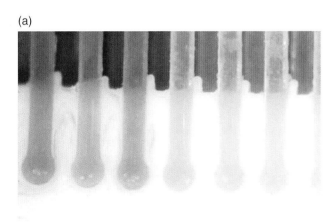

(b)

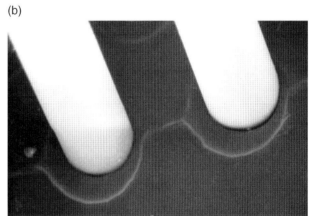

Figure 8-4 Filaments placed in the mold individually. This technique prevents gaps and holes almost completely. The bases of the filaments are round-shaped, which facilitates their mechanical fixation (a). Analysis with the scanning electron microscope showed a bulge located at one side of the filament base. The surrounding material is attached completely (b). From Wetzel *et al.* (2005). © 2005 American Dental Association. All rights reserved. Reprinted by permission.

Anchoring the tuft may also be achieved by forcing the bristles into the hot handle material during the manufacturing process. The strength of the hold is comparable to stapling although the process is slightly more expensive (Figure 8-3).

The bristle placement can alter the cleanliness of the brush or the ease in which the brush can be cleaned. Of the three main types of tuft anchors—staple set tufting, in-mold tufting, and individual in-mold placement—staple set tufts are the hardest to keep clean.

In-mold tufting is a manufacturing process where the tufts are welded together into a single bundle and inserted into a premade hole in the head of the brush. The space between the bristles is filled in with an injected material that fuses the tuft into place.

The individual in-mold placement of filaments allows for the most flexibility in brush head design. The bristles may all be of different lengths and caliber, that is, they needn't be inserted in tufts. See Figure 8-4.

Each individual filament is inserted into the head of the brush and secured by the cooling handle material. Manufacturing the brush like this is costly, however, the brush is cleaner and carries less bioburden (Wetzel *et al.* 2005). The bristles themselves may be coated with an antimicrobial.

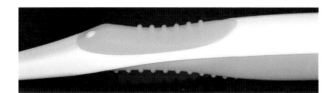

Figure 8-5 Example of a handle thumb rest and finger grip area on a toothbrush.

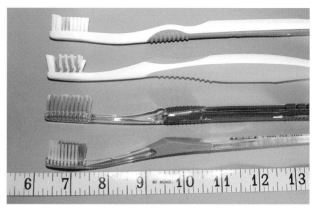

Figure 8-6 Toothbrushes with bristles at various planes with respect to the handles. In the toothbrush on the bottom, the bristle tips have been placed at the same plane as the handle.

Chlorhexidine has been used to decrease the bacterial load on the actual bristles, as have Triclosan and some metals like copper and silver. Each has exhibited some benefits however not long term (Turner *et al.* 2009). It appears that the coated bristles have no ability to keep the bacterial load down better than toothpaste (Quirynen *et al.* 2003). Other additions to the brush head make claims of better feel, better plaque removal, and even whitening. If the patient/client uses the brush longer and gets any clinical results there is no shame in allowing them to continue using it.

The handle

Toothbrush handles come in many configurations. The most popular stick handle works for most people, which is not to say that it is the only handle that works for everyone. When working with healthy children, teaching the use of a stick handle toothbrush is popular, and students find it easy to learn. Designs in toothbrush handles can be esthetically pleasing, which is highly important for some people, or the handle can be helpful in moving the bristles in the most desirable way.

The stick handle usually has a place for the thumb to rest. The thumb rest is a natural part of the handle/hand interface and can be used to help the user angle the bristles appropriately (Figure 8-5).

Education in the proper brushing technique is always a challenge and raises some interesting questions. For instance is it critical for a caregiver to work on the angle of the brush to reach the gumline, or is it more important to just brush the teeth regardless of the angulation? If the Bass technique is so superior how much time should be given to teach the method to a group of 9-year-old children, 15 year olds, or young adults?

The idea of the toothbrush doing more of the work is an idea that has fostered the designs of toothbrushes over the last century. A new toothbrush design focusing on the shape of the bristles in a convex shape intended the bristles to go into the sulcus without the person using the brush thinking through their process. The shape would allow the user to simply place the brush against the teeth, and they would automatically bend into the sulcus.

Comparing the flat head against the convex head did not support the new design (Staudt *et al.* 2001).

The neck of the toothbrush

It is generally agreed that a bend in the neck of the brush is helpful, and a contra angle is often employed. The main point is to find the best place for the bristle tips to be in relation to the handle of the brush. For instance in Figure 8-6, you can see the working end of the tufts are not on the same plane as the handle.

The toothbrush shown on the bottom is closest to that design. In speaking with toothbrush designers and manufacturers, they find that having the bristle tips on an even plane with the handle gives the user a feeling that they do not have to press as hard on the teeth. And this design feature is often a selling point to dental hygienists.

The neck of the brush can also be modified by the user at home or by the clinician in the treatment room before giving the brush to the patient/client. By warming the neck of the brush with hot tap water, the brush handle can be bent to customize it for the patient/clients (Figure 8-7). One basic modification to help achieve the angles needed to perform the modified Bass technique (Battaglia 2008) on the posterior and lower anterior teeth is to bend the neck twice so the bristle tips are still parallel to the handle, but lower.

Care of the toothbrush

The toothbrush may be a vector for pathogens (Saravia *et al.* 2008). The idea of bristles from different brushes touching one another and passing the bacteria back and forth is not unheard of. It is also interesting to note that a toothbrush near a flushing toilet has potential to be contaminated with fecal matter. Bacterium including

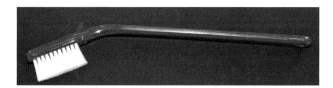

Figure 8-7 Heated with hot tap water, this brush handle is easy to bend.

Staphylococci, streptococci, Candida, Haemophilus, fungi, molds, *Corynebacterium*, pseudomonads, and coliforms are present on toothbrushes used for a few weeks (Taji and Rogers 1998; Malmberg *et al.* 1994). Oral biofilm harbors *E. coli* and other fecal bacteria, the source of which are likely toilets nearby that create aerosols when the lid is left up during flushing (Barker and Jones 2005). For the most part, the healthy human body is able to maintain a homeostasis in the presence of many pathogens. However, the contaminated toothbrush is most harmful to people with compromised immune systems. Whether induced by medical treatments such as chemotherapy (Ahmed *et al.* 2003; Danilatou *et al.* 2004) or as a function of systemic breakdown, toothbrushes and the oral health of the patient/client should be monitored closely by an experienced clinician.

Using a clean (that is, new) toothbrush frequently helps reduce bacteria in the mouth. Pai (2009) showed that using a new brush every day for 30 days reduced oral bacteria in healthy volunteers. For the person with a severely compromised immune system using a new toothbrush every day may be more helpful than any other method in reducing bacterial numbers to a less harmful level. At first glance it may sound expensive. The cost of bringing a person back to health after a bacteremia caused by oral bacteria far exceeds the cost of using a new brush every day. Pai suggested replacing a toothbrush at least monthly in *healthy* people.

One way to clean the brush for those who are not compromised is the use of the dishwasher (Figure 8-8).

For people with healthy gingival tissue, a regular wash cycle may be all that's necessary. Other popular ways of decontaminating the bristles are to use an antimicrobial mouthwash, an ultraviolet light (Figure 8-9), and ozone gas (Caudry *et al.* 1995; Boylan *et al.* 2008; Bezirtzoglou *et al.* 2008).

Caudry *et al.* (1995) showed that a 20-minute bath in a mouthwash containing essential oils killed bacteria normally associated with the toothbrush. The American Dental Association (ADA) recommends that people not store their brushes in an enclosed space, like a toothbrush head enclosure. The best defense against contaminated bristles, according to the ADA, is to let them completely air dry. However, some studies find remaining contaminants

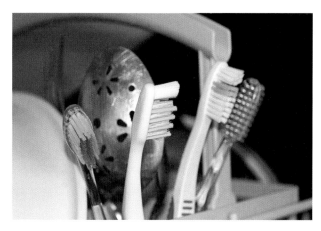

Figure 8-8 Toothbrushes being cleaned in a dishwasher.

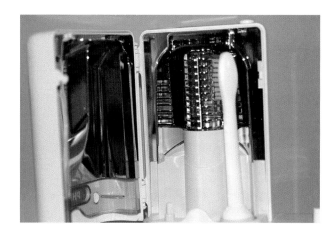

Figure 8-9 An example of a commercial UV light-sanitizing chamber for electric toothbrush heads.

after 24 hours of air drying. No mention is made of the humidity of the air in these studies. Given these parameters a person who is suffering an illness should use two toothbrushes concurrently to allow one to fully dry after soaking it in an acceptable mouthwash solution.

An immunocompromised person should ideally use a new brush every day, or at least one that has been disinfected between use. A pre-rinse with an acceptable mouthwash before brushing would be a good investment as well. Using toothpaste can reduce the bacterial load in the brush. For most people the traditional use of a toothbrush with toothpaste applied then rinsed off when finished will keep the brush free of pathogens, or at least most of the pathogens.

Toothpaste

A general discussion about toothpaste is warranted here in our discussion of plaque control. Avoiding the topic in the section on biofilm removal would leave a hole in the discussion because most people use toothpaste with their toothbrush, and many claims are made by toothpaste manufacturers. The current thinking is that it is the brush that reduces the biofilm and that toothpaste has little added effect (Paraskevas *et al.* 2007; Jayakumar *et al.* 2010).

Toothpaste has three main features: taste, abrasiveness, and fluoride delivery. It is commonly believed that the better the toothpaste flavor, the longer the brushing episode. The abrasives in the toothpaste, which are there to remove surface stains can also abrade tooth structure, especially dentin. Using the toothbrush as a fluoride delivery system is the best reason to use toothpaste.

The clinician should be aware of the patient's tolerances and preferences along with their clinical needs when recommending toothpaste. The fluoride concentration of the dentifrice is standardized at about 1,000 ppm fluoride. This has proven to be a relatively safe amount to use at home. The controversy around fluoride rages on though. (See Chapter 16.) In defense of fluoride, it works best when applied topically (Lynch *et al.* 2004).

The fluoride used in toothpaste is a pharmaceutical-grade drug that is intended to be used in the mouth and expectorated. Like aspirin and chocolate, the whole tube of toothpaste is not intended to be used at one time. Even a whole bag of candy will cause emesis in most children. The warning on the tube of toothpaste could be put on a whole list of products starting with chocolate cake. Patient/clients worried about fluoride in their toothpaste may be amenable to some of the other remineralization products on the market today (Rao *et al.* 2009).

There are two basic problems associated with toothpaste use: tooth abrasion and soft tissue sloughing. Tooth abrasion is commonly attributed to the toothbrush; however, many studies on the phenomenon show toothpaste to be the culprit (Kodaka *et al.* 1993; Wiegand *et al.* 2008; Franzò *et al.* 2010). Practically speaking, toothpaste abrasion occurs in two main ways. The most common way is to use too much toothpaste. A large stripe of toothpaste balancing on the tips of the bristles the length of the brush head is too much. Recommendations for toothpaste use follow:

1. People over 6 years of age a pea/pearl size amount.
2. People under 6 years of age a rice size amount, or a very thin smear.

When people load their brush with a TV commercial amount of paste and put the loaded brush in the same place at the same time over and over for years, a toll is taken on the enamel. If the tooth's root is visible at the margin of the tooth, the dentin will wear faster than the more mineralized enamel. This abrasive problem is also evident on the acrylic of a denture. To avoid this damage,

a smaller amount of toothpaste on the brush is called for and starting in a different location in the mouth is also helpful. Today toothpastes contain functional ingredients such as amorphous calcium phosphate (ACP), bio-active glass with ACP (NovaMin) and Recaldent (CPP-ACP). (See Chapter 18.) Although no studies to date have looked at abrasion with these toothpaste ingredients, it would seem that abrasion would be less when enamel-building components are present.

Baking soda in toothpaste has been erroneously thought to be very abrasive. It is not. Baking soda, or sodium bicarbonate, has very low abrasivity due its solubility (Muñoz *et al.* 2004).

In extreme cases of caries infection, the use of baking soda straight from the box may be indicated. Caries is a pH-mitigated disease. A quick lift to the alkaline from baking soda used as a tooth powder, or in a homemade mouth rinse, may be indicated. Some people like to use baking soda. The clinician can rest assured that the patient/client can retain enamel using this mild abrasive. Baking soda in toothpaste and chewing gum can help buffer acids and remove surface stains easily.

Along with the good flavor of the toothpaste, people like the foaming action which is the cause of the second problem with toothpaste—tissue sloughing. Some toothpaste companies advertise their toothpaste as having superior foaming and that the foam contributes to the overall cleaning ability of toothpaste. This may be true.

Sodium lauryl sulfate (SLS) is the most common foaming agent in toothpaste, and some people are very susceptible to tissue reactions to it. The damage may manifest as an aphthous ulcer or tissue sloughing (Herlofson *et al.* 1996). SLS is a detergent, or whetting agent, that penetrates bacterial cell walls and interferes with bacterial adhesion. Although it may irritate soft tissue in some people, SLS has also been shown to improve fluoride uptake in dental plaque (Nordström *et al.* 2009). Other foaming agents are available. Sodium lauroyl sarcosinate is another safe surfactant and cleansing agent that may be less caustic to those who have difficulty using SLS, and it is tolerated well by the groups of people that prefer natural foods.

Although toothpaste is the major culprit in enamel/root abrasion, the brush is not totally innocent. Using a toothbrush on enamel during the demineralization phase is thought to damage the tooth. Erosive foods and erosive (low pH) beverages particularly those containing citrus acid, trigger demineralization episodes, and brushing before remineralization takes place can affect the enamel negativity. Athletes are at risk because their sport drinks are usually a low pH and contain highly titratable citric acid. Compounding the low pH, exertion often requires mouth breathing, which decreases mouth moisture, therefore, the healing benefits of saliva are not fully realized (Sirimaharaj *et al.* 2002). The clinician should also be aware of this when tempted to polish teeth at the beginning of a dental procedure. Under the biofilm, one may find damaged enamel at the biofilm enamel interface. As most polishing pastes contain pumice, the damage to the enamel under the film may be irreversible. Some sources even recommend brushing the teeth before eating taking advantage of the hardest enamel and applying fluoride at the optimum time (British Health Foundation 2010).

Tooth erosion may also be attributable to GERD (Gastroesophageal Reflux Disease), bulimia, alcoholism, or the habit of swishing carbonated (carbonic acid) drinks before swallowing. (See Chapter 13.)

Interdental cleaning aids

Interdental brushes may be made similarly to the toothbrush. Bristles are placed into a handle, and the person running the brush moves the bristles between the teeth in an effort to remove the biofilm and food debris accumulated there (Figure 8-10).

Proper instruction of the use of the interdental cleaning aid has proven to be extremely beneficial. Tissue health improves, regardless of the aid used (Jackson *et al.* 2006).

The end tuft brush is an option that is often recommended when the embrasure space between the teeth is large or if the patient/client is wearing braces. The handles of the end tuft brushes are often larger and easier to manage than some of the thin handles. Handle design should be as important as bristles and head size when choosing an interdental aid.

End tuft brushes feature a small brush head making it easy to maneuver, particularly in the following instances:

- Between the buccinator muscle and the teeth
- Posterior embrasures from the buccal or the lingual
- Difficult-to-reach areas around orthodontic brackets
- Special maintenance concerns
  - implants
  - crowded teeth
  - bridges
  - crowns

The bristle tufts are often set in a circular pattern with shorter bristles on the outer ring, and taller bristles in the center. Instructions may include moving the bristles from the buccal or from the lingual or both. The design does not include a wire, which is a major feature in the inter-proximal brushes.

Interproximal brushes

Interproximal brushes are extremely versatile. The major architecture is a central wire twisted around nylon

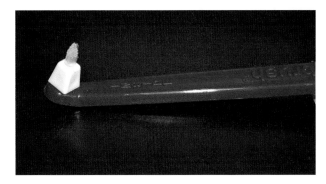

Figure 8-10 The 'Sulcabrush': an example of a specialized brush for cleaning the sulcus, gingival margins, and interproximal papillary areas.

filaments of varying lengths. Usually the filaments are very short. (See Figure 8-11.) This is where experience and education come in. There are many types of these little brushes with many attributes. Each patient/client must be evaluated for each type of brush. Those with titanium implants should use an interdental brush with a coated wire or refrain from using a wired brush as scratching the implant can increase the surface area for biofilm.

Manual dexterity

People who would benefit from using an interdental brush are often those with some type of dexterity limitation. A small brush with a small handle requiring a pinch-type grip may not be of value to certain patients.

Whitening brushes

Many people are obsessed with white teeth. They may have other glaring unfortunate body issues, and white teeth may be the only thing they can control. Darkening teeth is a sign of aging (Laskarin *et al.* 2006). It is unlikely that whitening brushes will contribute to increase the whiteness of teeth, however, if it helps to keep the patient/client motivated to clean their interdental spaces, it is money well spent.

Micro picks

A micro-interdental brush may be used as an alternative to floss for some (Yankell *et al.* 2002). Because of their size, the micro picks are very delicate and made to be disposable. The sticks have a flexible plastic pick, sometimes coated with silicon filaments, that easily adjusts for thorough and comfortable cleaning around all spaces, even in between tight teeth and hard to reach posterior teeth. These types of picks are often sold in small matchbook type containers, and individual picks are simply snapped off then discarded after use. Single usage keeps the brushes antibacterial and hygienic.

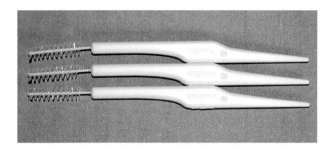

Figure 8-11 Interdental brush/pick. Some interdental brushes are one-piece plastic brushes, as shown here. Others are nylon bristles anchored in twisted wires.

Toothpicks, chew sticks (miswak)

Wood is a very good substitute for modern plastic or wire picks and brushes to clean teeth. When damp/wet, the softened cellulose fibers not only mechanically disturb plaque but the pressure from the wood pick or bristles and the capillary action of the cellulose can remove toxins from the biofilm.

Miswak sticks, obtained from the branches of the Miswak bushes in the Middle East to South and Southeast Asia, have been used as chew sticks for centuries to clean teeth (Figure 8-12).

The extract from the wood has been tested against a low pH oral environment and found to raise it (Sofrata *et al.* 2007); the wood itself has antimicrobial properties (Sofrata *et al.* 2008). The fact that it also contains fluoride makes this centuries-old plaque removal tool an excellent choice as an adjunct to, or replacement for, a toothbrush (al-Otaibi *et al.* 2004). The sticks are used on the teeth much like an eraser. The twig is softened in saliva, the outer bark is chewed off, and the fibrous core forms a brush, which lasts a few days. The 'brush' end of the twig is rubbed against the teeth and gingiva. Once the brush becomes abused looking, it is cut off, the bark removed once more, and fresh fibrous core filaments are exposed (Al-Otaibi *et al.* 2004). The Miswak chewing stick is a good alternative to a toothbrush and is sanctioned by the World Health Organization.

Nonfilament interdental cleaners

Sometimes the wire in the filament brushes is irritating to the gums or to the tooth itself. If the patient/client cannot maneuver the brush, or if the wire is a problem, a different interdental cleaning aid can be used to achieve biofilm removal. Many of these newer cleaning aids use less abrasive surfaces, such as velour, sponge, or floss woven into a fine mesh molded into a plastic stem. Some of these products may contain fluoride to provide extra protection to the tooth.

Denture brushes

The denture brush is made with thicker filaments than a traditional toothbrush. And most designs are aimed at providing the user with one single brush with which to brush all aspects of a complicated denture or partial denture design. The brush will remove soft deposits, not calculus. Studies have looked at the potential damage a stiff denture brush can make on the acrylic of the denture. Like teeth, it seems as though acrylic dentures can withstand the brush but have trouble with toothpaste. The best cleaning method for cleaning a denture is an effervescent tablet and a scrub with a denture brush and water.

Orthodontic brushes

People undergoing orthodontic treatment have very special needs. A common time for embarking on orthodontic treatment is at a time when children are not really ready to take care of themselves, and professional responsibility must prevail. That is to say that the clinician must take on more responsibility for oral cleanliness. This may mean that the patient may need to visit the clinician in very short intervals, perhaps even as often as every week.

The extra areas where the biofilm can hide harbor acidophiles, and adding acidic soft drinks and candies give these bacteria an ideal environment to proliferate. Toothbrushes made for brackets are still only as good as the user. A meta-analysis on power brushes versus manual brushes in people undergoing orthodontic treatment found neither to be better than the other (Kaklamanos and Kalfas 2008). Meta-analysis should not be the last word. If the person undergoing treatment is not fulfilling their obligation to remove their oral biofilm then the braces should be removed. This kind of statement is not easy to make, and there are not many orthodontists who can stomach this harsh treatment, but it has to be done. What good are straight teeth if they are totally without enamel? The decision to remove brackets and bands must be made swiftly. Giving the child 1 more month to shape up, or else, can easily suddenly be 18 months into treatment with disastrous results.

Special cases

The idea that "tooth brushing is easy," or that "everyone can do it" is not true or helpful. Many people have limitations due to physical or mental shortcomings or dental conditions. Those with Parkinson's disease, rheumatoid arthritis, or mixed dentition have special tooth brushing needs that can be warmly addressed by the dental health care provider. Handle modifications for those with dexterity problems range from home modifications to putting a tennis ball on the end of a brush handle for

(a)

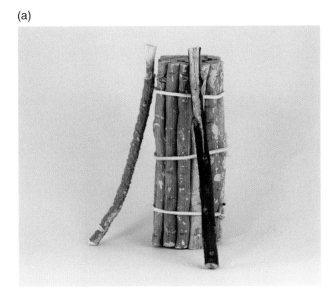

(b)

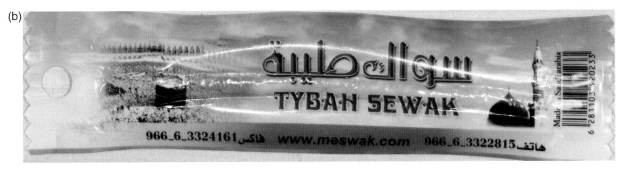

(c)

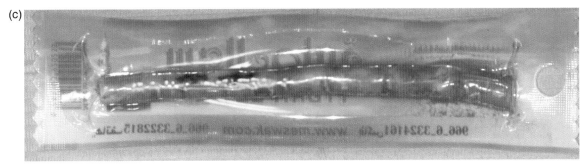

Figure 8-12 Examples of Miswak products sold in the Middle East. These are now being sold in North America in specialty shops. The sticks are available in bundles (a) or sold individually in hygienic wrappers (b and c).

example. This will have to be addressed with the caregiver or the patient/client him or herself. Studies looking at modifications are not helpful. Too many variables cannot be adjusted for when sending a person home with a toothbrush (de Mattos *et al.* 1998; Reeson and Jepson 2002).

Universally speaking, though, a few generalities can be made, such as the following:

1. Persons with Parkinson's disease rely on the weight of the item they're holding to stabilize the shaking hand. A tennis ball or bike grip will not work for them as well as a weighty power brush.

2. Persons with rheumatoid arthritis may need a molded handle created in the office with them present. A type of putty where their grip can be molded into the handle may be a working answer for people with this condition (de Mattos *et al.* 1998).

3. Patients with osteoarthritis have the peak dexterity and least amount of pain in the mid-afternoon (Read *et al.* 1981; Bellamy *et al.* 2002). Therefore, it may be

worthwhile to suggest the major oral hygiene be performed in the afternoon before dinnertime.

4. Children with mixed dentition, particularly those with erupting molars, do better on partially erupted molars with a power brush than a manual brush with longer bristles on the tip (Gonçalves *et al.* 2007).

5. Persons who have mental illnesses or autism may find toothbrushing or toothbrushes or even toothpastes incredibly distasteful or frightening. Alternatives such as xylitol, cranberry, probiotics, or mouth rinses may be necessary to improve hygiene in these groups. (See also chapters 6, 7, and 9.)

6. People who cannot care for their own teeth have better oral care if their caregiver has a higher dental IQ, so educating the caregiver on their own care is worthwhile.

Special design in toothbrushes

In an effort to make tooth brushing easier, more fun, more sanitary, more effective, or faster, some novelty toothbrushes often come to the forefront. The most popular unusual design is the triple-headed toothbrush. The goal of the design of these brushes is to address all three sides of the tooth in one motion, in effect cutting the time for brushing down by two-thirds (Azrak *et al.* 2004). These brushes are designed with different targets in mind: children, elderly (Miolin *et al.* 2007), mentally ill (Doğan *et al.* 2004), or infirm persons. Most of these brushes have shortcomings that may be difficult to overcome by the clinician. Although a traditional three-headed brush may seem like a good idea, the design may be great only for children. An older person or persons unable to perform their own oral hygiene may not be able to access the most vulnerable part of the tooth with it—the root. The clinician making recommendations must weigh the importance of removing all of the biofilm from all surfaces of all of the teeth and whether the person will use the brush at all. The roots may need to be coated with a glass ionomer or resin-modified glass ionomer to protect them if the brush and brusher will not or cannot access that area.

Another specialty design feature in toothbrushes is the colored bristle. Manufacturers use red or black bristles to hide bleeding. People who suddenly brush their teeth correctly are often alarmed when they see blood on the bristles. Masking the bleeding can help people brush their teeth with an appropriate amount of force and not become distressed and stop brushing altogether.

Inventors have created an electronic toothbrush that will clean all tooth surfaces, top and bottom, at once (Hydrabrush 2011).

This is a multi-headed brush that is designed to be bitten into, has bristles on the chewing side, and rests at a 45-degree angle on the lingual and buccal. It moves back and forth horizontally, much like the blades of an electric carving knife. The user bites into the brush heads and moves the tip of the machine from the anterior teeth to the posterior on one side and then from the anterior to the posterior teeth on the other side. This brush has already been shown to work as well as other powered toothbrushes already on the market (Patters *et al.* 2005).

Building a better mousetrap, or toothbrush, is an endeavor that many dentists and dental hygienists find enjoyable, if not profitable.

Manual versus power brushes

This question will never have a definitive answer. Again, the number of variables is overwhelming. The robotic studies of toothbrushes do not reflect the *in vivo* condition, and the *in vivo* studies cannot provide consistent results between users, or times of use. Many studies compare this brush and that one to the other one, and nearly all of the studies are mounted by the maker of the brush. In nearly all head-to-head toothbrush studies (no pun intended), the brush of the manufacturer that initiated the study wins the competition. If a toothbrush manufacturer were to embark on and pay for a study that did not show its brush to be superior, the research likely wouldn't be published.

A meta-analysis by the Cochrane Group has stated that there is lack of good research in this area. In a very public display in the year 2003, the group released their analysis of power toothbrush versus manual brush studies and found a very controversial outcome. The Cochrane Group tried to analyze unbiased research, which is code for independent research, that is, research not paid for by a company whose brush was studied. Only about 30 studies fit their criteria in a field of more than 300 potential papers. Less than 10% of the potential studies were used, conversely over 90% of the studies were discarded.

The trouble with meta-analysis in dentistry

Dentistry as a medical field is still a cottage industry. Dentists and dental hygienists practice with latitude unheard of in today's medical world. They create new and innovative products and often never mount a study to prove its worth. When studies are mounted, researchers had no incentive to look at previous studies and resemble a previous design. The following data are the Methods and Results sections of the abstract of Forrest and Miller (2004):

METHODS: Search strategies to identify published clinical trials on power toothbrushes were developed, and manufacturers were contacted for additional published and unpublished information. Trials were selected based on pre-established criteria; including whether they compared power versus manual toothbrushes used a randomized research design tested products in the general population without disabilities, provided data on plaque and gingivitis, and were at least 28 days in length. Six reviewers independently extracted information in duplicate. Indices for plaque and gingivitis levels were expressed as standardized mean differences for data distillation. Data distillation was accomplished using a meta-analysis, with a mean difference between power and manual toothbrushes as the measure of effectiveness.

RESULTS: Searches identified 354 trials, of which 29 met inclusion criteria. These trials involved 2,547 participants who provided data for meta-analysis. Results indicated that for both plaque and gingivitis, all types of power toothbrushes worked as well as manual toothbrushes, however only the rotating oscillating toothbrush consistently provided a statistically significant though modest benefit over manual toothbrushes in reducing plaque (7%) and gingivitis (17%). None of the battery powered toothbrush studies met the inclusion criteria.

As you can see, of the 354 trials identified that compared the toothbrush types, only 29 met the inclusion criteria. So if one brush reduced gingivitis by 23% in a 2-week study, it was not included. And studies that were 6 weeks long did not fit the inclusion criteria either. Notice too that none of the battery-powered toothbrushes met the inclusion criteria. That is not to say that battery-powered toothbrushes were not helpful in removing plaque or decreasing bleeding or healing gingivitis.

The comment about rotating oscillating brushes created quite a stir. Power brushes have been around in some form or fashion since the 1960s providing a wealth of research. Sonic brushes had only been in existence for little over a decade. Just because a meta-analysis is published, it cannot be more heavily weighted than other research in the dental field until more research is easier to combine.

As an example of how reviews of more recent studies can change our opinion of the best methods for oral hygiene, the Cochrane Oral Health Group carried a follow-up review of powered toothbrushes. Head-to-head (no pun intended) studies were compared, and it was concluded that no powered toothbrush was better than the other (Deacon *et al.* 2010).

Brushing time

The time it takes to brush a full complement of teeth is often a topic of conversation between clinicians and patient/clients. The recommended amount of time is 2 minutes, or 120 seconds, according to the toothbrush industry as evidenced by the prolific amount of timers on power brushes set at 2 minutes. The time is often divided up into quadrants, where the brush is used for 15 seconds each in the upper right buccal and lingual, upper left buccal and lingual; lower right buccal and lingual and lower left buccal and lingual. Although patients truly think that they brush for upward of 2 minutes, studies tell us that the average time a person brushes their teeth is about 33 seconds, only one-sixth the amount of time necessary to achieve plaque-free status.

Studies of uninstructed time for tooth brushing are old. Although the 1980s where hardly the dark ages, an entire generation has grown up and started a new generation in the interim. It may be time to look at how brushing times have changed over the nearly 30 years since the early studies were published.

The counting method may be a better way to teach tooth brushing as compared to timing. A set time for brushing does not ensure that all areas of the mouth are addressed equally or beneficially. This method suggests that each stroke be repeated to 10. For instance, in the modified Bass technique, the brush is placed in a location at the preferred 45-degree angle and the vibratory "stroke" be activated for a count of 10. And this counting method would be repeated as the person brushing moves around the mouth in a systematic fashion. The brush is moved just short of one heads length and the movement repeated to a count of 10, then moved again.

How best to teach brushing

The studies that look at how best to teach brushing are lacking. The main aspects to teaching this skill are show and tell in the treatment room, written directions, and video directions. Patients who have access to video instruction after the show and tell have the best results and best retention of the lesson. There are a number of tooth-brushing videos on YouTube, and it may be beneficial to find one to recommend to the patient/clients. It may also be worthwhile to videotape the patient/client instructions and email them or give the patient/client a device (on a CD, DVD, thumb drive, smart phone) to carry the personal instructions home with them. As more and more practices have their own Web site, an area of videos on biofilm removal may be a worthwhile endeavor.

A very low-tech way to motivate patient/clients to brush better is to use an automatic feedback system. Twice a year is not enough feedback to motivate people to make a change. Using disclosing solution at the office to teach people areas of inadequate toothbrushing is an example of an automatic feedback system. Asking them to use it at home can be very effective in creating change. Brushing until the disclosed biofilm is removed is a great way to give feedback. The opposite is also true, that is to use the disclosing solution after brushing.

The use of pH test strips may also contribute to better home care and adequate brushing. Using pH strips allows people to see when their oral pH changes and how brushing can make a change (Schäfer *et al.* 2003).

Fixed prosthesis biofilm removal

Fixed prostheses include implants, crowns, and bridges. They present a definite challenge for the patient/client with respect to biofilm management. Often the patient/client will not fully understand this type of restoration.

Implants

The Association of Dental Implant Auxiliaries (ADIA) (adiaonline.org) provides the following insight on implants:

> Implants are substitutes for teeth and they are today's best alternative to your natural teeth. They offer you a permanent or secure solution for replacing one or more teeth. They are made of biocompatible materials, just the same as hip implants or similar orthopedic devices, and function as anchors or support for traditional forms of dentistry, such as crowns, bridges or dentures. Many of our patients will tell you that implants have changed not only their smiles, their overall appearance but also even their lives! There are numerous other reasons to choose dental implants:
>
> Esthetically, they support teeth that look like real teeth.
> Functionally, dental implants feel and act like real teeth.
> With implants, you can eat and chew again without pain or irritation. Foods that were forbidden are now back in the diet.
> Implants eliminate the need for distasteful adhesives. There is no longer a need to use "glue" when your prosthesis is anchored to implants.
> Implants can actually improve the taste of food. With less plastic covering the roof of your mouth, you can enjoy natural sensations again.
> Lastly, implants can help maintain your bone structure and support your facial tissues. They can reduce or eliminate bone atrophy, which causes "shrinkage" or facial cosmetic changes.
>
> Are implants successful?
> Implants, as we know them today, have been in existence for at least twenty-five years. For the last ten years, however, success rates at many treatment centers are consistently over 95% with proper personal and professional care. Few forms of medical, orthopedic or dental treatment have such high success rates (Association of Dental Implant Auxiliaries (ADIA).

Implants should be cleaned the same as other teeth. They are susceptible to the same risks as natural teeth, except caries infections.

Floss can be a better adjunct to oral health in implants than regular teeth, as the implant is smoother and does not exhibit the rough surface that the natural tooth does. (See the sidebar.)

> To apply the Modified Bass Technique (aka Intrasulcular), the bristles of the brush are placed into the sulcus at a 45-degree angle, the bristles are mobilized in a vibration type movement, then swept toward to the occlusal portion of the tooth.

Crowns

Gold crowns and bridges are becoming popular once again. The human body tolerates this metal very well, and oral complications like itching, edema, redness, and pain are almost unheard of. These tissue reactions are histamine related. Porcelain fused to metal or other types of metal-based crowns usually contains an alloy that contains nickel. Nickel allergy can affect people of all ages. A nickel allergy usually develops after repeated or prolonged exposure to items containing nickel. Until the fixed prosthesis is placed, a patient/client may be only in contact to nickel in jewelry. When tissue response is less than optimal, the allergy question should be asked of the patient/client.

The esthetics of gold alloy was a negative feature years ago. Gold restorations vacillated between status symbol and ugly. The longevity of cast gold alloy restorations is a benefit, and if they can afford such restorations, educated patients sometimes prefer them to other options. Cast gold restorations were most popular from the 1930s to the 1970s. Esthetic options for their esthetics alone were not well received by the dental profession at that time.

In the early 1960s, the porcelain-fused-to-metal, or PFM, was reintroduced to the profession. Many dentists rejected the PFM restoration. Its acceptance started off slowly, as clinicians started to see more patient acceptance, and patients requested tooth-colored restorations. Dentists became increasingly comfortable with esthetics as an important deciding factor in restorative dentistry for anterior and posterior teeth. The profession's esthetic revolution began. By the early 1970s, many dentists were using esthetic materials in their crowns. Labs produced incredible artistic representations of enamel in crowns. Dental glasses evolved to where their beauty nearly matched the translucency and nuanced colors of natural teeth. Patients chose these restorations almost to the exclusion of cast gold restorations. That trend has continued through today (Christensen 2001).

These shifts are important to the clinician charged with maintaining them in a professional setting and for the patient/client. Regardless of the margin, the interface between the prosthesis and the tooth is cavernous to bacteria. Maintaining a low bacterial count is important so a biofilm cannot take hold there (Goodson et al. 2001).

Toothbrushing, interdental cleaning, and mouth rinsing are important to manage the biofilm around prosthesis. From a professional perspective, there are a number of things to consider when cleaning. Maintaining the cement or luting agent and maintaining the integrity of the material whether it is gold or glass are of high importance. The cement used to attach fixed prosthesis is difficult to manage and takes some practice. A new dental assistant may need time to become accustomed to removing it efficiently. If some cement remains, it can and does harbor biofilm, and the overhang must be removed. Some cements can be removed with an ultrasonic or sonic scaler, and there is a little device that attaches to the slow speed hand piece that removes overhangs.

When it is smooth, a clinician must still take care to use polishing materials that will not damage the cement or the finish of the final restoration. The clinician must also recommend home care products that will not harm the restoration. New polishing compounds are available to assure that the surface remains esthetically pleasing. When polishing using a rubber cup, these surfaces should be attended to with the lower abrasive polish before the more abrasive polish is used on the rest of the dentition.

Toothbrushing methods

Tooth brushing methods have been drilled into the heads of many a student of dentistry, dental hygienist, and dental assistant. It appears that the best approach to removing oral biofilm with a toothbrush is to use the modified Bass technique. Toothbrush development has focused on helping people achieve that ultimate 45-degree angle without having to maintain a 3.8 GPA in dental hygiene school.

Arguably the modified Bass technique is the best technique. The idea is to remove biofilm from the sulcus by directing the bristles into it and agitating. The movement of the bristle tips will break up the biofilm and loosen the biofilm from its mooring. Adding a little push toward the teeth before the sweeping motion increased plaque removal (Poyato-Ferrera et al. 2003).

Other brushing techniques include the Modified Stillman, Charter, rolling, and scrub. Each has advantages and disadvantages. The most important part of brushing is the ability and motivation of the person brushing.

An untrained person will naturally use a technique that looks like horizontal scrubbing, a rotary type motion similar to Fones technique, or an up and down type of motion sweeping over the mandibular and maxillary teeth (Leonard's technique) (Hiremath 2007). Many patients create an environment inhospitable to biofilm without damaging their tissue using these natural-type brushing motions. The modified Bass technique may be research based and a preferred method, but it is not the be-all end-all only technique. The clinician must keep in mind the talents of the patient/client (Morita et al. 1998).

Teaching brushing is an art in itself. The constant reinforcement of the intricacies is totally missing once the patient/client leaves the treatment room. A YouTube search for proper toothbrushing technique reveals more than 1,200 submissions (as of November 17, 2010). Many submissions have more than 100,000 views, and one has more than 1,000,000 views. Obviously there's a desire somewhere to brush better or teach better brushing. Presumably any hygienist or dentist who wants to offer reinforcement to their patients/clients can also upload their own video for their clientele. It seems that video of brushing is a very good way to teach it (Addy et al. 1999).

The use of a toothbrush and floss are the traditional means for removing the biofilm in North America. This is to say that there are other ways of removing the biofilm. As mentioned in other chapters of this text, the attachment of the biofilm to the tooth is quite interesting; it's not just a mechanical attachment. By recommending a brush and/or floss only, the clinician can miss many opportunities to educate the client/patient of other meaningful ways to manage the biofilm.

Cleaning the tongue

The surface of the tongue is enormously complex. In Chinese medicine, a person's overall health can be determined by looking at the tongue. In dependent populations, the state of the tongue can reveal the level of function (Kikutani et al. 2009). Biofilm grows on the tongue, not just the teeth. The dorsum of the tongue is a reservoir for microbes that contribute to enamel lesions, periodontal lesions, and halitosis (Van der Velden et al. 1986). Tongue cleaning can decrease plaque buildup on the teeth (Gross et al. 1975). As we know plaque to be a mixed biofilm, tongue cleaning has also shown a reduction in Candida infection.

The film on the tongue can be difficult to remove but should be part of every persons daily oral care regimen

(Chérel *et al.* 2008). Brushing the tongue with a manual (Figure 8-13) or power brush can be the easiest way to incorporate tongue cleaning to the daily routine

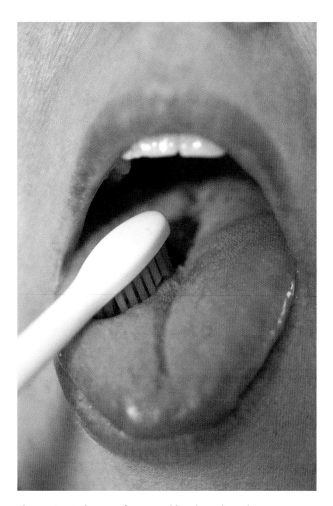

Figure 8-13 The use of a manual brush to clean the tongue.

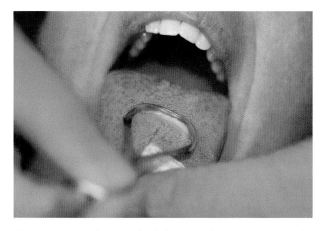

Figure 8-14 A photograph of the use of a tongue scraper for reaching to the posterior of the tongue to remove tongue deposits.

(Casemiro *et al.* 2008)). A scraping device intended for use on the tongue is also a viable method of removing the slime (Figure 8-14) (Pedrazzi *et al.* 2004).

Tongue cleaning at home may be avoided because of gagging by the patient/client using a regular toothbrush. The length of the toothbrush bristles may make this tool have too high a profile and touch the soft palate triggering reflexive action that is not exactly appealing. Gagging makes tongue cleaning intolerable. If people are complaining of gagging, they may find a brush made for tongue cleaning with a shorter bristle length to be helpful. Switching to a tongue scraper helps people with a gagging reflex. Professional tongue cleaning can be part of the prophylaxis appointment using an autocleaveable tongue cleaner.

Professional tongue cleaning with a Beaver Tail ultrasonic tip under low power and pressure can also reduce oral biofilm. Secondary to gagging is development of raw areas on the dorsum of the tongue. Using less pressure on the implement will allow the papillae to return to normal.

Dental floss

Dental floss is the dental hygienist's whip (Särner *et al.* 2010). Patients/clients are fully aware that they should floss because flossing is continually addressed as being sub-par by the dental hygienist. So ingrained in the dental community is the practice of flossing that when, in 2003, a published study on the efficacy of essential oil mouthwash and found it to be as good as flossing, the dental community was aghast. A lawsuit was brought about alleging breach of warranty, false advertising, and fraudulent business practices demanding that the mouthwash company stop misleading advertising. The judge in the case ordered that the advertising that one could stop flossing and rinse instead be stopped. New York judge, Denny Chin, stated in his decision, "Dentists and hygienists have been telling their patients for decades to floss daily. They have been doing so for good reason. The benefits of flossing are real—they are not a 'myth'" (MSNBC News 2010). Another class action suit alleging that the mouthwash advertisements were not in compliance with the original ruling, and the case was dismissed (Consumer Affairs 2010). Notwithstanding the judgment of a non-scientist, floss is not the only way to remove interproximal biofilm. The clinician must be aware of floss limitations, including manual dexterity and tooth anatomy (Zimmer *et al.* 2006). Manual dexterity is often cited as a reason a person cannot use dental floss (Marchini *et al.* 2006). Finger size alone can discourage some people from flossing their teeth.

Dental floss: the product

Arguably, the most over-demonstrated product in the dental appointment is floss. Every day hours are spent teaching patients how to use dental floss and why it is necessary to use daily. Flossing is a technical and difficult procedure that we ask our patients to do every day. Have you noticed that there are many names of ways to brush teeth (such as Bass, Stillman, Charter, and others)? People have given their names to using a brush this way or that; however, no one has been good enough at flossing to put their name on a particular technique. Perhaps wrapping your floss around the middle finger for anchoring is the MF technique, and anchoring the floss around the pinky finger the PF technique.

A YouTube phenomenon showing a monkey pulling a hair from her backside and using the stiff hair to clean between her teeth nearly went viral in 2010. Flossing is important and easy for many people, but as discussed in the section on brushing, not everyone can do it or do it well. Dental floss comes in a number of varieties. Thick and thin, flat and round, and coated with wax; made of Gore-tex; flavored; coated with fluoride, xylitol, or NovaMin; and colored. Flossers come ready to be strung up with floss, and some are already preloaded. Floss is a great product and efficient at removing biofilm from the interproximal tooth surfaces. Floss is also effective in decreasing microbiota from the mouth whether manually or automated (Hague and Carr 2007; Corby *et al.* 2008). Unfortunately most people do not use floss and will not use it regardless of how often it is taught to them. According to a bulleted list of dental statistics on the Canadian Dental Association Web site, 28% of adult Canadians floss up to five times a week.

If the clinician offers a lesson slightly different from the clinician before, the patient/client will be amazed and comment on how no one has shown them that before. Like periodontal charting, it's always new to them. So, as a warning, do not fall into that trap. Do not ask if someone has shown them before. That means they will have to admit that they have had a lesson and were not flossing in spite of it. Quite often the presence of papillary gingivitis, or bleeding on probing, is all one needs to observe to confirm that flossing has not been carried out.

If the clinician thinks the patient/client will benefit from using floss and together they find floss that will be used, great. The clinician must remember tooth anatomy, root structure, and honor the size of the bacterium. According to a recent review by the International Journal of Dental Hygiene (Berchier *et al.* 2008):

> The dental professional should determine, on an individual patient basis, whether high-quality flossing is an achievable goal. In light of the results of this comprehensive literature search and critical analysis, it is concluded that a routine instruction to use floss is not supported by scientific evidence.

Options for interdental cleaning include flossing, toothpicks, and interdental brushes. There are many ways to achieve the goal of less biofilm on the hard to reach tooth surfaces.

How to floss

There are many ways to anchor the floss. The most popular is to wrap it around the middle finger of each hand. An alternative that works well for children and people who find this type of wrapping uncomfortable is to knot a length of floss into a circle. (See Figure 8-15.)

Slide the floss gently between two teeth. Push the floss posteriorly to bend around the more distal tooth and move the floss up and down, in an effort to shave the biofilm from the mesial side of the distal tooth. Then, without removing the floss, gently bring the floss mesially taking care not to damage the papilla, and bend the floss around the distal of the more mesial tooth. Repeat the shaving motion. Lastly pop the floss out from between the two teeth. The floss user may unwind the floss from one anchor finger and put it through the embrasure. Wrap one round of floss onto the anchor finger with the less floss, usually the left side, and unwrap one round of floss off of the other anchor finger before gently sliding the floss between two other teeth.

A preloaded flosser is used similarly. These types of floss holders often have a very short span of floss (Figure 8-16). It should be used the same way. Gently slide the floss between two teeth, address the mesial of the distal tooth and then the distal side of the forward tooth.

Power flossers are effective for those who like power flossers.

The question of whether to brush first or floss first comes up often, and the upshot of studies trying to determine the better sequence is that it doesn't matter.

Floss may be made of a number of different materials. Mostly either a bundle of thin nylon filaments or a plastic (Teflon or polyethylene) ribbon often coated with wax, to make it easier for the patient/client to slip the string between the teeth. Some of these types of flosses are coated with flavorings as mint to entice the user to continue to floss and ignore the purple pulsing fingertips that comes with wrapping the string around the anchor fingers.

Woven floss is thought to remove more interproximal biofilm. Floss made with Gore-tex (for example, Glide) is popular in the USA. It is coated with wax for the opposite reason most floss is waxed. Gore-tex is so slippery that wax is added to slow it down as it snaps through the

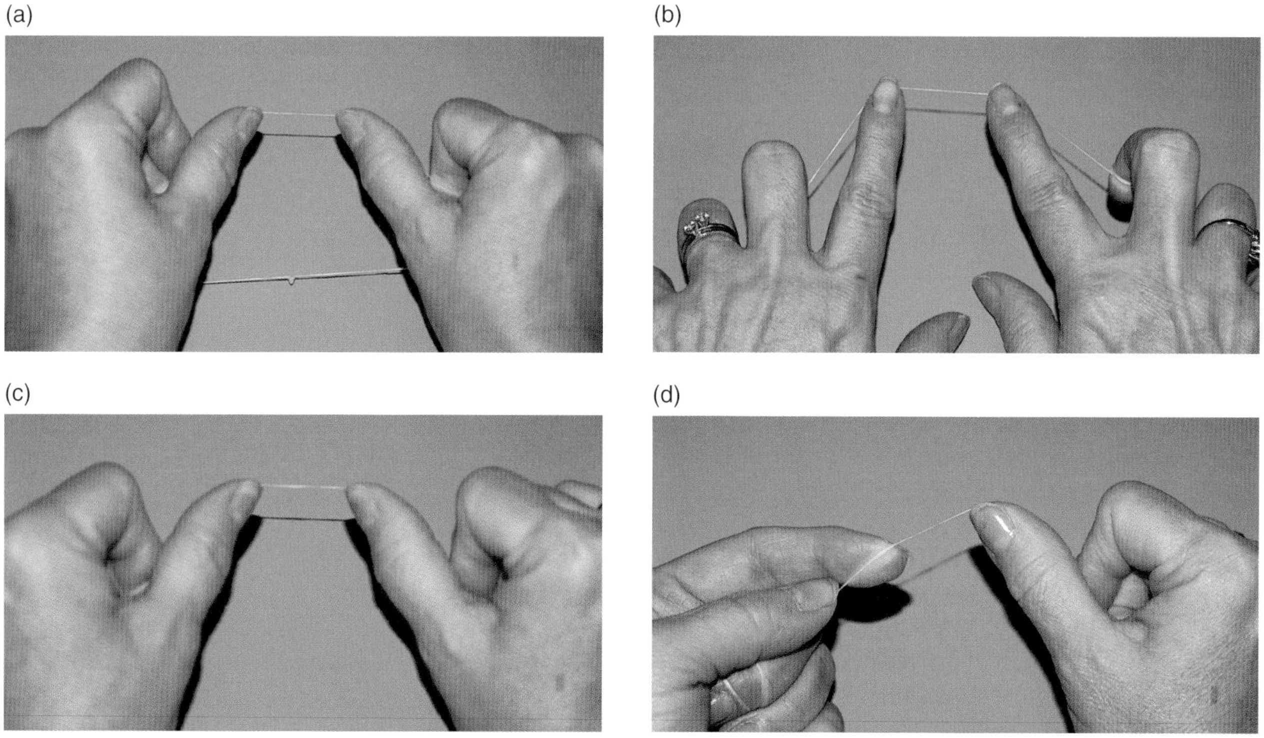

(a)

(b)

(c)

(d)

Figure 8-15 Flossing techniques. (a) Demonstrating the loop technique (alternate anchoring) for flossing. (b) With floss anchored to the middle finger, floss is stretched between the forefingers to access posterior teeth. (c) With floss anchored to the middle finger, floss is stretched between the thumbs to access teeth more anteriorly. (d) With floss anchored to the middle finger, floss is stretched between forefinger and thumb to access difficult areas of the mouth.

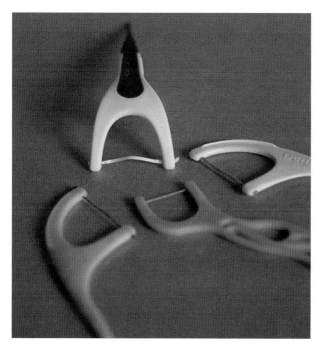

Figure 8-16 Preloaded flossers are loaded with different types of floss.

contact area. The wax is also helpful in removing deposits of food or biomaterial.

The waterjet

Times have changed with respect to oral irrigation at home. Early on people noticed that using a water jet device was helpful in creating and maintaining gingival health. When studies were done on just how the device was achieving this goal, researchers were saddened to find the results to be very lackluster. The plaque was still present after using the device. This finding shows the disregard that dentistry has for bacterium. The disclosed teeth still had disclosable plaque after using the jet device although it turned out that the plaque was devoid of living organisms (Barnes *et al.* 2005; Brady *et al.* 1973).

A water jet device has a number of aliases. It is very often just called a Waterpik, which, like Kleenex, is a trade name. Waterpik is the name of a water jet device made by Teledyne. The water jet device is also sometimes referred to as an oral irrigator. And although irrigation doesn't sound jet like, oral irrigation is most often referred to as a water jet device. Most early studies used

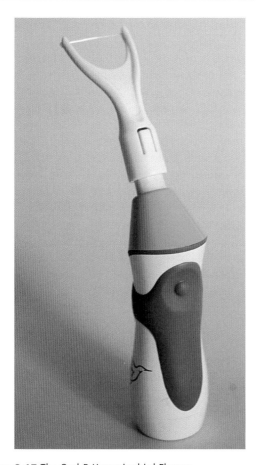

Figure 8-17 The Oral-B Hummingbird Flosser.

the Waterpik as the irrigator. Although today's studies use other models, the bulk of the research represents results obtained from the Waterpik irrigator. In this section, the term oral irrigation will be used and will reference the water jet in general.

How the oral irrigator works

Oral irrigation at home is worthwhile. It has shown benefits in reducing bleeding, gingivitis, and supragingival plaque (Barnes *et al.* 2005). Biofilm is very susceptible to changes in fluid dynamics. As an organism, the biofilm forms in areas of moving fluid, in this instance crevicular fluid. The biofilm adheres in this moving environment using the least possible adherence mechanism to survive. When the dynamics of the fluid change, the biofilm will change with it given enough time. In the case of a sonic toothbrush or an oral irrigator, the change in fluid dynamics is sudden and the microbes are, in effect, sucked out.

Dr. Bhaskar, periodontist and irrigator researcher, explained that the water moving across the opening of the pocket created a Venturi effect. To illustrate this more clearly, imagine a container of liquid lawn fertilizer

attached to a garden hose. The container has a lid with a hose attached, and on that lid are two other important pieces: a straw that dips down into the fertilizer, and a lever that directs the water across the opening of the straw or, closes the opening so water does not go across the opening of the straw.

As the water goes across the opening of the straw, suction is created and the fertilizer is drawn up the straw and into the stream of water from the hose. A mix is created with the water, and the mixture is expelled from the container and sprinkled onto the lawn.

Using the oral irrigator similarly will get the best results. Dr. Bhaskar recommended that the pressure be set at the highest tolerable pressure and increased until the highest possible pressure is reached. The water stream should be directed from the outside to the inside and allowed to pulse for a short time. One reservoir of water is enough for the whole mouth. The traditional tip should be directed at a 90-degree angle to the tooth. A special tip is created for a deeper irrigation. This tip is intended to be used at a 45-degree angle into the tissue. The design of the tip relieves the pressure so the tissue is unharmed.

The penetration of the water varies. Studies show a penetration of the fluid to travel at least half the distance of the pocket depth (Braun and Ciancio 1992). So to use a medicament is to achieve a level of penetration unseen by most other procedures. This delivery method is also found to be much better than direct application of a medicament using a syringe (Itic and Serfaty 1992).

Adding substances to the water of an oral irrigator is very tempting. Adding flavor or color may make using the machine easier to use longer. Although the cosmetics of using an oral irrigator may make a difference on a personal level, the studies that look at adding different products to the water continually point to clear water being the best thing to use in a home irrigator (Newman *et al.* 1994; Flemmig and Epp 1995). Povidone iodine is a favorite in periodontal medicine. Added to the reservoir of a home irrigator is helpful to reduce the pathogens (Hoang *et al.* 2003). Studies of this type were mainly conducted in the 1990s. The topic seems to have lost its allure as other studies on oral irrigation after the 1990s focus on microbiota on a microscopic level. The upshot is that plain water is not better or worse than adding something to the water. If it helps a person use the device then there are no contraindications.

Bacteremia

One reason oral irrigation took a while to catch on is that many people feared permanent damage if it was used incorrectly. This may be true. If the tip is aimed apically along the long axis of the tooth, tissue damage can occur. The urge is so great to operate it incorrectly that a tip modified to step down the pressure was developed to achieve patient comfort and safety. Bacteremia is a well-known event after dental procedures. It is also well known in dentistry that odontogenic bacteremia can occur during many orocentric activities from eating to toothbrushing (Daly *et al.* 2000; Lucas *et al.* 2008; Crasta *et al.* 2009; Lockhart *et al.* 2009). The bacteremia argument is a non-issue in discussions on oral irrigation when used correctly (Lucas and Roberts 2008).

Oral irrigation may be recommended for persons undergoing orthodontic treatment. The pulsing water will remove food and biofilm from the teeth and around the brackets and bands. A special tip created for this application shows a reduction in plaque and bleeding (Sharma *et al.* 2008).

Mouthwashes and mouth rinses

The ideal mouthwash

An ideal mouthwash should have the following characteristics:

- Nontoxic
- Palatable
- Limited absorption
- Substantive
- Bactericidal and bacteria specific
- Penetrate biofilm
- Low induced drug resistance

Introduction

In an effort to disrupt bacterial biofilm in hard to reach places, patients/clients will often try to use a mouthwash. Oral health care clinicians are in a position to educate them on the best one to use for each situation and achievable goals of the patient. For fresh breath only, a mouth spray may be all that's needed. A quick squirt from a pocket size container may help make a client's breath fresh enough for an intimate conversation. If the goal is to augment oral health, a whole different conversation may be embarked on. The nature of the biofilm makes mouthwash choices important.

Most studies are focused on the amount of planktonic bacteria floating freely in the mouth. This kind of action is worthwhile, and fewer numbers of volatile bacteria in the environment can make for a more constrained growth in the biofilm. However, in an effort to promote good oral health, the use of mouthwashes to penetrate and disrupt the biofilm as an adjunct to mechanical

methods of biofilm management has been studied (Gunsolley 2006).

The ingredients in most of the mouthwashes/rinses include the use of alcohol. As discussed in Chapter 1, alcohol mouthwashes/rinses have been accused of increasing the risk for oral cancer. That risk may be exaggerated (La Vecchia 2009). Although alcohol is used primarily to keep other antibacterial ingredients dissolved, it may have some antibacterial properties itself (Pan *et al.* 2010).

Most clinical studies on mouthwash effectiveness have been directed at antibacterial and antigingivitis effects and conducted by the manufacturer. Rinses have little effect against caries. The controversy rages over which is the best mouthwash to use. The best option is the one the patient will use. This simple fact cannot be overemphasized. Taste and tissue response are minor considerations compared to the antibacterial effect; the goal is to destroy the biofilm that is otherwise unreachable by mechanical action (Hioe and van der Weijden 2005). The main reasons for using a mouthwash can be itemized in two categories, for the patient/client and for the professional clinician. The patient/client will often be seeking a mouthwash that is most effective in producing fresh breath and a clean mouth as an adjunct to toothbrushing or as a stand-alone home care procedure. A clinician who is more interested in how effective the rinse is in controlled oral bacteria may instruct a patient to use a rinse as a pretreatment infection control measure (Fine *et al.* 1992; Fine *et al*, 1993; Fischman 1994; Feres *et al.* 2010). Table 8-1 summarizes suggested instructions to the client/patient on how to rinse prior to a dental hygiene appointment.

Essential oils

This is a large category. Essential oil (EO) is easily tolerated by the health conscience, therefore, EO rinses are popular. From health food stores, to the corner drug store or even gasoline station, EO mouthwashes are prolific. The essential oils cause the burning sensation, not the alcohol. Effective mouth rinsing (Table 8-2) is a technique that should be learned and should not be simplified because of the strong taste of the rinse.

EO mouth rinses act on the bacterial cell walls and inhibit enzyme activity. Other studies show that EOs inhibit aggregation with the early colonizers of the biofilm, pioneer species. In studies looking at EO mouth rinses as a stand-alone oral hygiene measure, they appear to perform well (Stoeken *et al.* 2007).

Studies comparing mouthwashes with different active ingredients, essential oil mouthwashes seem to compare favorably with chlorhexidine. Researchers often find this type of antiseptic rinse to be superior to the cetylpyridinium chloride rinses (Amini *et al.* 2009).

The effect of EOs on hard and soft tissue of the mouth has been looked at as well as what the effect of this type of mouthwash has had on man-made prosthetic material. Studies that evaluate the safety of prosthetic materials intended to approximate the dimensions of the tooth prove again that there are no good materials when contrasting them to enamel. In short, there's no filling like no filling. The combination of ingredients in the EO mouthwash has shown that there is damage to the man-made material. So, care must be taken when recommending this type of mouthwash to patient/clients (Almeida *et al.* 2010). A good relationship with the patient/client's dental history is important. Most people will have no idea what type of material is used as a prosthetic material to repair caries lesions.

Pretreatment of the pockets with an antimicrobial mouthwash before periodontal treatment may also be helpful in reducing bacteremia in patients undergoing treatment for periodontal disease. This can be done by filling a lavage bottle with an acceptable irrigant, like EO (Fine *et al.* 2010, Morozumi *et al.* 2010), and flushing around all the teeth using the lower power setting on the ultrasonic unit.

Recommending EO mouthwashes after periodontal therapy is also helpful in reducing the bacteria that are associated with the periodontal infection (Cavalca Cortelli *et al.* 2009).

Cetylpyridinium chloride

Cetylpyridinium chloride (CPC) mouthwash is studied in two main concentrations. Both have been shown to be beneficial in reducing plaque even in combination with different brushing activities (Witt *et al.* 2006).

Table 8-1 How to use a mouthwash

Step	Instructions
1.	Take a prescribed amount of the fluid into the mouth ● Cap full ● One half ounce
2.	Hold fluid in the mouth, lips together, teeth with adequate free way space
3.	Force fluid through interdental spaces ● With lips together balloon cheeks, then suck them in alternately several times
4.	Divide the mouth into three parts: anterior, left, and right ● With lips together rinse the front first ● Then move fluid to the left side and move fluid by activating buccinators and massater ● Lastly move fluid to the right side and move the fluid by activating buccinators and massater
5.	Remove fluid from the mouth as directed ● Open lips and let fluid drain into sink or container ● Spit into container using force ● Swallow

Adapted from Wilkins (1994).

Table 8-2 How to gargle

Step	General steps	Details
1.	Read before starting	● If using a commercial mouthwash, read the directions to see how much mouthwash to rinse with. ● If mixing your own, use about one ounce or one shotglass of the mixture.
2.	Place in mouth	● Start by taking an amount of the liquid into the mouth. ● If less than the recommended amount, gargle as many times as it takes to use the whole dose.
3.	Tilt back	● Let the liquid go through your mouth. ● Tilt your head back letting liquid settle at the back of your throat, closing the throat so you don't swallow. ● It should feel as if you're about to swallow the liquid.
4.	'Gargle'	● Slowly let out a breath through your throat. ● The air mixes with the liquid causing the liquid to bubble and churn around the tonsillar area. ● Try to make a sound while letting the liquid churn (gargling noise). ● Part the lips, slightly, to avoid spillage. Gargle for 5 to 10 seconds, then close your lips and tilt your head forward to let the liquid flow away from your throat into your mouth.
5.	Repeat	● Breathe in through the nose then tilt your head back and repeat five to six times before spitting the liquid into a cup or the sink. ● Don't swallow your gargling liquid. Neither salt water nor commercial mouthwashes are intended to be ingested, especially by children who might end up swallowing too much fluoride.

CPC mouthwash compares favorably with EO mouthwash. The CPC mouthwash can be recommended for patient/clients who may have small children at home or who have a problem with alcohol (Witt *et al.* 2005; Mankodi *et al.* 2005).

It appears that CPC mouthwashes are safe to dental prosthetic materials, but there may be a lack of synergy between the ingredients in toothpastes and CPC mouthwashes. The recommendation is to rinse after toothpaste or wait up to 60 minutes before using the CPC rinse (Sheen 2003; White *et al.* 2008).

Detergent rinses

There is still only one mouthwash that advertises itself as a pre-brushing rinse. The active ingredient has not been proven to increase health (Angelillo *et al.* 2002).

Triclosan

Triclosan has the unique distinction of being in the news the most often. For various reasons this ingredient is one that really has its ups and downs. The research shows us that triclosan as an ingredient is safe for humans and effective against oral pathogens. It is not as effective as chlorhexidine (Arweiler *et al.* 2001).

Chlorhexidine

Using chlorhexidine (CHX) in a mouthwash or a varnish can reduce biofilm. (See Chapter 10.) CHX binds to the bacterial cell membrane breaking it down. Chlorhexidine also binds to the pellicle, which interferes with the adherence of the early colonizers slowing the growth of the biofilm (Sekino *et al.* 2003).

CHX kills bacteria and yeast. This finding intrigued researchers investigating cariology. At one time in the early 2000s, CHX was recommended as a good mouthwash to use sporadically against caries infections. In 2008 Young and Featherstone *et al.* (2008) removed this recommendation from the CAMBRA protocol for children with caries infection.

Chlorhexidine is still the "go-to" mouthwash when comparing different active ingredient mouthwashes and rinses.

However, there are some concerns about its biocompatibility with other oral care products, especially SLS-containing toothpastes (Owens *et al.* 1997).

Fluoride

The use of fluoride in dentistry is nearly abusive. The idea that fluoride can remineralize and heal teeth as a stand-alone ingredient is, still today, an exploitation of the science to where the truth is barely recognizable. The adage, a little is good so a lot is better, has all but stymied dental research. A 2010 PubMed search using the string

"*fluoride caries*," limiting for English and current 5 years revealed 873 articles. Using the search string "*calcium phosphate enamel*" under the same limitations revealed only 127. Scientists are still spending time and money researching questions about fluoride when time may be better spent looking for alternatives. If fluoride was the final answer, no one would have issues with caries.

All of this is not to say that fluoride is not worthwhile. Low doses and long duration are important in the fluoride mouth rinse. (See Chapter 16.)

Xylitol

The recipe for xylitol mouthwash giving the best results is still being developed. The amount of xylitol needed to be effective at reducing biofilm and increasing health has yet to reach the university study level. Small xylitol product companies don't have the resources needed to mount such a study. So the true health benefits of a xylitol mouthwash may yet be discovered. Chronic wound studies using xylitol reveals some useful information that may translate to the oral cavity (Dowd *et al.* 2009). Xylitol helps to penetrate the film that blocks antibiotics from entering. The penetration allows antibiotics or other bactericidal products, like lactoferrin (found in healthy saliva) and white blood cells from the infection control mechanism of the body, access to the microbes, which can help kill them. The decrease in slime production from the *Streptococcus* species allows oxygen into the wound, which stimulates healing. Xylitol has been shown to interfere with biofilm quorum sensing decreasing the film further. This combination—desliming and oxygenization—allows the body's defenses to heal the wound (Biesbrock *et al.* 2007). Xylitol is proving to be an important ingredient for periodontal infections, which is in fact a micro wound, and finding xylitol in more mouthwashes in the future or using xylitol confections may help increase or establish oral health. A homemade xylitol mouth rinse is simple to make for home use (Table 8-3). (Chapter 9 contains more information on xylitol.)

A word of warning when reading research papers on the effectiveness of any topical antimicrobial intended for oral use. The majority of the studies show the effects of the tested product on planktonic bacteria, virus, or yeast. That is to say they measure the effects on bacteria that may be in a homogeneous biofilm, often called a colony. A true biofilm is multispecies, where the cohabitants communicate and live in a very different way than they did in the outside. Often the biofilm in the study will be described as *Streptococcus mutans* biofilm or *Lactobacillus* biofilm. This requires clinicians to use caution in reading too much into the study for use in clinical decision making.

Table 8-3 Homemade mouthwashes

Mouthwash	Ingredients and instructions
Isotonic sodium chloride	<ul><li>1/2 teaspoon salt</li><li>1 cup warm water</li><li>Mix</li><li>Use PRN as directed<ul><li>Rinse or gargle for 30 to 60 seconds</li><li>Expectorate or let fall from mouth</li></ul></li><li>Save mixture, use until gone or within 24 hours</li></ul>
Hypertonic sodium chloride	<ul><li>1/2 teaspoon salt</li><li>1/2 cup warm water</li><li>Mix</li><li>Use PRN as directed<ul><li>Rinse or gargle for 30 to 60 seconds</li><li>Expectorate or let fall from mouth</li></ul></li><li>Save mixture, use until gone or within 24 hours</li></ul>
Sodium bicarbonate	<ul><li>1/2 teaspoon baking soda</li><li>1 cup water (may be ozonated)</li><li>Mix</li><li>Use PRN after meals and before bed<ul><li>Rinse *and* gargle for 30 to 60 seconds</li><li>Expectorate or let fall from mouth</li></ul></li><li>Save remaining mixture to use again for up to 24 hours</li></ul>
Sodium chloride-sodium bicarbonate	<ul><li>1/2 teaspoon sodium chloride</li><li>1/2 teaspoon sodium bicarbonate</li><li>1 cup warm water</li><li>Mix</li><li>Use PRN as directed<ul><li>Rinse or gargle for 30 to 60 seconds</li><li>Expectorate or let fall from mouth</li></ul></li><li>Save mixture and use until gone or within 24 hours</li></ul>
Hydrogen Peroxide	<ul><li>Full strength<ul><li>1/2 ounce</li><li>Rinse or gargle for 30 to 60 seconds</li><li>Expectorate or let fall from mouth</li></ul></li></ul>
Xylitol mouth rinse	<ul><li>1 cup water</li><li>1 teaspoon granular xylitol</li><li>Mix with teaspoon</li><li>Use throughout the day<ul><li>Rinse and gargle for 30 seconds</li><li>Swallow</li></ul></li></ul>

Partially adapted from Alvarez (1998).

Dental health care providers are just getting used to the idea of incorporating mouthwash or mouth rinsing to their patient/clients. Those who are not already recommending mouthwash as an adjunct should become more familiar with the continually growing body of research supporting this practice. Many practitioners recommend simple homemade formulations for effective mouth rinsing (Table 8-3).

Conclusion

Do we need to brush, floss, and rinse? Yes, unfortunately the idea of being free from the tyranny of brush and floss is not in the future. It is important for a clinician to remove the idea of brush and floss as the only way to eliminate the surge of dental disease. It is *not* the only way. Establishing a mindset of biofilm reduction as opposed to biofilm removal should be the clinician's goal. This simple change from the time honored and disrespectful idea of removing all traces of biofilm is more accurate and opens synaptic channels in the clinician's mind to find alternatives to oral health preservation. The use of different sizes, colors, and shapes of toothbrushes is important only if the patient will use it more frequently. The color matters to the individual running the brush. The handle design is there for the benefit of the user, not the clinician. The brush that works well for the clinician may not work at all for a particular patient/client. This egocentric method of product recommendation should not enter into the oral hygiene recommendations for patient/clients. Many options should be made available from the clinic, or a trading system put into place with a nearby shop. Perhaps it's even time for a dental hygiene shop where only hygiene products are dispensed. No matter the circumstances, the best tool to use is the one the patient/client will use. And that tool may be a weekly appointment with a dental hygienist.

References

Adachi, M., Ishihara, K., Abe, S. *et al.* (2007) Professional oral health care by dental hygienists reduced respiratory infections in elderly persons requiring nursing care. *International Journal of Dental Hygiene*, 5, 69–74.

Addy, M., Renton-Harper, P., Warren, P. (1999) An evaluation of video instruction for an electric toothbrush. Comparative single-brushing cross-over study. *Journal of Clinical Periodontology*, 26, 289–293.

Ahmed, R., Hassall, T., Morland, B. *et al.* (2003) Viridans streptococcus bacteremia in children on chemotherapy for cancer: an underestimated problem. *Pediatric Hematology and Oncology*, 20, 439–444.

Alaki, S.M., Burt, B.A., Garetz, S.L. (2008) Middle ear and respiratory infections in early childhood and their association with early childhood caries. *Pediatric Dentistry*, 30, 105–110.

Almeida, G.S., Poskus, L.T., Guimarães, J.G. *et al.* (2010) The effect of mouthrinses on salivary sorption, solubility and surface degradation of a nanofilled and a hybrid resin composite. *Operative Dentistry*, 35, 105–11.

al-Otaibi M. (2004) The miswak (chewing stick) and oral health. Studies on oral hygiene practices of urban Saudi Arabians. *Swedish Dental Journal*, Suppl. (167), 2–75.

Al-Otaibi, M., Al-Harthy, M., Gustafsson, A. *et al.* (2004) Subgingival plaque microbiota in Saudi Arabians after use of miswak chewing stick and toothbrush. *Journal of Clinical Periodontology*, 31, 1048–1053.

Alvarez, K.H. (1998) Oral Infection Control. In: *William and Wilkins' Dental Hygiene Handbook*. (Ed. K.H. Alvarez), p. 209, Williams and Wilkins, Baltimore MD.

Amini, P., Araujo, M.W., Wu, M.M. *et al.* (2009) Comparative antiplaque and antigingivitis efficacy of three antiseptic mouthrinses: a two week randomized clinical trial. *Brazilian Oral Research*, 23, 319–325.

Angelillo, I.F., Nobile, C.G., Pavia, M. (2002) Evaluation of the effectiveness of a pre-brushing rinse in plaque removal: a meta-analysis. *Journal of Clinical Periodontology*, 29, 301–309.

Arweiler, N.B., Henning, G., Reich, E. *et al.* (2001) Effect of an amine-fluoride-triclosan mouthrinse on plaque regrowth and biofilm vitality. *Journal of Clinical Periodontology*, 29, 358–363.

Association of Dental Implant Auxiliaries (ADIA). (2011) Frequently asked questions. [online] available at http://adiaonline.org/patient-information.php.

Azrak, B., Barfaraz, B., Krieter, G. *et al.* (2004) Effectiveness of a three-headed toothbrush in pre-school children. *Oral Health and Preventive Dentistry*, 2, 103–9.

Barker, J. and Jones, M.V. (2005) The potential spread of infection caused by aerosol contamination of surfaces after flushing a domestic toilet. *Journal of Applied Microbiology*, 99, 339–347.

Barnes, C.M., Russell, C.M., Reinhardt, R.A. *et al.* (2005) Comparison of irrigation to floss as an adjunct to tooth brushing: effect on bleeding, gingivitis, and supragingival plaque. *Journal of Clinical Dentistry*, 16, 71–77.

Battaglia, A. (2008) The Bass technique using a specially designed toothbrush. International Journal of Dental Hygiene, 6, 183–187.

Bellamy, N., Sothern, R.B., Campbell, J. *et al.* (2002) Rhythmic variations in pain, stiffness, and manual dexterity in hand osteoarthritis. *Annals of Rheumatic Diseases*, 61, 1075–1080.

Berchier, C.E., Slot, D.E. *et al.* (2008) The efficacy of dental floss in addition to a toothbrush on plaque and parameters of gingival inflammation: a systematic review. *International Journal of Dental Hygiene*, 6, 265–279.

Berry, A.M. and Davidson, P.M. (2006) Beyond comfort: oral hygiene as a critical nursing activity in the intensive care unit. *Intensive and Critical Care Nursing*, 22, 318–328.

Bezirtzoglou, E., Cretoiu, S.M., Moldoveanu, M. *et al.* (2008) A quantitative approach to the effectiveness of ozone against microbiota organisms colonizing toothbrushes. *Journal of Dentistry*, 36, 600–605.

Biesbrock, A.R., Bartizek, R.D., Gerlach, R.W. (2007) Oral hygiene regimens, plaque control, and gingival health: a two-month clinical trial with antimicrobial agents. *Journal Clinical Dentistry*, 18, 101–105.

Boylan, R., Li, Y., Simeonova, L. *et al.* (2008) Reduction in bacterial contamination of toothbrushes using the Violight ultraviolet light activated toothbrush sanitizer. *American Journal of Dentistry*, 21, 313–317.

Brady, J.M., Gray, W.A., Bhaskar, S.N. (1973) Electron microscopic study of the effect of water jet lavage devices on dental plaque. *Journal Dental Research*, 52, 1310–1313.

Braun, R.E., Ciancio, S.G. (1992) Subgingival delivery by an oral irrigation device. *Journal of Periodontology*, 63, 469–472.

British Health Foundation (2010) Brush Before Breakfast Advises the British Health Foundation. [online] available at http://www.emaxhealth.com/79/1063.html.

Buehlmann, M., Frei, R., Fenner, L. *et al.* (2008) Highly effective regimen for decolonization of methicillin-resistant Staphylococcus aureus carriers. *Infection Control and Hospital Epidemiology*, 29, 510–516.

Carvalho, Rde, S., Rossi, V., Weidlich, P. *et al.* (2007) Comparative analysis between hard- and soft-filament toothbrushes related to plaque removal and gingival abrasion. *Journal of Clinical Dentistry*, 18, 61–64.

Casemiro, L.A., Martins, C.H., de Carvalho, T.C. *et al.* (2008) Effectiveness of a new toothbrush design versus a conventional tongue scraper in improving breath odor and reducing tongue microbiota. *Journal of Applied Oral Science*, 16, 271–274.

Caudry, S.D., Klitorinos, A., Chan, E.C. (1995) Contaminated toothbrushes and their disinfection. *Journal of the Canadian Dental Association*, 61, 511–516.

Cavalca Cortelli, S. Cavallini, F., Regueira Alves, M.F. *et al.* (2009) Clinical and microbiological effects of an essential-oil-containing mouth rinse applied in the "one-stage full-mouth disinfection" protocol—a randomized doubled-blinded preliminary study. *Clinical Oral Investigation*, 13, 189–194.

Chai, J., Chu, F.C., Chow, T.W. *et al.* (2006) Influence of dental status on nutritional status of geriatric patients in a convalescent and rehabilitation hospital. *International Journal of Prosthodontics*, 19, 244–249.

Chérel, F., Mobilia, A., Lundgren, T. *et al.* (2008) Rate of reformation of tongue coatings in young adults. *International Journal of Dental Hygiene*, 6, 371–375.

Christensen, G.J. (2001) Cast gold restorations. Has the esthetic dentistry pendulum swung too far? *Journal of the American Dental Association*, 132, 809–811.

Claydon, N., Addy, M., Scratcher, C. *et al.* (2002) Comparative professional plaque removal study using 8 branded toothbrushes. *Journal Clinical Periodontology*, 2002, 29, 310–316.

Consumer Affairs (2010) Court Dismisses Latest Listerine Suit: More controversy over claim that mouthwash is 'as effective as floss.' [online] available at http://www.consumeraffairs.com/news04/2010/03/listerine.html#ixzz18DbE1tp2.

Corby, P.M., Biesbrock, A., Bartizek, R. *et al.* (2008) Treatment outcomes of dental flossing in twins: molecular analysis of the interproximal microflora. *Journal of Periodontology*, 79, 1426–1433.

Cortelli, S.C., Cortelli, J.R., Aquino, D.R. *et al.* (2010) Self-performed supragingival biofilm control: qualitative analysis, scientific basis and oral-health implications. *Brazilian Oral Research*, 24 Suppl 1, 43–54.

Crasta, K., Daly, C.G., Mitchell, D. *et al.* (2009) Bacteraemia due to dental flossing. *Journal of Clinical Periodontology*, 36, 323–332.

Daly, C., Mitchell, D., Grossberg, D. *et al.* (1997) Bacteraemia caused by periodontal probing. *Australian Dental Journal*, 42, 77–78.

Danhauer, J.L., Johnson, C.E., Corbin, N.E. (2010) Bruccheri KG. Xylitol as a prophylaxis for acute otitis media: systematic review. *International Journal of Audiology*, 10, 754–761.

Danilatou, V., Mantadakis, E., Galanakis, E. *et al.* (2003) Three cases of viridans group streptococcal bacteremia in children with febrile neutropenia and literature review. *Scandanavian Journal of Infectious Diseases*, 35, 873–876.

Deacon, S.A., Glenny, A.M., Deery, C. *et al.* (2010) Different powered toothbrushes for plaque control and gingival health. *Cochrane Database Systematic Reviews*, 12, CD004971.

De Marchi, R.J., Hugo, F.N., Hilgert, J.B. *et al.* (2008) Association between oral health status and nutritional status in south Brazilian independent-living older people. *Nutrition*, 24, 546–553.

de Mattos Mda, G., Pinelli, L.A., Ribeiro, R.F., *et al.* (1998) Fabrication of an acrylic resin device used to increase the size of toothbrush handles. *Journal of Prosthetic Dentistry*, 79, 361–2.

Doğan, M.C., Alaçam, A., Aşici, N., *et al.* (2004) Clinical evaluation of the plaque-removing ability of three different toothbrushes in a mentally disabled group. *Acta Odontologia Scandinavica*, 62, 350–354.

Dowd, S.E., Sun, Y., Smith, E. *et al.* (2009) Effects of biofilm treatments on the multi-species Lubbock chronic wound biofilm model. *Journal Wound Care*, 18, 508, 510–12.

Dumitrescu, A.L. and Kawamura M. (2010) Involvement of psychosocial factors in the association of obesity with periodontitis. *Journal of Oral Science*, 52, 115–124.

Feres, M., Figueiredo, L.C., Faveri, M. *et al.* (2010) The effectiveness of a preprocedural mouthrinse containing cetylpyridinium chloride in reducing bacteria in the dental office. *Journal of the American Dental Association*, 141, 415–422.

Fine, D.H., Furgang, D., Korik, I. *et al.* (1993) Reduction of viable bacteria in dental aerosols by preprocedural rinsing with an antiseptic mouthrinse. *American Journal of Dentistry*, 6, 219–221.

Fine, D.H., Furgang, D., McKiernan, M. *et al.* (2010) An investigation of the effect of an essential oil mouthrinse on induced bacteraemia: a pilot study. *Journal of Periodontology*, 37, 840–847.

Fine, D.H., Mendieta, C., Barnett, M.L. *et al.* (1992) Efficacy of preprocedural rinsing with an antiseptic in reducing viable bacteria in dental aerosols. *Journal of Periodontolog*, 63, 821–824.

Fischman, S.L. (1994) A clinician's perspective on antimicrobial mouthrinses. *Journal of the American Dental Association*, 125 Suppl 2, 20S–22S.

Flemmig, T.F., Epp, B., Funkenhauser, Z. *et al.* (1995) Adjunctive supragingival irrigation with acetylsalicylic acid in periodontal supportive therapy. *Journal of Clinical Periodontology*, 22, 427–433.

Forrest, J.L. and Miller, S.A. (2004) Manual versus powered toothbrushes: a summary of the Cochrane Oral Health Group's Systematic Review. Part II. *Journal of Dental Hygiene*, 78, 349–354.

Franzò, D., Philpotts, C.J., Cox, T.F. *et al.* (2010) The effect of toothpaste concentration on enamel and dentine wear in vitro. *Journal of Dentistry*, 38, 974–979.

Glassman, P. and Subar, P. (2010) Creating and maintaining oral health for dependent people in institutional settings. *Journal of Public Health Dentistry*, 70 Suppl 1, S40–S48.

Gonçalves, A.F., de Oliveira Rocha, R., Oliveira, M.D. *et al.* (2007) Clinical effectiveness of toothbrushes and toothbrushing methods of plaque removal on partially erupted occlusal surfaces. *Oral Health and Preventive Dentistry*, 5, 33–37.

Goodson, J.M., Shoher, I., Imber, S. *et al.* (2001) Reduced dental plaque accumulation on composite gold alloy margins. *Journal of Periodontal Research*, 36, 252–259.

Gross, A., Barnes, G.P., Lyon, T.C. (1975) Effects of tongue brushing on tongue coating and dental plaque scores. *Journal Dental Research*, 54, 1236.

Grossi, S.G., Skrepcinski, F.B., DeCaro, T. *et al.* (1997) Treatment of periodontal disease in diabetics reduces glycated hemoglobin. *Journal of Periodontology*, 68, 713–719.

Gunsolley, J.C. (2006) A meta-analysis of six-month studies of antiplaque and antigingivitis agents. *Journal of the American Dental Association*, 137, 1649–1657.

Hague, A.L., Carr, M.P. (2007) Efficacy of an automated flossing device in different regions of the mouth. *Journal of Periodontology*, 78, 1529–1537.

Herlofson, B.B., Barkvoll, P., Bartizek, R. *et al.* (1996) The effect of two toothpaste detergents on the frequency of recurrent aphthous ulcers. *Acta Odontologia Scandinavica*, 54, 150–153.

Hioe, K.P., van der Weijden, G.A. (2005) The effectiveness of self-performed mechanical plaque control with triclosan containing dentifrices. *International Journal of Dental Hygiene*, 3, 192–204.

Hiremath, S.S. (2007) Oral hygiene aids. In: *Textbook of Preventive and Community Dentistry*, (Ed. S.S. Hiremath), 2nd Edn. p. 416, Elsevier, Haryana, India.

Hoang, T., Jorgensen, M.G., Keim, R.G. *et al.* (2003) Povidone-iodine as a periodontal pocket disinfectant. *Journal Periodontal Research*, 38, 311–317.

Hyrdrabrush. (2011) 30 Second Smile: Little effort, big results. [online] Available at http://www.hydrabrush.com.

Itic, J. and Serfaty, R. (1992) Clinical effectiveness of subgingival irrigation with a pulsated jet irrigator versus syringe. *Journal of Periodontology*, 63, 174–181.

Jackson, M.A., Kellett, M., Worthington, H.V., Clerehugh, V. (2006) Comparison of interdental cleaning methods: a randomized controlled trial. *Journal of Periodontology*, 77, 1421–1429.

Jayakumar, A. Padmini, H. Haritha, A. *et al.* (2010) Role of dentifrice in plaque removal: a clinical trial. *Indian Journal of Dental Research*, 21, 213–217.

Kaklamanos, E.G. and Kalfas, S. (2008) Meta-analysis on the effectiveness of powered toothbrushes for orthodontic patients. *American Journal of Orthodontics and Dentofacial Orthopedics*, 133(2), 187.e1–14.

Kikutani, T., Tamura, F., Nishiwaki, K., *et al.* (2009) The degree of tongue-coating reflects lingual motor function in the elderly. *Gerodontology*, 26, 291–296.

Kodaka, T., Kuroiwa, M., Kobori, M. (1993) Scanning laser microscopic surface profiles of human enamel and dentin after brushing with abrasive dentifrice in vitro. *Scanning Microscopy*, 7, 247–254.

Kokubu, K., Senpuku, H., Tada, A. *et al.* (2008) Impact of routine oral care on opportunistic pathogens in the institutionalized elderly. *Journal of Medical and Dental Science*, 55, 7–13.

La Vecchia, C. (2009) Mouthwash and oral cancer risk: an update. *Oral Oncology*, 45, 198–200.

Laskarin, M., Brkić, H., Pichler, G. (2006) The influence of age on tooth root colour changes. *Collegium Antropologicum*, 30, 807–810.

Limeback, H. (1998) Implications of oral infections on systemic diseases in the institutionalized elderly with a special focus on pneumonia. *Annals of Periodontology*, 3, 262–275.

Lockhart, P.B., Brennan, M.T., Thornhill, M. *et al.* (2009) Poor oral hygiene as a risk factor for infective endocarditis-related bacteremia. *Journal of the American Dental Association*, 140, 1238–1244.

Lucas, V. and Roberts, G.J. (2000) Odontogenic bacteremia following tooth cleaning procedures in children. *Pediatric Dentistry*, 22, 96–100.

Lucas, V.S., Gafan, G., Dewhurst, S. *et al.* (2008) Prevalence, intensity and nature of bacteraemia after toothbrushing. *Journal of Dentistry*, 36, 481–487.

Lynch, R.J., Navada, R., Walia, R. (2004) Low-levels of fluoride in plaque and saliva and their effects on the demineralisation and remineralisation of enamel; role of fluoride toothpastes. *International Dental Journal*, 54(5 Suppl 1), 304–309.

Makiura, N., Ojima, M., Kou, Y. *et al.* (2008) Relationship of Porphyromonas gingivalis with glycemic level in patients with type 2 diabetes following periodontal treatment. *Oral Microbiology and Immunology*, 23, 348–351.

Malmberg, E., Birkhed, D., Norvenius, G. (1994) Microorganisms on toothbrushes at day-care centers. *Acta Odontologia Scandinavica*, 52, 93–98.

Mankodi, S., Bauroth, K., Witt, J.J. *et al.* (2005) A 6-month clinical trial to study the effects of a cetylpyridinium chloride mouthrinse on gingivitis and plaque. *American Journal of Dentistry*, 18 Spec No., 9A–14A.

Marchini, L., Vieira, P.C., Bossan, T.P., *et al.* (2006) Self-reported oral hygiene habits among institutionalised elderly and their relationship to the condition of oral tissues in Taubaté, Brazil. *Gerodontology*, 23, 33–37.

Miolin, I., Kulik, E.M., Weber, C. *et al.* (2007) Clinical effectiveness of two different toothbrushes in the elderly. *Schweizer Monatsschrift fur Zahnmedizin,* 117, 362–367.

Mojon, P., Budtz-Jørgensen, E., Rapin, C.H. (1999) Relationship between oral health and nutrition in very old people. *Age and Ageing,* 28, 463–468.

Morita, M., Nishi, K., Watanabe, T. (1998) Comparison of 2 tooth-brushing methods for efficacy in supragingival plaque removal. The Toothpick method and the Bass method. *Journal Clinical Periodontology,* 25, 829–831.

Morozumi, T., Kubota, T., Abe, D., *et al.* (2010) Effects of irrigation with an antiseptic and oral administration of azithromycin on bacteremia caused by scaling and root planing. *Journal of Periodontology,* 81, 1555–1163.

MSNBC News (2010) Listerine No Replacement for Flossing? [online] available at http://www.msnbc.msn.com/id/6799764/ns/health-health_care/.

Muñoz, C.A., Stephens, J.A., Proskin, H.M., *et al.* (2004) Clinical efficacy evaluation of calcium, phosphate, and sodium bicarbonate on surface-enamel smoothness and gloss. *Compendium of Continuing Education in Dentistry,* 25(9 Suppl 1), 32–39.

Mylonas, A.I., Tzerbos, F.H., Mihalaki, M. *et al.* (2007) Cerebral abscess of odontogenic origin. *Journal of Craniomaxillofacial Surgery,* 35, 63–67.

Newman, M.G., Cattabriga, M. Etienne, D. *et al.* (1994) Effectiveness of adjunctive irrigation in early periodontitis: multi-center evaluation. *Journal of Periodontology,* 65, 224–229.

Nishiyama, Y., Inaba, E., Uematsu, H. *et al.* (2010) Effects of mucosal care on oral pathogens in professional oral hygiene to the elderly. *Archives of Gerontology and Geriatrics,* 51, e139–e143.

Nordström, A., Mystikos, C., Ramberg, P., *et al.* (2009) Effect on de novo plaque formation of rinsing with toothpaste slurries and water solutions with a high fluoride concentration (5,000 ppm). *European Journal of Oral Science,* 117, 563–567.

O'Connell, P.A., Taba, M., Nomizo, A. *et al.* (2008) Effects of periodontal therapy on glycemic control and inflammatory markers. *Journal of Periodontology,* 79, 774–783.

Ogata, J., Minami, K., Miyamoto, H., *et al.* (2004) Gargling with povidone-iodine reduces the transport of bacteria during oral intubation. *Canadian Journal of Anesthesiology,* 51, 932–936.

Owens, J., Addy, M., Faulkner, J. *et al.* (1997) A short-term clinical study design to investigate the chemical plaque inhibitory properties of mouthrinses when used as adjuncts to toothpastes: applied to chlorhexidine. *Journal of Clinical Periodontology,* 24, 732–737.

Pai, V. (2009) Effect of a single-use toothbrush on plaque microflora. *Indian Journal of Dental Research,* 20, 404–406.

Pan, P.C., Harper, S., Ricci-Nittel, D., *et al.*(2010) In-vitro evidence for efficacy of antimicrobial mouthrinses. *Journal of Dentistry,* 38 Suppl 1, S16–S20.

Panchabhai, T.S., Dangayach, N.S., Krishnan, A. *et al.* (2009) Oropharyngeal cleansing with 0.2% chlorhexidine for prevention of nosocomial pneumonia in critically ill patients: an open-label randomized trial with 0.01% potassium permanganate as control. *Chest,* 135, 1150–1156.

Paraskevas, S., Rosema, N.A., Versteeg, P. *et al.* (2007) The additional effect of a dentifrice on the instant efficacy of toothbrushing: a crossover study. *Journal of Periodontology,* 78, 1011–1016.

Patters, M.R., Bland, P.S., Shiloah, J., *et al.* (2005) Comparison of the Hydrabrush powered toothbrush with two commercially-available powered toothbrushes. *Journal of the International Academy of Periodontology,* 7, 80–89.

Paula, V.A., Modesto, A., Santos, K.R. *et al.* (2010) Antimicrobial effects of the combination of chlorhexidine and xylitol. *British Dental Journal,* 209, E19.

Pedrazzi, V., Sato, S., de Mattos Mda, G. (2004) Tongue-cleaning methods: a comparative clinical trial employing a toothbrush and a tongue scraper. *Journal of Periodontology,* 75, 1009–1012.

Pobo, A., Lisboa, T., Rodriguez, A., *et al.* (2009) RASPALL Study Investigators. A randomized trial of dental brushing for preventing ventilator-associated pneumonia. *Chest,* 136, 433–439.

Powers, J., Brower, A., Tolliver, S. *et al.* (2007) Impact of oral hygiene on prevention of ventilator-associated pneumonia in neuroscience patients. *Journal of Nursing Care Quality,* 22, 316–321.

Poyato-Ferrera, M., Segura-Egea, J.J., Bullón-Fernández, P. (2003) Comparison of modified Bass technique with normal toothbrushing practices for efficacy in supragingival plaque removal. *International Journal of Dental Hygiene,* 1, 110–114.

Quirynen, M., De Soete, M., Pauwels, M., *et al.* (2003) Can toothpaste or a toothbrush with antibacterial tufts prevent toothbrush contamination? *Journal of Periodontology,* 74, 312–322.

Rao, S.K., Bhat, G.S., Aradhya, S. *et al.* (2009) Study of the efficacy of toothpaste containing casein phosphopeptide in the prevention of dental caries: a randomized controlled trial in 12- to 15-year-old high caries risk children in Bangalore, India. *Caries Research,* 43, 430–435.

Read, P.W., Fernandes, L., Harris, P. *et al.* (1981) Dental study in patients with rheumatoid arthritis. *Rheumatology Rehabilitation,* 20, 108–112.

Reeson, M.G. and Jepson, N.J. (2002) Customizing the size of toothbrush handles for patients with restricted hand and finger movement. *Journal of Prosthetic Dentistry,* 87, 700.

Saravia, M.E., Nelson-Filho, P. *et al.* (2008) Viability of Streptococcus mutans toothbrush bristles. *Journal of Dentistry for Children (Chicago),* 75, 29–32.

Särner, B. Birkhed, D. Andersson P. *et al.* (2010) Recommendations by dental staff and use of toothpicks, dental floss and interdental brushes for approximal cleaning in an adult Swedish population. *Oral Health and Preventive Dentistry,* 8, 185–189.

Scannapieco, F.A., Bush, R.B., Paju, S. (2003) Associations between periodontal disease and risk for nosocomial bacterial pneumonia and chronic obstructive pulmonary disease. A systematic review. *Annals of Periodontology,* 8, 54–69.

Schäfer, F., Nicholson, J.A., Gerritsen, N. *et al.* (2003) The effect of oral care feed-back devices on plaque removal and attitudes towards oral care. *International Dental Journal,* 53, 404–408.

Sekino, S., Ramberg, P., Uzel, N.G., *et al.* (2003) Effect of various chlorhexidine regimens on salivary bacteria and de novo plaque formation. *Journal of Clinical Periodontology,* 30, 991–925.

Sharma, N.C., Lyle, D.M., Qaqish, J.G., *et al.* (2008) Effect of a dental water jet with orthodontic tip on plaque and bleeding in adolescent patients with fixed orthodontic appliances. *American Journal of Orthodontic Dentofacial Orthopedics,* 133, 565–567.

Sheen, S., Eisenburger, M., Addy, M. (2003) Effect of toothpaste on the plaque inhibitory properties of a cetylpyridinium chloride mouth rinse. *Journal of Clinical Periodontology,* 30, 255–260.

Sirimaharaj, V., Brearley Messer, L., Morgan, M.V. *et al.* (2002) Acidic diet and dental erosion among athletes. *Australian Dental Journal,* 47, 228–236.

Sofrata, A., Lingström P, Baljoon M, Gustafsson A. (2007) The effect of miswak extract on plaque pH. An in vivo study. *Caries Research,* 41, 451–454.

Sofrata, A.H., Claesson, R.L., Lingström, P.K. *et al.* (2008) Strong antibacterial effect of miswak against oral microorganisms associated with periodontitis and caries. *Journal of Periodontology,* 79, 1474–1479.

Sripriya, N. and Shaik Hyder Ali, K.H. (2007) A comparative study of the efficacy of four different bristle designs of tooth brushes in plaque removal. *Journal of the Indian Society of Pedodontics and Preventive Dentistry,* 25, 76–81.

Staudt, C.B., Kinzel S., Hassfeld S. *et al.* (2001) Computer-based intraoral image analysis of the clinical plaque removing capacity of 3 manual toothbrushes. *Journal of Clinical Periodontology,* 28, 746–752.

Stoeken, J.E., Paraskevas, S., van der Weijden, G.A. (2007) The long-term effect of a mouthrinse containing essential oils on dental plaque and gingivitis: a systematic review. *Journal of Periodontology,* 78, 1218–1228.

Taji, S.S. and Rogers, A.H. (1998) ADRF Trebitsch Scholarship. The microbial contamination of toothbrushes. A pilot study. *Australian Dental Journal,* 43, 128–130.

Tantipong, H., Morkchareonpong, C., Jaiyindee, S. (2008) Randomized controlled trial and meta-analysis of oral decontamination with 2% chlorhexidine solution for the prevention of ventilator-associated pneumonia. *Infection Control and Hospital Epidemiology,* 29, 131–136.

Turner, L.A., McCombs, G.B., Hynes, W.L. *et al.* (2009) A novel approach to controlling bacterial contamination on toothbrushes: chlorhexidine coating. *International Journal of Dental Hygiene* 7, 241–245.

Van der Velden, U., Van Winkelhoff, A.J., Abbas, F. *et al.* (1986) The habitat of periodontopathic micro-organisms. *Journal of Clinical Periodontology,* 13, 243–248.

Wetzel, W.E., Schaumburg, C., Ansari, F. *et al.* (2005) Microbial contamination of toothbrushes with different principles of filament anchoring. *Journal of the American Dental Association,* 136, 758–765; quiz 806.

White, D.J., Barker, M.L., Klukowska, M. (2008) In vivo antiplaque efficacy of combined antimicrobial dentifrice and rinse hygiene regimens. *American Journal of Dentistry,* 21, 189–196.

Wiegand, A., Schwerzmann, M., Sener, B., *et al.* (2008) Impact of toothpaste slurry abrasivity and toothbrush filament stiffness on abrasion of eroded enamel—an in vitro study. *Acta Odontologia Scandinavica,* 66, 231–235.

Wilkins, E. (2008) *Clinical Practice of the Dental Hygienist* (Ed. E.M. Wilkins), 7th edn, pp. 338. Lippincott Williams and Wilkins, Philidelphia PA.

Wilnes, E.M. (1994) Interdental care and chemotherapy. In: *Clinical Practice of the Dental Hygienist* (Ed. E.M. Wilnes), 7th edn, pp. 365. Williams and Wilkins, Philadelphia, USA.

Witt, J., Bsoul, S., He, T. *et al.* (2006) The effect of toothbrushing regimens on the plaque inhibitory properties of an experimental cetylpyridinium chloride mouthrinse. *Journal of Clinical Periodontology,* 33, 737–742.

Witt, J.J., Walters, P., Bsoul, S. *et al.* (2005) Comparative clinical trial of two antigingivitis mouthrinses. *American Journal of Dentistry,* 18 Spec No., 15A–17A.

Yamanaka, A., Kimizuka, R., Kato, T. *et al.* (2004) Inhibitory effects of cranberry juice on attachment of oral streptococci and biofilm formation. *Oral Microbiology and Immunology.* 19, 150–154.

Yankell, S.L., Shi, X., Emling, R.C. (2002) Efficacy and safety of BrushPicks, a new cleaning aid, compared to the use of Glide floss. *Journal of Clinical Dentistry,* 13, 125–129.

Zhang, J.H., Dong, Z., Chu, L. (2010) Hydrogen sulfide induces apoptosis in human periodontium cells. *Journal of Periodontal Research,* 45, 71–78.

Zimmer, S., Kolbe, C., Kaiser, G. *et al.* (2006) Clinical efficacy of flossing versus use of antimicrobial rinses. *Journal of Periodontology,* 77, 1380–1385.

Zimmer, S. Oztürk M., Barthel, C.R. *et al.* (2011) Cleaning efficacy and soft tissue trauma after use of manual toothbrushes with different bristle stiffness. *Journal of Periodontology,* 82, 267–271.

9

The role of sugar alcohols, xylitol, and chewing gum in preventing dental diseases

Peter Milgrom and Kiet A. Ly

Introduction

In ordinary usage, sugar generally implies household table sugar; scientifically, it is known as sucrose. Like other naturally occurring sweet substances in its class, sucrose is a saccharide, meaning sugar, but more accurately, it is a carbohydrate.

Carbohydrates are organic compounds consisting of carbon, hydrogen, and oxygen molecules. They are divided into four groups: monosaccharide (mono = one, 3–6 carbon molecule, simple sugars); disaccharides (di = two units); oligosaccharides (oligo = several); or polysaccharides (poly = many, dozens to thousands). Monosaccharides such as glucose also called dextrose (grape or corn sugar) and fructose (fruit sugar), and disaccharides including lactose, maltose, and particularly sucrose are ubiquitous in the human diet especially in processed foods and snacks. These two classes of carbohydrates are readily fermentable by the oral bacteria such as mutans streptococci that are implicated in the development of dental caries and are highly cariogenic. Frequent or excessive consumption of these carbohydrates, especially between meals, leads to serious tooth decay and numerous health problems, for instance obesity and diabetes.

The epidemic of these dental and health problems have created a multi-billion dollar industry for "sugar substitutes" popularly known as "sugar-free" sweeteners. The most commonly used are sugar alcohols and intense sweeteners, which can be naturally occurring or artificially produced. These "sugar-free" sweeteners are low to non-cariogenic and are lower in or have no caloric values.

Sugar alcohols such as sorbitol, maltitol, mannitol, erythritol, and xylitol are widely found in foodstuff and are classified as nutritive sweeteners. They generally have one-third to two-thirds the caloric content of sucrose. Sugar alcohols are less sweet than sucrose except for xylitol, which has similar sweetness but only 60% of the caloric content (Table 9-1). Chemically, sugar alcohols are saccharide with hydroxyl groups, which lend them the term alcohol or poly-"ols." They are found naturally but can also be produced through chemical processes.

Intense sweeteners such as aspartame, saccharin, sucralose, and acesulfame are classified as non-nutritive sweeteners. They have negligible to no caloric values. However, their sweetness is several to hundreds of times that of sucrose. All intense sweeteners are artificially produced.

Dental caries, sugar alcohols, and xylitol

Mutans streptococci and dental caries

Oral mutans streptococci, specifically *Streptococcus mutans* and *Streptococcus sobrinus*, make up a primary group of bacteria implicated in the cause of tooth decay (Loesche 1986). These bacteria thrive in acidic environment and on fermentable carbohydrates such as sucrose, fructose, and glucose. They produce large amounts of lactic acid, a by-product of their fermentation process, which helps them flourish. They also produce extracellular polysaccharides or glucan-binding proteins that promote adhesion and formation of dental plaque on tooth surfaces (Gibbons and van Houte 1973; Kandelman 1997), thereby enhancing their ability to harbor and multiply. Acidic environment on the plaque-enamel interface can tip the scale of the enamel demineralization/remineralization equilibrium favoring demineralization leading to the development of cavity formation and dental caries or cavities.

Comprehensive Preventive Dentistry, First Edition. Edited by Hardy Limeback.
© 2012 John Wiley & Sons, Ltd. Published 2012 by John Wiley & Sons, Ltd.

Table 9-1 Properties of cariogenic and non-cariogenic sweeteners

Sweetener	Nutritive value (Calories/gram/m)	"Sugar-free" label	Sweetness*
Cariogenic sugars			
sucrose	4	no	1.0
glucose	4	no	0.7
fructose	4	no	1.5
galactose	4	no	0.2
Non-cariogenic sugars			
Sugar alcohols/Polyols			
xylitol	2.4	yes	1.0
sorbitol	2.6	yes	0.6
mannitol	1.6	yes	0.5
maltitol	2.1	yes	0.9
lactitol	0.02	yes	0.4
erythritol	0.02	yes	0.8
isomalt	2.0	yes	0.5
hydrogenated starch hydroxylate	3.0	yes	0.4–0.9
Artificial sweeteners			
Aspartame[†] (NutriSweet®, Equal)	0.0	yes	180
Saccharin (Sweet'N Low)	0.0	yes	300
Sucralose (SPLENDA®)	0.0	yes	600
Acesulfame potassium (Sunett)	0.0	yes	200

*Sucrose (table sugar) is the standard for sweetness comparison and is given the sweetness value of "1."
[†]Aspartame is technically a nutritive sweetener. Because of its intense sweetness, however, it is used in such small amounts that its nutritive value is negligible.

Sugar alcohols

Sugar alcohols, as a class, are low- to non-acidogenic. That is, they do not produce an acid environment when consumed because they are poorly fermented by acidogenic bacteria (Edwardsson *et al.* 1977). These characteristics lend them their very low- to non-cariogenic property (Van Loveren 2004). Therefore, their consumption contributes little if any to the development of tooth decay. National panels such as that from the 1989 UK COMA (Committee on Medical Aspects of Food Policy) report recommend that "food manufacturers produce 'sugars-free' alternatives to existing sugar-rich products, particularly those for children."

Sorbitol and xylitol well studied

Among the sugar alcohols, sorbitol and xylitol and their roles in oral health have been extensively studied. Clinical studies support the non-cariogenic property of sorbitol and polyols in general. (For review see Deshpande and Jadad 2008). On the other hand, research has shown that xylitol actively protects against tooth decay by reducing plaque and the level of mutans streptococci in saliva and plaque. (For review see Söderling 2009). These properties

significantly limit the level of lactic acid produced by these cariogenic bacteria, lactic acid that would have caused demineralization of tooth enamel leading to cavities formation. Overall, studies where xylitol and sorbitol were included, independently or in combination, have shown that 100% xylitol products had greater reductions in caries and/or mutans streptococci levels than a combination of xylitol and sorbitol, which in turn was better than sorbitol alone. (For reviews see Ly *et al.* 2008 and Milgrom 2009).

Xylitol in focus

Xylitol is a 5-carbon polyol, a pentatol, produced commercially from natural sources such as birch and beech trees and corncobs. Xylitol was discovered in the late 1800s and later found to occur naturally in plants and fruits and in mammalians including human metabolism, which produces several grams per day. It was not until the European sugar shortage during WWII that catapulted xylitol into mass production as a substitute sweetener for sugar. Xylitol was found to be more slowly absorbed than sugar and caused little spikes in blood sugar or insulin levels after consumption (Montague *et al.* 1967; Spitz *et al.* 1970). For these reasons, xylitol was first used in the medical arena as parenteral nutrition in intravenous infusions in place of IV Dextrose and as sugar replacement in diabetic foods. Exploration of xylitol's dental properties began at the turn of the 1970s.

Like other polyols, xylitol has been used primarily as a sugar-free sweetener in foods and confectionary products but less so because xylitol is more costly to produce at this time. However, as research reports continue to confirm the active protective effects of xylitol against plaque build-up, mutans streptococci, and tooth decay (Ly *et al.* 2008; Milgrom *et al.* 2009; Söderling 2009), there has been a rapid rise in xylitol oral health products such as chewing gum, lozenges, mints, and toothpaste. The market demand generally pushes for development of technologies that would improve production and reduce cost to meet the market demand.

Xylitol side effects and safety

The main side effects of xylitol, as with other polyols in its class, are laxative symptoms, which are dose dependent and range from stomach upset, cramps, and bloating to loose stools and osmotic diarrhea (Wang and van Eys 1981). These symptoms generally resolve by themselves or with the removal of the polyol from the diet. The side effects threshold for xylitol is about 50 grams per day, a threshold higher than that for mannitol or sorbitol. This amount is several times that needed for the use of xylitol in dental caries prevention. Habituation to polyols occurs where frequent prolonged use raises the tolerance level (Wang and van Eys 1981).

Xylitol is safe for use with children. Clinical studies where young children consumed up to 18 g of xylitol and/or sorbitol, alone or in combination, reported similar laxative symptom experience as controls (Akerblom *et al.* 1982; Forster *et al.* 1982; Milgrom *et al.* 2009).

Xylitol is non-fermentable

Xylitol is not readily fermented (metabolized) into energy sources by mutans streptococci. However, xylitol does compete with sucrose for the bacteria's cell-wall transporter and is absorbed and accumulated intracellularly by cariogenic bacteria. Inside the cell, xylitol competes with sucrose as a substrate for the fermentation process, the energy production steps necessary for cell growth and replication. However, unlike the fermentation of sucrose, which yields net energy, produces lactic acid by-products, and promotes cell growth, the cariogenic bacteria expend energy attempting to metabolize xylitol but yield no net energy or lactic acid in the process (Trahan *et al.* 1985). The intermediate substrates for producing high-energy compounds are consumed and not reproduced during xylitol fermentation. The result is a net loss of energy and needed intermediate substrates.

Furthermore, xylitol out competes sucrose as the substrate for fermentation thus the cariogenic bacteria continue to try and metabolize xylitol. This has been referred to as the "futile cycle" (Pihlanto-Leppala *et al.* 1989; Söderling and Pihlanto-Leppala 1989). As a result, mutans streptococci replication is limited and their levels fall. Even when growth of mutans streptococci is not reduced, xylitol interferes with components of the cell wall of the bacteria resulting in reduced aggregation at the tooth surface and less tooth decay.

Xylitol selects for non-virulent mutans streptococci

Long-term habitual consumption of xylitol has been suggested to select for mutans streptococci strains that have adapted mechanisms to ferment xylitol for energy. However, these "mutated" mutans streptococci strains appear to have low virulent level (Trahan *et al.* 1992). The acquisition of less mutans streptococci and less virulent strains in children whose mothers habitually consume xylitol may play an important role in the reduction in risk of developing tooth decay in those children (Milgrom *et al.* 2009; Söderling 2009).

Turku sugar studies—first to explore xylitol dental effects

Numerous studies have evaluated the effectiveness of xylitol in reducing tooth decay. Among the first was the Turku Sugar Studies conducted in Finland at the turn of the 1970s. The initial studies comparing various sugars and sugar alcohols found that xylitol reduced plaque formation (Mäkinen and Scheinin 1971; Scheinin and Mäkinen 1971). Subsequently, a series of studies was designed and conducted to elucidate various effects of xylitol on parameters such as oral flora and reduction of cariogenic pathogens like *S. mutans* and *S. sobrinus* (Turku VIII and XX) (Larmas *et al.* 1976a; Larmas *et al.* 1976b); biochemical properties in saliva and plaque (Turku VII) (Mäkinen and Scheinin 1976a); and the lack of effect in reducing salivary and plaque pH (Turku XXI) (Söderling *et al.* 1976); and human metabolic tolerance after long-term regular consumption of xylitol (Turku XIII) (Mäkinen and Scheinin 1976b). Two studies in this series evaluated tooth decay as the end point. These studies are discussed below.

Turku sugar studies—dietary substitution of sucrose with xylitol

This study involved 125 adults averaging 27.5 years who were assigned to one of three groups. Two groups had an almost complete substitution of sucrose by fructose or xylitol in their regular diet for 2 years. Participants were asked not to change their dietary pattern but to replace food products with one of the 100 products specifically developed for the study that contained the sweetener they were assigned to. Examples of products included sweetener for coffee, tea, and cooking, sweetened soft drinks, juices, soup, and jams, more than 30 different pastries and sweets, a variety of marinated herring, pickles, mustards, and a number of cough and medicine mixtures. Groups were blinded to the type of sweetener the products contained. Average individual monthly intake of sweeteners for the sucrose group was 2.2 Kg, compared to 2.1 Kg for fructose, and 1.5 Kg for xylitol. The highest daily amount of sweetener consumed varied from 200–400 g. At the end of the study, the mean increments of decayed, missing, and filled tooth surfaces (DMFS) were 7.2 in the sucrose-group, 3.8 in the fructose-group, and 0.0 in the xylitol-group. The results showed substitution of sucrose for xylitol resulted in a huge reduction of caries increment compared to sucrose. Fructose was found to be less cariogenic than sucrose (Turku I and V) (Scheinin *et al.* 1974; Scheinin *et al.* 1976).

Turku sugar studies—xylitol versus sucrose chewing gum

In this study, 102 participants, mostly dental and medical students, were assigned to consume either sucrose or xylitol chewing gum, 4 to 5 times per day for 1 year. Each stick of chewing gum contained 1.5 g of sucrose or xylitol. Participants maintained normal dietary and oral hygiene habits. They were instructed to consume 3 to 7 sticks of chewing gum at spaced out intervals and to keep a complete log of consumption. At the end of the year, the sucrose group consumed on average 4 pieces of chewing gum per day, and the xylitol group consumed 4.5 pieces. The sucrose group had a mean increment in decay, missing, filled tooth surfaces (DMFS) of 2.9 compared to 1.0 in the xylitol group (Scheinin *et al.* 1975). Following the Turku Studies, a number of xylitol field trials were conducted among children to replicate and confirm these findings. These studies include those conducted by the World Health Organization in Hungary, French Polynesia, and Thailand.

Ylivieska study—xylitol long-term effects

The Ylivieska study, also conducted in Finland in the early 1980s among 11 to 12 year olds, showed that the consumption of 7 to 10 g/day of xylitol in chewing gum over a 2- and 3-year period increased the efficacy of caries reduction by 30 to 60% beyond the regular use of topical fluoride (Isokangas 1987). The study also showed a reduction in *S. mutans* level among the xylitol chewing gum group (Mäkinen *et al.* 1989). More importantly,

a follow-up of the participants 2 to 3 years after discontinuation of the study suggested that children in the xylitol group continued to develop less new tooth decay and that the preventive effect was greatest among teeth that were erupting during the study period (Isokangas *et al.* 1989).

Xylitol field studies confirmed xylitol effectiveness

In the mid 1980s, a 2-year school-based xylitol chewing gum study was conducted among elementary schoolchildren in low socioeconomic areas of Montreal, Canada. A total of 574 third graders, aged 8 and 9 years, from 13 schools participated. Among these, 274 participants completed the baseline, 12-month, and 24-month dental examinations. The schools were assigned to one of two experimental groups: 65% xylitol (1.1 g xylitol per stick) or 15% xylitol (0.3 g xylitol per stick), or to the no chewing gum control group. Chewing gum was distributed 3 times a day by the teachers who also supervised the 5-minute chewing period. After 2 years, the average DMFS increments were 6.1, 2.4, and 2.1, for the no gum control, and the xylitol 15% and 65% chewing gum groups, respectively. This equates to a caries increment reduction of about 60% (Kandelman and Gagnon 1987; Kandelman and Gagnon 1990). The xylitol doses used in this study, about 1 to 3 g per day, were relatively low compared to previous studies yet still showed xylitol effect. Other studies using low-dose xylitol in the form of chewing gum or hard candies failed to show the benefits of xylitol (Petersen and Razanamihaja 1999; Machiulskiene *et al.* 2001; Oscarson *et al.* 2006).

At the turn of the 1990s, a more complex study design evaluating xylitol and/or sorbitol chewing gum and dental caries in permanent teeth was conducted in Belize. The 40-month study included 1,277 fourth graders (mean age 10.2 years) who were randomized into one of nine groups: four 100% xylitol groups with the dose ranging from 4.3 to 9.0 g/day divided into 3 to 5 frequency of consumption; two xylitol-sorbitol groups (8.0 to 9.7 g/day); a sorbitol (9.0 g/day) group; a sucrose group; and a control (no gum) group. Study gums chewed during school hours were under supervision but were unsupervised on non-school days. The study reported that the 100% xylitol pellet chewing gum resulted in the highest caries reduction when compared to control (no gum). Furthermore, groups consuming higher xylitol dose had greater caries reduction than similar but lower dose xylitol gum. Xylitol-sorbitol mixed chewing gum had lesser but still significant reduction followed by sorbitol compared to control. Not surprisingly, the sucrose gum group fared worse than the control group (Mäkinen *et al.* 1995).

The same group of researchers conducted a second study to evaluate xylitol and/or sorbitol chewing gum and dental caries in primary dentition. Participants were 510 6-year-old children from a rural district of Belize where the caries rate was known to be high. Participants were assigned to 1 of 7 groups: the no-gum group; two (stick or pellet gums) sorbitol groups; two xylitol groups; and two xylitol-sorbitol groups. Chewing gum consumption was supervised and occurred 5 times per school day and was unsupervised on non-school days. The study observed the strongest reduction in mutans streptococci and caries risk in the group receiving xylitol pellet chewing gum (Mäkinen *et al.* 1996).

Other more recent studies, particularly those using similar xylitol doses and frequencies as the above studies, have shown support for these findings and have been reviewed (Deshpande and Jadad 2008; Milgrom *et al.* 2009; Söderling 2009). Overall, these reviews suggest efficacy is associated with dose and frequency of use where greater reduction is seen with higher xylitol dose and frequency of consumption.

Xylitol dose and frequency of use for efficacy

A research team at the University of Washington in the US set out to design a series of studies to determine the minimum dose and frequency of xylitol consumption needed for efficacy. The first study of the series, the xylitol dose response study, aimed to determine the minimal dose of consumption needed for xylitol to reduce salivary and plaque *S. mutans*, a surrogate marker of tooth decay. Participants were randomly assigned to one of four groups consuming the following: control (sorbitol); 3.4 g xylitol chewing gum; 6.9 g xylitol chewing gum; or 10.3 g xylitol chewing gum. Control gums were use to fill in gaps so that all groups consumed the same number of chewing gum pieces per day, divided into 4 chewing periods. The study found significant reduction in plaque *S. mutans* level after 5 weeks and 6 months of exposure compared to sorbitol control. The results also suggested a plateau effect between 6.4 g and 10.3 g per day. Furthermore, the 3.4 g per day group showed a small but not statistically significant reduction (Milgrom *et al.* 2006).

The second study of the series evaluated the response of *S. mutans* to varying frequencies (0, 2, 3, and 4) of xylitol chewing gum consumption at a standard daily dose (10.3 g/day). The study found a linear increase in *S. mutans* reduction to increasing frequency of xylitol consumption. However, dosing frequency of less than 3 times per day showed small and non-statistically significant benefit (Ly *et al.* 2006).

At this time, there is general agreement in the literature that a xylitol dose of 5 to 10 g/day divided into 3 or more frequencies of consumption are needed for chewing gum, lozenges, or mints for therapeutic effects. However, it appears that different xylitol delivery vehicles (different products) have different oral bioavailability that may affect the dose and frequency of exposure needed for effectiveness. A clinical trial in toddlers showed xylitol syrup 4 g twice per day reduced tooth decay (Milgrom *et al.* 2009). Similarly, studies have reported that fluoride toothpaste containing 10% xylitol reduce tooth decay more than fluoride toothpaste alone (Sintes *et al.* 1995; Sintes *et al.* 2002). The daily xylitol exposure totaled only about 0.2 g/day for the toothpaste studies. These studies are discussed below.

Xylitol syrup

In a study conducted in the Republic of the Marshall Islands, toddlers averaging 15 ± 3 months of age were assigned to one of three groups. Each group received a total of 3 unit doses of sorbitol and/or xylitol. Two groups received an 8-g/day dose of xylitol divided into 2 or 3 unit doses, and a control group was given 1 xylitol unit dose of 2.7 g/day. The non-xylitol unit dose contained 2.0 g of sorbitol plus an intense sweetener. All unit doses were packaged in 8 mL tubes and matched in sweetness using an intense sweetener. Syrups were squirted onto the teeth and gum of the toddlers by their mother or primary care taker. The study reported 52% of toddler in the control xylitol low-dose group developed tooth decay after about 12 months compared to 40% and 24% for toddlers in the 8 g/day divided into 3 unit doses and 2 unit doses, respectively. The prevented fraction was determined to be 50% and 70%, respectively (Milgrom *et al.* 2009).

Xylitol toothpaste

Two large studies using 10% xylitol fluoride toothpaste showed reduction in tooth decay. The first study involved 2,630 school children aged 8–10 years attending 17 schools in the San Jose, Costa Rica metropolitan area. Participants were followed for 3 years. Children were randomly assigned to use a 0.243% NaF toothpaste with or without 10% xylitol and instructed to brush with their assigned toothpaste for 1 minute, twice daily—once in school and once at home or twice at home when not in school. After brushing, children expectorated and thoroughly rinsed with water. Toothpaste applications were done by or under supervision of teachers or mothers. After 3 years, the 10% xylitol toothpaste group showed a 12% decrease in increments of decayed/filled surfaces compared to the non-xylitol toothpaste (Sintes *et al.* 1995).

In the second study by the same investigators but using a different toothpaste base (0.836% sodium monofluorophosphate in a dicalcium phosphate dihydrate base) with or without 10% xylitol, 3,394 school children aged 7–12 years at 28 public schools in the central plateau of Costa Rica participated. Similar instructions as above were given to the children. Decayed, filled surfaces/decayed, filled teeth (DFS/DFT) increments over the 30-month study period were 1.3/0.7 for the 10% xylitol compared to 1.5/0.8 for the non-xylitol group (Sintes et al. 2002). It is worth noting that both toothpaste studies were sponsored by the Colgate-Palmolive Company and neither are currently available. There has been a proliferation of xylitol-containing toothpastes available in North America through the internet. None have been thoroughly tested and demonstrated to be efficacious. Some do not contain fluoride.

Numerous other xylitol products—do they work?

Most studies have involved xylitol chewing gums, and a few involved lozenges, hard candies, mints, gummy bears, and syrup. These studies consistently showed efficacy at a xylitol dose of 5 to 10 g/day. Smaller dose studies using chewing gum or hard candies have yielded conflicting results. Yet, the xylitol toothpaste studies reported effectiveness even though the amount of daily xylitol exposure was less than 1 g per day. There remains much skepticism over these findings. Further research is needed for this product.

In response to the findings overall, numerous multi-national and regional confectionary and oral health vendors have produced and marketed a host of xylitol chewing gums, mints, lozenges, and toothpastes to improve oral health and reduce tooth decay (Table 9-2 and Table 9-3).

There are numerous other xylitol oral health products being marketed as well such as xylitol teeth wipes for infants, xylitol mouthwash, xylitol floss, etc. These products have not been clinically evaluated for efficacy. Research suggests that different xylitol products may have different oral bioavailability for topical effects on teeth surfaces. Thus, it is conceivable that these products work. However, these products and any new xylitol product made need to be studied via a stringent research protocol in order to demonstrate their effectiveness. Until the product has been studied, it would be unwise to suggest that the use of those products would improve oral health.

Xylitol and other health conditions

Although the focus of this chapter is limited to xylitol and oral health, it is worth noting that xylitol is also marketed for a list of other health conditions. Most notable is in nutrition and dietetics foods, particularly for diabetics. This finding is attributed to xylitol's low caloric content and glycemic index, less than 1/10th that of sucrose. Thus, its consumption causes little insulin response (Natah et al. 1997). There is exciting recent work that suggests xylitol, when combined with other agents, may speed the healing of diabetic ulcers and bed sores because of its ability to disrupt cell wall functions and reduce bacterial aggregation at wound sites. There are also claims that xylitol reduces osteoporosis and ear and sinus infections, but there are too few studies to lend support to these claims. Nevertheless, entrepreneurs seize the opportunities to produce and market products such as xylitol nasal spray to prevent sinus infections and allergies or promote consumption of xylitol foodstuff to reduce the risk of osteoporosis and aging.

Maternal xylitol consumption and *S. mutans* level and caries in their children

Studies have also shown children whose mothers consumed xylitol chewing gum in the perinatal period had lower *S. mutans* levels. This is a viable caries prevention strategy for clinicians who treat children with Early Childhood Caries. Söderling and colleagues recruited mother-infant pairs into a 2-year study and randomized the pair into one of three groups: xylitol chewing gum, chlorhexidine varnish, or fluoride varnish. Mothers with high levels of mutans streptococci ($>10^5$ CFU) were selected. Mothers received varnish treatments at 6, 12, 18, and 24 months after delivery or were asked to chew xylitol gum beginning at 3 months after delivery. Average gum chewing was 4 times per day totaling 6–7 g per day. Children did not receive any treatment. At 2 years of age, only 10% of children whose mother were in the xylitol chewing gum group had detectable mutans streptococci level compared to 29% and 49% in the chlorhexidine and fluoride groups, respectively (Söderling et al. 2000). At the 5-year caries assessment follow-up, children in the xylitol group had 71% less tooth decay compare to the varnish groups (Isokangas et al. 2000). At the 6-year follow-up, children in the xylitol group continue to show lower levels of mutans streptococci (Söderling et al. 2001).

In a similar 1-year study but using chewing gum beginning at 6 months postpartum, mothers with high levels of mutans streptococci were randomized into one of three groups: xylitol, chlorhexidine/xylitol, or fluoride. The reference group was mothers with low or medium mutans streptococci counts who received no intervention. The study reported 10% of 18-month-old children of mothers in the xylitol chewing gum group harbored mutans streptococci compared to 16% and 28% in the chlorhexidine/xylitol and fluoride group,

Table 9-2 Xylitol-containing gums, their xylitol content, and preventive potential

Products[†]	Xylitol (grams per piece)	Pieces 5 (10) g/day	Preventive Potential[††]
Gums			
Epic—Xylitol gum (various flavors)	1.00	5 (10)	Yes
Clen-Dent/Xponent gum (various flavors)	0.67	8 (15)	Yes
Eco-Dent "Between Dental Gum" (various flavors)	0.70	7 (14)	Yes
Fazer XyliDent and xylitol gums	0.66	8 (15)	Yes
Fennobon Oy "XyliMax Gum"	1.00	5 (10)	Yes
Leaf Jenkki Professional Gum	0.71	7 (14)	Yes
Leaf Jenkki Classic Gum (various flavors)	0.36		
Leaf Frozen Gum (various flavors)	0.35–0.39		
Lotte—Xylitol Gum (various flavors)	0.83	6 (12)	Yes
Omnii "Theragum"	0.70	7 (14)	Yes
Spry Xylitol gum (various flavors)	0.75	7 (13)	Yes
Tundra Trading "XyliChew Gum"	0.80	7 (13)	Yes
Xylimax chewing gum	1.00	5 (10)	Yes
Vitamin Research "Unique Sweet Gum"	0.72	7 (14)	Yes
Altoids sugar-free chewing gum	1 of 3 polyols (1.0)	NC[†††]	Maybe
B-FRESH Gums (various flavors)	1 of 2 polyols (1.0)	NC	Maybe
Arm & Hammer "Dental Care Baking Soda Gum"	2 of 3 polyols (1.0)	NC	No
Arm & Hammer "Advance White Icy Mint Gum"	2 of 3 polyols (1.0)	NC	No
Biotene "Dental Gum" and "Dry Mouth Gum"	2 of 2 polyols (1.0)	NC	No
Starbucks "After Coffee Gum"	2 of 4 polyols	NC	No
Trident® fusion flavors	4 of 4 polyols (1.0)	NC	No
Stride gum (various flavor)	3 of 3 polyols (1.0)	NC	No
Trident For Kids Gum	3 of 3 polyols (1.0)	NC	No
Wrigley "Orbit Sugar-Free Gum"	4 of 4 polyols (1.0)	NC	No
Fennobon "XyliDent Gum"	NC	NC	NC
Ford Gum "Xtreme Xylitol Gums"	NC	NC	NC
Wrigley "Everest Mint Gum"	NC	NC	NC

[†]Product list is not exhaustive. Xylitol market is rapidly changing and new xylitol containing products appear frequently, and products formulation and xylitol content may have changed.

[††]"Yes," "No," or "Maybe" is based on the potential a person is willing to consume two to three pieces, three to five times per day to meet the effective dose range of 5 to 10 grams per day. Products with potential for effectiveness but the xylitol dose is either unknown but is among the first polyol in the ingredients list are assigned "Maybe."

[†††]N/C = Not Certain. Information cannot be derived from internet vendor, or market packaging, or not successful in obtaining information from vendors' information representatives.

respectively. In the reference group, 10% of the children had detectable mutans streptococci (Thorild *et al.* 2003). At 3 years of age, 13% of the children in the xylitol group had medium to high counts of salivary mutans streptococci with a decayed, extracted, filled surfaces (defs) of 0.1 compared to 16% with defs of 0.2 for chlorhexidine/xylitol group, and 22% with defs of 0.4 for the fluoride group. The reference group had results between the xylitol and chlorhexidine/xylitol groups (Thorild *et al.* 2004). At 4 years of age, the mean defs was 0.4 for the xylitol group, 0.7 for the chlorhexidine/xylitol group, and 1.4 for the fluoride group (Thorild *et al.* 2006).

Chewing gum in the control of dental caries

Chewing gum culture then and now

Chewing gum is commonly thought of as part of American culture popularized during World War II when it was included in US GI rations (Redclift 2004). Chewing gum is now a worldwide phenomenon. The first USA patent for a chewing gum was issued in 1869 to Dr. W.F. Semple, a dentist in Ohio (Imfeld 1999). Yet, chewing non-food items and gummy substances for pleasure can be traced to ancient Greek culture and throughout the Middle East and Mayan Indians in the

Table 9-3 Xylitol-containing mints, candies, oral health products, and their xylitol content

Products[†]	Xylitol (grams per piece)	Pieces 5 (10) g/day	Preventive Potential[††]
Mints & Candies			
Clen-Dent/Xponent "Mints"	0.67	8 (15)	Yes
Epic "Xylitol Mints"	0.50	10 (20)	Yes
Leaf Läkerol Dents Lozenges	50% by wt		
Leaf Läkerol Pastilles (various flavors)	50% by wt		
Lotte Xylitol Mint (various flavors)	0.83 g		
Smart Sweet Fragmints	0.50	10 (20)	Yes
Spry "Mints":	0.50	10 (20)	Yes
Spry SparX Candies	0.5 g		
Tundra Trading "XyliChew Mints"	0.55	9 (18)	Yes
VitaDent "Mints"/ "Unique Sweet Mints"	0.5	10 (20)	Yes
Xylimax Mints	1.0		
SMINT "Mints"	<0.20	30 (50)	No
Brown & Haley "Zingos Caffeinated Peppermints"	2 of 2 polyols	NC[†††]	No
Oxyfresh "Breath Mints"	2 of 2 polyols	NC	No
Starbucks "After Coffee Mints"	2 of 2 polyols	NC	No
Xleardent "Mints"	NC	NC	No
Oral Hygiene			
Biotene "Dry Mouth Toothpaste" (±Calcium)	10%		
Biotene "First Teeth" Infant Toothpaste	1 of 2 polyols		
Crest "Multicare Cool Mint Toothpaste"	10%		
Epic toothpaste without fluoride	25%		
Epic toothpaste with fluoride	35%		
Squigle "Enamel Saver Toothpaste"	36% (0.24% sodium fluoride)		
Tooth Builder® Toothpaste	36% (Fluoride Free)		
XyliWhite Toothpaste (fluoride free)	25%		
Biotene "Oral Balance" Dry mouth gel	2 of 2 polyols		
Rembrandt toothpaste "For Canker Sore"	only sweetener (fourth ingredient)		
Spry Infant "Tooth Gel"	N/C only polyol (no fluoride)		
Spry toothpaste "MaxXylitol and Aloe"	N/C only polyol (no fluoride)		
Tom's of Maine "Baking Soda" Toothpaste line	N/C (varies in ingredient list)		
Tom's of Maine "Natural Toothpaste" line	N/C (varies in ingredient list)		
Tom's of Maine "Sensitive Toothpaste" line	N/C (varies in ingredient list)		
Epic "Mouthwash"	25%		
Biotene "Mouthwash"	1 of 2 polyols		
Gerber "Tooth & Gum Cleanser"	2 of 2 polyols (sixth ingredient)		
Now Foods "XyliWhite" Mouthwash	only sweetener (second ingredient)		
Oxyfresh "Mouthrinse"	only sweetener (second ingredient)		
Rembrandt "Dazzling Breathdrops"	only sweetener (second ingredient)		
Spry "Oral Rinse"	1 of 2 polyols (no fluoride)		
Tom's of Maine "Natural Mouthwash" line	N/C (varies in ingredient list)		

[†]Product list is not exhaustive. Xylitol market is rapidly changing and new xylitol-containing products appear frequently, and products formulation and xylitol content may have changed.

[††]"Yes," "No," or "Maybe" is based on the potential a person is willing to consume two to three pieces, three to five times per day to meet the effective dose range of 5 to 10 grams per day. Products with potential for effectiveness, but the xylitol dose is either unknown but is among the first polyol in the ingredients list are assigned "Maybe."

[†††]N/C = Not Certain. Information cannot be derived from internet vendor, or market packaging, or were not successful in obtaining information from vendors' information representatives.

early centuries A.D. (Redclift 2004). Today, chewing gum is a worldwide multi-billion dollar industry with more than half a million tons consumed annually (Imfeld 1999).

Originally, chewing gums were sweetened with sucrose; thus, they contributed to tooth decay. Today, the majority of chewing gum in the US and more than half of the chewing gums in the world are sweetened with sugar-free sweeteners such as polyols and/or intense sweeteners. Studies showed these sugar substitutes do not lead to clinically relevant acid production (Imfeld 1999), and they are accepted as non-cariogenic by the US Food and Drug Administration (FDA) and food and drug regulatory bodies in numerous countries all over the world.

Chewing gums have been studied and used as delivery vehicles for a host of dental protective substances such as calcium, bicarbonate, carbamide, chlorhexidine, fluoride, and polyol sweeteners and for medicinal substances such as nicotine, methadone, aspirin, antihistamines, antifungals, caffeine, and vitamins. The use of polyol-sweetened chewing gum, particularly xylitol, alone or in combination with other dental protective substances in oral health prevention programs, especially for high-risk populations, may have significant impact in reducing tooth decay and improving the oral health of the world's children. Interest has peaked particularly because tooth decay in young children is rising as availability of processed food and beverage products high in fermentable carbohydrates are increasingly readily available and are inexpensive.

Chewing gum effects on oral health

Chewing gum consists typically of a sweetener, gum base, flavoring, and aromatic agent. There are numerous claims for the effects of chewing gum. For example, chewing gum cleans food debris from teeth and plaque, stimulates salivary flow, raises saliva and plaque pH, and reduces gingivitis and periodontitis. These effects are generally based on the mechanics of chewing and the increase in salivary flow in response to mastication.

A review critically evaluated the chewing gum effects and applications and concluded that the mechanical act of mastication (gum chewing) is a potent stimulator of salivary flow, that chewing gum after meals stimulates saliva flow with increased concentration of bicarbonate resulting in elevated plaque pH and enhanced acid buffering capacity, and promotes enamel remineralization. However, the latter effect is lost when sucrose-based chewing gum is consumed. In contrast, little evidence supported gum chewing to reduce gingivitis or as being effective in removing plaque, particularly in interproximal areas where oral hygiene is most important (Imfeld 1999).

Clearly, sucrose chewing gum promotes tooth decay, sugar-free chewing gum does not, and the mastication process may be protective. On the other hand, sugar-free chewing gums containing appropriate amounts of dental protective substances, alone or in combination, have been used in Scandinavia and have the potential for wide usage in preventive oral health programs to improve oral health and reduce tooth decay.

Chewing gum as a delivery vehicle for fluoride, minerals, alkalinizing agents, and chlorhexidine

In the 1960s, fluoride-containing chewing gum was introduced as an alternative to fluoride tablets for populations not served by fluoridated water systems or fluoridated salt distribution schemes. It was shown to reduce demineralization and enhance remineralization of enamel (Hattab et al. 1989; Lamb et al. 1993; De Los Santos et al. 1994). However, other topical fluorides became readily available and overshadowed fluoride chewing gum.

Also in the 1960s, chewing gum was explored for the delivery of minerals such as calcium and phosphate. Studies of various forms of calcium phosphates reported enhanced acid-buffering capacity and decreased demineralization (Richardson et al. 1972; Chow et al. 1994). Chewing gum containing xylitol and calcium lactate has also been shown to enhance remineralization of enamel compared to chewing gum containing only xylitol or no gum at all (Suda et al. 2006). Similarly, bicarbonate has been used to effectively alkalinize saliva and plaque (Imfeld 1983; Nilner et al. 1991). Other researchers using various forms of market available bicarbonate chewing gum reported an increase in salivary pH and reduction of dental plaque and gingivitis (Kleber et al. 2001; Sharma et al. 2001; Anderson and Orchardson 2003). The latter effects are particularly important for patients with dry mouth. The antiseptic, chlorhexidine (CHX), has been used in mouth rinses to treat gingivitis and periodontitis. It has also been used as a short-term substitute for mechanical brushing. Chewing gums containing CHX are found to minimize the undesirable staining and bitter taste effect of CHX while maintaining similar effectiveness against gingivitis and periodontitis to that of CHX mouth rinses. Several studies showed that chewing CHX gum twice daily with no other oral hygiene measures was as effective in inhibiting plaque growth as rinsing with CHX (0.2%) twice a day (Ainamo et al. 1990; Smith et al. 1996; Yankell and Emling 1997).

The potential use of these dental protective chewing gums in targeted oral health programs that span from toddlers to the elders can have a profound impact on reduction of oral diseases. These chewing gums are available in the market. However, it is unclear if the marketed oral health products contain adequate amounts of dental protective substances for efficacy. Furthermore, there are no clear guidelines for amount, frequency, and length of use of these dental protective chewing gum products for clinical efficacy. More research is needed to address questions of clinically effective amount, frequency, and length of use.

Polyol chewing gum and dental caries

Polyol sweeteners have been used as substitutes for sucrose and fructose in food, confectionary products, and chewing gum for several decades. Polyol sweeteners are regulated by the FDA, and many are classified as GRAS (Generally Recognized As Safe) or approved as food additives. In the late 1990s, the US FDA authorized the claim that "sugar alcohols" present in the food "does not promote," "may reduce the risk of," or "useful [or is useful] in not promoting" dental caries. This Code of Federal Regulation (21CFR101.80) was updated in 2010. The Canadian Food and Drug Regulations permit similar claims: "won't cause cavities," "does not promote tooth decay," "does not promote dental caries," or "non-cariogenic" as do numerous European and Asian countries. Consequently, polyol sweeteners are found in numerous foods, confectionary goods, and other products such as chewing gum marketed to promote better oral health.

Numerous clinical studies have evaluated the non-cariogenic to caries protective effects of xylitol and/or sorbitol chewing gums. Overall, the studies suggest that habitual use of chewing gum containing xylitol totaling 5 to 10 g per day resulted in reduction of mutans streptococci levels and/or tooth decay. Greater reduction is observed with higher xylitol doses and higher frequencies of consumption. The studies also suggested that the combination of xylitol and sorbitol in chewing gum is more effective than sorbitol alone but not as effective as xylitol alone (Ly et al. 2006).

Potential applications of dental chewing gum for children at high risk for caries

Topical fluorides are the mainstays for primary prevention of tooth decay in children. They include fluoride toothpaste, water fluoridation, fluoride tablets, and professionally applied fluoride gel, foam, and varnish. Unless intensely provided and minimally dependent on usage by children, topical fluorides are limited in their effectiveness against virulent dental caries. Sealants are primarily used to protect molars of children nearing their teen years. But by then, a large number of children already suffer from tooth decay. Dietary changes have been difficult to achieve. Effective strategies to modify children's diets are not readily applicable, nor are they typically effective without significant effort.

Given the popularity of chewing gum throughout the world, especially among children, the use of dental protective chewing gum products containing Chlorhexidine or polyols, especially xylitol, is attractive as an adjunct to other preventive practices. The research studies discussed in this chapter have shown that xylitol chewing gum can reduce plaque, mutans streptococci, and tooth decay. There is agreement for effective dose and frequency of their use. Therefore, it behooves us not to exploit these characteristics of xylitol for the primary prevention of tooth decay in children.

Xylitol chewing gum acceptability among children

Xylitol chewing gum is readily available. Most xylitol clinical and field studies worldwide including those in the US have used chewing gum and have shown chewing gum to be well accepted by school-age children. However, the American Academy of Pediatrics classifies chewing gum among products with choking risk. Following that logic and other concerns, teachers and school officials actively discourage chewing gum consumption in day care and schools. In a study examining the acceptance of xylitol chewing gum regimen by preschoolers and teachers in a Head Start program, the researchers found that children readily accepted the xylitol chewing gum. However, teachers' acceptance was low because of concern of class disruption and indiscriminate disposal of chewing gum (Autio and Courts 2001). Yet, xylitol chewing gum studies in various school settings in several countries have not reported these problems or choking concerns. In these studies, children were guided in gum chewing and taught proper disposal of consumed chewing gum with great success.

Xylitol chewing gum and public health programs

Xylitol chewing gum has being used in non-research-oriented population-based oral health prevention programs. For instance, in 1991, 15% of boys and 35% of girls consumed xylitol chewing gum daily. In 1992, Finland initiated the "Smart Habits" xylitol campaign where consumption of xylitol chewing gum was widely promoted. The program was geared at children and teens with the aim of improving oral health and reducing dental caries. Children were given xylitol chewing gum to chew in the classroom and were taught to discard used chewing gum in wastebaskets. The program promoted the use of xylitol chewing gum over gum with other sweeteners. Subsequently, other xylitol-containing products such as lozenges and hard candies also became accepted by teachers, parents, and children as part of their "Smart Habits" program. Several years later, as part of a national survey, similarly age children were asked about their xylitol chewing gum consumption habits. The survey report that nearly half of boys and 57–69% of girls (ages 11–15) consumed xylitol chewing gum on a daily basis. Less than 1% chewed sugar gum (Honkala *et al.* 1999).

The US Army Dental Command (DENCOM) recognizes the potential benefits of xylitol for their troops. DENCOM implemented its "Look for Xylitol First" initiative. The objective was to train all members of the dental care team on the positive benefits of xylitol and to teach their patients (troops) how to be smart consumers and evaluate products for their xylitol content. The US Army also began including xylitol chewing gum in MRE (Meals Ready to Eat) rations. The overall goal was to reduce tooth decay among their troops especially those deployed who often neglect oral hygiene while in the field.

For many years now, the use of xylitol chewing gum is widely accepted in Scandinavian countries and routinely promoted by their public health systems. Consumption of xylitol products regularly after a meal has become a common habit in the everyday life of the Finnish. Similarly, the Canadian Children's Oral Health Initiative suggests "the promotion of products containing xylitol for the parents or caregivers of infants ages 0-2-1/2 years." In 2008, The European Food Safety Authority (EFSA) has approved a health claim specifying that "xylitol chewing gum reduces the risk of caries in children" (EFSA Journal 2008). Similar claim is permitted for use in Japan. Xylitol chewing gum has been actively promoted in Japan, China, Korea, Thailand, and the Philippines and has captured more than 50% of the chewing gum market in many of these countries.

Conclusion

Chewing gums containing protective substances have been shown to be effective and to have the potential for significant impact in improving oral health toward Healthy People 2010 and WHO Global Oral Health goals. Xylitol chewing gum stands out among the rest because dose and frequency of use is known. Numerous national dental associations in Europe, Asia, North America, and South America including the American Academy of Pediatric Dentistry have endorsed the use of xylitol-containing products for caries prevention. Xylitol chewing gum has been successfully implemented as a population-based program in Finland and by The U.S.

Army. Its use for oral health prevention is widely promoted in several countries in Europe and Asia. Perhaps it is time for school officials, policy makers, and national pediatrics and dental associations to seriously consider the potential public health benefits of xylitol chewing gum for children and push for development of policies and/or programs to promote and include xylitol chewing gum use in the armament with topical fluorides as primary prevention modalities to maximally reduce the current world epidemic of tooth decay in children.

References

Ainamo, J., Nieminen, A., Westerlund, U. (1990) Optimal dosage of chlorhexidine acetate in chewing gum. *Journal of Clinical Periodontology*, 17, 729–733.

Akerblom, H.K., Koivukangas, T., Puukka, R., *et al.* (1982) The tolerance of increasing amounts of dietary xylitol in children. *International Journal of Vitamin and Nutrition Research.* Supplement, 22, 53–66.

Anderson, L.A. and Orchardson, R. (2003) The effect of chewing bicarbonate-containing gum on salivary flow rate and pH in humans. *Archives Oral Biology*, 48, 201–204.

Autio, J.T. and Courts, F.J. (2001) Acceptance of the xylitol chewing gum regimen by preschool children and teachers in a Head Start program: a pilot study. *Pediatric Dentistry*, 23, 71–74.

Chow, L.C., Takagi, S., Shern, R.J., *et al.* (1994) Effects on whole saliva of chewing gums containing calcium phosphates. *Journal of Dental Research*, 73, 26–32.

De Los Santos, R., Lin, Y. T., Corpron R.E., *et al.* (1994) In situ remineralization of root surface lesions using a fluoride chewing gum or fluoride-releasing device. *Caries Research*, 28, 441–446.

Deshpande, A. and Jadad, A.R. (2008) The impact of polyol-containing chewing gums on dental caries: a systematic review of original randomized controlled trials and observational studies. *Journal of the American Dental Association*, 139, 1602–1614.

Edwardsson, S., Birkhed, D., Mejàre B. (1977) Acid production from Lycasin, maltitol, sorbitol and xylitol by oral streptococci and lactobacilli. *Acta Odontologica Scandinavica*, 35, 257–263.

European Food Safety Authority (EFSA). (2008) *The EFSA Journal*, 852, 12–15.

Förster, H., Quadbeck, R., Gottstein, U. (1982) Metabolic tolerance to high doses of oral xylitol in human volunteers not previously adapted to xylitol. *International Journal of Vitamin and Nutrition Research.* Supplement, 22, 67–88.

Gibbons, R.J. and van Houte, J. (1973) On the formation of dental plaques. *Journal of Periodontology*, 44, 347–360.

Hattab, F.N., Green, R.M., Pang, K.M., *et al.* (1989) Effect of fluoride-containing chewing gum on remineralization of carious lesions and on fluoride uptake in man. *Clinical Preventive Dentistry*, 11, 6–11.

Imfeld, T. (1983) [Nutrition and dental caries. Non-cariogenic between-meal snacks and sweets: a marketplace for small and average-size businesses in the food industry. An interview with Dr. med. dent. T. Imfeld]. *Swiss Dentistry*, 4, 6–10.

Imfeld, T. (1999) Chewing gum—facts and fiction: a review of gum-chewing and oral health. *Critical Revues in Oral Biology and Medicine*, 10, 405–419.

Isokangas, P. (1987) Xylitol chewing gum in caries prevention. A longitudinal study on Finnish school children. *Proceedings of the Finnish Dental Society*, 83(Suppl 1), 1–117.

Isokangas, P., Söderling, E., Pienihäkkinen, K., *et al.* (2000) Occurrence of dental decay in children after maternal consumption of xylitol chewing gum, a follow-up from 0 to 5 years of age. *Journal of Dental Research*, 79, 1885–1889.

Isokangas, P., Tiekso, J., Alanen P., *et al.* (1989) Long-term effect of xylitol chewing gum on dental caries. *Community Dentistry and Oral Epidemiology*, 17, 200–203.

Kandelman, D. (1997) Sugar, alternative sweeteners and meal frequency in relation to caries prevention: new perspectives. *British Journal of Nutrition*, 77 (Suppl 1), S121–S128.

Kandelman, D. and Gagnon, G. (1987) Clinical results after 12 months from a study of the incidence and progression of dental caries in relation to consumption of chewing-gum containing xylitol in school preventive programs. *Journal of Dental Research*, 66, 1407–1411.

Kandelman, D. and Gagnon, G. (1990) A 24-month clinical study of the incidence and progression of dental caries in relation to consumption of chewing gum containing xylitol in school preventive programs. *Journal of Dental Research*, 69, 1771–1775.

Kleber, C.J., Davidson, K.R., Rhoades, M.L. (2001) An evaluation of sodium bicarbonate chewing gum as a supplement to toothbrushing for removal of dental plaque from children's teeth. *Compendium of Continuing Education in Dentistry*, 22, 36–42.

Lamb, W.J., Corpron, R.E., More, F.G., *et al.* (1993) In situ remineralization of subsurface enamel lesion after the use of a fluoride chewing gum. *Caries Research*, 27, 111–116.

Larmas, M., Makinen, K.K., Scheinin, A. (1976a) Turku sugar studies. VIII. Principal microbiological findings. *Acta Odontologica Scandinavica*, 34, 285–328.

Larmas, M., Scheinin, A., Gehring, F., *et al.* (1976b) Turku sugar studies XX. Microbiological findings and plaque index values in relation to 1-year use of xylitol chewing gum. *Acta Odontologica Scandinavica*, 34, 381–396.

Loesche, W.J. (1986) Role of Streptococcus mutans in human dental decay. *Microbiology Revues*, 50, 353–380.

Ly, K.A., Milgrom, P., Roberts M.C., *et al.* (2006) Linear response of mutans streptococci to increasing frequency of xylitol chewing gum use: a randomized controlled trial [ISRCTN43479664]. *BMC Oral Health*, 6, 6.

Ly, K.A., Milgrom, P., Rothen, M. (2006) Xylitol, sweeteners, and dental caries. *Pediatric Dentistry*, 28, 154–163; discussion 192–198.

Ly, K.A., Milgrom, P., Rothen, M. (2008) The potential of dental-protective chewing gum in oral health interventions. *Journal of the American Dental Association*, 139(5): 553–63.

Machiulskiene, V., Nyvad, B., Baelum V. (2001) Caries preventive effect of sugar-substituted chewing gum. *Community Dentistry and Oral Epidemiology*, 29, 278–288.

Mäkinen, K.K., Bennett, C.A., Hujoel, P.P., *et al.* (1995) Xylitol chewing gums and caries rates: a 40-month cohort study. *Journal of Dental Research*, 74, 1904–1913.

Mäkinen, K.K., Hujoel, P.P., Bennett, C.A. (1996) Polyol chewing gums and caries rates in primary dentition: a 24-month cohort study. *Caries Research*, 30, 408–417.

Mäkinen, K.K. and Scheinin, A. (1971) The effect of the consumption of various sugars on the activity of plaque and salivary enzymes. *International Dentistry Journal*, 21, 331–339.

Mäkinen, K.K. and Scheinin, A. (1976a) Turku sugar studies VII. Principal biochemical findings on whole saliva and plaque. *Acta Odontologica Scandinavica*, 34, 241–283.

Mäkinen, K.K. and Scheinin, A. (1976b) Turku sugar studies XIII. Effect of the diet on certain clinico-chemical values of serum. *Acta Odontologica Scandinavica*, 34, 371–380.

Mäkinen, K.K., Söderling, E., Isokangas, P., *et al.* (1989) Oral biochemical status and depression of Streptococcus mutans in children during 24- to 36-month use of xylitol chewing gum. *Caries Research*, 23, 261–266.

Milgrom, P., Ly, K.A., Roberts, M.C., *et al.* (2006) Mutans streptococci dose response to xylitol chewing gum. *Journal of Dental Research*, 85, 177–181.

Milgrom, P., Ly, K.A., Rothen, M. (2009) Xylitol and its vehicles for public health needs. *Advances in Dental Research*, 21, 44–47.

Milgrom, P., Ly, K.A., Tut, O.K., *et al.* (2009) Xylitol pediatric topical oral syrup to prevent dental caries: a double-blind randomized clinical trial of efficacy. *Archives of Pediatrics and Adolescent Medicine*, 163, 601–607.

Montague, W., Howell, S. L., Taylor, K.W. (1967) Pentitols and the mechanism of insulin release. *Nature*, 215(5105), 1088–1089.

Natah, S.S., Hussien, K.R., Tuominen, J.A., *et al.* (1997) Metabolic response to lactitol and xylitol in healthy men. *American Journal of Clinical Nutrition*, 65, 947–950.

Nilner, K., Vassilakos, N., Birkhed, D. (1991) Effect of a buffering sugar-free lozenge on intraoral pH and electrochemical action. *Acta Odontologica Scandinavica*, 49, 267–272.

Oscarson, P., Lif Holgerson, P., Sjöström, I., *et al.* (2006) Influence of a low xylitol-dose on mutans streptococci colonisation and caries development in preschool children. *European Archives of Paediatric Dentistry*, 7, 142–147.

Petersen, P.E. and Razanamihaja, N. (1999) Carbamide-containing polyol chewing gum and prevention of dental caries in schoolchildren in Madagascar. *International Dental Journal*, 49, 226–230.

Pihlanto-Leppälä, A., Söderling, E., Mäkinen, K. (1989) Uptake of 14C-xylitol by xylitol-cultured Streptococcus sobrinus ATCC 27352 and Streptococcus mitis ATCC 36249 in vitro. *Proceedings of the Finnish Dental Society*, 85, 423–428.

Redclift, M.R. (2004) *Chewing gum: the fortunes of taste*. Routledge, New York.

Richardson, A.S., Hole, L.W., McCombie F., *et al.* (1972) Anticariogenic effect of dicalcium phosphate dihydrate chewing gum: results after two years. *Journal of the Canadian Dental Association*, 38, 213–218.

Scheinin, A. and Mäkinen, K.K. (1971) The effect of various sugars on the formation and chemical composition of dental plaque. *International Dental Journal*, 21, 302–321.

Scheinin, A., Mäkinen, K.K., Tammisalo, E., *et al.* (1975) Turku sugar studies XVIII. Incidence of dental caries in relation to 1-year consumption of xylitol chewing gum. *Acta Odontologica Scandinavica*, 33, 269–278.

Scheinin, A., Mäkinen, K.K., Ylitalo, K. (1974) Turku sugar studies. I. An intermediate report on the effect of sucrose, fructose and xylitol diets on the caries incidence in man. *Acta Odontologica Scandinavica*, 32, 383–412.

Scheinin, A., Mäkinen, K.K., Ylitalo, K. (1976) "Turku sugar studies. V. Final report on the effect of sucrose, fructose and xylitol diets on the caries incidence in man." *Acta Odontologica Scandinavica*, 34, 179–216.

Scientific Opinion of the Panel on Dietetic Products, Nutrition and Allergies on a request from LEAF Int, Leaf Holland and Leaf Suomi Oy on the scientific substantiation of a health claim related to xylitol chewing gum/pastilles and reduce the risk of tooth decay. *The EFSA Journal* (2008) 852, 1–16.

Sharma, N.C., Galustians, J.H., Qaqish, J.G. (2001) An evaluation of a commercial chewing gum in combination with normal toothbrushing for reducing dental plaque and gingivitis. *Compendendium of Continuing Education in Dentistry*, 22, 13–17.

Sintes, J.L., Elias-Boneta, A. Stewart, B., *et al.* (2002) Anticaries efficacy of a sodium monofluorophosphate dentifrice containing xylitol in a dicalcium phosphate dihydrate base. A 30-month caries clinical study in Costa Rica. *American Journal of Dentistry*, 15, 215–219.

Sintes, J.L., Escalante, C., Stewart, B., *et al.* (1995) Enhanced anticaries efficacy of a 0.243% sodium fluoride/10% xylitol/silica dentifrice: 3-year clinical results. *American Journal of Dentistry*, 8, 231–235.

Smith, A.J., Moran, J., Dangler L.V., *et al.* (1996) The efficacy of an anti-gingivitis chewing gum. *Journal of Clinical Periodontology*, 23, 19–23.

Söderling, E., Isokangas, P., Pienihäkkinen, K., *et al.* (2000) Influence of maternal xylitol consumption on acquisition of mutans streptococci by infants. *Journal of Dental Research*, 79, 882–887.

Söderling, E., Isokangas, P., Pienihäkkinen, K., *et al.* (2001) Influence of maternal xylitol consumption on mother-child transmission of mutans streptococci: 6-year follow-up. *Caries Research*, 35, 173–177.

Söderling, E. and Pihlanto-Leppala, A. (1989) Uptake and expulsion of 14C-xylitol by xylitol-cultured Streptococcus mutans ATCC 25175 in vitro. *Scandinavian Journal of Dental Research*, 97, 511–519.

Söderling, E., Rekola, M., Mäkinen, K.K., *et al.* (1976) Turku sugar studies XXI. Xylitol, sorbitol-, fructose- and sucrose-induced physico-chemical changes in saliva. *Acta Odontologica Scandinavica*, 34, 397–403.

Söderling, E.M. (2009) Xylitol, mutans streptococci, and dental plaque. *Advances in Dental Research*, 21, 74–78.

Spitz, I.M., Rubenstein, A.H., Bersohn, I., *et al.* (1970) Metabolism of xylitol in healthy subjects and patients with renal disease. *Metabolism*, 19, 24–34.

Suda, R., Suzuki, T., Takigichi R. *et al.* (2006) The effect of adding calcium lactate to xylitol chewing gum on remineralization of enamel lesions. *Caries Research*, 40, 43–46.

Thorild, I., Lindau, B., Twetman S. (2003) Effect of maternal use of chewing gums containing xylitol, chlorhexidine or fluoride on mutans streptococci colonization in the mothers' infant children. *Oral Health and Preventive Dentistry*, 1, 53–57.

Thorild, I., Lindau, B., Twetman S. (2004) Salivary mutans streptococci and dental caries in three-year-old children after maternal exposure to chewing gums containing combinations of xylitol, sorbitol, chlorhexidine, and fluoride. *Acta Odontologica Scandinavica*, 62, 245–250.

Thorild, I., Lindau, B., Twetman S. (2006) Caries in 4-year-old children after maternal chewing of gums containing combinations of xylitol, sorbitol, chlorhexidine and fluoride. *European Archives of Paediatric Dentistry*, 7, 241–245.

Trahan, L., Bareil, M., Gauthier, L., *et al.* (1985) Transport and phosphorylation of xylitol by a fructose phosphotransferase system in Streptococcus mutans. *Caries Research*, 19, 53–63.

Trahan, L., Söderling, E., Dréan, M.F., *et al.* (1992) Effect of xylitol consumption on the plaque-saliva distribution of mutans streptococci and the occurrence and long-term survival of xylitol-resistant strains. *Journal of Dental Research*, 71, 1785–1791.

Van Loveren, C. (2004) Sugar alcohols: what is the evidence for caries-preventive and caries-therapeutic effects? *Caries Research*, 38, 286–293.

Wang, Y.M. and van Eys, J. (1981) Nutritional significance of fructose and sugar alcohols. *Annual Review of Nutrition*, 1, 437–475.

Yankell, S.L. and Emling, R.C. (1997) Efficacy of chewing gum in preventing extrinsic tooth staining. *Journal of Clinical Dentistry*, 8, 169–172.

10

Preventing dental disease with chlorhexidine

Hardy Limeback and Ross Perry

Introduction

Caries and periodontal disease are asymptomatic, chronic, low-grade bacterial infections. These infections cause a slowly progressive destruction of tissue. Given this nature of the two major dental diseases, dental research has been pursuing an effective and safe antimicrobial strategy to reduce and then minimize the infection. A key focus of this search for an antimicrobial approach to disease prevention has been chlorhexidine, a widely used, broad spectrum antiseptic. This chapter reviews the development and status of chlorhexidine products and treatment regimens in dental prevention, and more specifically its use in managing adult caries.

Chlorhexidine in the current armamentarium of the dental professional

Chlorhexidine is used primarily in managing gingivitis and adult caries, and currently it has minimal application to pediatric and adolescent dental disease. A recent study found that about one in five American dental professionals prescribe for their adult patients a dilute (0.12% w/v) chlorhexidine mouth rinse to manage their caries (Riley et al. 2010). This 0.12% chlorhexidine mouth rinse is approved in North America for the prevention of gingivitis, but there are no published studies supporting its use in caries management; however, it is the only available chlorhexidine oral care product in the US. Given the limited availability of chlorhexidine dosage forms in the US to prevent adult caries, dental professionals use fluoride in gels, rinses, and varnishes as the primary defense. For childhood caries topical fluorides are the first line of defense. (See Chapter 16.)

Since 2001, however, five assessments have concluded that the evidence base for fluoride in adult caries

prevention is limited. The first review by the National Institutes of Health concluded that useful studies of preventive treatments (primarily fluoride) were based on children only and that there was no satisfactory evidence about the prevention of primary or secondary caries in adults (National Institutes of Health 2001). Brunton and Kay (2003) reached the same conclusion in 2003 as did Twetman et al. in 2004. Most recently, the same observation was made by Griffin et al. in 2007, although this systematic review claimed that water fluoridation has a preventive effect on adult caries. Spolsky et al. in 2007 also reported that controlled clinical trials of fluoride varnish in adults have yet to be undertaken.

In the absence of firm, conclusive evidence about both chlorhexidine and fluoride in managing adult caries, dental professionals have relied on both patient and professional mechanical cleanings of the tooth surface to prevent caries. For the majority of patients who are at low risk of caries, this mechanical control of the biofilm is sufficient to prevent the onset or progression of this disease most of the time. However, mechanical controls for the high-risk adult patient (who experiences most of the caries in the population), often have limited if any effect at the root surface and around existing restorations (Chalmers 2006).

This is due to the nature of the dental biofilm in high-risk adult patients. After careful brushing and professional cleaning, approximately 100,000 bacteria per square millimeter will remain in the tubules, surface indentations, and adjacent soft tissue near the root surface (Love and Jenkinson 2002). This residual film facilitates the recolonization of the tooth surface in such a way that viable counts of bacteria return to pre-treatment levels within 3 to 7 days.

Comprehensive Preventive Dentistry, First Edition. Edited by Hardy Limeback.
© 2012 John Wiley & Sons, Ltd. Published 2012 by John Wiley & Sons, Ltd.

Chlorhexidine: antibacterial mechanism

Chlorhexidine is a cationic chlorophenyl bisbiguanide, which was first used as an anti-plaque agent in 1969 (Seymour *et al.* 1999). The drug's bactericidal action at the cell wall of the bacteria is facilitated by electrostatic forces between the negatively charged cells and the net positively charged chlorhexidine molecules (Rölla and Melsen 1975). Having gained access to the cell membrane, chlorhexidine disorients its lipoprotein structure, destroying the osmotic barrier of the bacteria. Cell permeability increases, and intracellular components such as potassium ions leak through the damaged membrane. A secondary action of chlorhexidine is to cause intracellular coagulation, which effectively slows down the rate of cell-content leakage. This cytoplasmic coagulation is responsible for the bactericidal effect of chlorhexidine and is directly dependent on the concentration of the drug.

The literature generally accepts that the bacterial outer envelope is responsible for the different microbial responses to chlorhexidine. Chlorhexidine is thought to damage the cell wall and outer membrane and promote its own uptake so that it can reach its target site at the cell cytoplasmic membrane and within the cell cytoplasm. The literature also suggests there are several target sites within the bacterial cell for chlorhexidine such as the cytoplasmic membrane and cytoplasmic constituents (Table 10-1). It is unlikely that the mode of action of chlorhexidine involves specific inhibition of a particular enzyme system (Maillard 2002).

The conventional view is that chlorhexidine is retained on oral surfaces by reversible electrostatic binding to acid protein groups such as phosphates, sulfates, and carboxyl ions, which exist extensively in the oral tissues (Gjermo 1989). Calcium ions in saliva are able to displace chlorhexidine from the carboxyl-binding sites. This displacement is comparatively slow and may help to explain the prolonged bacteriostatic effect of the drug in the mouth. Further, chlorhexidine can displace calcium ions that are bound to the sulfated glycoproteins of bacterial plaque. Seymour suggests three possible mechanisms for the inhibition of bacterial plaque by chlorhexidine:

- The blocking of acidic groups of salivary glycoproteins will reduce the plaque's adsorption to hydroxyapatite and the formation of the acquired pellicle.
- The ability of bacteria to bind to tooth surfaces may be reduced by the adsorption of chlorhexidine to the extracellular polysaccharides of bacterial capsules or glycocalyces.
- Chlorhexidine may compete with calcium ions for acidic agglutination factors in plaque (Seymour 1999).

Table 10-1 Bacterial targets of chlorhexidine

Target site	Mechanism(s)
Outer layers	
Outer membrane*	Increased permeability
Cytoplasmic membrane	Increased permeability
	Adenosine triphosphate synthesis
	Inhibition of enzyme activity
Cytoplasmic constituents	General coagulation

* gram-negative bacteria.
Source: J. Maillard, Bacterial target sites for biocide action," *Journal of Applied Microbiology Symposium Supplement*, v. 92, 2002, pp. 16S–27S.

The pharmacology of chlorhexidine

Chemical structure

Because chlorhexidine is a symmetrical, long-chain nitrogen-rich polymer (a bisguanide) with two chlorobenzene rings at opposite ends (Figure 10-1), it usually is more soluble as a digluconate. It precipitates readily out of aqueous solution unless it is combined with molecules such as gluconate, acetate, or hydrochloride. The molecule, in relation to other constituents (for example, gluconate, calcium on the enamel surface), can take on many forms in three dimensions and can even self-aggregate to form micelles (Heard and Ashworth 1968).

Chlorhexidine is available in different salts. The most common salt in oral care products is chlorhexidine digluconate, but chlorhexidine acetate is also used. These salts do not materially differ in terms of pharmacology or toxicology but rather in terms of their solubility and formulation properties. There is some basis to believe that the chlorhexidine acetate salt may cause less staining of dentition than chlorhexidine digluconate.

Pharmacology

The key pharmacological features of chlorhexidine are summarized in Table 10-2 and include the following:

- Limited systemic absorption after oral and topical applications.
- Low toxicity.
- A retention in the mouth, which is influenced by sucrose and pH.
- No evidence of permanent resistance by cariogenic microorganisms from long-term chronic dosing with chlorhexidine. Any minor degree of resistance, as evidenced by increasing MIC levels, is reversed rapidly on withdrawal of the drug.

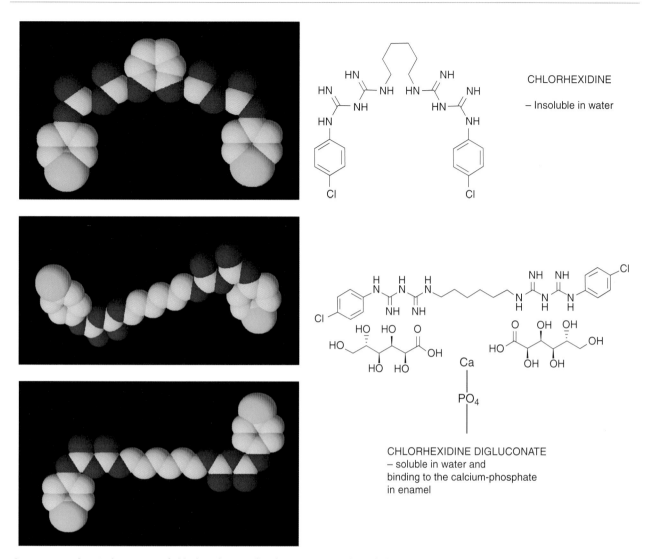

CHLORHEXIDINE

– Insoluble in water

CHLORHEXIDINE DIGLUCONATE
– soluble in water and
binding to the calcium-phosphate
in enamel

Figure 10-1 Chemical structure of chlorhexidine. Molecular structure ©chemBlink Inc. Source: http://www.chemblink.com.

The safety record of chlorhexidine in medical and dental use

Severe allergic reactions have been reported in the literature from the use of chlorhexidine both topically and on catheters during anesthesia and surgery. Garvey *et al.* (2001) reviewed adverse reactions to chlorhexidine recorded by the Danish Medicines Agency between 1968 and 2000 and found 26 reports. Of these, five anaphylactic shocks were reported, two from oral application, one from cutaneous application, and two in connection with anesthesia. A similar review of reactions in the Netherlands between 1983 and 1994 showed six cases of anaphylactic shock to chlorhexidine, all in connection with urological procedures. In Japan, nine cases of anaphylaxis to chlorhexidine were reported in the period 1967 to 1984, all of which related to the mucous membranes. In the UK from 1965 to 1996, a total of 182

reactions to chlorhexidine were recorded, of which two were anaphylactic shock.

Based on these reports, Garvey *et al.* (2001) submit that allergy to chlorhexidine has several features in common with latex allergy: it probably needs to get through broken skin or mucous membranes for sensitization to occur; it causes mild non-specific allergic reactions on some occasions but also has the potential to cause more serious reactions. Reactions in humans to chlorhexidine can be both immediate and delayed-type hypersensitivity.

By contrast to these serious adverse reactions in surgical patients, reports on sensitivities to chlorhexidine in the general population show that they are rare. For example, in a survey of 104 hospitals workers in Denmark, all of which had routine exposure to chlorhexidine, none tested positive to chlorhexidine. Testing was for both delayed-type allergy and

Table 10-2 Overview of key pharmacological features of chlorhexidine

Feature	Evidence
Method of action	Chlorhexidine is adsorbed onto the cell walls of microorganisms, which causes leakage of intracellular components. At low concentrations, chlorhexidine is bacteriostatic, and at higher concentrations, chlorhexidine is bactericidal (Seymour 1999).
Toxicity	The oral LD_{50} for chlorhexidine gluconate are 2,515 and 2,547 mg/kg body weight (bw) in male and female mice (Alderly Park strain), 2,270 and 2,000 mg/kg bw in male and female Wistar rats and greater than 3,000 mg/kg bw in male and female Alderly Park rats (European Agency for the Evaluation of Medicinal Products 1996). Adult humans have consumed 2 gm daily for a week without any untoward symptoms (Senior 1973).
Carcinogenesis, mutagenesis and developmental toxicity	Carcinogenesis was not observed in a drinking water study in rats where the highest dose of chlorhexidine used was 38 mg/kg of bw per day. This dose is at least 500 times the amount that would be ingested from the recommended human daily dose of 0.012% w/v chlorhexidine oral rinse (Peridex package insert, Procter & Gamble, US).
	The U.S. Environmental Protection Agency (EPA) has reported that a battery of mutagenicity studies of chlorhexidine diacetate were negative for mutagenic effects (U.S. E.P.A., Registration Eligibility Decision, *Chlorhexidine Diacetate* 1996).
	The EPA has concluded that the developmental toxicity no-observed-effect-level (NOEL) is equal to or greater than the highest dose tested, 62.5 mg/kg/day, and the maternal toxicity NOEL is 15.63 mg/kg/day U.S. E.P.A., Registration Eligibility Decision, *Chlorhexidine Diacetate* 1996).
Pharmacology	Studies using humans and animals have shown that chlorhexidine gluconate is poorly absorbed from the gastrointestinal tract. In humans, the mean plasma level of chlorhexidine gluconate reached a peak of 0.206 mcg per gram 30 minutes following an oral dose of 300 mg (Rushton 1977).
	In oral dosing studies in rats (5–50 mg/kg bw), dogs (0.5–5 mg/kg1 bw), marmosets (6.6–7.3 mg/kg bw), and rhesus monkeys (5.5 mg/kg bw) using 14C-labelled chlorhexidine, oral bioavailability was estimated to be less than 1% European Agency for Evaluation of Medicinal Products 1996).
	Human volunteers were given an oral dose of 0.07 mg/kg bw ^{14}C-labeled chlorhexidine in gelatin capsules. No radioactivity was detected in blood samples (the limit of detection (LOD) was 0.005 μg/ml). 0.3% of the dose was recovered from urine and 81.9% from feces (Winrow 1973).
	Parachloroaniline, a degradation product of chlorhexidine, which is known to be excreted from the kidneys, was not found. In humans, about 98% of the dose of chlorhexidine was excreted within 1.5 weeks. The rate of excretion after a single dose and after a long period of dosing did not appear to change (Case 1977).
	No chlorhexidine was detected in the blood of human infants washed in a 4% chlorhexidine solution (LOD 0.1 μg/ml). Studies in adult volunteers failed to detect chlorhexidine in blood samples after a single topical application of 5% solution of ^{14}C-labeled chlorhexidine to 50 cm^2 of skin (LOD 0.005 μg/ml) (Case 1977).
Microbial re effects and resistance	At concentrations greater than 100 μg/ml, chlorhexidine is bactericidal and between 1–100 μg/ml is bacteriostatic (European Agency for Evaluation of Medicinal Products 1996). Human studies of daily use of chlorhexidine over 12 to 24 months showed no permanent change in resistance of *Streptococcus mutans* (Gronroos *et al.* 1995).

immediate-type allergy. The authors of this survey submit that for sensitization and allergic reactions to chlorhexidine to occur, exposure needs to be either (a) repeated within a short time, (b) more prolonged as in a lubricant jelly left in the urethra after urinary catheterization, or (c) more intense as in exposure directly into a vein during central venous cannulation or surgical incision (Garvey *et al.* 2003).

In another survey of 565 patients referred to a Danish department of dermatology for investigation of skin complaints between 1999 and 2000, five (0.9%) tested positive on a prick test with chlorhexidine at 0.5% (Garvey *et al.* 2001). In another survey of 58 full-time neonatal nurses in a New York hospital, four reported skin reactions to hand washing daily over 7 months with an antiseptic soap containing 2% chlorhexidine

Table 10-3 Summary of chlorhexidine dental products

Product	Concentration of chlorhexidine	Indication (status)	Approved in
Rinse	0.12% w/v	Gingivitis (prescription)	US, Canada
	0.2% w/v	Gingivitis, oral hygiene (over the counter)	European Union
Gel	1.0% w/w	Gingivitis, oral hygiene, high risk caries (over the counter)	European Union
Subgingival wafer	1.0% w/w	Adjunct to scaling and root planning (prescription)	US, Canada, European Union
Coating or varnish	1.0% w/v	Reduction of S. mutans, sensitivity (medical device)	US, Canada, European Union
	10.0% w/v	To prevent caries in high risk adults (prescription or pharmacy only)	Canada, European Union

gluconate. These reactions were dry, cracking skin, which developed gradually (Cimiotti 2003).

The long-term safety experience with chlorhexidine in the oral cavity is impressive. In a survey of dentists in Norway, in which the 0.2% w/v chlorhexidine mouth rinse and the 1.0% w/w chlorhexidine dental gel had been available for nearly 20 years, the following side effects were found: 77% of dentists indicated chlorhexidine stained the teeth, dental restorations, and the oral mucosa; 12% reported a bitter taste experienced by the patients; and 6% indicated that patients complained of disturbances such as dry mouth and oral ulcerations (Albander *et al.* 1994).

Oral dosage forms of chlorhexidine

For dental use, chlorhexidine is primarily delivered via a mouth rinse, a gel, a subgingival wafer, and a supragingival coating or varnish (Table 10-3). The concentrations of chlorhexidine in these dosage forms, and the therapeutic indications differ significantly and by country. Chlorhexidine has been more widely used by European dentistry where a majority of dental practices routinely advise their patients to use chlorhexidine rinse and gel at home to supplement their oral hygiene. In North America, chlorhexidine has had more limited use, primarily because of tradition and because the drug approval authorities have required more rigorous assessment of efficacy via randomized controlled trials.

Of particular importance is the range of therapeutic indications for various chlorhexidine products. In North America, dental professionals have used the dilute chlorhexidine rinse since the late 1980s for gingivitis but have commonly expanded the use of this product for caries management. Among all chlorhexidine products, however, only the 10% chlorhexidine coating has a specific indication for the professional use in preventing caries in high-risk adult patients.

Chlorhexidine and fluoride

Fluoride does not interfere with the antimicrobial effects of chlorhexidine but may interfere with the binding sites of chlorhexidine on the tooth surface. The surfactants in toothpaste, such as sodium lauryl sulphate, may precipitate chlorhexidine gluconate. Even at low concentrations such as 0.05%, chlorhexidine is incompatible with bicarbonates, chlorides, citrates, phosphates, sulfates, and most dyes, ingredients that might be found in toothpastes. Insoluble compounds of calcium, magnesium, and zinc can reduce its activity, but organic matter does not affect it (AHFS Drug Information 2005).

Chlorhexidine mouth rinses for plaque and gingivitis control

Chlorhexidine formulated in mouth rinses has been effectively used over 40 years to reduce dental plaque and the gingivitis that it causes (Löe and Schiott, 1970). Many studies show that it reduces plaque indices by about 60% and, subsequently, it shows that gingivitis indices were reduced by about one-third. In the late 1980s, the drug approval authorities in North America approved under prescription a 0.12% w/v chlorhexidine rinse for the prevention of gingivitis, and subsequently the American Dental Association issued its seal of approval to this product.

The adoption of this rinse by the dental profession in North America has been protracted. Currently a minority of dental practices issue prescriptions to their patients for the home use of this chlorhexidine rinse. The product has two disadvantages. It can stain the teeth and yield an objectionable taste, and secondly, its preventive effects can be limited by patient non-compliance. Studies show that only a minority of adults will complete their

Table 10-4 Alternative formulations claiming the prevention of gingivitis

Ingredient	Usual vehicle	Properties	Effectiveness
Essential oils	mouth rinse (such as Listerine)	Antiseptic	effective in reducing plaque and gingivitis, but vehicle controls (26% alcohol) not tested
Sanguinaria	mouth rinse (also dentifrices, such as Viadent in the US and Perioguard in the UK)	Alkaloid with antibacterial properties	needs to be combined with toothpaste containing sanguinaria associated with leukoplakia (Mascarenhas *et al.* 2001)
triclosan	usually combined with copolymer rinses and dentifrices (such as Colgate Total)	antiseptic anti-inflammatory	not long lasting better performance as a rinse when combined with zinc citrate
Stannous fluoride	primarily toothpastes	combination of tin and fluoride appears to be antibacterial	"Dentifrices with stannous fluoride had statistically significant, but marginally clinically significant, evidence of an antiplaque effect; however, there was both a statistically and clinically significant antigingivitis effect." (Gunsolley 2006)
Cetylpyridinium chloride (CPC)	mouth rinse	amphiphilic quaternary compound antibacterial by reducing surface tension	not long lasting but does seem to reduce plaque (Herrera 2009)

prescription medications. Moreover, the rate of prescription may be affected by the minimal professional fees associated with its use.

The 0.12% chlorhexidine oral rinse does not cause permanent bacterial resistance and does not cause any adverse effect on the oral flora (Santos 2003). About one-third of the active ingredient is retained in the oral cavity, attaching to teeth and soft tissues. It is poorly absorbed in the GI tract and is considered safe to use except in those patients who have an allergy to the chemical. There are no studies to show its safe use during pregnancy or lactation. It is possible that its suspected cytotoxicity effects may have accounted for the few minor complaints experienced by patients using chlorhexidine gluconate rinses. According to the National Institutes of Health (NIH), these include "aphthous ulcers, grossly obvious gingivitis, trauma, ulceration, erythema, desquamation, coated tongue, keratinization, geographic tongue, mucocele, and short frenum. Each occurred at a frequency of less than 1.0%. Among post marketing reports, the most frequently reported oral mucosal symptoms associated with this rinse are stomatitis, gingivitis, glossitis, ulcer, dry mouth, hypesthesia, glossal edema, and paresthesia. Minor irritation and superficial desquamation of the oral mucosa have also been noted. There have been cases of parotid gland swelling and inflammation of the salivary glands (sialadenitis) reported in patients using Peridex" (NIH 2001).

One of the effects that chlorhexidine has is the inhibition of metallo-matrix proteinases (MMP) in dentin. (Gendron *et al.* 1999). This may improve long-term bonding of composites by inhibiting the breakdown of the collagen matrix at the bonding surface, and this may also provide added antimicrobial activity to improve the resistance of dentin restorations to further recurrent decay (Carrilho *et al.* 2007).

Alternatives to chlorhexidine mouth rinses for controlling plaque and gingivitis

Some alternative formulations have been used to control plaque and gingivitis. These formulations are over-the-counter formulations and include the essential oils in alcohol, cetylpyridinium chloride (CPC) in alcohol, sanguinarine, stannous fluoride, and triclosan (Table 10-4). The reduction of gingivitis may be statistically significant in some studies but not often clinically significant. In many cases the reduction is not supported by well-controlled clinical trials (Adams and Addy 1994; Paraskevas 2005).

Although the essential oil mouthwashes (Listerine) can be effective adjuncts to daily oral hygiene programs and in some cases have been shown to be almost as effective as chlorhexidine (Gunsolley 2010), some authors believe that the alcohol content and low pH are a concern for a mouthwash that is used routinely (Brecx *et al.*

2003). Chlorhexidine still outperforms all other anti-plaque agents (Jones 1997; Paraskevas 2005) and is quite often used as the positive control in testing other anti-plaque and anti-gingivitis products.

Chlorhexidine and caries prevention

The evidence for the effectiveness of chlorhexidine in the prevention and control of caries is mixed. Six studies (five of which were controlled) have been published on the reduction of caries in adults with various dosage forms and regimens of chlorhexidine (Katz et al. 1982, Keltjens et al. 1990; Joyston-Bechal et al. 1992; Shaeken et al. 1991; Powell et al. 1999; Brailsford et al. 2002). Four of the controlled studies reported statistically significant reductions in adult caries. The one controlled study that failed to show statistically significant reductions in adult caries (Powell et al. 1999) involved a minimal dosing regimen (0.12% rinse once a week). The sixth adult study of irradiated head and neck cancer patients was uncontrolled for ethical reasons; however, this study showed a negative caries increment (DMFT) in treated patients over 1 year (Joyston-Bechal et al. 1992).

Several systematic reviews and even meta-analyses have been published. Van Rijkom (1996) reviewed the early studies, mostly on chlorhexidine varnishes and concluded that chlorhexidine treatment inhibited caries by nearly half. It was also concluded that "Multiple-regression analysis showed no significant influence on the prevented fractions or the variables 'application method,' 'application frequency,' 'caries risk,' 'fluoride regime,' 'caries diagnosis,' and 'tooth surface.'" Twetman in 2004 concluded that the evidence for chlorhexidine's ability to inhibit fissure caries or root surface caries was inconclusive. However, that was based on only a select few studies. Zhang et al. (2006) selected 14 clinical studies where chlorhexidine varnish was compared to vehicle controls or no treatment. Although only eight studies met their criteria for inclusion in their systematic review, they concluded that professional application of chlorhexidine every 3–4 months had a 'moderate' caries inhibiting effect, but this effect disappeared after 2 years, and there was no evidence of effectiveness with longer intervals between applications.

A review by Autio-Gold (2008) concluded that mouth rinses were not very effective in controlling caries. Chlorhexidine gels were better at controlling S. mutans counts, but the most effective treatment in terms of controlling MS bacteria was with chlorhexidine varnishes. The most recent review of the chlorhexidine literature was published in 2010 (James et al. 2010). Based on 12 clinical studies that satisfied inclusion criteria, it was reported that two split-mouth clinical trials and one trial on primary teeth showed promising reduction in caries. The other clinical studies, however, showed no statistically significant difference in caries increment. The quality of the majority of the trials was poor and only four of the studies were considered to be free of bias (Bratthall et al. 1995; Haukali and Poulsen 2003; Du et al. 2006; Ersin et al. 2008). Looking at just those studies, the authors concluded that there was not enough evidence to show that chlorhexidine is an effective agent for preventing caries.

It can be concluded, then, from the published studies conducted to date, that the evidence for the effectiveness of chlorhexidine for the control of caries is equivocal. This does not mean that the idea of using bacteriostatic agents in controlling the bacteria that cause caries should be abandoned—quite the contrary. The studies clearly show that chlorhexidine controls mutans streptococci (MS) growth. In patients with very high MS and lactobacilli counts, it makes sense to add chlorhexidine as a preventive agent in the fight to control caries in high-risk patients. Obviously, more well-conducted clinical trials are required.

New developments in chlorhexidine varnish technology

Although the rinses and gels with chlorhexidine were the original delivery systems for this antimicrobial agent, the varnish system has been the more recent focus of research and product development. The varnish format provides distinct benefits over other dosage forms:

- Varnishes can deliver a higher concentration of chlorhexidine to the tooth surface because they are professionally applied only to the hard tissues; in turn, this improves the sustained release of the agent against the re-emerging biofilm and extends the period of time when demineralization takes place.
- Varnishes can include a matrix or delivery agent that promotes the substantivity of chlorhexidine on the tooth surface; for example, in Prevora, which is described below, research showed that a natural organic matrix of Sumatra benzoin provided more prolonged antimicrobial action to chlorhexidine.
- Varnishes assure a higher level of patient compliance.
- Varnishes minimize side effects and in particular the staining of the teeth.
- Varnishes encourage professional adoption as they generate fees during their use.

The concentration of chlorhexidine in a varnish format ranges from 1–40% (Table 10-5). The treatment approach and treatment regimen also vary. Two varnishes are used only at the site of emerging caries while the third varnish, Prevora, is applied to the entire dentition.

Table 10-5 Four chlorhexidine varnishes in North America and Europe

Brand name	Manufacturer	CHX Concentration	Indication
Cervitec	Ivoclar	1%	tooth sensitivity (North America) and reduction of *S. mutans* (EU)
Prevora	CHX Technologies	10%	To prevent caries in high risk adults (Canada, Ireland, UK, EU)
BioC	Biodent BV, Nijmegen, The Netherlands	20%	to reduce *S. mutans* (Europe)
EC40	Biodent BV,	35%	to reduce *S. mutans* (Europe)

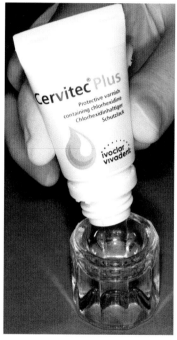
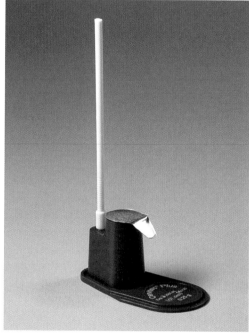

Figure 10-2 Chlorhexidine Varnish (Cervitec). This varnish, used in Europe for years, is now available in North America through Ivoclar in tube form (left) or single doses. It has been approved for treating sensitive teeth but not caries.

Only one varnish, Prevora, has been approved by regulatory authorities to prevent caries in high-risk adults. The others have limited indications. This is because only Prevora has submitted well-controlled randomized controlled data to the regulatory authorities to support its claims of efficacy (Figure 10-2).

The Prevora antibacterial tooth coating

Prevora is a high-strength (10% w/v) formulation of chlorhexidine acetate, which is applied by the dental professional to the full dentition of the adult patient who is at risk of (more) cavities. Prevora's unique contribution to caries prevention is its comprehensive base of clinical evidence and, accordingly, a relevant indication or label claim for prevention of caries, issued by the North American and European regulatory authorities. Four randomized controlled clinical trials have been conducted with Prevora

on a range of age groups and risk levels (Table 10-6). These studies yield much information on how chlorhexidine works, who will benefit from antimicrobial therapy and why, and to what extent prevention of caries can be delivered professionally to those groups who are most at risk.

The therapeutic indication of Prevora— prevention of caries in high-risk adults

This indication has been issued by regulatory authorities in Canada, Ireland, and the United Kingdom, and by the European Commission. The US Food and Drug Administration is expected to review Prevora for a similar indication. No other product, chlorhexidine or otherwise, has been awarded this approved use.

The significance of a new preventive treatment for adult caries is illustrated in Table 10-7. Root caries becomes the most common dental disease at mid-life.

Table 10-6 Randomized controlled clinical trials of Prevora

Study population	Controls	Period of treatment and observation	% reduction in mean increment (p value)
Older adults with dry mouth	Placebo, sham	12 months	All caries = 24.5% (0.03) Root caries = 40.8% (0.02)
Younger adults with 1+ cavity	Placebo	13 months	Coronal caries = 43.1% (0.02) High risk patients, all caries = 58.1% (0.005) High risk patients, coronal caries – 69.9% (0.0009)
At-risk young adolescents	Placebo, positive control (fluoride varnish), negative control (visiting the family dentist)	3 years	Female per protocol population, all caries at p <0.05 A<P = 20% A<Fluoride varnish = 31% A<Family dentist = 28%
Early childhood caries population of infants 4 to 6 months of age at baseline	Placebo	18 months (only the mothers of these children were treated)	No difference in mean increment active versus placebo but reduction in the numbers of infants with severe levels of ECC by 35% (0.02)

Table 10-7 Prevalence of conditions at mid life

	Chronic condition	Prevalence in US at mid life (ages 45–64) (affected)	# of treatments in development
1.	Chronic joint symptoms—arthritis	29–35%	60+
2.	Hypertension	29%	17
3.	Root caries	20–30%	1 (Prevora)
4.	Mental illness	14%	30+
5.	Heart disease (all types)	13%	20+

Sources: CDC, National Center for Health Statistics, *Vital Health Statistics*, Series 10, Number 22, Summary of Health Statistics for US Adults: National Health Interview Survey, 2002.
CDC, Trends in oral health status: US, 1988–1994, and 1999–2004, Vital and Health Statistics, Series 11, #248.

Not only is caries the third most common chronic disease in an aging population (Table 10-7), it is the fifth most expensive disease to treat, and compared to other major diseases where there are a number of new treatments in development, has comparatively few treatments in the approval pipeline. In the US, the prevalence of root caries increases dramatically with age (Figure 10-3).

Adult caries is clustered in the high-risk subpopulations. For example, among Canadians aged 50+, over a 3-year period of observation, 13.6% of the population had 42.6% of all cavities (Hawkins *et al.* 1997). In Prevora's study of younger adults, 15% of participants had 43% of all cavities over 13 months. These high-risk adults tend to have a complex of socio-economic and behavioral factors. They tend to have lower household income, no dental insurance, are smokers, have poor general health, and practice poor oral health behavior with irregular visits to the dental office (CDC 2007; Griffin *et al.* 2009). High-risk adults commonly start any treatment plan with multiple cavities.

Most dental practices have a number of high-risk adult patients, and the prospects are for these numbers to increase, as people age (Fure 2004). In 2011, the first of the 75 million US baby boomers will begin to retire, with a near-complete dentition. Studies show that as the general population ages, more people become uninsured and attend the dental office less regularly (AHRQ, MEPS 2007), follow multiple-medication use (Gu *et al.* 2010), experience significant gingival recession (Albandar and Kingman 1999), undergo periodontal maintenance care

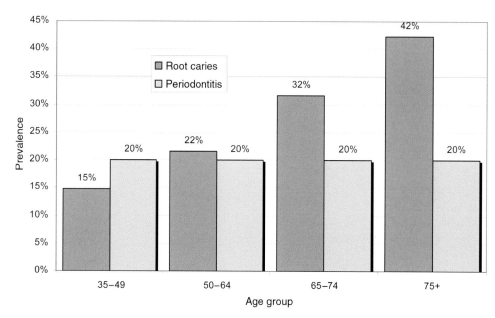

Figure 10-3 Prevalence of Root Caries and Periodontitis by Age Group. Sources: CDC 2007. Trends in the oral health status: US, 1988–1994 and 1999–2004. Vital Health Statistics. Series 11, #248, and Albandar and Kingman 1999.

(Reiker *et al.* 1999), and consume snacks more frequently (Schactele *et al.* 1985). All of these factors render the aging baby boomers at increasing risk for caries.

In the other major chronic diseases, hypertension or arthritis, high-risk patients receive intensive treatment involving multiple strategies and medications. More than one-third of American adults with high blood pressure take more than two drugs for their condition (Gu *et al.* 2006). For the third most common chronic adult disease, caries, many American adults also reportedly receive a wide range of preventive treatments including a variety of dosage forms of fluoride administered in the office and at home, as well as chlorhexidine rinse (Riley *et al.* 2010). A recent survey found that about one in four dental patients receive these additional preventive measures, often in both the dental office and at home (Riley *et al.* 2010). However, unlike hypertension and arthritis where there are a number of FDA-approved treatments, adult dental caries has no professional preventive treatment approved by the FDA. This reflects the absence of reliable evidence for existing adult caries preventive treatments.

The Prevora treatment plan

The high-risk adult patient receives four applications of Prevora in the first 8 weeks of the treatment plan and a single treatment at approximately month 6. At the end of the first year, the Prevora patient is assessed for the risk of further caries, and treatments may be continued accordingly. An individual application takes approxi-

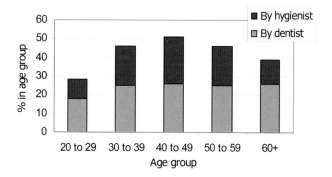

Figure 10-4 Prevalence of gingival recession in Canada. Source: CHX Technologies, On-line survey 2007.

mately 20 minutes including set-up and patient consultation, and involves no special equipment. The general procedures for Prevora treatment follow:

1. Conduct a risk assessment of the adult patient for caries. Caries is a predictable, slowly progressive disease that provides good opportunities to the dental professional to evaluate disease risk. The primary risk factors for adult caries follow:
    *   A recent history of this disease. This applies to both coronal and root caries (Powell 1998; Ritter *et al.* 2010). Essentially, an adult with several caries at the start of the treatment plan is highly likely to experience more caries in the near term. This is because restoration at specific sites leaves infectious biofilm on other tooth surfaces, and because the high-risk adult follows home-care hygiene

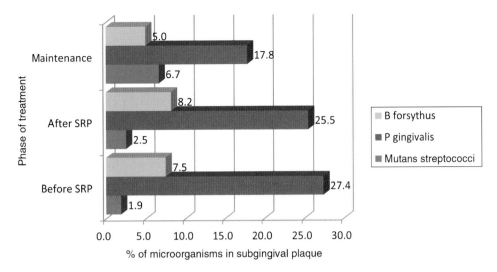

Figure 10-5 Mean percentage of microorganisms in the subgingival plaque of patients undergoing periodontal treatment. Source: Van der Reijden *et al.* 2001. Mutans streptococci in subgingival plaque of treated and untreated patients with periodontitis. J Clin Periodontol., 28: 686–691.

measures that cannot manage the re-emergence of the biofilm post prophylaxis.

- Extensive gingival recession at more than one site. A survey of Canadian dental patients found that a majority at mid-life have been told by their dental professional that they have receding gums (Figure 10-4). One American study reported that among older patients, those with at least one site of gum recession ≥4 mm had a 4.5 times greater chance of experiencing root caries in the next 3 years than those with less recession (Lawrence *et al.* 2004).

2. A dry mouth resulting from multiple medication use. As the dental population ages, multiple-medication use becomes more common. In Canada, for example, half of seniors take three or more different medications, and 27% take five or more drugs daily (Statistics Canada 2006). Studies show that multiple-medication use, and in particular use of certain types of medications (for example, a combination of anti-hypertensives and psychiatric medication) are associated with higher rates of root caries (Rindal *et al.* 2005; Singh *et al.* 2006).

3. Ongoing periodontal maintenance care. As the number of older patients grows, routine scaling and root planing has become an expanding service performed by the dental hygiene team. Does maintenance scaling and root planing bring any caries risks for your older patients? Research studies report these important facts:

- Patients undergoing routine scaling have a higher chance for root caries. In one study conducted

over 4 years, 66% of patients experienced the disease of root caries (Rivald and Hamp 1981).

- In a second study, 82% experienced root decay over a 22-year follow-up period (Reiker *et al.* 1999).

What explains this apparent increased risk for root decay? Changes in the subgingival microbial population including *Streptococcus mutans*, the bacteria that causes root decay. The presence of *Streptococcus mutans* below the gum line of periodontal maintenance patients was first documented in the mid 1980s (Loesche *et al.* 1985). A 2001 study (Figure 10-5) shows that *Streptococcus mutans* increases significantly after scaling (Van der Reijden *et al.* 2001).

4. Patients past mid-life. Dental caries, as measured by dental restoration, has declined in prevalence among adolescents and younger adults over the past 25 years. By contrast, for adults over the age of 45, the mean number of restored teeth has grown steadily since the late 1970s.

The incidence and prevalence of dental caries increases with age. One longitudinal survey of community dwelling Swedes in their 60s, 70s, and 80s found that the attack rate of dental caries in those over 80 is more than three times that of those in their 60s (Figure 10-6).

CDC data corroborate increasing prevalence for root caries with age (Figure 10-7).

The US Census Bureau projects that Americans age 65+ currently comprise 13% of the total population but by 2020, American seniors will constitute 16.1% of the population. The number of American seniors will grow from 40.2 million in 2010 to 54.8 million in 2020.

At the root caries prevalence rate of 32% for young American seniors, reported by the CDC, within the 10 years (2010–2020), there will be an estimated 17.5 million American seniors experiencing this disease. Slightly fewer American seniors will experience coronal decay.

In summary, there are good reasons for clinical and practice management, to conduct a risk assessment of the adult patient for caries. Hygiene teams perform a similar risk assessment of the adult patient for periodontal disease (for example, pocket depth, bleeding on probing, attachment loss), and periodontal disease is a much less prevalent condition than caries as the population ages. The risk assessment for adult caries takes less than 3 minutes, and may involve a simple standard form that notes the disease indicators and risk factors to be recorded at the dental visit and also provides some commentary for the dental professional to consult with the patient (Figure 10-8).

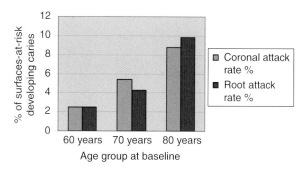

Figure 10-6 Caries prevalence in Swedes between 60 and 80 years of age (in the mid 1990s). Source: Fure 1998.

If your patient is at high-risk, here is what to do and say:

- Empathize with your patient but report to them in objective terms their risk status and its implications. A patient at high risk has a high probability of more disease in the near-term and should consider more preventive care.
- Provide informed consent to the patient about his/her treatment options, including the following:
  - Taking a chance without more prevention
  - Entering the Prevora treatment plan, the only proven and approved preventive program for adult caries
  - Following another preventive plan
- Explain to the patient the financial and health costs of each alternative.

The role of informed consent with the prevora treatment plan

Prevora is the first proven and approved preventive treatment for adult caries; therefore, it creates a new imperative for providing informed consent of the adult patient. This is because Prevora creates a viable treatment option for the adult caries patient. Informed consent is an important ethical concept to health care delivery, but it is also critical to the patient-professional relationship and the motivation of the patient to pursue better oral health. As in medicine, patients are more willing to take preventive action and treatment when they know their health status.

In seeking informed consent from the patient with regard to caries management, there are a number of points to consider:

- The patient wants to know their oral health status, as is evident from the acceptance to risk assessment in periodontal care.

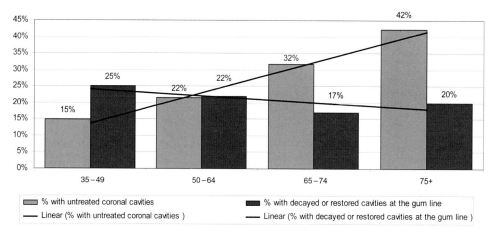

Figure 10-7 Prevalence of cavities by type and by age in the US, 1994–2004. Source: CDC, Trends in oral health status: US, 1988–1994 and 1999–2004, Vital Health Statistics, Series 11, #248, April 2007.

- The patient expects his/her dental professional to evaluate his/her risks of more disease; surveys routinely show that this is one of the main reasons for attending the dental office.
- The patient has become informed of their oral health status independent of the dental professional. A recent UK survey of patients receiving medical care found that only 20% of the information obtained by the patient to his/her condition was sourced from the medical professional (eMC Medicine Guides 2011).
- Surveys of Canadian and UK adult dental patients report that more than 4 in 10 know that caries is associated with a bacterial infection, and more than half are aware of the linkages between oral health and systemic health (CHX Technologies and Denplan Ltd. 2009).
- The patient is highly motivated to maintain or improve their oral health. That is why they visit the dental office. One survey of Canadian dental patients found, for example, that 2 in 10 adult patients were sufficiently motivated to purchase more preventive care than they would change dentists (Ipsos Reid 2008).

Accordingly, the risk assessment process in managing adult caries is not only a necessary legal requirement to satisfy informed consent, but also is an essential component of improving the patient interface and client satisfaction.

The procedures to administer Prevora

When the patient consents to purchasing more preventive care, the dental professional sets up the treatment plan with Prevora. This consists of four treatments in the first 8 weeks of the plan, followed by a single treatment at the next semi-annual recall appointment. At the end of the first year of the treatment plan, the dental professional conducts another risk assessment to evaluate if further treatments with Prevora are required.

The actual procedures to apply Prevora are readily learned from the Web site (www.prevora.com), involve no special equipment, and take less and less time with familiarity. The Prevora appointment should last no longer than 20 minutes once the dental professional gets confident with the administration of this antibacterial coating. The steps in applying Prevora follow:

1. Assemble the required supplies with two vials of Prevora (Stage 1 + Stage 2), flour of pumice and rubber cup, unwaxed floss, cotton rolls for isolation of the quadrant, and two or more mini-brushes.

Assessing Your Adult Patient's Risks for Coronal and Root Caries

The following disease indicators and risk factors are important to your patient's chances for developing new cavities. Adult caries is a predictable disease, which your patients would prefer to avoid.

Note the condition of your adult patient for these factors. One disease indicator or two or more risk factors at this visit mean your patient is at high risk of (more) cavities.

Disease indicators	Yes	No
3 or more cavities at the start of the treatment plan		
A long history of cavities, including crowns and implants		
Risk factors		
2 or more sites of recession ≥ 4mm		
A chronic dry mouth		
Undergoing periodontal maintenance care		
Risk calculation o 1 or more disease indicators? o 2 or more risk factors?		

Figure 10-8 Sample risk assessment form for adult caries.

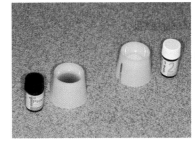

1. Assemble required supplies
   - Tooth brush
   - Examination kit (mirror, explorer)
   - Pumice, rubber cup, slow speed hand-piece
   - Cotton rolls, microbrushes
   - Cheek spreaders

2. Dispense Prevora solutions
   - Phase 1 (chlorhexidine gluconate)
   - Phase 2 (resin)

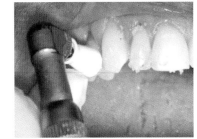

3. Rubber cup polish with pumice to remove plaque

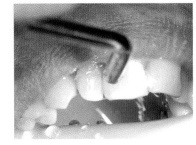

4. Rinse thoroughly

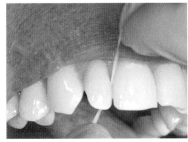

5. Floss

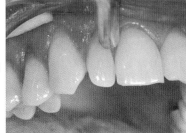

6. Dry

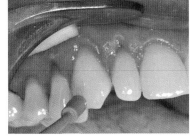

7. Apply phase 1

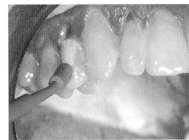

8. Apply phase 2

Figure 10-9 Steps for applying Prevora chlorhexidine coating. Photographs courtesy of Dr. Stephen Hendry, Kitchener ON, Canada.

2. Dispense the two phases of Prevora. Conduct a prophylaxis using flour of pumice and unwaxed floss. A shorter prophylaxis can be conducted at the second, third, and fourth applications as the patient will have noticeably less plaque accumulation.

3. Isolate the first quadrant with cotton rolls and air dry. Dip the first mini-brush into the open vial of Prevora Stage 1, dab the brush at all interproximal sites in the quadrant, and then apply a thin coat of Stage 1 on all supra-gingival tooth surfaces in this quadrant. Then air dry. Dip the second mini-brush into the open vial of Prevora Stage 2 and apply a thin coat of Stage 2 on the same tooth surfaces that received Prevora Stage 1. Then air dry. Repeat these steps in the other three quadrants. Advise the patient of the post-treatment instructions using the leaflet provided in the box of Prevora (Figure 10-9).

The efficacy and safety of Prevora

Two randomized, placebo-controlled, double-blinded, prospective, multi-center studies of adults at varying levels of risk of caries have been conducted with Prevora. These studies have been submitted and reviewed by drug approval authorities in Canada and the European Union, and have been the basis for Prevora's unique indication to prevent caries in high-risk adults. These studies have also been submitted to the Food and Drug Administration

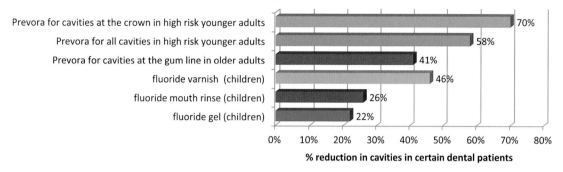

Preventing tooth decay in adults and children
(% reduction in cavities reported from controlled studies)

Figure 10-10 Efficacy of Prevora in reducing caries. Sources: CHX Technologies, Clinical Study Reports #001 and #006 and Anusavice 2005.

for its review. Both studies were conducted under investigational license with the FDA and were approved by local ethics committees. The studies were also conducted according to good clinical practice.

These studies found Prevora to significantly reduce annual caries increment compared to placebo (Figure 10-10). The preventive effect observed over 1 year and five applications of Prevora ranged from 41% (p = 0.02) at the root surface of older adults with medication-induced xerostomia, to 70% (p = 0.0005) at the coronal surfaces of high risk uninsured adults with multiple cavities at the start of the treatment plan. The preventive effect ranged with disease risk. Study participants in the active stage of the disease and with multiple cavitated lesions experienced the highest level of protection during the study period; by contrast, for those patients at lower risk (for example, only one cavitated lesion or with no lesions at baseline), there was little to no preventive effect. Hence, it is important to recommend Prevora only to those patients at high risk.

Prevora's preventive effect in high-risk adults is significantly superior to fluoride's effect in preventing caries in children. In terms of safety, in these controlled adult studies, there were no related serious adverse events such as hospitalization or deaths attributed to Prevora. Related adverse events were primarily limited to the oral cavity and included temporary stinging of the oral mucosa and a short bitter taste. These occurred at the rate of 8 per 100 treatments and were attributed to misapplication of the medication to the soft tissues. Observations of tooth discoloration were very rare.

Other evidence of Prevora's preventive effect in other high risk populations

Two other randomized controlled clinical trials have been completed with Prevora. The first study involved at-risk young adolescents and a 3-year period of treatment

and observation; the controls in this study were placebo, a negative control (going to the family dentist), and a positive control (fluoride varnish and diet counselling at the study's dental center). In this study, participants who followed the protocol experienced significant prevention with Prevora if they were female: 31% fewer caries compared to fluoride varnish, 28% fewer compared to visiting their family dentist, and 20% fewer compared to placebo. The compliant male participants experienced no preventive effect from Prevora; this medication worked no better than fluoride varnish or receiving regular family dental care.

The gender effect of Prevora in this adolescent study is attributed to significant differences in the diet of female adolescents from their male counterparts, as well as significant differences in oral hygiene behavior. From parallel surveys of nutrition and oral care, males consumed more sweets, drank more acidic beverages more frequently, and brushed their teeth less often. Because of this behavior, no preventive program was effective. In this context, it becomes important to counsel the Prevora patient to limit the sugars in their diet and to maintain good oral hygiene. Prevora is no substitute for proper conventional oral preventive measures.

The final randomized controlled study of Prevora tested its ability to reduce early childhood caries (ECC), the most common and expensive pediatric disease in America. Caries is a transmittable infection involving cross-infection of bacteria from the mother to the child at an early age. The pathogen *Streptococcus mutans* requires hard surfaces to colonize and prosper but has been found in edentulous infants. In this study, mothers of infants 4 to 6 months old and without teeth were treated with Prevora to minimize the transmission of cariogenic microorganisms from their mouths to their infants at the point of the first teeth erupting. The mothers received four applications in the first month and single applications at their next two semi-annual recall appointments. The primary objective was to evaluate if the infants in the Prevora group of mothers had fewer cavities at 24 months of age than those whose mothers had received placebo.

This mother-children study found there was no difference in the mean number of cavities in the infants between Prevora and placebo groups, but there was a significant reduction in the number of children in the Prevora group with severe forms of this disease. The Prevora group had significantly fewer infants with five or more cavities at 24 months of age. Reduction of severe forms of ECC is clinically and economically important as those with numerous cavities are the first to receive restorative care under general anesthesia in the operating room.

The context for considering chlorhexidine products for caries management

The growing movement toward evidence-based dental care has called into question the proof and utility of many conventional dental procedures and dental products, particularly as they pertain to prevention of caries. For example, as a result of the evidence-based movement, it is now known that there is a paucity of just how effective topical fluoride is in preventing adult caries. This is the conclusion of four reviews of the research literature, starting with the consensus conference by the National Institutes of Health in 2001 (NIH 2001; Brunton and Kay 2003; Twetman et al. 2004; American Dental Association 2006). Likewise, it is apparent that the restorative approach to managing adult caries is problematic and can be ineffective and temporary particularly at the root surface and for high-risk patients. For example, over 60% of dental restorations in adults replace those that have failed or that are challenged by recurrent decay (The University of York, NHS Centre for Reviews and Dissemination 1999). Studies show that at 2 years, less than half of the composite root restorations and less than 20% of glass ionomer root restorations were intact (Levy and Jensen 1990; Hu et al. 2005). Studies of restorations placed by community dentists in the UK found that the mean age of all restorations (crown and root) at the time of replacement was between 6.8 and 8.3 years for amalgam, between 4.5 and 5.7 years for composites, and between 3.8 and 3.9 years for glass ionomer (Wilson et al. 1997; Burket et al. 2001). Similar replacement spans were reported for Norwegian and Swedish dentists (Mjor et al. 1997; Mjor et al. 2000).

It is in this context of the lack of evidence about the efficacy of both fluoride and restorative care in controlling adult caries that the literature on chlorhexidine should be considered. The individual studies and the meta-analysis performed by many found some significance for this antimicrobial. In particular, the controlled studies of Prevora in high-risk adults show a highly significant benefit for this coating.

What guidance can the dental professional draw from these overviews of the literature, particularly in light of the Prevora studies described above? These observations are pertinent:

- Caries prevention is highly influenced by patient selection and dosage form. Chlorhexidine at high concentration and professionally applied to those at high risk is highly effective. Accordingly, it is necessary to conduct a simple and accurate risk assessment of the patient prior to considering the preventive alternatives.
- The evidence from studies that have been reviewed and approved by drug approval authorities such as the European Medicines Agency is of the highest quality and has undergone the most rigorous assessment. Products with a specific therapeutic indication or label claim for caries prevention issued by the regulatory authorities (and not by dental associations) have demonstrated a statistically significant and clinically significant preventive effect in a generalizable population. Dental professionals are not used to examining products for their indicated or approved use because there have been very few uses, if any, for in-office use. Rather, to date dental professionals have taken anecdotal evidence or studies in the literature as guidance.
- Study design and endpoints are critical to study outcomes and conclusions. In adult caries, for example, studies should use cavitated lesions and highly calibrated examiners, and a study population reflective of the clustered set of patients experiencing the disease.

The prospects for continued innovation in chlorhexidine products and in more preventive dental care

The main sponsor for commercial development of new products in medicine is the pharmaceutical industry, not government funding agencies. The major pharmaceutical companies have been responsible for developing and introducing new oral care products via their consumer divisions, but their pharmaceutical research has tended to focus on conventional medical diseases such as cardiovascular disease, inflammatory disease, cancer, and infectious diseases. Over the past 20 years, the new preventive products introduced for professional use have been limited to periodontal disease (for example, Periostat, Actisite, Arestin) rather than caries. These new periodontal products were developed by small, research-intensive companies and were subsequently marketed by the consumer divisions of multinational pharmaceutical companies.

Despite being the third most common chronic disease in adults, caries remains relatively unaddressed to the pharmaceutical industry for several reasons:

- Caries at the pre-cavitated stage is difficult to diagnose reliably and consistently; in turn, this raises the sample size of controlled studies and extends the period of observation. Both dramatically increase the cost of conducting such studies.
- Caries is a slowly progressing disease, so controlled studies are protracted unless a high-risk population can be recruited and retained.
- Caries is a biofilm-based disease that is modulated by lifestyle and by socioeconomic factors. These realities can present both technological and marketing risks to a comprehensive clinical program of a new treatment.
- Caries studies need to access the cluster of the population that has aggressive forms of this disease. Recruiting and retaining high-risk patients can be problematic because the individuals tend to infrequently visit the dental office.
- Adult caries is currently managed primarily by restoration, not by prevention. In adult patients, spending on restoration exceeds that of spending on prevention. This pattern is based largely on the emphasis of reimbursement systems for dental groups, the absence of an effective and approved preventive treatment plan, and conventions and inertia in the dental professionals. None of these factors encourage large capital commitments to conducting long-term clinical trials.
- Studies conducted by academic investigators commonly do not meet the standards imposed by regulatory authorities to approve any therapeutic claims. Drug development is a complex process requiring management not only of clinical aspects but also pre-clinical and manufacturing aspects of product development. It also requires regulatory expertise. Typically, these are beyond the resources and scope of the independent investigator.
- Lastly, both chlorhexidine and fluoride are generic active ingredients that cannot be patented. This requires innovation on the delivery systems of these ingredients, which can be problematic to patent and to develop.

So, on the face of it, the prospects of more new preventive products for adult caries beyond Prevora appear to be limited.

There have emerged, however, some developments that favor not only innovation but also adoption of new preventive products by the dental profession. These forces are resident in the aging population, in the movement toward health care consumerism, and in the overlap that has developed between oral disease and overall health. Another force encouraging adoption and change in the dental office has been the decline in dental attendance during the recession of 2008–2010 and subsequently, the onset of government austerity measures that have affected the subsidies for dental care in certain countries.

The rapidly aging population in the industrial economies imparts change to health care delivery in general and, specifically to how dentistry is valued and purchased. Past the age of 60 in many countries, the dental patient starts to pay for his/her dental services mostly out-of-pocket. An individual receiving subsidies on dental care acts differently from one who pays directly for these services. In business terms, the "value proposition" for dentistry changes from one of relative disinterest by the patient to what is provided in the dental office, to one that prefers choice and justification and that seeks cost containment and prevention. Dentistry is no longer in the golden era of generous third-party reimbursement, and no longer has the income growth in the population that supported lifestyle dental services such as cosmetics and whitening.

There is some evidence that the older dental patient is already questioning the value proposition of conventional dental services as shown by increasing infrequent attendance from age 40, and a significant drop off in semi-annual attendance after age 70 (Figure 10-11).

Although the economic and demographic landscape is changing profoundly for dentistry, perhaps the most fundamental change has been the thirst for information by what are called "health care consumers." For example, a 2006 survey of Canadian workers reported that only 39% would unquestionably follow their doctor's recommendations; 61% would look up information, question their doctor, and seek second opinions according to what they learned (Sanofi Aventis 2006). This is particularly true for women, for those over age 50, and for those with higher incomes. Another survey in the UK showed that only a small part of the patient's information on their health is sourced from the doctor (http://www.medicines.org.uk/guides/pages/surveyresults). Many dental professionals recognize this more assertive and sophisticated adult dental patient from their day-to-day experience.

Encouraging this movement of the health care consumer in the dental office is the information that is publicly available on the connection between oral disease and systemic health. This information is known by more than 40% of adults in the UK and Canada.

The literature associating periodontal disease and systemic medical conditions is well developed compared to that connecting caries and medical conditions. This may be attributed to the physiological and immunological attributes of periodontal disease, but another factor is

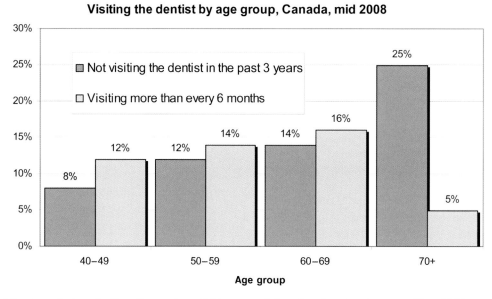

Figure 10-11 Attendance in dental offices. Source: Ipsos Reid, survey of Canadian dental patients age 40+, 2009.

that the periodontal research community is more active in the biology of its disease, seems to be comparatively well funded, and is relatively uninterested in the surgical approach to disease management. Yet there are a number of studies in caries research that link this disease to others, particularly in the case of root caries.

There have been 11 large, longitudinal population studies since 1989 showing that non-periodontal dental diseases and tooth loss are associated with increased risk of atherosclerosis, coronary heart disease, and cerebrovascular disease (Holm-Pedersen 2005). Four studies have linked root caries to overall health:

- In 1996, it was found that older adults with ≥two new root lesions were four times more likely to die during a 3- to 5-year follow-up period, than those with fewer than two root lesions (Mauriello *et al.* 1996). A subsequent study in 1999 by the same researchers extended and confirmed these findings (Muariello *et al.* 1999).
- In 2005, a Swedish study of persons aged ±80 living in the community found that those with ≥three active root caries had more than twice the odds of cardiac arrhythmias than those without root caries. The odds did not change significantly after adjusting for age, xerogenic medications, and number of teeth. There was no association between periodontal disease and arrhythmia.
- In 2006, a study of Americans aged 52–74 found that the incidence of heart attack over a 6-year period was 4.7% among the root caries group versus 2.4% for those without root caries (Mauriello *et al.* 2006). Regression analysis ruled out confounding factors

such as periodontal pocketing, race, age, sex, and the usual risk factors such as smoking, income, diabetes, hypertension, and low-density lipoprotein. This research group also ranked root caries among the important risk factors for coronary heart disease. The explanation of the significant relationship between caries and other medical conditions remains unclear in the literature although recent studies have reported a large presence of *Streptococcus mutans* in the ather-omatous plaque of patients with advanced coronary disease (Nakano *et al.* 2009).

From the patients' perspective, however, the scientific details of these associations are certainly not understood but remain emotive and consequential. To the layman, the mouth is part of the body. The patient also understands if he/she has had tooth decay or is at risk of this disease because the major risk factors are simple and readily self diagnosed. Many adult patients can tell if they have a dry mouth, if they have receding gums, and if they are undergoing periodontal care.

Importantly, studies conducted by the Food and Drug Administration found that patients are good at making a self-diagnosis of a disease. When a patient asked about an advertised drug or treatment at a medical office, for example, 88% of the time they had the condition that the drug treated. And 80% of doctors believed their patients understood what condition the drug treated and agreed with the diagnosis (Lewis 2003).

To conclude, there will be continued innovation in new chlorhexidine products if the patients demand a new value proposition of more preventive care, and in turn, make the dental professional provide these new products and services. In the industrial economies, commonly half of the patients in the waiting room are baby boomers who are paying directly for their services and are experiencing caries often for the first time. An aging, uninsured dental patient starting to experience root caries seems to be the most pressing force for more adult dental prevention.

Overall conclusions

Various preventive products have incorporated chlorhexidine as their active ingredient to impact the biofilm at the gingival margin, in the periodontal pocket, and on the tooth surface. The concentrations, treatment regimens, and therapeutic label claims for these chlorhexidine products vary substantially. One product, a 10% chlorhexidine coating under the brand Prevora, has been approved for the prevention of caries in high-risk adults.

Editor's disclosure

Ross Perry is the president of CHX Technologies, the maker of Prevora. His contribution to this chapter is based on an extensive experience with the development, marketing research and product testing of this new drug for dentistry that targets root caries.

Dr. Limeback has no financial interest in CHX Technologies.

References

Adams, D. and Addy, M. (1994) Mouthrinses. *Advances in Dental Research*, 8, 292–301.

AHFS Drug Information. (2005) Copyright, 1959–2010, Selected Revisions January 2005. American Society of Health-System Pharmacists, Inc., 7272 Wisconsin Avenue, Bethesda, Maryland 20814.

AHRQ, MEPS. (2007) Chartbook No. 17, dental use, expenses, dental coverage, and changes, 1996 and 2004.

Albandar, J.M., Gjermo, P., Preus, H.R. (1994) Chlorhexidine use after two decades of over-the-counter availability. *Journal of Periodontology*, 65, 109–112.

Albandar, J. and Kingman, A. (1999) Gingival recession, gingival bleeding and dental calculus in adults 30 years of age and older in the U.S., 1988–1994. *Journal of Periodontology*, 70, 30–43.

American Dental Association. (2006) Professionally-applied topical fluoride: evidence-based clinical recommendations. *Journal of the American Dental Association*, 137, 1151–1159.

Anusavice, K.J. (2005) Present and future approaches for the control of caries. *Journal of Dental Education*, 69, 538–554.

Arends, J., Duschner, H., Ruben, J.L. (1997) Penetration of varnishes into demineralized root dentine in vitro. *Caries Research*, 31, 201–205.

Autio-Gold, J. (2008) The role of chlorhexidine in caries prevention. *Operative Dentistry*, 33, 710–716.

Brailsford, S.R., Fiske, J., Gilbert, S., *et al.* (2002) The effects of the combination of chlorhexidine/thymol- and fluoride-containing varnishes on the severity of root caries lesions in frail institutionalised elderly people. *Journal of Dentistry*, 30, 319–324.

Bratthall, D., Serinirach, R., Rapisuwon, S., *et al.* (1995) A study into the prevention of fissure caries using an antimicrobial varnish. *International Dental Journal*, 45, 245–254.

Brecx, M., Netuschil, L., Hoffmann, T. (2003) How to select the right mouthrinses in periodontal prevention and therapy. Part II. Clinical use and recommendations. *International Journal of Dental Hygiene*, 1, 188–194.

Brunton, P. and Kay, E. (2003) Prevention. Part 6: Prevention in the older dental patient. *British Dental Journal*, 195, 237–241.

Carrilho, M.R., Geraldeli, S., Tay, F., *et al.* (2007) In vivo preservation of the hybrid layer by chlorhexidine. *Journal Dental Research*, 86, 529–533.

Case, D. (1977) Safety of Hibitane 1. Laboratory experiments. *Journal of Clinical Periodontology*, 4, 66–72.

Center for Disease Control. (2007) Trends in oral health status. Vital Health Statistics, Series 11, #248, April.

Chalmers, J.M. (2006) Minimal intervention dentistry: part 2. Strategies for addressing restorative challenges in older patients. *Journal of the Canadian Dental Association*, 72, 435–440.

CHX Technologies and Denplan Ltd., Patient surveys 2006–2009.

Cimiotti, J. (2003) Adverse reactions associated with an alcohol-based hand antiseptic among nurses in a neonatal intensive care unit. *American Journal of Infection Control*, 31, 43–48.

Du, M.Q., Tai, B.J., Jiang, H., *et al.* (2006) A two-year randomized clinical trial of chlorhexidine varnish on dental caries in Chinese preschool children. *Journal of Dental Research*, 85, 557–559.

eMC Medicine Guides. (2011) Data Pharm Communications. What information do people want about their medicines? Survey analysis. [online] available at http://www.medicines.org.uk/guides/pages/surveyresults.

Ersin, N.K., Eden, E., Eronat, N., *et al.* (2008) Effectiveness of 2-year application of school based chlorhexidine varnish, sodium fluoride gel, and dental health education programs in high-risk adolescents. *Quintessence International*, 39, e45–e51.

European Agency for Evaluation of Medicinal Products, Committee for Veterinary Medicinal Products, Chlorhexidine: Summary Report EMEA/MRL/107/96, June 1996.

Faria, G., Cardoso, C.R., Larson, R.E., *et al.* (2009) Chlorhexidine-induced apoptosis or necrosis in L929 fibroblasts: A role for endoplasmic reticulum stress. *Toxicology and Applied Pharmacology*, 234, 256–65.

Fure, S. (1998) Five-year incidence of caries, salivary and microbial conditions in 60-, 70- and 80-year-old Swedish individuals. *Caries Research*, 32, 166–174.

Fure, S. (2004) Ten-year cross-sectional and incidence studies of coronal and root caries and some related factors in elderly Swedish individuals. *Gerodontology*, 21, 130–140.

Garvey, L., Roed-Petersen, J., Menné, T., *et al.* (2001) Danish anaesthesia allergy centre—preliminary results. *Acta Anaesthesiology Scandindavica*, 45, 1204–1209.

Garvey, L.H., Roed-Petersen, J., Husum, B. (2001) Anaphylactic reactions in anaesthetised patients—four cases of chlorhexidine allergy. *Acta Anaesthesiology Scandindavica*, 45, 1290–1294.

Garvey, L.H., Roed-Petersen, J., Husum, B. (2003) Is there a risk of sensitization and allergy to chlorhexidine in health care workers? *Acta Anaesthesiology Scandindavica*, 47, 2003, 720–724.

Gendron, R., Grenier, D., Sorsa T., *et al.* (1999) Inhibition of the activities of matrix metalloproteinases 2, 8 and 9 by chlorhexidine. *Clinical Diagnosis and Laboratory Immunology*, 6, 437–439.

Gent, J.F., Frank, M.F., Hettinger, T.P. (2002) Taste confusions following chlorhexidine treatment. *Chemical Senses*, 27, 73–80.

Gjermo, P. (1989) Chlorhexidine and related compounds. *Journal of Dental Research*, 68, 1602–1608.

Griffin, S.O., Barker, L.K, Griffin, P.M., et al. (2009) Oral health needs among adults in the United States with chronic diseases. *Journal of the American Dental Association*, 140, 1266–1274.

Griffin, S.O., Regnier, E., Griffin, P.M., et al. (2007) Effectiveness of fluoride in preventing caries in adults. *Journal of Dental Research*, 86, 410–415.

Grönroos, L., Mättö, J., Saarela, M., et al. (1995) Chlorhexidine susceptibilities of mutans streptococcal serotypes and ribotypes. *Antimicrobial Agents and Chemotherapy*, 39, 894–898.

Gu, Q., Dillon, C.F., Burt, V.L. (2010) Prescription drug use continues to increase: U.S. prescription drug data for 2007–2008. *NCHS Data Brief*, 42, 1–8.

Gu, Q., Paulose-Ram, R., Dillon, C., et al. (2006) Antihypertensive medication use among US adults with hypertension. *Circulation*, 113, 213–21.

Gunsolley, J.C. (2006) A meta-analysis of six-month studies of antiplaque and antigingivitis agents. *Journal of the American Dental Association*, 137, 1649–1557.

Gunsolley, J.C. (2010) Clinical efficacy of antimicrobial mouthrinses. *Journal of Dentistry*, 38 Suppl 1, S6–10.

Haukali, G. and Poulsen, S. (2003) Effect of a varnish containing chlorhexidine and thymol (Cervitec) on approximal caries in 13- to 16-year-old school children in a low-caries area. *Caries Research*, 37, 185–189.

Hawkins, R.J., Jutai, D.K., Brothwell, D.J., et al. (1997) Three-year coronal caries incidence in older Canadian adults. *Caries Research*, 31, 405–410.

Heard, D.D. and Ashworth, R.W. (1968) The colloidal properties of chlorhexidine and its interaction with some macromolecules. *Journal of Pharmacy and Pharmacology*, 20, 505–512.

Herrera, D. (2009) Cetylpyridinium chloride containing mouth rinses and plaque control. *Evidence Based Dentistry*, 10, 44.

Holm-Pedersen, P., Avlund, K., Morse, D.E., et al. (2005) Dental caries, periodontal disease, and cardiac arrhythmias in community-dwelling older persons aged 80 and older: is there a link? *Journal of the American Geriatric Society*, 53, 430–437.

Hu, J.Y., Chen, X.C., Li, Y.Q., et al. (2005) Radiation-induced root surface caries restored with glass-ionomer cement placed in conventional and ART cavity preparations: results at two years. *Australian Dental Journal*, 50, 186–190.

Ipsos Reid. (2008) Survey of attitudes to professional dental care amongst Canadian adults age 40+.

James, P., Parnell, C., Whelton, H. (2010) The caries-preventive effect of chlorhexidine varnish in children and adolescents: a systematic review. *Caries Research*, 44, 333–340.

Joyston-Bechal, S., Hayes, K., Davenport, E.S., et al. (1992) Caries incidence, mutans streptococci and lactobacilli in irradiated patients during a 12-month preventive programme using chlorhexidine and fluoride. *Caries Research*, 26, 384–390.

Katz, S. (1982) The use of fluoride and chlorhexidine for the prevention of radiation caries. *Journal of the American Dental Association*, 104, 164–170.

Keltjens, H.M., Schaeken, M.J., van der Hoeven, J.S., et al. (1990) Caries control in overdenture patients: 18-month evaluation on fluoride and chlorhexidine therapies. *Caries Research*, 24, 371–375.

Kuyyakanond, T. and Quesnel, L.B. (1992) The mechanism of action of chlorhexidine. *FEMS Microbiology Letters*, 79, 211–215.

Lawrence, H.P., Hunt, R.J., Beck, J.D. (1995) Three-year root caries incidence and risk modeling in older adults in North Carolina. *Journal of Public Health Dentistry*, 55, 69–78.

Lessa, F.C., Aranha, A.M., Noguira, I., et al. (2010) Toxicity of chlorhexidine on odontoblast-like cells. *Journal of Applied Oral Science*, 18, 50–58.

Levy, S.M. and Jensen, M.E. (1990) A clinical evaluation of the restoration of root surface caries. *Special Care Dentistry*, 10, 156–160.

Lewis, C. (2003) The impact of direct-to-consumer advertising. FDA Consumer Magazine, March–April.

Löe, H., Schiott C.R., Karring G., et al. (1976) Two years oral use of chlorhexidine in man. I. General design and clinical effects. *Journal of Periodontal Research*, 11, 135–44.

Loesche, W.J., Syed, S.A., Schmidt, E., et al. (1985) Bacterial profiles of subgingival plaques in periodontitis. *Journal of Periodontology*, 56, 447–456.

Love, R.M. and Jenkinson, H.F. (2002) Invasion of dentinal tubules by oral bacteria. *Critical Revues in Oral Biology and Medicine*, 13, 171–183.

Mascarenhas, A.K., Allen, C.M., Loudon, J. (2001) The association between Viadent use and oral leukoplakia. *Epidemiology*, 12, 741–743.

Maillard, J.Y. (2002) Bacterial target sites for biocide action. *Symposium Series (Society for Applied Microbiology)*, 31, 16S–27S.

Mauriello, S.M., Elter, J.R., Moss, K., et al. (2003) Relationship of Incident Root Caries and Mortality in Older Adults. The 32nd Annual Meeting and Exhibition of the American Association of Dental Research. Abstract 0652. San Antonio, Texas.

Mauriello, S.M., Moss, K.L., Beck J.D. (2006) Root caries prevalence and incident myocardial infarction. The ADEA/AADR/CADR Meeting & Exhibition. *International Association of Dental Research*. Abstract 1471, Orlando, Florida.

Mauriello, S., et al. (1999) Root caries incidence as a risk predictor for mortality. IADR Abstract 3582, *Journal of Dental Research* 78.

Nakano, K., Nemoto, H., Nomura, R., et al. (2009) Detection of oral bacteria in cardiovascular specimens. *Oral Microbiology and Immunology*, 24, 64–68.

National Institutes of Health (2001) Consensus statement: Diagnosis and management of dental caries throughout life, available at http://consensus.nih.gov/cons/115/115.

Paraskevas, S. (2005) Randomized controlled clinical trials on agents used for chemical plaque control. *International Journal of Dental Hygiene*, 3, 162–178.

Powell, L.V., Persson, R.E., Kiyak, H.A., et al. (1999) Caries prevention in a community-dwelling older population. *Caries Research*, 33, 333–339.

Powell, L.V. (1998) Caries prediction: a review of the literature. *Community Dentistry and Oral Epidemiology*, 26, 361–371.

Ravald, N. and Hamp, S. (1981) Prediction of root surface caries in patients treated for advanced periodontal disease. *Journal of Clinical Periodontology*, 8, 400–414.

Reiker, J., van der Velden, U., Barendregt, D.S., et al. (1999) A cross-sectional study into the prevalence of root caries in periodontal maintenance patients. *Journal of Clinical Periodontology*, 26, 26–32.

Riley, J.L. 3rd, Gordan, V.V., Rindal, D.B., et al. (2010) Dental PBRN Collaborative Group. Preferences for caries prevention agents in adult patients: findings from the dental practice-based research network. *Community Dentistry and Oral Epidemiology*, 38, 360–70.

Rindal, D.B., Rush, W.A., Peters, D., et al. (2005) Antidepressant xerogenic medications and restoration rates. *Community Dentistry and Oral Epidemiology*, 33, 74–80.

Ritter, A.V., Shugars, D.A., Bader, J.D. (2010) Root caries risk indicators: systematic review of risk models. *Community Dentistry and Oral Epidemiology*, 38, 383–397.

Rölla, G. and Melsen, B. (1975) On the mechanism of plaque inhibition by chlorhexidine. *Journal of Dental Research (spec issue B)*, 54, 57–62.

Rushton, A. (1977) Safety of Hibitane. II. Human experience. *Journal of Clinical Periodontology*. 4, 73–79.

Russell, A.D. (1986) Chlorhexidine: antibacterial action and bacterial resistance. *Infection*, 14, 212–215.

Santos, A. (2003) Evidence-based control of plaque and gingivitis. *Journal of Clinical Periodontology*, 30 (Suppl 5), 13–16.

Schachtele, C.F., Rosamond, W.D., Harlander, S.K. (1985) Diet and aging: current concerns related to oral health. *Gerodontics*, 1, 117–24.

Schaeken, M.J., Keltjens, H.M., Van Der Hoeven, J.S. (1991) Effects of fluoride and chlorhexidine on the microflora of dental root surfaces and progression of root-surface caries. *Journal of Dental Research*, 70, 150–3.

Schaeken, M.J., van der Hoeven, J.S., Hendriks, J.C. (1989) Effects of varnishes containing chlorhexidine on the human dental plaque flora. *Journal of Dental Research*, 68, 1786–1789.

Senior, N. (1973) Some observations on the formulation and properties of chlorhexidine, *Journal of the Society of Cosmetic Chemists*, 24, 259–278.

Seymour, R.A., Meechan, J.G., Yates M.S., *et al.* (1999) *Pharmacology and Dental Therapeutics*, pp. 187–189, Oxford University Press, Oxford, UK.

Singh, M.L., Papas, A.S., Biesbrock, A.R. (2006) Root caries increment in a medication-induced saliva hypofunction population. *The ADEA/AADR/CADR Meeting & Exhibition. International Association of Dental Research*. Abstract 1472, Orlando, Florida.

Spolsky, V., Black, B., Jenson, L. (2007) Products—old, and emerging. *Canadian Dental Association Journal*, 35, 724–737.

Statistics Canada (2006) Seniors' health care use, v16 (Cat. # 82–003).

Twetman, S. (2004) Antimicrobials in future caries control? A review with special reference to chlorhexidine treatment. *Caries Research*, 38, 223–229.

Twetman, S., Petersson, L., Axelsson, S., *et al.* (2004) Caries-preventive effect of sodium fluoride mouthrinses: a systematic review of controlled clinical trials. *Acta Odontologica Scandinavica*, 62, 223–230.

The University of York, NHS Centre for Reviews and Dissemination (1999) Dental restoration: what type of filling? Effective Health Care.

US Census Bureau. Projections of 2008, Table 2 and 3.

Van der Reijden, W.A., Dellemijn-Kippuw, N., Stijne-van Nes, A.M., *et al.* (2001) Mutans streptococci in subgingival plaque of treated and untreated patients with periodontitis. *Journal of Clinical Periodontology*, 28, 686–691.

Van Leeuwen, M.P., Slot, D.E., Van der Weijden, G.A. (2011) Essential oils compared to chlorhexidine with respect to plaque and parameters of gingival inflammation: a systematic review. *Journal of Periodontology*, 82, 174–194.

van Rijkom, H.M., Truin, G.J., van't Hof, M.A. (1996) A meta-analysis of clinical studies on the caries-inhibiting effect of chlorhexidine treatment. *Journal of Dental Research*, 75, 790–795.

Wilson, N.H., Burke, F.J., Mjör, I.A. (1997) Reasons for placement and replacement of restorations of direct restorative materials by a selected group of practitioners in the United Kingdom. *Quintessence International*, 28, 245–248.

Winrow, M. (1973) Metabolic studies with radio-labeled chlorhexidine in animals and man. *Journal of Periodontal Research*, 8 (Suppl 12), 45–48.

Zhang, Q., van Palenstein-Helderman, W.H., van't Hof, M.A., *et al.* (2006) Chlorhexidine varnish for preventing dental caries in children, adolescents and young adults: a systematic review. *European Journal of Oral Science*, 114, 449–455.

11

Ozone in the prevention of dental diseases

Hardy Limeback and Amir Azarpazhooh

Introduction

After every electrical storm with lightning, the air just seems to 'smell' a little different. The ancient Greeks noticed this odor after lightning strikes and called it ozein for scent. But Native American Indians had always known about that smell. It was an odor that would predict better outcomes in their attempt to catch fish. This interesting observation has been carried down over many generations to this day. The cooler, oxygen-rich water at the surface brought the fish to the surface. In 1785, Van Marum noticed a characteristic odor near his electrifier when electric sparks were passed, and in 1801, Cruickshank observed the same odor at the anode during water electrolysis. Then, in 1840, Christian Friedrich Schoenbein (1799–1868) discovered an "electric and pungent smell" while working with a voltaic pile in the presence of oxygen and named it ozone. He considered ozone not only to be an oxidant but also a disinfectant (Bocci 2010).

Ozone is a naturally occurring molecule that exists in the form of a gas in the stratosphere in the layer known as the 'ozone layer.' It is a simple molecule of three oxygen atoms in an unstable, highly reactive, cyclic tri-atomic configuration (Figure 11-1).

In the stratosphere, which is between 16 and 48 kilometers (10 and 30 miles) above the earth's surface, intense electrical energy such as lightning splits up oxygen molecules (O_2) to form individual oxygen atoms that combine with other O_2 molecules to form ozone (O_3) gas (Bocci 2010, pp. 1–2).

$$3\,O_2 = 2\,O_3 - 68,400 \text{ cal.}$$

OR

$$O_2 + UV\ (<242\ nm) = O + O$$
$$2\,O_2 + 2O = 2\,O_3$$

Ozone molecules occur at levels between 1 and 10 parts per million (ppm) in the stratosphere, and these concentration levels are protective of life on earth because the ozone absorbs harmful UV-C and UV-B ultraviolet light. Although both oxygen and ozone together absorb 95 to 99.9% of the sun's ultraviolet radiation, only ozone absorbs the most energetic ultraviolet light (UV-C and UV-B). When ozone reacts with ultraviolet light, it reverts back to oxygen. Without the action of the ozone layer, UV-C and UV-B rays from the sun, which are extremely damaging to DNA, would slowly destroy life on the planet. Ozone is also a greenhouse gas so it plays a role in keeping the planet warm (Wang et al. 1993). About 90% of the ozone in the earth's atmosphere is found in the stratosphere. Therefore, ozone has a critical role in ecological framework for life on the earth's surface. The other 10% of ozone in the in the atmosphere occurs in the troposphere, and when it occurs at ground level it is harmful to human life because of its irritation to eyes and lung tissues. When ozone is produced as a result of polluting processes, nitrogen oxide and sulphur-containing chemicals combine with the ozone to produce the characteristic mixtures of harmful gases found in 'smog.' Smog is the result of industrial and automobile combustion reactions, and the interaction of sunlight with polluted air, especially in hot summer months. The California and the US

Comprehensive Preventive Dentistry, First Edition. Edited by Hardy Limeback.
© 2012 John Wiley & Sons, Ltd. Published 2012 by John Wiley & Sons, Ltd.

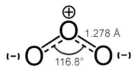

Figure 11-1 Ozone Gas-Molecular Formula. Ozone (O$_3$) is a gas at room temperature and is an unstable tricyclic molecule of three oxygen atoms. (Source: Ben Mills, Odell, UK).

Table 11-1 Stability of ozone related to temperature

Temperature	Time to reach 50% concentration
−50°C	3 months
20°C	40 minutes
30°C	25 minutes

Source: Bocci 2005, p. 5.

Environmental Protection Agency (EPA) have set upper limits of ozone at ground level to protect human health.

The permissible concentration of ozone, to which workers may be exposed, is 0.1 ppm over 24 hours. The short-term exposure limit was 0.3 ppm for 15 minutes. A concentration of 10 ppm of ozone in air is generally accepted as Immediately Dangerous to Life or Health (IDLH). Ozone can be detected by its odor at a concentration of about 0.04 ppm (Lippmann 1993).

Ozone: is it a disinfectant or medicine?

The "Dr. Jekyll and Mr. Hyde" protective/harmful dual role that ozone plays in the atmosphere is reflected in its role as a medicinal treatment. At high exposures, ozone can be harmful to human health. But at low exposures, ozone can treat infections through its disinfection properties. It also has immune-boosting properties.

Ozone, because it has a paired number of electrons in the external orbit, is far more reactive than oxygen and can generate some of the radical oxygen species (ROS) produced by oxygen during mitochondrial respiration. Phagocytes produce anion superoxide, hydrogen peroxide (H$_2$O$_2$), and hypochlorous acid (HClO) catalyzed by myeloperoxidase. The relevance of the ROS in normal processes in humans is evident by the production of H$_2$O$_2$ in almost all cells by the nicotinamide adenine dinucleotide phosphate (NADPH)-oxydase isoenzymes. Ozone generates a great variety of oxidized molecules that are not long lived at all (Bocci *et al.* 2009). However, the powerful oxidizing ability of ozone at high concentrations that makes it a potential cytotoxic agent for lungs also makes it ideal as an oxidizing gas for the neutralization of contaminants in polluted air. Ozone is sometimes used to 'clean' contaminated air. Ozone generators, for example, are used to remove the smoke smell from rooms after fires and the musty smell of mold in humid buildings. Since high-energy electrical potential is really all that is required to convert oxygen to ozone, many devices now exist with the basic design of a high electrical energy transformer to convert air to ozone and other oxides.

Ozone decomposes readily, but this reaction is temperature sensitive. The colder the temperature, the longer ozone persists as a molecule, either as a gas or in aqueous solution. This is illustrated in Table 11-1.

Ozone is an effective anti-microbial agent capable of killing bacteria, fungi, protozoa, and viruses as well. Some microorganisms survive at higher concentrations of ozone, but ozone up to 1 µg ml^{-1} can eliminate *E. coli*, *Pseudomonas aeruginosa*, and *Serratia marcescens*, as well as *Candida albicans*. Staphylococcae are killed with 3–5 µg ml^{-1}. Ozone concentrations over 5 µg ml^{-1} will eradicate most microorganisms in a few seconds.

As a disinfectant agent in either the gaseous or aqueous phases, ozone has a variety of uses. It has been used in the drinking water industry as a disinfectant for over 100 years. In France, Paris was the first to ozonate its drinking water, and now more than 3,000 municipalities around the world use ozone to clean their water and sewage. Compared to chlorine, ozone can act more rapidly in lower concentration with no adverse side effects such as altered taste and odor.

Ozone gas is difficult to manage; however, ozone dissolved in pure water or in oils such as olive oil can be handled much more easily by the general practitioner. Using ozone in the aqueous phase makes it suitable for topical applications, as a soaking solution to disinfected dental instruments, or as a solution to disinfect medical and dental tubing and parts. If ozone is properly administered in the dental office, it can be a useful therapeutic agent with little or no side effects.

Mode of action of ozone

When ozone gas is bubbled through aqueous solutions, it dissolves and immediately reacts with organic molecules. Ozone rapidly decomposes through a complex series of chain reactions once in solution. In the aqueous phase, ozone reacts with single electron donors to generate the O$_3^{\cdot-}$ radical ion.

$$X: + O_3 \rightarrow X^+ + O_3^{\cdot-}$$

This radical ion receives a proton in aqueous solutions and forms HO$_3^{\cdot}$,

$$O_3^{\cdot-} + H^+ \rightarrow HO_3^{\cdot}$$

which decomposes to a more powerful oxidant of hydroxyl radical

$$HO_3 \rightarrow \cdot OH + O_2$$

(Grootveld *et al.* 2004). Hydroxyl (OH·) radicals are among the most reactive oxidizing species. They readily react with double bonds and break them down (Hems *et al.* 2005). This oxidizing action is also responsible for the 'bleaching' effect of ozone on colored compounds.

Ozone breaks down the cell walls and cytoplasmic membranes of bacteria and fungi. It attacks glycoproteins, glycolipids, and other amino acids, and once inside the cell, it blocks the enzymatic control system of the cell. This results in increases in membrane permeability, and the cell ceases to function because it no longer can maintain its intracellular electrolyte balance. More ozone can then penetrate into the cell, and this causes further destruction and cell death (Nagayoshi *et al.* 2004; Arita *et al.* 2005).

The oxidation of many organic molecules involved in the caries process disrupts the function of cariogenic bacteria, eliminating many in the process. For example, ozone can decarboxylate pyruvic acid, a potent caries-producing bacterial acid, into acetic acid, a much less potent cariogenic acid (Abu Naba'a 2004). Ozone acts much more quickly than chlorine, and the higher the ozone concentration, the more effective the disinfecting dose.

Effects of ozone on human health

Humans are exposed to ozone generated at home and in the workplace on a daily basis. Ozone is given off during electric arc welding and electroplating, from X-ray generators, by high voltage electrical equipment, during photoengraving, from electrostatic air cleaners, from indoor ultraviolet sources, and even from photocopying machines. Natural pollution sources of ozone are formed locally in air from lightning and in the stratosphere by ultraviolet radiation. At sea level, the ozone concentration is about 0.05 to 0.08 ppm (Logan 1989).

Ozone has a pungent smell, which most humans can detect when it is present at very low levels (for example, 50 parts per billion [ppb]). Exposure to high concentrations of ozone can cause significant irritation and damage to lung tissue (McDonnell *et al.* 1983), eyes, and skin (Bocci 2004). Table 11-2 summarizes the exposure concentrations, duration of exposure, and expected reactions that occur from these exposures.

In order to avoid producing toxic side products in machines that are designed to make ozone from air, Bocci (2010, p.11) recommends that only medical-grade ozone be used. Ozone should be produced from pure oxygen under controlled conditions, where the rate of flow, concentration, and total dose can be carefully regulated. Ozone generators for manufacturing medical-grade ozone are designed to allow the passage of pure oxygen (from O_2 tanks connected to the ozonator) through high voltage tubes that create a high enough energy field to produce a mixture of about 5% ozone and 95% oxygen. When air is used as the source of gas, the nitrogen gas in air is converted to toxic nitrogen oxide mixtures.

Ozone dose calculations

Knowing how much ozone to use in the treatment of oral tissues is key to avoiding toxicity. Therefore, some basic calculations are presented here for the reader so that comparisons between systems delivering ozone can be made (Ozone Solutions 2011).

Table 11-2 Effect of ozone on human tissue

Ozone exposure	Time of exposure	Effect
0.10 ppm	7 hours	Pulmonary edema, congestion, non-productive cough, possible
0.35 ppm	1 hour	Haemorrhage
0.35 ppm	2 hours	Increased respiratory rate and tidal volume
0.5 ppm	12 weeks (3 hours/day, 6 days/week)	Significant changes in lung function
2.0 ppm	2 hours	Respiratory distress with dyspnea, cyanosis, and pulmonary edema—causes a sense of pressure in the chest, temporary exhilaration followed by depression and a decrease in lung capacity
5–10 ppm	Brief exposure Inhaled more than 1 hour	Increase in pulse, respiratory effort May cause pulmonary edema and death
Mild to moderate exposures to gas Moderate exposure to ozone in aqueous solutions		Eye irritation Skin irritation, burns

Physical properties, standard conditions

Density of ozone: $2.14 \, kg/m^3$

Molecular weight of ozone: 48

Density of oxygen: $1.43 \, kg/m^3$

Molecular weight of oxygen: 32

Density of air: $1.29 \, kg/m^3$

Density of water: $1,000 \, kg/m^3$

Ozone concentration in water

$1 \, mg/L = 1 \, ppm \, O_3 = 1 \, g \, O_3/m^3$ water {by weight}

Ozone concentration in air by volume

$1 \, g \, O_3/m^3 = 467 \, ppm \, O_3$

$1 \, ppm \, O_3 = 2.14 \, mg \, O_3/m^3$

Ozone concentration in air by weight

$100 \, g \, O_3/m^3 = 7.8\% \, O_3$ (approximate)

$1\% \, O_3 = 12.8 \, g \, O_3/m^3$ (approximate)

$1\% \, O_3 = 6,051 \, ppm$ ozone

$7.8\% \, O_3 = 467 \, ppm$

Ozone concentration in oxygen by weight

$100 \, g \, O_3/m^3 = 6.99\% \, O_3$ (approximate)

$1\% \, O_3 = 14.3 \, g \, O_3/m^3$ (approximate)

$1\% \, O_3 = 6,678 \, ppm$ ozone

$6.99\% \, O_3 = 467 \, ppm$

For example, the HealOzone unit delivers gas at a rate of 615 cc/min.

The concentration of the gas is 2,100 ppm ozone in air.

$1 \, ppm \, O_3 = 2.14 \, mg \, O_3/m^3$ air

$2,100 \, ppm \, O_3 = 4,494 \, mg \, O_3/m^3$ air

$1 \, L = 0.001 \, m^3$

$4,494 \, mg \, O_3/m^3 = 4.494 \, mg \, O_3/L$

Rate of delivery = 615 cc/min = 0.615 L/min

Dose delivered = $4.494 \, mg \, O_3/L \times 0.615 \, L/min = 2.764 \, mg \, O_3/min = 0.046 \, mg \, O_3/sec$

A 10-second application would deliver 0.46 mg ozone to the surface.

The new HealOzone ×4 unit is designed to function with pure oxygen delivered by attaching oxygen tanks to the unit, and this will allow a great production of ozone (HealOzone 2011).

Why ozone is safe to administer to most human tissues

We have learned how ozone destroys the cell membranes of microorganisms and breaks down biological organic molecules. Paradoxically, mammalian host tissues and cells are not damaged by ozone, at least not at therapeutic levels. The primary reason that toxicity to blood, biological fluids, and internal organs can be totally avoided is that mammalian systems are equipped with extensive anti-oxidative mechanisms. The antioxidant system is made up of scavenger components, such as albumin, vitamins C and E, uric acid, bilirubin, cysteine, ubiquinol, alpha-lipoic acid, and intracellular antioxidants, such as glutathione (GSH), thioredoxin, and enzymes (superoxide dismutase [SOD]; glutathione peroxidise [GSH-Px], glutathione reductase [GSH-Rd], glutathione transferase [GSH-T], catalase, etc.), and proteins such as transferrin and caeruloplasmin, able to chelate free iron and copper that, otherwise, can favor the formation of hydroxyl radicals (Bocci 2010).

The host immune system responding to invading bacteria will generate antibodies directed toward pathogenic antigens, and interestingly the mechanisms involved in antibody inactivation of pathogens is now believed to involve the production of endogenous ozone that the antibodies themselves generate (Wentworth *et al.* 2002). Ozone in medicine can improve oxygen metabolism and improve the antioxidant defence mechanism (Bocci and Paulesu 1990; Bocci *et al.* 1993a, 1993b). Activated leukocytes have been shown to produce ozone (Babior *et al.* 2003; Nieva and Wentworth 2004).

Thus, our own bodies use ozone as a defense mechanism against invading microorganisms. Obviously, providing addition ozone to help our own defense mechanisms to ward off infection is the goal of ozone therapy in medicine and dentistry, as long as practitioners are not exposing the body to toxic levels of the highly reactive molecule.

Ozone use in medicine

The first ozone generator was developed in 1857 by German electrical engineer Werner von Siemens. In 1870, C. Lender used this ozone generator for purifying blood in Germany. The first potential medical application of ozone was described by Dr. Charles J. Kenworthy, in "Ozone," a report published by the Florida Medical Association (Grootvelt *et al.* 2004). During World War I, ozone was used for treating gaseous post-traumatic

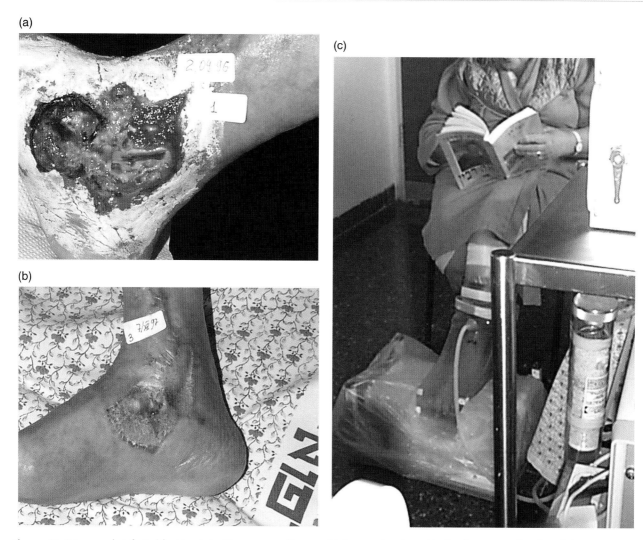

Figure 11-2 A severely infected foot healed with ozone gas therapy. (a) A wound at the ankle that is so severely infected that amputation might be considered. (b) Results of multiple ozone gas applications using medical ozone applied through (c) an air-tight plastic bag. These photographs clearly demonstrate the power of ozone gas in eliminating microorganisms that interfere with healing. This foot would likely have been amputated above the infection, but it was saved after ozone gas therapy. Photos courtesy of N. Calderon, MD, and T Kaufman, MD. Division of Plastic Surgery, Bnai-Zion University Medical Center, Haifa, Israel. (Forwarded by Dr. Fadi Sabbah DDS, Lebanon)

gangrene, infected wounds, mustard gas burns, and fistulas in German soldiers (Bocci 2005).

There are four primary routes for the medical administration of ozone:

1. Autohemotherapy, which is removing 200 ml (as in major autohemotherapy) or 5–10 ml (as in minor autohemotherapy) of blood from patient and treating it with oxygen and ozone and infusing the mixture back to patient.
2. Rectal insufflation (enema) of the mixture of oxygen/ozone.
3. Oxygen bagging, which involves exposing the mixture of oxygen/ozone to the skin by pumping it to an airtight bag around the area to be treated.

Figure 11-2 shows the remarkable results that can be obtained with ozone bagging.

4. Externally applied ozonated olive or sunflower oils (Oleozón).

Ozone therapy was accepted as an alternative medicine in the USA from 1880 until 1932. To date, ozone therapy has been a recognized treatment modality in 16 countries (Grootveld *et al.* 2004). Its use has been investigated in treatment of ocular diseases such as optic neuropathies, glaucoma, central retinal vein obstructions, and degenerative retinal diseases. It can react with blood components and positively affect oxygen metabolism, cell energy, the immunomodular property, antioxidant defense system, and microcirculation (Bocci 2010).

Ozone therapy is being used in many countries. For over 4 decades, 70% of 10,000 German doctors have used some kind of ozone therapy. The leader in the field in Germany in terms of experience with ozone machines and their use is the company "Dr. J. Hänsler GmbH Germany" (www.ozonosan.de) that makes the "Ozonosan system." This company was started by Dr. J. Hänsler, and now is directed by his daughter Renate Viebahn-Hänsler, PhD. Ozone therapy became so popular among German medical practitioners that the German "Medical Society for the Use of Ozone in Prevention and Therapy" was founded in 1971 as a non-profit organization. Sister societies joined from Switzerland, Austria, and Italy. The "European Cooperation of Medical Ozone Societies" (EuroCoop) formed in 2002. Its aim has been to standardize ozone therapy and ensure its safe use by competent doctors, trained by the component organizations. The eventual goal is to have a uniform European Standard Qualification Program for ozone practitioners. In 2006 two associations joined the EuroCoop: the Egyptian Ozone Association starting with the first scientific congress in Cairo in February 2006, and the Turkish Ozone Association, organizing their first International Medical Ozone Congress in Istanbul June 16–18, 2006.

Application of ozone in dentistry

Three main routes of administration of ozone have been used in dentistry: administering the gas directly to oral tissues, in aqueous solution (distilled water), or in oils. Dr. E.A. Fisch, born at the turn of the 20th century, was the first dentist to use ozonated water in his practice. An older German surgeon, Dr. Erwin Payr, used it in surgery and reported his results at the 59th Congress of the German Surgical Society in Berlin (Bocci 2005, p. 2). Ozonated water is used to inhibit infections, promote hemostasis, and enhance local oxygen supply (Baysan et al. 2000).

Effect of ozone on oral microorganisms and oral cells

Nagayoshi et al. (2004) examined the effect of ozonated water on oral microorganisms and dental plaque. After treating the dental plaque samples with 4 ml of ozonated water for 10 seconds, no microorganisms were detected. They also stained bacterial cells and conducted fluorescence microscopic analysis to estimate the effect of ozonated water on Streptococcus mutans. Their results revealed that S. mutans cells were killed instantaneously in ozonated water. They found that ozonated water significantly inhibited the accumulation of experimental dental plaque and remarkably decreased the number of viable S. mutans. They concluded that ozonated water was effective for killing gram-positive and gram-negative oral microorganisms and oral C. albicans in pure culture. In addition, ozonated water had a strong bactericidal activity against the bacteria in plaque biofilm and therefore might be useful to control oral infectious microorganisms in dental plaque.

In another study (Nagayoshi et al. 2004) researchers examined the effect of ozonated water against Enterococcus faecalis and S. mutans infections in dentin of freshly extracted bovine incisors. After treating with ozonated water, the number of Colony Forming Units (CFU) of bacteria in the infected dentin chips was significantly decreased. Also, fluorescence microscopic analysis showed an increase of membrane permeability of S. mutans cells, meaning that ozonated water has a strong bactericidal effect against bacteria invading dentinal tubules of root canals. When the dentin chips were subjected to ozonated water irrigation and sonication, ozonated water had nearly the same antimicrobial activity as 2.5% sodium hypochlorite (NaOCl). They also compared the cytotoxicity of ozonated water and NaOCl against L-929 mouse fibroblasts and found that L-929 fibroblasts were significantly damaged by 2.5% NaOCl, in contrast to ozonated water. They concluded that ozonated water had nearly the same antimicrobial activity as 2.5% NaOCl during irrigation, especially when combined with sonication, and showed a low level of cytotoxicity against cultured cells and therefore, its application might be useful for root canal irrigation.

In contrast to these findings, in a study by Hems et al. (2005), NaOCl was found to be superior to ozonated water in killing E. faecalis in broth culture and in biofilms. They evaluated the bactericidal potential of ozonated water and gaseous ozone against Enterococcus faecalis. The antibacterial efficacy of ozone was tested against both broth and biofilm cultures. Ozone was sparged for 30, 60, 120 and 240 s, through overnight broth cultures of E. faecalis and compared with those that were centrifuged, washed, and resuspended in water. They found significant reductions of bacteria in the unwashed (2 log10 reductions) and washed (5 log10 reductions) broth cultures following 240 seconds of ozone applications. They found that ozone had an antibacterial effect on planktonic E. faecalis cells. However, it was not effective against E. faecalis cells in a biofilm unless they were displaced into the surrounding medium by agitation. They also showed that ozone had little effect when embedded in biofilms, and its antibacterial efficacy was not comparable with that of NaOCl. Also, gaseous ozone had no effect on the E. faecalis biofilm.

Huth et al. (2008) showed that higher concentrations of ozone are required to eliminate Enterococcus faecalis,

Table 11-3 Ozone in preventive dentistry: Disinfecting dentures

Author, Date	Ozone Source	Experiment	Results
Estrela *et al.* 2006	Ozone gas from pure oxygen bubbling with flow rate at 7 g/h ozone (1.2%) into the microbial suspensions	Bacterial cultures sonicated 20 seconds in ultrasonic solutions (distilled water vinegar/distilled water and Endozime AWpluz) treated with ozone gas	– Eliminated *S. aureus*
Arita *et al.* 2005	Flowing ozonated water (2 or 4 mg/l) for 1 minute	Heat-cured acrylic resins cultured with *C. albicans*, and treated with or in combination with ultrasonication	– Reduced *C. albicans* on dentures
Murakami *et al.* 2002	10 ppm ozone (bubbled through water)	Methicillin-resistant *Staphylococcus aureus* and T1 phage added to denture cleaning tank	– Elimination of methicillin-resistant *Staphylococcus aureus* in 10 minutes and 90% reduction of virus in 40 minutes
Oizumi *et al.* 1998	20 mg/hour ozone gas versus 1 ppm ozone in water	*Streptococcus mutans, Staphylococcus aureus*, and *Candida albicans* tested for susceptibility	– Gas eliminated microorganisms in 3 minutes – More effective than the ozonated water

Candida albicans, Peptostreptococcus micros, and *Pseudomonas aeruginosa.* She and her colleagues developed a biofilm model to simulate the bacterial deposits in root canals. Ozone gas was produced from 1 to 53 gm/m³ and tested on the bacteria, along with NaOCl (sodium hypochlorite, at 5.25% and 2.25%), chlorhexidine digluconate (at 0.2%) and 3% hydrogen peroxide. Ozone was as effective at killing bacteria as the NaOCl but more effective than hydrogen peroxide.

Kamali *et al.* (2003) showed a significant difference in the number of *Mutans streptococci* (MS) in the saliva and plaque before and after ozone treatment. Ozone had effectively penetrated into the lesions and killed the majority of microorganisms. In a different study (Hedberg *et al.* 2003), 20 seconds of the application of ozone gas reduced the growth of lactobacilli significantly.

The application of ozone to dental tissues being restored might prevent recurrent decay. This was tested in an *in vitro* experiment to test the effect of the HealOzone device on MS in teeth that were restored (Polydorou *et al.* 2006). Dentin chips that were infected with MS for 2 days were bonded with various bonding systems. The antimicrobial effect of the bonding systems combined with 80 seconds of the ozone treatment was significantly better than the 40 seconds of ozone treatment.

Ozone for disinfecting dentures

As part of a comprehensive preventive dentistry program for patients, especially those at high risk for oral infections, or those living in long-term care homes,

ozone is useful for the disinfection of partial and full dentures. Dental clinics that have ozonators can set up denture baths for disinfecting dentures, and long-term care homes could add this technology to their daily routine. It is inexpensive and more effective than many denture cleansers. Some preliminary studies have been conducted (Table 11-3).

Table 11-4 summarizes the studies that have been conducted to examine the effect of ozone on caries. *In vivo* clinical trials are needed where outcomes such as the prevalence of oral infections can be monitored.

Ozone instruments designed for dentistry

The HealOzone unit

Even though ozone has been used in medicine and dentistry for years, based on the leadership of medical pioneers such as Dr. Velio Bocci, methods to apply ozone to oral tissues were not commercially available. This changed with the development of the HealOzone unit (HealOzone 2130C-KaVo Dental, Biberach, Germany), which was the system used in most published clinical trials on caries reversal. CurOzone developed the HealOzone system in conjunction with Professor Edward Lynch in the UK. It was used in numerous studies and applications by Professor Lynch's research group. After amassing a large body of literature, published and unpublished, Professor Lynch wrote the first book on the subject (Lynch 2004).

The HealZone unit is a self-contained portable machine that produces ozone at a fixed concentration of 2,100 ppm ozone ± 5% at a flow rate of 615 cc min.

Table 11-4 Ozone in preventive dentistry: Ozone and caries

Author, Date	Ozone Source	Experiment	Results
Abu Naba'a *et al. 2003*	HealOzone for 10 seconds	– Patients examined at 3, 6, 9, and 12 months using photography and DIAGNOdent	41 (28.5%) of control teeth had white spot lesions. 13 (9%) ozone-treated teeth had white spot lesions ($p < 0.01$).
Holmes 2003	Healozone (40 seconds) applied to root caries lesions	– 6- and 18-month Recall—reversal of lesions monitored clinically – Double blinded Air vehicle control	– 100% reversal of ozone-treated root caries, whereas 37% of control caries progressed ($p < 0.01$)
Nagayoshi *et al.* 2004	10 minutes flushing (30 ml/minute) 4 mg/L of ozonated water with ultrasonication	Bovine dentin slices contaminated with *S. faecalis* and *S. Mutans*. – Viability in tubules measured with "Live-Dead" stain and fluorescent microscope	– Significant decrease in bacterial viability (same as sodium hypochlorite) but less cyctotoxicity to fibroblasts
Baysan and Lynch 2004	HealOzone (10 or 20 seconds) applied to root caries	'Biopsy' taken at baseline and after treatment	– Ozone gas reduced micro-organisms and arrested or reversed the majority of the root lesions
Huth *et al.* 2005	HealOzone (40 seconds)	– Early coronal caries on molars monitored for 3 months with DIAGNOdent	Significantly more caries reversal or reduced caries progression with ozone in caries high risk patients – Results not significant with the whole group
Polydorou *et al.* 2006	HealOzone (ozone gas from air 2,100 ppm at 615 cc/minute) 40- or 80-second exposure	Dentin chips infected with *S. mutans* bonded, then tested for remaining microbes	80 sec. exposure to ozone is more anti-bacterial in dentin than 40 sec.
Dahnhardt *et al.* 2006	HealOzone (20 seconds) applied to open carious lesions	– Hardness measured and reversal monitored with the DIAGNOdent at 4, 6, 8 months	– Hardness improved with ozone treatment but no significant reversal of root caries as measured by DIAGNOdent (Note: This instrument does not detect changes in mineralization, only bacterial staining.)
Baysan and Lynch 2007	HealOzone (10 seconds) applied to root caries	– Compared to root sealant (positive control) or no treatment control – Recalls at 1, 3, and 6 months – Root caries progression assessed clinically	– 38.1% of the ozone gas-treated root lesions became hard (compared to zero for the controls $p < 0.001$)
Kronenberg *et al.* 2009	HealOzone (duration not reported)	– 26 month-split mouth study – HealOzone, versus Cervitec – Fluor Protector versus no treatment control	– ozone did not prevent new lesions but the Chlorxidine-fluoride treatment significantly reduced white spot lesions
Kshitish and Laxman 2010	Ozonated water (0.041 ppm) delivered using a modified needle attached to an irrigation device, "Kent ozone dental jet TY-820"	– Subgingival ozonated water irrigation versus 0.2% chlorhexidine gluconate (Cavitron ultrasonic device) – 10-minute applications at baseline – Plaque, gingival, and bleeding indices and microbiology assessed at 7 days – Split mouth design	The ozonated water performed better than the chlorhexidine in reducing disease indices, both failed to reduce bacteria significantly but ozone had better antifungal activity.

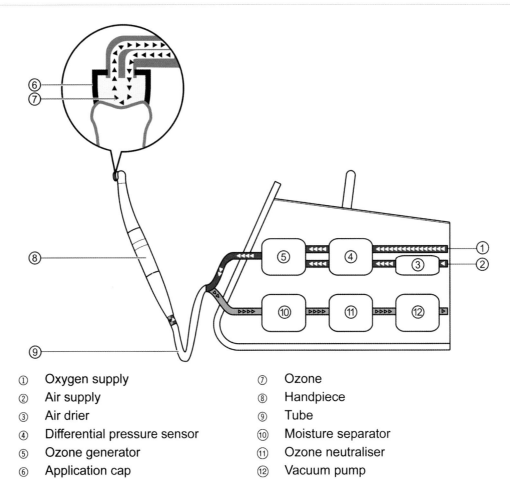

①	Oxygen supply	⑦	Ozone
②	Air supply	⑧	Handpiece
③	Air drier	⑨	Tube
④	Differential pressure sensor	⑩	Moisture separator
⑤	Ozone generator	⑪	Ozone neutraliser
⑥	Application cap	⑫	Vacuum pump

Figure 11-3 The HealOzone and its basic parts.

When it was developed for use in dentistry, the heal-Ozone unit was made to conform to all European Union legislation covering medical devices (CE: 93/42/EWG [EEC]). The HealOzone unit is now being used in many countries, and has been introduced to North America, where Health Canada has approved its use. However, the US Food and Drug Administration (FDA) is still evaluating ozone generators for direct application by dentists to tissues in the mouth.

The HealOzone is a portable machine with a built-in vacuum pump that pulls air through the ozone generator (producing a flow rate of 615 cc/minute as mentioned) to supply ozone to the handpiece. Disposable silicon cups of varying sizes are attached to the handpiece for the purpose of creating a seal with the tissue in contact. The vacuum pump draws air through the ozone generator and to the tip of the handpiece where ozone is expressed but immediately sucked back by the vacuum. A break in the seal is detected by the machine, and the ozone generator is turned off. At the end of the programmed exposure, the machine purges the ozone in the silicon tip, handpiece, and handpiece line to the machine. The ozone that is returned to the machine during the treatment and during the purging is sent to an ozone neutralizer (containing manganese II ions) that converts the ozone back to oxygen.

Figure 11-3 shows an illustration of the HealOzone unit's basic parts and how it functions.

Figure 11-4 shows a HealOzone unit on the countertop of a dental operatory.

Figure 11-5 shows the new HealOzone X4 unit, which is a next generation unit by CurOzone (distributed by Kavo). The X4 model has four modes of operations. The first mode is the previous ambient air mode and the endodontics mode, which produces $4.7\,gm/m^3$ for surface application and about $7\,gm/m^3$ in the endodontic function, all using ambient air. The next mode, which uses the 110 L oxygen tank attached at the rear, produces approximately $34\,gm/m^3$ in the regular mode and about $32\,gm/m^3$ in the endodontics mode. The oxygen tank has about 200 thirty-second treatments until it needs to be replaced. It is connected with a quick connect coupling and has a pressure reducer for safety purposes. The software indicated to the operator whether the tank is

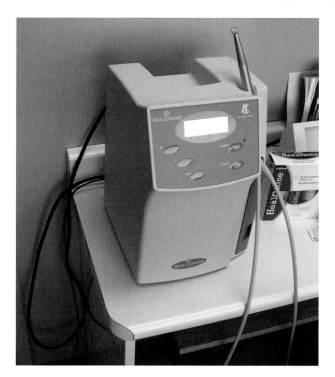

Figure 11-4 The HealOzone unit in the dental office.

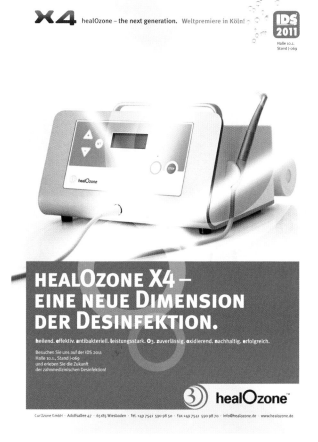

Figure 11-5 The HealOzone X4.

half full or nearly empty. These warning modes can be stored in the computer software. There is also a feature to connect a hospital main supply line, to avoid changing tanks frequently.

Other ozone units used in dentistry

There have been other units developed for the administration of ozone to dental tissues, but these have yet to be marketed in North America (Table 11-5).

Ozone in the management of incipient caries

Studies *in vivo* have been conducted to test the efficacy of ozone in the management of incipient caries. Abu Naba'a *et al.* (2004) conducted a split-mouth randomized clinical trial with 90 participants who had at least two primary pit or fissure lesions (without cavitation) in their permanent posterior teeth. The test surfaces were treated with ozone, the controls were not. About one-third of the teeth received sealants. Caries progression and regression were measured by change in clinical severity scores, mean log(e) DIAGNOdent readings, and mean log(e) ECM (electric caries meter) scores at baseline, 1, 3, 6, 9, and 12 months. The results seemed promising with an ozone group showing statistical improvement at the first and second recall appointment but then they significantly fell at the follow-up recalls. Ozone did not affect sealant retention. The study also showed a significant decrease in anxiety from the treatment and patients' acceptability of the therapy.

Huth *et al.* (2005) carried out a split-mouth randomized controlled clinical study to evaluate the effect of 40-second ozone gas (HealOzone) on the reversal of incipient fissure caries on 57 pairs of contra-lateral permanent molars. There was more caries reversal in the ozone-treated lesions within the group of patients at high current caries risk. However, there was no statistically significant difference between the groups when the whole study population was examined. Despite some study design problems, the results seemed promising. Also, it should be noted that the majority of the clinical studies that are reviewed depend upon findings produced by the DIAGNOdent and Electric Caries Meter. Although the validity and reliability of these devices have been extensively tested, they have not yet replaced visual, tactile, and radiographic detection as a routine method of early caries diagnosis.

Kronenberg *et al.* (2009) failed to show in a 26-month split-mouth clinical trial that the HealOzone reduced white spot lesions in patients undergoing orthodontic therapy. The positive control (Cervitec chlorhexidine

Table 11-5 Ozone units available for dentistry in some countries

Name of Unit	Manufacturer/distributor	Features
Medozons-BM/CM SV System	ORIGINAL DENTAL, Ltd B.A.U. Str., Beirut-Lebanon P.O. Box. 14-6410 www.originaldental.com Email: originaldental@gmail.com	– Electrical transformer – Built-in ozone destructor – Handpiece and silicon tips
OzonyMed	REDEE 62-704 Kowale Pańskie 35, Poland www.redee.eu Email: info@redee.eu	– Variety of plasma handpieces
Prozone	W&H Dentalwerk Bürmoos GmbH Ignaz-Glaser-Straße 53, Postfach 1 5111 Bürmoos, Austria www.wh.com Email: office@wh.com	– Air source – Dehydration chamber – Handpiece and plastic tips – Ozone concentration at the tip not known
OZONYTRON®XP	MIO International OZONYTRON® GmbH Hechtseetrasse 16 Rosenheim Germany83022 E-Mail: info@ozonytron.com	– 3 ozone generators (plasma, electrical) – Hollow needles available – "Full-Mouth-Disinfection" is possible with the third external ozone generator using a full tray set up and the OZONYTRON®OZ.
Dr. Katz Ozonator	Corporate Address Dr. Harold Katz LLC 750 N. Highland Ave. Los Angeles, CA 90038 Fax: 1-323-993-8327	– Simple ozonator – Not meant for direct application to tissues – Uses air to make ozone for bubbling through water to make disinfecting solutions
DOU120 Ozone generator	Longevity Resources Web site: www.ozonegenerator.com Email: info@ozonegenerator.com	– Ozone generator that uses oxygen tanks – No handpiece – Makes ozonated liquids for dental treatment

varnish in combination with Fluor Protector fluoride varnish) produced a significant reduction in white spot lesions.

Ozone in the management of open caries

Dahhardt *et al.* (2006) evaluated the efficacy of ozone gas on the reversal of caries in open single-surface lesions. After removing caries from the large lesions dentin 20 seconds of ozone gas (HealOzone) was administered to the 'leathery' and the hardness to the dentin was followed. Smaller lesions were left untreated as the control group. Comparing the differences between test and control teeth over time, the DIAGNOdent values improved, however the improvement was not statistically significant. Moreover, the use of ozone resulted in an average reduction of 13% of the DIAGNOdent values immediately after the ozone treatment. Finally, with the use of a questionnaire, it was found that the level of fear was

reduced prior to the second session and following the last session by 82% and 93%, respectively.

Treating root caries with ozone

After developing and testing the HealOzone system and testing its antibacterial properties (Baysan *et al.* 2000), the HealOzone was tested further by measuring survival of microorganisms on root surfaces with root caries and monitoring to see if it was possible to reverse the lesions. Baysan and Lynch (2004) were successful in showing that not only did the HealOzone reduce surface bacteria, but it encouraged remineralization. In their *in vitro* study, they assessed the antimicrobial effect of aqueous ozone on primary root carious lesions (PRCL). They harvested 40 soft PRCLs from freshly extracted teeth and removed half of the lesions on each sample with a sterile excavator. The remaining lesion was exposed to ozonated water for a period of either 10 or 20 seconds (0.069 or 0.138 ml of ozone, respectively). A significantly reduced microbiological count (p < 0.001) was observed in the ozone-treated groups compared with the control groups. They also used 40 sterile saliva-coated glass beads to demonstrate the specific antimicrobial efficacy of 10 seconds of ozone gas (HealOzone, KaVo) on *S. mutans* and *S. sobrinus*. The glass beads were randomly divided into two groups for each microorganism: ozone and control. They found a significant (p < 0.0001) reduction in ozone-treated samples for both microorganisms compared with the control samples.

Nagayoshi *et al.* (2004) subsequently, and independently, showed that ozonated water can kill bacterial but it was not cytotoxic to fibroblasts.

In an *in vivo* setting, Baysan *et al.* (2007) conducted a split-mouth randomized clinical trial. They included 79 participants, at least 18 years old, with either two or four primary root carious lesions (PRCL). The included lesions were leathery (severity index two) and accessible to treatment. The lesions were randomized with equal numbers of intervention and control, in each mouth in a way that each participant had equal numbers of intervention and control lesions (two or four in total):

1. Cleaning, 10 seconds of ozone gas, and reductant solution (containing xylitol and fluoride). The intervention was repeated at 1 month (with no ozone), 3 months, and 6 months (both with ozone for 10 seconds).
2. Reductant only (applied for 5 seconds), repeated after 1 month and 3 months.
3. Ozone and sealant. Ozone therapy was applied at 3 months. Sealants were reapplied if it was a partial or complete defect.
4. Sealant only.

For all groups, caries progression and regression were measured by the change in clinical severity scores, mean log (e) DIAGNOdent readings, and mean log (e) ECM scores. They also recorded further dental interventions, pain, patient satisfaction, and adverse events.

Their results showed that in the 6-month follow-up, the mean changes in ECM readings were significantly higher (that is, better remineralization) in the ozone-treated group than in the control group (5.62 versus 4.92, respectively). Also, DIAGNOdent measurements in the 6-month follow-up were significantly lower (that is, better remineralization) in the ozone-treated group than in the control group (10.9 versus 46.4, respectively). In 12 months 47% of PRCLs became hard in the ozone group, while none became hard in the control group (p < 0.001). Fifty-two percent of lesions reversed from a

severity index of 2 to 1 in the ozone group compared with 11.6% in the control group (p < 0.001).

Caution should however be used when interpreting the effects of ozone on the 'reversal' of caries for two reasons. First, as presented in Chapter 2, the DIAGNOdent likely measures the fluorescence of the porphyrins produced by bacteria-contaminating mineralized tissues. This instrument fails to detect artificial caries and is not very good at monitoring the reversal of white post lesions. Secondly, ozone has a bleaching effect and may, therefore, destroy some of the porphyrins that are left behind by bacteria. Alternative caries detection methods should really be employed when measuring caries reversal under the influence of ozone gas. Fortunately, more researchers also employed the tradition clinical methods of tactile and visual aids to diagnose caries.

Holmes (2003) was the first to conduct a double-blind, randomized clinical trial to evaluate the effect of ozone gas, combined with the daily use of a remineralizing patient kit, on the clinical severity of non-cavitated leathery PRCLs using 89 subjects (age range 60–82). Each subject had two leathery PRCLs (a total of 178 lesions), which were randomly assigned for treatment with ozone gas (40 seconds at 2,100 ppm ± 10%) or air. Lesions were clinically recorded at baseline, 3, 6, 12, and 18 months as soft, leathery, or hard. He found that at 3 months, 69% of lesions in the ozone group had become hard, and none had deteriorated. In the control group, after 3 months, 4% had become worse (p < 0.01). At the 6-month recall, 8% of lesions treated with ozone remained leathery, and the rest had become hard. In contrast, in the control group, 11% of lesions had become worse, and only one lesion had become hard (p < 0.01). At the 12-month recall, in the ozone group, only two lesions remained leathery, and the rest had hardened. Over the same period, in the control group, 21 lesions had become worse, one remained hard, and the rest remained leathery (p < 0.01). At the 18-month recall, in the ozone group, all of the lesions had arrested, while in the control group, 37% of the lesions had become worse, one had reversed, and the rest remained leathery (p < 0.01).

Finally, it is worth mentioning that as an added benefit to using ozone to reduce the risk for dental caries, ozone may be an important adjunct in the prevention of periodontal disease. A recent publication in India suggested that ozone could be used to reduce periodontal disease risk, but more studies are needed. The study summary is also shown in Table 11-4, although the study did not address the prevention of caries (Kshitish and Laxman 2010).

Some dentists have already developed strategies to administer ozone safely to the periodontal tissues.

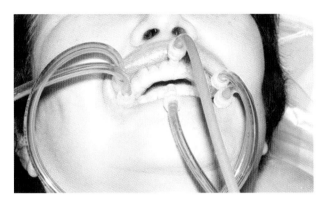

Figure 11-6 Periodontal therapy using a custom tray and ozone gas. Courtesy of Dr. Bill Domb Uplands, CA, USA.

In Figure 11-6, a patient has been fitted with a custom tray that has been custom fitted with silicon inlet and outlet silicon tubing. Medical ozone gas, made from pure oxygen, is injected in the intake port, and high volume suction is used in the exit ports to remove the ozone safely. In this way, ozone gas is administered to all of the diseased periodontal tissues at the same time.

Systematic reviews on ozone in clinical dentistry

In 2004, the Cochrane Library hosted a systematic review to assess the effectiveness of ozone gas in arresting or reversing the progression of dental caries. The authors included three relevant randomised controlled trials (Abu Naba'a, Abu Naba'a Pilot, and Baysan studies as discussed above) with a combined total of 432 randomised lesions from 137 participants. They evaluated these studies at high risk of bias and concluded that reliable evidence is lacking that the application of ozone gas to the surface of decayed teeth stops or reverses the decay process and that there is not enough high quality evidence to support the use of ozone gas in a primary care setting.

Brazzelli *et al.* (2006) conducted a systematic review to assess the effectiveness of ozone gas (HealOzone, KaVo) for the management of pit and fissure caries, and root caries. They reached a similar conclusion to that of the Cochrane Library. They also constructed a Markov model to explore possible cost-effectiveness aspects of HealOzone in addition to current management of dental caries over a 5-year period. They found that treatment using current management plus HealOzone cost more than current management alone for non-cavitated pit and fissure caries (£40.49 versus £24.78), but cost less for non-cavitated root caries (£14.63 versus £21.45). They stated that current evidence is insufficient to conclude that it is a cost-effective addition to the management and treatment of occlusal and root caries.

Conclusion

There have been hundreds of articles written on the benefit of ozone treatment in medicine. It was only a matter of time that ozone would be developed for the treatment of dental caries and periodontal disease. After all, these are both infectious diseases, and controlling the growth of the bacteria responsible for caries and periodontitis is a laudable goal. We have reviewed in this chapter the current evidence of how ozone has been applied to dental tissues in an attempt to reverse caries or at least arrest them. So far we can conclude the following:

1. The clinical studies identified focused on the application of ozone gas in the management of primary occlusal and root carious lesions. Despite the good evidence in *in vitro* settings, and despite a handful of promising clinical trials, the clinical application of ozone in caries reversal has not achieved strong level of efficacy and cost-effectiveness.
2. There is good evidence of *in vitro* biocompatibility of aqueous ozone with human oral epithelial cells, gingival fibroblast cells, and periodontal cells.
3. There is conflicting evidence of antimicrobial efficacy of ozone in *in vitro* settings; however, there is some evidence that ozone (in both gaseous or aqueous phase) is a potentially effective disinfectant agent.

In conclusion, there will likely be new instruments designed to administer ozone gas in a safe and effective way to dental tissues. There is still a need for the highest level of evidence, that is, well-designed, double-blind randomized clinical trials with adequate sample size, limited or no loss to follow-up, and carefully standardized methods of measurement and analysis in order to justify the use of ozone as the primary treatment modality in dentistry. Until such time that ozone can be proven to be more effective and less costly to administer than other preventive therapies, it remains as an adjunct therapy in dentistry. The likelihood that this modality of care will become routine in dentistry is based on the growing body of evidence that it is a safe and useful tool for dentistry. Since the dental hygiene profession traditionally applies preventive therapy to mineralized tissues, this therapy may even be appropriate for dental hygienists to administer.

References

Abu Naba'a, L., Al Shorman, H., Holmes, J., *et al.* (2004) Evidence-based research into ozone treatment in dentistry: an overview. In: *Ozone: The Revolution in Dentistry.* (Ed. E. Lynch). pp. 73–115. Quintessence Publishing Co., London.

Arita, M., Nagayoshi, M., Fukuizumi, T., *et al.* (2005) Microbicidal efficacy of ozonated water against Candida albicans adherng to acrylic denture plates. *Oral Microbiology & Immunology*, 20, 206–210.

Babior, B.M., Takeuchi, C., Ruedi, J., *et al.* (2003) Investigating antibody-catalyzed ozone generation by human neutrophils. *Proceedings of the National Academy of Science USA*, 100, 3031–3034.

Baysan, A. and Lynch, E. (2007) Clinical reversal of root caries using ozone: 6-month results. *American Journal of Dentistry*, 20, 203–208.

Baysan, A. and Lynch, E. (2004) Effect of ozone on the oral micro biota and clinical severity of primary root caries. *American Journal of Dentistry*, 17, 56–60.

Baysan, A., Whiley, R.A., Lynch, E. (2000) Antimicrobial effect of a novel ozone-generating device on micro-organisms associated with primary root carious lesions in vitro. *Caries Research*, 34, 498–501.

Bocci, V. (2010) *Ozone. A new Medical Drug.* Springer, The Netherlands.

Bocci, V. (2004) Ozone as Janus: this controversial gas can be either toxic or medically useful. *Mediators of Inflammation*, 13, 3–11.

Bocci, V., Borrelli, E., Travagli, V., *et al.* (2009) The ozone paradox: ozone is a strong oxidant as well as a medical drug. *Medicinal Research Reviews*, 29, 646–682.

Bocci, V., Luzzi, E., Corradeschi, F., *et al.* (1993a) Studies on the biological effects of ozone: 3. An attempt to define conditions for optimal induction of cytokines. *Lymphokine Cytokine Research*, 12, 121–126.

Bocci, V., Luzzi, E., Corradeschi, F., *et al.* (1993b) Studies on the biological effects of ozone: 4. Cytokine production and glutathione levels in human erythrocytes. *Journal of Biological Regulators and Homeostatic Agents*, 7, 133–138.

Bocci, V. and Paulesu, L. (1990) Studies on the biological effects of ozone: 1. Induction of interferon gamma on human leukocytes. *Haematologica*, 75, 510–515.

Brazzelli, M., McKenzie, L., Fielding, S., *et al.* (2006) Systematic review of the effectiveness and cost-effectiveness of HealOzone for the treatment of occlusal pit/fissure caries and root caries. *Health Technology Assessment*, 10, iii–iv, ix–80.

Broadwater, W.T., Hoehn, R.C., King, P.H. (1973) Sensitivity of three selected bacterial species to ozone. *Applied Microbiology*, 26, 391–393.

Dahnhardt, J.E., Jaeggi, T., Lussi, A. (2006) Treating open carious lesions in anxious children with ozone: a prospective controlled clinical study. *American Journal of Dentistry*, 19, 267–270.

Ebensberger, U., Pohl, Y., Filippi, A. (2002) PCNA-expression of cementoblasts and fibroblasts on the root surface after extraoral rinsing for decontamination. *Dental Traumatology*, 18, 262–266.

Estrela, C., Estrela, C.R., Decurcio Dde, A., *et al.* (2006) Antimicrobial potential of ozone in an ultrasonic cleaning system against Staphylococcus aureus. *Brazilian Dental Journal*, 17, 134–138.

Grootveld, M., Baysan, A., Sidiiqui, N., *et al.* (2004) History of the clinical applications of Ozone. In: *Ozone: The revolution in Dentistry.* (Ed. E. Lynch). pp. 23–30. Quintessence Publishing Co., London.

HealOzone. (2011) The next generation healOzone X4. [online] available at http://www.healozone.de/en/healozone.html.

Hedberg, L., Larsson, E., Pettersson, A., *et al.* (2003) The efficiency of an ozone delivery system (KaVo HealOzone™) as lactobacilli eliminator in vitro. Institute of Odontology, Karolinska Institute, Huddinges Sweden. http://www.ki.se/odont/news/index_en.html.

Hems, R.S., Gulabivala, K., Ng, Y.L., *et al.* (2005) An in vitro evaluation of the ability of ozone to kill a strain of Enterococcus faecalis. *International Endodontic Journal*, 38, 22–29.

Holmes, J. (2003) Clinical reversal of root caries using ozone, double-blind, randomised, controlled 18-month trial. *Gerodontology*, 20, 106–114.

Huth, K.C., Paschos, E., Brand, K., *et al.* (2005) Effect of ozone on non-cavitated fissure carious lesions in permanent molars: a controlled prospective clinical study. *American Journal of Dentistry*, 18, 223–228.

Huth, K.C., Quirling, M., Maier, S., *et al.* (2009) Effectiveness of ozone against endodontopathogenic microorganisms in a root canal biofilm model. *International Endodontic Journal*, 42, 3–13.

Kamali, A., Kajnas, E., Andersson, E., *et al.* (2003) The efficiency of the ozone anticaries agent in reducing Mutans Streptococci. Institute References 292 of Odontology, Karolinska Institute, Huddinges Sweden. http://www.ki.se/odont/news/index_en.html.

Kim, J.G., Yousef, A.E., Dave, S. (1999) Application of ozone for enhancing the microbiological safety and quality of foods: a review. *Journal of Food Protection*, 62, 1071–1087.

Kronenberg, O., Lussi, A., Ruf, S. (2009) Preventive effect of ozone on the development of white spot lesions during multibracket appliance therapy. *Angle Orthodontics*, 79, 64–69.

Kshitish, D. and Laxman, V.K. (2010) The use of ozonated water and 0.2% chlorhexidine in the treatment of periodontitis patients: a clinical and microbiologic study. *Indian Journal of Dental Research*, 21, 341–348.

Lippmann, M. (1993) Health effects of tropospheric ozone: review of recent research findings and their implications to ambient air quality standards. *Journal of Exposure Analysis and Environmental Epidemiology*, 3, 103–129.

Logan, J.A. (1989) Ozone in rural areas of the United States. Journal of Geophysics Research, 94, 8511–8532.

Lynch, E. (2004) *Ozone: The revolution in Dentistry.* Quintessence Publishing Co., London.

McDonnell, W.F., Horstman, D.H., Hazucha, M.J., *et al.* (1983) Pulmonary effects of ozone exposure during exercise: dose-response characteristics. *Journal of Applied Physiology*, 54, 1345–1352.

Moseley, R., Waddington, R.J., Embery, G. (1997) Degradation of glycosaminoglycans by reactive oxygen species derived from stimulated polymorphonuclear leukocytes. *Biochimica Biophysica Acta*, 1362, 221–231.

Murakami, H., Mizuguchi, M., Hattori, M., *et al.* (2002) Effect of denture cleaner using ozone against methicillin-resistant Staphylococcus aureus and E. coli T1 phage. *Dental Materials Journal*, 21, 53–60.

Nagayoshi, M., Fukuizumi, T., Kitamura, C., *et al.* (2004) Efficacy of ozone on survival and permeability of oral microorganisms. *Oral Microbiology and Immunology*, 19, 240–246.

Nagayoshi, M., Kitamura, C., Fukuizumi, T., *et al.* (2004) Antimicrobial effect of ozonated water on bacteria invading dentinal tubules. *Journal of Endodontics*, 30, 778–781.

Nieva, J. and Wentworth P. Jr. (2004) The antibody-catalyzed water oxidation pathway—a new chemical arm to immune defense? *Trends in Biochemical Sciences*, 29, 274–278.

Oizumi, M., Suzuki, T., Uchida, M., *et al.* (1998) In vitro testing of a denture cleaning method using ozone. *Journal of Medical and Dental Sciences*, 45, 135–139.

Ozone Solutions. (2011) Ozone Conversions. [online] available at http://www.ozonesolutions.com/Ozone_Conversions.html.

Polydorou, O., Pelz, K., Hahn P. (2006) Antibacterial effect of an ozone device and its comparison with two dentin-bonding systems. *European Journal of Oral Sciences*, 114, 349–353.

Rickard, G.D., Richardson, R., Johnson, T., *et al.* (2004) Ozone therapy for the treatment of dental caries. *Cochrane Database of Systematic Reviews*, 3, CD004153.

Solomon, S. (1999) Stratospheric ozone depletion: a review of concepts and history. *Reviews of Geophysics*, 37, 275–316.

Waddington, R.J., Moseley, R., Embery, G. (2000) Reactive oxygen species: a potential role in the pathogenesis of periodontal diseases. *Oral Diseases*, 6, 138–151.

Wang, W.-C., Zhuang, Y.-C., Bojkov, R.D. (1993) Climate implications of observed changes in ozone vertical distributions at middle and high latitudes of the Northern Hemisphere, *Geophysics Research Letters*, 20, 1567–1570.

Wentworth, P., Jr., McDunn, J.E., Wentworth, A.D., *et al.* (2002) Evidence for antibody-catalyzed ozone formation in bacterial killing and inflammation. *Science*, 298(5601), 2195–2199.

12

Protection of the dentition

Hardy Limeback

Sports dentistry and protective mouthguards

Historical perspective

Severe trauma to the orofacial complex can result in devastating injuries that can result in life-long oral complications. Certain sporting activities, where there is frequent bodily contact, carry higher risk for oral injuries than others. Mouthguards, composed primarily of a soft, pliable material covering one dentition, usually the maxillary dentition, were first introduced in boxing in the 1920s (Knapik *et al.* 2007). During the early years athletes engaged in contact sports such as rugby, football, and hockey did not wear any protective equipment for the face until the 1960s. A concerted effort was made by the American Dental Association (ADA 1960) to promote the introduction of mouthguards into contact sports in the 1960s. In 1962, the National Alliance Football Rules Committee introduced mandatory mouthguards for football in high school and junior college, and this rule was reinforced by the NCAA (National Collegiate Athletic Association) in 1973 (Kumamoto and Maeda 2004). Orofacial injuries dropped significantly. In 1974, the NCAA made them mandatory for ice hockey, field hockey, and lacrosse. US hockey adopted a mandatory mouthguard policy in 1975. Most amateur athletic associations now require mouthguards, but it seems that the professional leagues, where influential role models compete, still leave it up to the individual athlete (ADA Council on Access, Prevention and Interprofessional Relations; ADA Council on Scientific Affairs 2006).

The extent of the problem

Some studies have estimated that nearly one-third of all injuries to the dentition is from sporting activities (Borssen and Holm 1997; Chisick *et al.* 2000). More than 5 million teeth are avulsed each year as a result of sports injuries and trauma (Gutmann and Gutmann 1995). Trauma to the orofacial complex in sports is a worldwide problem and has been documented in other countries (Rodd and Chesham 1997; Borssen and Holm 1997; Love *et al.* 1998; Levin *et al.* 2003; Petersen *et al.* 2005). In the 1940s and 1950s, dental injuries represented 23–54% of all football injuries (Knapik *et al.* 2007). In a 1950s study, out of 4,000 college football players there were 733 chipped or fractured teeth (Vanet 1951).

In those days it was mostly male athletes who got injured in the mouth, and this seems to hold true today. Football and rugby still have the highest prevalence of orofacial injury at 54% (Kumamoto and Maeda 2003), and males appear to be at greater risk than females in contact sports but that simply reflects the greater participation of men in heavy contact sports (Wisniewski *et al.* 2004). That is changing quickly as more and more women get involved in team contact sports; the incidence of injuries to females will climb proportionately. The risk of an individual acquiring and sustaining an orofacial injury is 10% (Flanders 1995). Approximately 80% of all dental injuries in sports occur to the maxillary incisors (Gutmann *et al.* 1995; Bastone *et al.* 2000).

Although it is obvious that mouthguards help prevent orofacial injuries in contact sports, accidents do happen in other sports. For example, in basketball and soccer, there are more facial injuries than in football, where face shields

Comprehensive Preventive Dentistry, First Edition. Edited by Hardy Limeback.
© 2012 John Wiley & Sons, Ltd. Published 2012 by John Wiley & Sons, Ltd.

and mouthguards are now mandatory (ADA 2005). In basketball 14–34% of the injuries to the athletes are in the orofacial area (Flanders and Bhat 1995; Cornwall *et al.* 2003; Levin *et al.* 2003). One survey of dentists showed that the highest incidence of oral injury was in biking and baseball, two non-contact sports where mouthguards are normally not worn (Soporowski *et al.* 1994).

"Impact" of dental trauma

There are several consequences from craniofacial injuries that result from trauma to the facial complex. These include psychosocial and economic. Children with damaged and untreated anterior teeth were 20 times more likely to report a negative impact on quality of life (Cortes *et al.* 2002). The children surveyed reported embarrassment, avoidance of social contact, and trouble eating. This observation was confirmed in Brazilian children (Ramos-Jorge *et al.* 2007; Bendo *et al.* 2010). Cost estimates have been made in terms of life-long dental costs related to dental trauma. In Ontario, Locker and Maggira's 2004 estimate for the province of Ontario for direct and indirect costs related to all dental trauma, including sports injuries, ranged between $3.2 to almost $5 million. This translates to a cost to Americans that would range up to $25 million (Locker and Maggiria 2004).

Trauma to just one anterior tooth can result in failure of the pulp tissue to survive, and when that happens, the tooth, over a lifetime, can cost thousands of dollars to replace (Pennington *et al.* 2009). It is estimated that in Australia, the cost related to sport injuries to the maxillofacial region is about $1.4 billion annually, and up to half of the injuries are preventable (Newsome *et al.* 2010).

Although less common, mandibular fractures, dentoalveolar fractures, and temporomandibular joint injuries can also occur in sports. These injuries may require long-term care and result in extended health problems. This is likely to contribute to a decrease in general health (with associated increased medical, economic and societal cost, and work or school absenteeism). Cost estimates from more severe sports injuries such as broken jaws are lacking in the literature, but hockey fans know all too well the economic costs to the entire team when a player is injured and has to sit out part of the season.

Types of traumatic dental injuries to teeth

The categories of traumatic injuries to an individual tooth and the corresponding characteristics associated with these injuries are presented in Table 12-1.

These injuries are depicted with illustrations in Figure 12-1 (A to H). A maxillary incisor, the most common tooth to be injured, is used as an example in the figure.

The different fracture categories listed in Table 12-1 are similar (Figures 12-2–12-5) but not identical to those presented by Diangelis and Bakland (1998).

In addition to trauma to single or multiple teeth, there are possible injuries to the mandible and maxilla.

Table 12-1 Types of traumatic injuries to an individual tooth and the corresponding characteristics

Category (according to Figure 12-1)	Type of injury	Characteristic
A	ENAMEL FRACTURE	cracks, chips, fractures—dentin not affected
B	CROWN FRACTURE (no pulp exposure)	enamel fracture with underlying dentin involved but no pulp exposure
C	CROWN FRACTURE (with pulpal involvement)	A complicated fracture involving enamel, dentin, and exposure of the pulp
D	ROOT FRACTURE	horizontal or vertical root fracture (crown is still intact)
E	CROWN-ROOT FRACTURE	fracture that extends through the enamel, dentin, and involves the root
F	LUXATION	
	1. Concussion	• Trauma (sensitive to percussion) but no other signs or symptoms
	2. Subluxation	• Increased mobility but no displacement
	3. Lateral luxation	• Anter-distal or mesio-distal displacements
	4. Extrusive luxation	• Partial displacement out of the socket with or without mobility
	5. Intrusive luxation	• Tooth has been forced apically and is firmly embedded in bone
G	AVULSION	Complete displacement of a tooth from its socket
H	FRACTURE OF THE ALVEOLAR PROCESS	Bone fracture: blood supply may be compromised if apical damage affects the vasculature

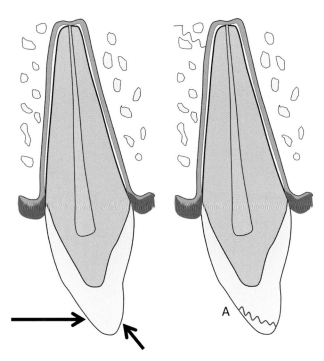

Figure 12-1 A. Enamel fracture. The arrows on the left diagram indicate the direction of the likely blows to the tooth. The injury from the anterior could be from a blow by a ball or another hard object (such as an elbow). The arrow showing a blow from below can be due to a mandibular incisor that is in contact with the maxillary incisor (for instance, during end to end occlusion) when the trauma is a blow to the chin and there is no mouthguard to cushion the blow. The result is enamel fracture (red wavy line) in the diagram on the right.

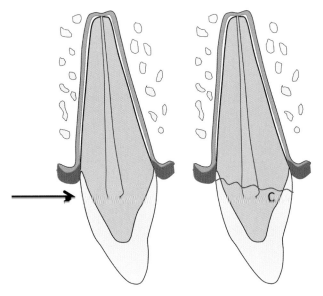

Figure 12-1 C. Crown fracture with pulpal involvement. The blow to the tooth is usually more directed at the gingival margin (left diagram) resulting in a complex fracture with the pulpal tissue exposed (right diagram). This can be very painful, and the tooth will require emergency root canal therapy. Restoration of the tooth will be complex if the fracture is close to the alveolar ridge and a restoration encroaches on the biological width (Golberg *et al.* 2000).

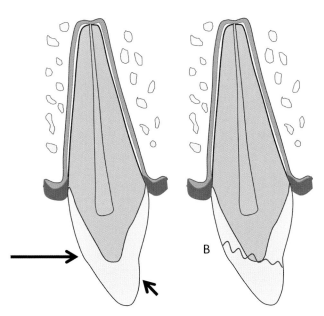

Figure 12-1 B. Crown fracture. No pulp exposure. This injury is a little more severe than in Figure 12-1A (enamel fracture) in that dentin is involved. The tooth is usually sensitive to cold air. The directional arrows of the blows are the same as in Figure 12-1A.

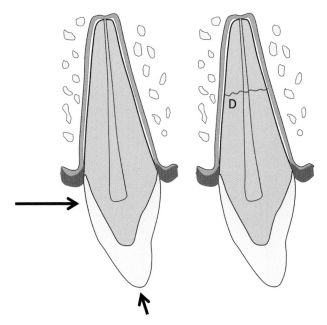

Figure 12-1 D. Root fracture. The direction of the trauma to the tooth can come from a direct hit to tooth or even the periodontium from the anterior, or from an upward blow directly onto the incisal edge of the tooth. Depending on the direction of the trauma, the root can fracture near the apex or closer to the crown. Either way the prognosis to save the tooth with root canal therapy is guarded.

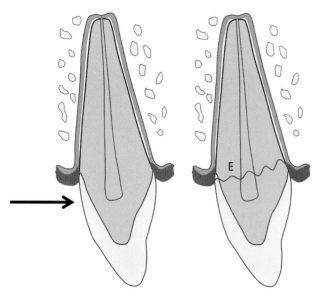

Figure 12-1 E. Crown-root fracture. This is a more complex fracture than in Figure 12-1C and will likely result in the extraction of the remaining root structure.

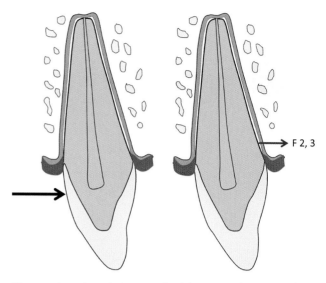

Figure 12-1 F2 and F3. Lateral subluxation. The trauma from the anterior to the periodontium or tooth does not fracture the tooth but causes it to move lingually by injuring the periodontal ligament (breaking collagen fibers at the facial) and compressing alveolar bone on the lingual. This usually results in a mobile tooth.

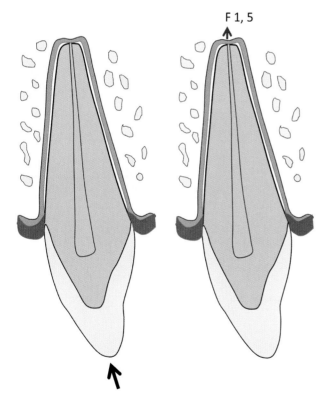

Figure 12-1 F1 or F5. Intrusive luxation. Trauma from a direct blow to the incisal edge can result in simple 'tooth concussion' or more serious damage with compressed bone and soft tissues resulting in symptoms and mobility.

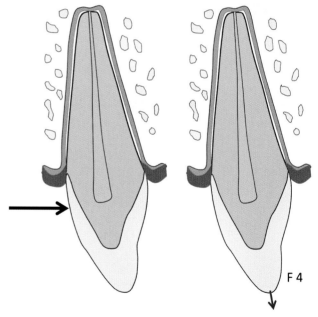

Figure 12-1 F4. Extrusive luxation. The trauma to the tooth (from an anterior blow to the dentition) causes the tooth to extrude slightly from its socket. Periodontal fibers have been torn, and the tooth may or may not be in the same occlusion as before.

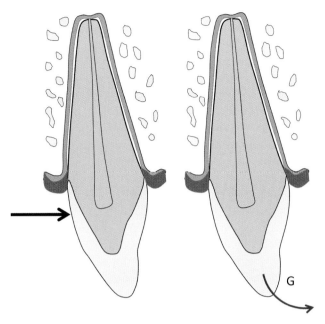

Figure 12-1 G. Avulsion. In this case the trauma to the tooth or the periodontium is severe enough to totally avulse the tooth. There are many approaches to handling this dental emergency that will not be discussed in this text.

(a)

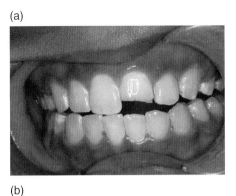

(b)

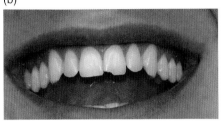

Figure 12-2 Example of two enamel fractures (Category A from Figure 12-1). Photo in 9(a) courtesy of Dr. Sundeep Patel, Winnipeg, Manitoba, Canada.

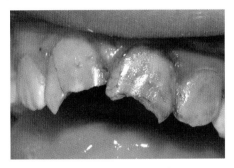

Figure 12-3 Example of Category B of Figure 12-1 (crown fracture with pulpal involvement). Courtesy of Dr. Robert Zaichick, Belleville, Ontario, Canada.

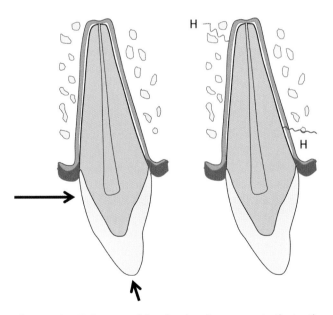

Figure 12-1 H. Fracture of the alveolus. Any trauma to the tooth that is not severe enough to fracture the tooth could potentially still injure the alveolar bone. In this case two fractures of bone are depicted: one at the crest of the bone in response to trauma from the facial, and one at the apex, in response to trauma from the incisal.

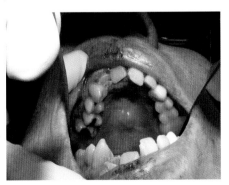

Figure 12-4 Example of Categories E and F from Figure 12-1. This is a not a photograph of a dental injury related to sports. However, it illustrates the type of complex injury that can occur from such a direct blow from the incisal direction. The patient is in her eighties, and one of the author's patients, who lost her balance and injured her teeth after hitting her face on a sidewalk. The intruded maxillary incisors were extruded orthodontically and restored with composite resin. The central incisor, however, ended up with lateral root resorption and apical osteitis.

(a)

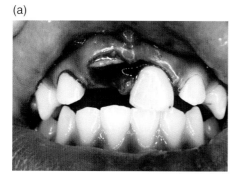

(b)

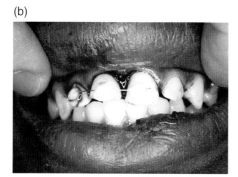

Figure 12-5 Example of a basketball injury leading to intrusive luxation (Category F) and lateral luxation toward the palate (also Category F). This picture of a 12-yr-old male, seen in the emergency department of a hospital in Memphis, TN, is courtesy of Dr. Robert Shoun, a pediatric dentist in South Carolina. The teeth, still present in the sockets (a) were repositioned and splinted (b) to allow the patient to occlude.

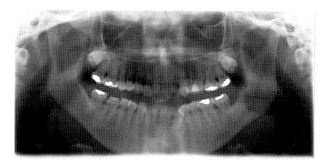

Figure 12-6 Panoramic radiographic of a fractured mandible.

Figure 12-6 shows a panoramic radiographic image of a fractured mandible.

Nearly a third of all mandibular fractures are caused by trauma during sports (Emshoff *et al.* 1997).

Current recommendations

The ADA (2004) recommends that mouthguards be used in both contact and non-contact individual sports. (See Table 12-2.)

The American Medical Association and the American Academy of Pediatrics endorse the use of mouthguards.

The Canadian Academy of Sport Medicine has a position statement on head injuries and concussions in soccer in which they call for mouthguards to be worn during participation in soccer for protection of the dentition and the possible role in concussion prevention. The American Academy for Sports Dentistry recommends the use of properly fitted mouthguards and is in favour of mandates for their use in all collision and contact sports for practices and games (see below).

The Academy of General Dentistry recommends "that players participating in basketball, softball, wrestling, soccer, lacrosse, rugby, in-line skating and martial arts, whether for an athletic competition or leisure activity, wear mouthguards while competing" (Academy of General Dentistry 2007). In Canada, the Canadian Dental Association has a position statement that encourages dentists to counsel patients about orofacial protection and encourages organized activities to develop safety protocols to minimize the risk of orofacial injury (Canadian Dental Association 2005).

Sports dentistry

The definition of 'sports dentistry,' according to the Academy for Sports Dentistry, follows: "'Sports Dentistry' involves the prevention and treatment of orofacial athletic injuries and related oral diseases, as well as the collection and dissemination of information on dental athletic injuries and the encouragement of research in the preventive of such injuries" (Academy for Sports Dentistry 2011). In 1983, the Academy for Sport Dentistry (ASD) was formed to basically help people help athletes at risk to orofacial injury from their sport. It is an organization that does not limit itself to dentists but was open to physicians, educators, dentists, hygienists, dental technicians, and even the trainers. The organization is basically there to share and disseminate knowledge about dental injuries in sports and to encourage research in this field. It is an international organization of about 600 members. Each year the organization holds meetings with workshops to train individuals on the fabrication of high quality mouthguards for competitive athletes.

The ASD has guidelines on how to become a 'team dentist'

The following criteria are needed to meet the qualifications of the position of a Team Dentist" (Academy for Sports Dentistry 2011b):

- Be a licensed dentist in compliance with the dental practice act of his/her state.
- Be a member in good standing of the Academy for Sports Dentistry (ASD)

Table 12-2 Sports where mouthguards are recommended

Contact sports (Most athletes wear mouthguards or face protection.)	Non-contact sports (Some athletes wear mouthguards.)	Individual sports (Mouthguard use is not common.)
boxing, martial arts, wrestling football, rugby ice hockey lacrosse	basketball handball, squash, racquetball soccer water polo volleyball baseball, softball	bicycling equestrian acrobatics gymnastics inline skating, skateboarding skiing, surfing shot putting, weightlifting skydiving*

*It is understandable that the ADA would recommend mouthguard use while skydiving, perhaps to avoid injury to the dentition during parachute landings, but it is hard to imagine even the best-fitting custom-made mouthguard staying in place while sky-diving enthusiasts are free falling. The air velocity is extreme. Furthermore, if an accident should occur and the main and reserve parachutes do not open, protecting his teeth is probably not going to be the primary concern of the skydiver!

- Attend and complete the ASD Team Dentist course
- Complete a minimum of 15 credit hours of continuing education in sports dentistry-related subjects every 3 years
- Acquire the knowledge and expertise to educate health care professionals, certified athletic trainers, coaches, athletes, and parents on the benefits and methods of prevention of sports-related oral facial injuries and oral diseases
- Be proficient in the fabrication and delivery of properly fitted mouthguards including impression techniques and establishment of occlusion
- Be well versed in the diagnosis and treatment of orofacial trauma including but not limited to:
  - Oral-facial first aid resulting from contusions, lacerations
  - Emergency/immediate treatment of dental luxations, avulsions, and tooth fractures
  - Identification of maxillary and mandibular fractures
  - Identification and treatment of TMJ injuries and dislocations
  - Identify medical complications of head trauma
  - Be familiar with doping issues and the effects of illicit and performance-enhancing drugs
  - Establish a support team of dental specialists and auxiliary staff
  - Cooperate with the other members of the sports medicine team to ensure the health and well-being of the athletes

These criteria were approved by the Academy for Sports Dentistry Board of Directors December 5, 2009.

The ASD also set down guidelines on how to make a 'properly fitted mouthguard.'

An athletic mouthguard is a resilient device or appliance placed inside the mouth to reduce injuries particularly to the teeth and surrounding structures.

For optimal safety and well-being of athletes competing in the twenty-first century, the Academy for Sports Dentistry has adopted the position that the single word "mouthguard" must be replaced by the term "a properly fitted mouthguard."

In contact sports, it is critical that the mouthguard provides protection from direct and indirect impact. It must fit accurately, stay in position during impact, and redistribute the impact's energy. The criteria for the fabrication or adaptation of a properly fitted mouthguard must include the following considerations:

1. Pertinent medical history
2. Dental status that considers:
   a. Dental caries
   b. Periodontal status
   c. Developmental occlusion
   d. Orthodontic or prosthodontic appliances
   e. Congenital/pathological conditions
   f. Jaw relationships
3. Demographic factors
4. Type of sport played

The fitting of a mouthguard is best accomplished under the supervision or direction of a dentist. The athlete and/or parents should always be advised of the special design for the "properly fitted mouthguard," and the end product should have the following properties and considerations:

1. It should be fabricated to adequately cover and protect both the teeth in the arch, and the surrounding tissues.

2. It should be fabricated on a stone model taken from an impression of the athlete.

3. It needs to have adequate thickness in all areas to provide for the reduction of impact forces. In particular, a minimum of 3-mm thickness in the occlusal/labial area is needed.

4. It should have a seated equilibrated occlusion that is balanced for even occlusal contact. This helps to provide for the ideal absorption of impact energy.

5. The mouthguard needs to have a fit that is retentive and not dislodged on impact.

6. Speech considerations need to be addressed equal to the demands of the playing status of the athlete.

7. The mouthguard should be made of a material that meets FDA approval.

8. The properly fitted mouthguard should be routinely and professionally examined for fit and function. Frequency of routine inspection is dependent on factors such as the athlete's age, the demand of the sport that the athlete is engaged in, and the willingness of the athlete to properly care for the appliance. The frequency of the inspection should be determined by the dental professional for each individual situation and athlete.

The guidelines were approved by the Academy for Sports Dentistry Board of Directors on April 5, 2010.

Sports dentistry and dental traumatology

Sports dentistry is still a relatively young special interest area in dentistry. The first World Congress on Sports Dentistry and Dental Traumatology was held in June 2001 in Boston, Massachusetts, USA. It was the culmination of the convergence of two organizations: the International Association of Dental Traumatology (IADT) and the International Academy for Sports Dentistry (IASD). The IADT had a journal (Endodontics and Dental Traumatology) that published articles on the clinical treatment modalities that focused primarily on traumatic injuries to the teeth and their supporting structures. Now known simply as "Dental Traumatology," this journal is now the official publication of both the IADT and the IASD.

Reasons for slow adaptation in sports

Despite evidence that mouthguards can prevent dental injury, compliance has been a stumbling block. In one study, parents didn't even know that their children could benefit from wearing mouthguards (Gardiner and Renalli 2000). A survey conducted in Canada of young teens indicated that the main reason for non-compliance with mouthguard use was a lack of advice by parents and coaches, and lack of comfort (breathing, speech, esthetics).

This is not surprising since nearly 70% of mouthguard users wore the over-the-counter stock trays or 'boil and bite' mouthguards. Studies have shown that custom-fitted mouthguards do not interfere with breathing or lung physiology during heavy competition (Gebauer et al. 2011). Over 50% of the children reported that they had never been told to wear a mouthguard by parents and/or coaches, and 40.7% believed that they did not need to wear one during sporting activities (Fakhruddin et al. 2007).

Professional athletes could play an important part as role models for young people by wearing mouthguards, but many continue to go without mouthguard protection, often with dire consequences. In fact, when they are no longer mandated to wear mouthguards, nearly one-third of them stop wearing them when they reach professional status. In professional ice hockey, there are still many players with missing front teeth. It seems to be a rite of passage for the ice hockey player. In other professional sports, such as basketball and soccer (European football), there are some great role models, but they seem to be the exception.

In the National Collegiate Athletic Association (NCAA), officials are supposed to charge a time out to the team when a a player is not wearing a mouthguard. They can also assess a 5-yard penalty if time-outs have been exhausted. Lancaster and Ranalli (1993) found that officials were unlikely to enforce these penalties for mouthguard violations. The officials stated that it was up to the coaches to enforce mouthguard usage (Lancaster and Ranalli 1993).

Since coaches have the most influence on players' attitudes about mouthguards, they should be the ones to turn to for getting better compliance in young athletes (Gardiner and Ranalli 2000). It is hard to convince coaches that they can make a difference (Berg et al. 1998). But Gardiner and Ranalli (2000) in their survey of 89 coaches regarding attitudinal barriers feel that success in increased compliance lies with the coaches and that three-quarters of them would take action with players who do not wear their mouthguards.

For individual sporting competitions, where mandatory mouthguard use is not in place, compliance is more of a problem. It is not common to see a gymnast wearing a mouthguard, or an equestrian insert a mouthguard after putting on her helmet prior to mounting her horse. Mouthguards are rarely worn by professional skateboarders, bicycle racers, or downhill skiers, but that could be because they have adopted the helmet as the primary protective gear to protect their head from serious injury if they fall. However, as more and more professionals don their helmets before attempting difficult stunts or taking part in individual races, young people who look up to them will be more likely to wear a helmet for their own individual sporting activities. A helmet, even one with full face coverage, does not protect the individual athlete from damage to the dentition should he or she sustain a blow to the chin where the teeth could fracture because of traumatic occlusion. Thus, mouthguards have become mandatory along with helmets with full-face protection in amateur contact sports for the child athlete in contact sports such as football and ice hockey.

Evidence of effectiveness

NCAA basketball athletes who wore custom mouth guards had significantly less dental trauma and oral injuries (1.16 injuries per 1,000 athletic exposures) than players who did not (3.00 injuries per 1,000 athletic exposures) (Labella *et al.* 2002). Studying Hawaiian intermediate and high school athletes, Beachy (2004) found that there were no reported injuries to the teeth of athletes who wore mouthguards. Cohort studies were conducted on young high school and elementary rugby players that showed that the students benefitted from wearing mouthguards (Morton and Burton 1979; De Wet *et al.* 1981). Marshall *et al.* (2004) found a protective effect of mouthguards, but their studies did not have the power to show statistical significance.

In a systematic review, Knapik *et al.* (2007) found that there was only one interventional study conducted to test the effectiveness of mouthguards. In that interventional study, Finch *et al.* (2005) randomly assigned trained Australian rugby players to a test group of mouthguard users and a control group of non-users and followed them prospectively. It was found that the mouthguard users had an orofacial injury rate of 1.8 injuries per 1,000 hours of play, whereas the control group had a rate of 4.4 per 1,000 hours of play. This difference had a statistical significance of p <0.01. Knapik's review concluded there was evidence for the benefit of mouthguards, but studies of the highest quality (interventional studies such as the one conducted by Finch) were few and far between. According to Kapnik:

> "Despite these issues, meta-analyses indicated that the risk of an orofacial injury during sports was 1.6–1.9 times higher when a mouthguard was not worn."

Mouthguard design

The ideal mouthguard design

The ideal mouthguard should have the following qualities:

1. The mouthguard, ideally, should be custom made to fit the wearer's own mouth, covering all the teeth, with careful attention to detail (well adapted to teeth and gum tissues and the bite in occlusion). It is usually a maxillary guard. Comfort is very important since the participating athlete does not want to be distracted by pain in the oral cavity while 'concentrating on the game.'

2. The mouthguard should be made of approved resilient and flexible materials that are easily cleaned. Ideally the guard should be pressure laminated and be 3-mm thick. The mouthguard should be durable and long lasting, especially since mouthguards can be expensive. Pressure-laminated mouthguards are the most durable and long lasting.

3. The mouthguard should stay in place even when dislodging forces are administered (rough play, heavy contact, purposeful tongue and lip movements).

4. The mouthguard should provide high-impact energy absorption, protecting the teeth from significant traumatic blows and helping stabilize the mandible through cushioned occlusion.

5. Ideally, mouthguards should be colored to suit individual needs. In certain ice hockey leagues, clear mouthguards are not permitted because the danger they pose to other skaters; if someone loses one on the ice and a skater does not see it, there is a risk that the skater might have an accident skating over it.

Stock mouthguards

Basic stock mouthguards are sold in sporting good stores and do not require a custom fitting. However, they are ill-fitting, uncomfortable, and have the least protection of available mouthguards. Since they are so loose, the wearer has to clench in order to avoid having the mouthguard dislodge during rough play. This interferes with breathing. It is more than likely that the stock mouthguard routinely dislodges during play (Greasley *et al.* 1998).

Figure 12-7 shows an example of a stock mouthguard. There is obviously little in the way of retention. The lips are meant to keep the appliance in place. Breathing is through the small opening, and there is a tab that can be used to secure the mouthguard to the cage of a helmet. If both lips extend beyond the border of the anterior guard, the mouthguard will likely be dislodged, unless of course the athlete is clenching when he or she is injured. This form of mouthguard is least likely to protect the dentition from injury.

Mouth-formed mouthguards ('boil and bite')

'Boil and bite' mouthguards are popular over-the-counter mouthguards that the user warms in hot water and fits to his own teeth. They are more comfortable and fit better to the teeth than the stock mouthguards. They range in

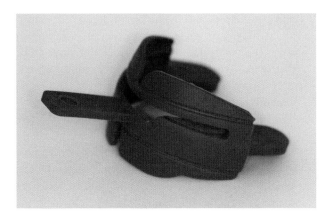

Figure 12-7 A stock mouthguard.

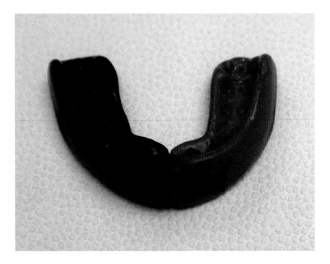

Figure 12-8 A 'boil and bite' over-the-counter mouthguard. This more expensive model (approximately $20) fits well in the mouth with good retention and adequate thickness. It is difficult to chew through this type of mouthguard.

price, and the more expensive ones are better fitting and more resilient (Figure 12-8) than the previous, less expensive models (Ranalli 2000).

For example, there are shell-liner mouthguards that consist of polyvinyl chloride outer shells that fit loosely over the dentition and an inner lining of plasticized acrylic gel or silicone rubber (Chalmers 1998; Biasca et al. 2002). This appliance is less commonly available and usually bulkier than a boil-and-bite mouthguard.

In the less expensive models (one material only), if the user does not follow instructions and allows the posterior teeth to contact during the 'molding' step, the posterior area might end up too thin and not be protective at all. Inexpensive models have shown to be easily perforated with constant chewing forces. The boil-and-bite mouthguards generally do not cover the posterior teeth that well (Kuebker et al. 1986). One

study reported that they did not perform any better than the stock mouthguards (DeYoung et al. 1994). In of a group of hockey players on a 'skating' treadmill, one study showed that the bulky homemade mouthguards actually interfered with breathing efficiency (Delaney and Montgomery 2005). Considering how lucrative professional hockey is, any advantage one player has over the other will be considered extremely important.

Custom-made mouthguards (vacuum formed)

Custom-made mouthguards are preferred over the over-the-counter, home stock, or home-fitted mouthguard. However, a custom fitting requires the help of a dentist or dental hygienist, but in some cases, the athlete can take impressions of his teeth at home and send the impression to laboratory technicians who make the mouthguard in their own facility and return it to the athlete in the mail. The basic principle is that mouthguard materials of varying resistance and thickness are vacuum formed over a stone model of the dentition.

Custom-fitted mouthguards provide superior comfort and fit compared with the previously mentioned mouthguards. The athlete can be secure in the feeling that the mouthguard will not dislodge easily from the mouth when the teeth are not clenched. Usually a custom-fitted mouthguard is retentive because of the suction it creates when air is expelled between the mouthguard material and the dental tissues (when the mouthguard is tightly in place). When the air seal is compromised (for example, a change in the dentition, such as what occurs in growing children in the mixed dentition phase), the mouthguard has less retention. Echlin et al. (2005) reported four studies that concluded that the custom-fabricated mouthguards provided superior protection to the stock and mouth-formed mouthguards. The custom-made mouthguard also has a longer life span than the other mouthguards, which may be more likely to harden or tear over time. Although custom-fitted mouthguards are bound to be more expensive than over-the-counter mouthguards because of the labor involved, they are often covered by private dental insurance plans.

Single-layered, vacuum-formed mouthguards

One of the most common mouthguards made in dental offices is the vacuum-formed mouthguard using only a single unit of thermoplastic material that is applied to a stone model of the dentition using a vacuum former machine and a 'suck-down' procedure that sucks a heated and softened thermoplastic material onto the dentition.

The materials commonly used on mouthguards are polyvinyl acetate-polyethylene or ethylene vinyl acetate (EVA) copolymer, polyvinylchloride (PVC), latex rubber, acrylic resin, and poly-urethane (Knapik 2007), with EVA copolymers being the most popular mostly because of the ease of fabrication. The European Union has criticized the use of PVCs because of the presumed link to the production of phthalates (used in polyvinyl chloride production) and chronic conditions (Fontelles and Clark 2005).

Pressure-laminated mouthguards

Pressure-laminated mouthguards are considered to be the best kind to make for athletes. They provide the best fit, comfort, retention, and protection. The pressure lamination process allows for the production of a thicker and more resilient mouthguard. The following steps are involved in the production of pressure-laminated mouthguards, which are more involved than the vacuum-formed procedures (Padilla 2005):

1. A high quality impression of the mouth is taken. Care is taken to avoid bubbles and to get a record of the vestibule areas. Often a high quality impression material is preferred over alginate.

2. A stone cast model is poured with hard stone, allowed to set, and trimmed without passing the highest point of the vestibular border marked with a pencil.

3. The model is lubricated then placed in a positive pressure lamination machine for mouthguard fabrication (for example, the Dreve Drumomat, the Erkodent Erkopress, or the Biostar by Scheu Dental).

4. The first 3-mm layer of colored ethylene vinyl acetate is applied, and the machine's heater and pressure chamber will pressure laminate the first layer onto the cast model.

5. After cooling and trimming the first layer, identification labels are added and a second clear layer is pressure laminated onto the first layer. The thickness of the second layer can vary depending on the needs of the sport.

6. The final mouthguard is trimmed, polished, and tried in the mouth for fit and comfort. The occlusion is adjusted and balanced so that all posterior teeth occlude. This is done by warming the posterior of the mouthguard and asking the patient to occlude gently. Ideally the thickness of the mouthguard in the posterior is no less than 3 mm.

Factors affecting fit

The following factors affect the fabrication and fit of a mouthguard:

- Residual moisture on the working model. It is important to use dry cast models and a silicone spray when making a vacuum-formed mouthguard. Water interferes with the cooling and hardening of the EVA sheet.

- Air entrapment in the pressure-lamination process. This will interfere with the sealing of the layers, which will hasten the deterioration of the mouthguards where the layers peel apart.

- Extension of the mouthguard against the frenum and improper trimming to suit vestibular spaces will lead to dislodgement when the lips and cheeks are active. Proper trimming of the mouthguard is essential (Vastardis 2005).

Double-layered pressure-laminated mouthguards (for example, Pro-form mouthguards)

Laboratory-processed professional-grade Pro-form mouthguards are usually made for amateur athletes looking for better mouthguards than the single-layered 'suck-down' type vacuum-formed mouthguards. The Pro-form offers a level of protection, retention, comfort, and fit, without interfering with speech or breathing during play. Pro-form mouthguards are better in fit and retention than boil-and-bite mouthguards. They are also more durable. Pro-form sports mouthguards reduce tooth injuries by distributing the stress of impact to the entire length of the tooth. The double layer of laminated vinyl has the extra lingual plate imbedded behind the incisors. Tensile strength, softness, compression percentage, and uniform density are all important characteristics of mouthguard materials. Pro-form maintains these characteristics using a heat-/pressure-laminating process. Tensile strength of the laminate is excellent due to the laminate's two layers of materials making up the mouthguard. Density is maintained at the pressure-laminating process so shrinkage of the mouthguard is uniformly controlled. Figure 12-9 shows an example of a Proform mouthguard fabricated for a young athlete still in mixed dentition. As the dentition matures, replacement mouthguards have to be made.

Custom double- and triple-laminated mouthguards

There are several laboratories and services that provide professionally fabricated, custom-fitted, pressure-laminated mouthguards. A custom-made multiple-layered mouthguard can be modified for full contact sports by laminating two or three layers of EVA material to achieve the necessary thickness. Artistic patterns can be added to customize the mouthguards for team or individual sports. (See Figure 12-10.)

(a)

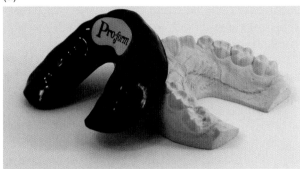

(b)

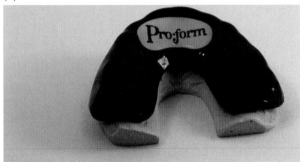

Figure 12-9 Pressure laminated 'Pro-form' custom mouthguard for an 8-year-old hockey player. (a) The cast model and black mouthguard. Note the red outline as a guide for the laboratory. (b) Fit of the mouthguard is checked prior to insertion.

Can mouthguards reduce the incidence of concussions in sports?

A concussion is the result of trauma to the brain. There is now consensus as to what defines a concussion. Concussions, which are also known as 'mild traumatic brain injuries,' have the following five features (Halstead and Walter 2010):

1. There was either a direct blow to the head, face, or neck or elsewhere on the body with an "impulsive" force transmitted to the head.
2. There is a rapid onset of short-lived impairment of neurologic function that resolves spontaneously.
3. Neuropathological changes can occur, but the acute clinical symptoms reflect a functional disturbance not structural injury.
4. There is a graded set of clinical symptoms that may or may not involve loss of consciousness. After the injury, clinical and cognitive symptoms typically resolve and follow a sequential course. In a small percentage of cases, post-concussive symptoms may be prolonged.
5. There are no abnormalities with standard structural neuroimaging.

In high school sports, the concussion rates varied from 0.05 per 1,000 athlete exposures in baseball, volleyball, and boys' basketball, to 0.28 to 1.03 per 1,000 athlete exposures in boys' lacrosse, girls' soccer, and football (Halstead and Walter 2010). Loss of consciousness may occur and after regaining consciousness, the athlete might have the following signs and symptoms: headache, nausea, vomiting, balance and visual problems, fatigue, sensitivity to noise, impaired mental function (concentration, memory, confusion), feeling irritable and emotional, drowsiness, sleeping more than usual or not being able to sleep. Theoretically, mouthguards should be able to help protect the cranium from serious impact during contact sports. There are some studies to show that there is some basis for these theories:

- Opening the condylar space. Mouthguards, especially the 3-mm-thick pressure-laminated types, open the condylar space. When a properly fitted and balanced custom-made mouthguard is in place, there is a forward/downward displacement of the mandible, thus opening the space between the glenoid fossa and the condylar head. This reduces the risk for traumatic impact of the condyl with the glenoid fossa (Stenger *et al.* 1964).
- Force dissipation. Mouthguards absorb the energy from a blow to the mandible or directly to the face. Forces to the cranium are dissipated through cushioning effects and dampening of the energy transmission. The entire dentition serves to spread out the forces of the blow. There is less force transmitted through the temporomandibular joint (Chapman 1986; Tekeda *et al.* 2005).
- Reduction of rotational forces. A blow to the mandible from below can be transmitted through the midfacial skeleton, forcing the skull to rotate backward. If the mouthguard is clenched, the user tenses the neck muscles, which stabilizes the skull and reduces brain trauma (Porter and O'Brian 1994). It is important, however, to have evidence from 'field' studies to show that mouthguards do indeed reduce concussions. There are some studies, but they did not all show positive results (De Wet 1981; McNutt 1989; Benson and Meeuwisse 2005). According to Benson *et al.* (2009), who did a systematic review of 51 studies, there was no strong evidence that mouthguards reduced the rate of concussion risk. These authors did, however, conclude that full facial protection in ice hockey may reduce concussion severity as measured by time lost from competition. A more recent review of the literature on mouthguards and concussions reported that there was no strong evidence that mouthguards reduce concussion rates in rugby players (Cusimano *et al.* 2010).

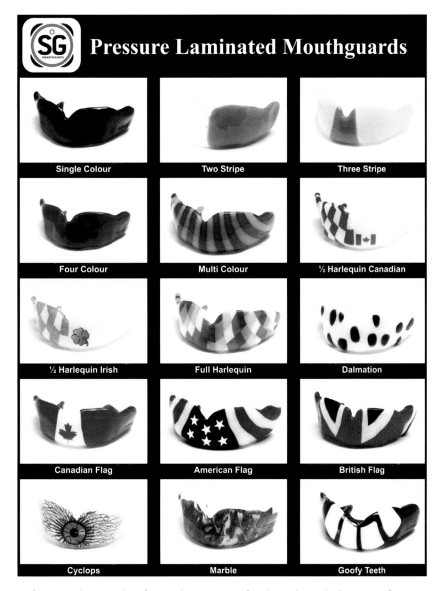

Figure 12-10 A selection of pressure-laminated professional-type custom-fitted mouthguards. (Courtesy of Smartguards, Mississauga, ON).

The Academy for Sports Dentistry continues to emphasize today that there have been no independently peer-reviewed published scientific research that "either supports or refutes the wearing of any type of mouthguard or oral appliance for concussion prevention, or athletic performance and strength enhancement" (ASD Web site).

Do mouthguards increase athletic performance?

We often observe weight lifters clench their teeth during extreme excursion when lifting heavy weights. It has been proposed that athletes can focus more on their task if the act of clenching their teeth, which must distract them, can be 'cushioned' with special custom-fitted mouthguards. Anecdotal reports that athletes perform better with certain brands of mouthguards in place, has given rise to companies that promote mouthguards specifically for improving athletic performance. There is also the idea that placing the jaw in an optimum position in relation to the rest of the skeleton, improves postural stability and improves repeated tasks. This was actually shown in a clinical study (Bracco *et al.* 2004). When famous athletes advertise the fact that they feel that the mouthguards have helped them 'improve their game,' amateur athletes and even young athletes who will never become professional athletes, become interested in the concept. For example, the Pure Power Mouthguard (PPM) is a new mouthguard system that requires optimal neuromuscular positioning of the mandible in a splint that combines the maxillary and mandibular mouthguards in a predetermined alignment.

An intriguing study on 13 volunteers showed that even wearing a boil-and-bite mouthguard could affect visual and auditory reaction times, even if only slightly (Garner and Miskimin 2009), supposedly by removing clenching pressures on the TMJ, which is directly inferior to the auditory canal and lateral to the eye sockets. Obviously, more rigorous clinical trials are required because the evidence that mouthguards improve athletic performance is sparse in terms of clinical trials (Von Arx et al. 2008). Despite supportive testimonials from athletes, the lack of evidence of effectiveness, and perhaps because these special mouthguards can cost upward of $2,000, the company that makes Pure Power Mouthguards, owned by a dentist in Truro Nova Scotia in Canada, ended up in receivership.

Do mouthguards increase the risk of oral or systemic infections?

There have been case reports of infected mouthguards causing systemic illnesses in athletes (Glass et al. 2007). In one case cellulitis in the leg of a high school football player was caused by the same oral bacterium that was found in large numbers in the mouthguard. In another case, a junior football player developed asthma from the mold that harboured in the mouthguard. A prospective study of athletes wearing boil-and-bite mouthguards was conducted by Glass et al. (2009) who not only found several microorganisms that grew in the mouthguards, but the poor-fitting mouthguards also caused various oral lesions, such as hyperkeratosis and ulcers.

There has been little else published in the literature about whether contaminated mouthguards pose a health risk to the wearer. Using bleach solutions to disinfect the mouthguards is contraindicated because oxidizing agents will prematurely break down the mouthguard material, reducing its resilience and possibly increasing the risk for dental injury. It is assumed that since it has been shown that wet toothbrushes allow the growth of large numbers of microorgasims, which can be controlled using 0.12 % chlorhexidine digluconated rinses (Mehta et al. 2007), soaking mouthguards in the same solution overnight would control the growth of not only bacteria on the mouthguards but yeast as well. (See Chapter 10 on chlorhexidine.)

References

Academy of General Dentistry. (2007) Mouthguards fight "weekend warrior" syndrome. [online] available at http://www.agd.org/public/oralhealth/Default.asp?IssID=331&Topic=S&ArtID=1326.

Academy for Sports Dentistry. (2011a) What is sports dentistry? [online] available at http://www.academyforsportsdentistry.org/Home/tabid/38/Default.aspx. Accessed March 14, 2011.

Academy for Sports Dentistry. (2011b) Qualifications of a team dentist. [online] Available at http://www.academyforsportsdentistry.org/Organization/PositionStatement/tabid/58/Default.aspx.

Academy for Sports Dentistry. (2011c) A properly fitted mouthguard. [online] Available at http://www.academyforsportsdentistry.org/Organization/PositionStatement/tabid/58/Default.aspx.

ADA Council on Access, Prevention and Interprofessional Relations; ADA Council on Scientific Affairs. (2006) Using mouthguards to reduce the incidence and severity of sports-related oral injuries. *Journal of the American Dental Association*, 12, 1712–20; quiz 1731.

American Dental Association. (1960) Resolution 39-1960-H: Mouth protectors. *Transactions*, 233–234.

American Dental Association. (2004) The importance of using mouthguards: tips for keeping your smile safe. *Journal of the America Dental Association*, 135, 1061.

American Dental Association. (2005) *Current Policies adopted 1954–2004. Orofacial protectors.* American Dental Association, p. 184. Chicago, IL.

Bastone, E.B., Freer, T.J., McNamara, J.R. (2000) Epidemiology of dental trauma: a review of the literature. *Austrian Dental Journal*, 45, 2–9.

Beachy, G. (2004) Dental injuries in intermediate and high school athletes: a 15-year study at Punahou School. *Journal of Athletic Training*, 39, 310–315.

Bendo, C.B., Paiva, S.M., Torres, C.S., et al. (2010) Association between treated/untreated traumatic dental injuries and impact on quality of life of Brazilian schoolchildren. *Health and Quality of Life Outcomes*, 8, 114.

Benson, B. and Meeuwisse, W. (2005) The risk of concussion associated with mouthguard use among professional ice hockey players. *Clinical Journal of Sport Medicine*, 15, 395.

Benson, B.W., Hamilton, G.M., Meeuwisse, W.H., et al. (2009) Is protective equipment useful in preventing concussion? A systematic review of the literature. *British Journal of Sports Medicine*, 43 (Suppl 1), i56–i67.

Berg, R., Berkey, D.B., Tang, J.M., et al. (1998) Knowledge and attitudes of Arizona high-school coaches regarding oral-facial injuries and mouthguard use among athletes. *Journal of the American Dental Association*, 129, 1425–1432.

Biasca, N., Wirth, S., Tegner, Y. (2002) The avoidability of head and neck injuries in ice hockey: an historical review. *British Journal of Sports Medicine*, 36, 410–427.

Borssen, E. and Holm, A.K. (1997) Traumatic dental injuries in a cohort of 16-year-olds in northern Sweden. *Endodontics and Dental Traumatology*, 13, 276–280.

Bracco, P., Deregibus, A., Piscetta, R. (2004) Effects of different jaw relations on postural stability in human subjects. *Neuroscience Letters*, 356, 228–230.

Canadian Academy of Sport Medicine, Delaney, J.S. and Frankovich, R. (2004) *Head injuries and concussions in soccer. Position statement.* The Academy, Ottawa, Canada.

Canadian Dental Association. (2005) *CDA position on prevention of traumatic oral facial injuries.* Canadian Dental Association, Ottawa, Canada.

Chalmers, D.J. (1998) Mouthguards. Protection for the mouth in rugby union. *Sports Medicine*, 25, 339–349.

Chapman, P.J. (1986) The bimaxillary mouthguard: a preliminary report of use in contact sports. *Australian Dental Journal*, 31, 200–206.

Chisick, M.C., Richter, P., Piotrowski, M.J. (2000) Put more "bite" into health promotion: a campaign to revitalize health promotion in the Army Dental Care System. Part I. The mouthguard, sealant, and nursing caries initiatives. *Military Medicine*, 165, 598–603.

Cornwell, H., Messer, L.B., Speed, H. (2003) Use of mouthguards by basketball players in Victoria, *Australia. Dental Traumatology*, 19, 193–203.

Cortes, M.I., Marcenes, W., Sheiham, A. (2002) Impact of traumatic injuries to the permanent teeth on the oral health-related quality of life in 12–14-year-old children. *Community Dentistry and Oral Epidemiology*, 30, 193–198.

Cusimano, M.D., Nassiri, F., Chang, Y. (2010) The effectiveness of interventions to reduce neurological injuries in rugby union: a systematic review. *Neurosurgery*, 67, 1404–1418.

de Wet, F., Badenhorst, M., Rossouw, L. (1981) Mouthguards for rugby players at primary school level. *Journal of the Dental Association of South Africa*, 36, 249–253.

Delaney, J.S. and Montgomery, D.L. (2005) Effect of noncustom bimolar mouthguards on peak ventilation in ice hockey players. *Clinical Journal of Sport Medicine*, 15, 154–157.

DeYoung, A.K., Robinson, E., Godwin, W.C. (1994) Comparing comfort and wearability: custom-made vs. self-adapted mouthguards. *Journal of the American Dental Association*, 125, 1112–1118.

Diangelis, A.J. and Bakland, L.K. (1998) Traumatic dental injuries: current treatment concepts. *Journal of the American Dental Association*, 129, 1401–1414.

Echlin, P.S., Upshur, R.E., Peck, D.M., et al. (2005) Craniomaxillofacial injury in sport: a review of prevention research. *British Journal of Sports Medicine*, 39, 254–263.

Emshoff, R., Schöning, H., Röthler, G., et al. (1997) Trends in the incidence and cause of sport-related mandibular fractures: a retrospective analysis. *Journal of Oral and Maxillofacial Surgery*, 55, 585–592.

Fakhruddin, K.S., Lawrence, H.P., Kenny, D.J., et al. (2007) Use of mouthguards among 12- to 14-year-old Ontario schoolchildren. *Journal of the Canadian Dental Association*, 73, 505 a–e.

Finch, C., Braham, R., McIntosh, A., et al. (2005) Should football players wear custom fitted mouthguards? Result from a group randomized controlled trial. *Injury Prevention*, 11, 242–246.

Flanders, R.A. (1995) Project Mouthguard. *Illinois Dental Journal*, 64, 67–69.

Flanders, R.A. and Bhat, M. (1995) The incidence of orofacial injuries in sports: a pilot study in Illinois. *Journal of the American Dental Association*, 126, 491–496.

Fontelles, J.B. and Clarke, C. (2005) Directive 2005/84/EC of the European Parliament and of the Council of 14 December 2005 amending for the 22nd time Council Directive 76/769/EEC on the approximation of the laws, regulations and administrative provisions of the Member States relating to restrictions on the marketing and use of certain dangerous substances and preparations (phthalates in toys and childcare articles). *Official Journal of the European Union* 48, 40–43.

Gardiner, D.M. and Ranalli, D.N. (2000) Attitudinal factors influencing mouthguard utilization. *Dental Clinics of North America*, 44, 53–65.

Garner, D.P. and Miskimin, J. (2009) Effects of mouthpiece use on auditory and visual reaction time in college males and females. *Compendium of Continuing Education in Dentistry*, 30 Spec No 2, 14–17.

Gebauer, D.P., Williamson, R.A., Wallman, K.E., et al. (2011) The effect of mouthguard design on respiratory function in athletes. *Clinical Journal of Sport Medicine*, 21, 95–100.

Glass, R.T., Conrad, R.S., Rieger Wood, C., et al. (2009) Protective athletic mouthguards: do they cause harm? *Sports Health: A Multidisciplinary Approach*, 1, 411–415.

Glass, R.T., Wood, C.R., Bullard, J.W., et al. (2007) Possible disease transmission by contaminated mouthguards in two young football players. *General Dentistry*, 55, 436–440.

Goldberg, P.V., Higginbottom, F.L., Wilson, T.G. (2001) Periodontal considerations in restorative and implant therapy. *Periodontology 2000*, 25, 100–109.

Greasley, A., Imlach, G., Karet, B. (1998) Application of a standard test to the in vitro performance of mouthguards. *British Journal of Sports Medicine*, 32, 17–19.

Gutmann, J.L. and Gutmann, M.S. (1995) Cause, incidence, and prevention of trauma to teeth. *Dental Clinics of North America*, 39, 1–13.

Halstead, M.E. and Walter, K.D. (2010) Council on Sports Medicine and Fitness. American Academy of Pediatrics. Clinical report—sport-related concussion in children and adolescents. *Pediatrics*, 126, 597–615.

Knapik, J.J., Marshall, S.W., Lee, R.B., et al. (2007) Mouthguards in sport activities: history, physical properties and injury prevention effectiveness. *Sports Medicine*, 37, 117–144.

Kuebker, W.A., Morrow, M., Cohen, P.A. (1986) Do mouth-formed mouth guards meet the NCAA rules? *Physician and Sportsmedicine*, 14, 69–74.

Kumamoto, D.P. and Maeda, Y. (2004) A literature review of sports-related orofacial trauma. *General Dentistry*, 52, 270–280.

Labella, C.R., Smith, B.W., Sigurdsson, A. (2002) Effect of mouthguards on dental injuries and concussions in college basketball. *Medicine & Science in Sports and Exercise*, 34, 41–44.

Lancaster, D.M. and Ranalli, D.N. Comparative evaluation of college football officials' attitudes toward NCAA mouthguard regulations and player compliance. *Pediatric Dentistry*, 15, 398–402.

Levin, L., Friedlander, L.D., Geiger, S.B. (2003) Dental and oral trauma and mouthguard use during sport activities in Israel. *Dental Traumatology*, 19, 237–242.

Locker, D. and Maggirias, J. (2004) Costs of traumatic dental injury in Ontario. Health measurement and epidemiology report. Toronto (ON): Community Dental Health Services Research Unit, Faculty of Dentistry, University of Toronto.

Love, R.M., Carman, N., Carmichael, S., et al. (1998) Sport-related dental injury claims to the New Zealand Accident Rehabilitation & Compensation Insurance Corporation, 1993–1996: analysis of the 10 most common sports, excluding rugby union. *New Zealand Dental Journal*, 94, 146–149.

Marshall, S.W., Loomis, D.P., Waller, A.E., et al. (2005) Evaluation of protective equipment for prevention of injuries in rugby union. *International Journal of Epidemiology*, 34, 113–118.

McNutt, T., Shannon, S., Wright, J., et al. (1989) Oral trauma in adolescent athletes: a study of mouth protectors. *Pediatric Dentistry*, 11, 7–11.

Mehta, A., Sequeira, P.S., Bhat, G. (2007) Bacterial contamination and decontamination of toothbrushes after use. *New York State Dental Journal*, 73, 20–22.

Morton, J.G. and Burton, J.F. (1979) An evaluation of the effectiveness of mouthguards in high-school rugby players. *New Zealand Dental Journal*, 75, 151–153.

Neussl, A. (2008) Mouthguards in the American Hockey League *Journal of Dental Hygiene*, 5, 44–44(1).

Newsome, P., Owen, S. Reaney, D. (2010) The dentist's role in the prevention of sports-related oro-facial injuries. *International Dentistry SA*, 12, 50–60.

Padilla, R.R. (2005) A technique for fabricating modern athletic mouthguards. *Journal of the California Dental Association*, 33, 399–408.

Pennington, M.W., Vernazza, C.R., Shackley, P., et al. (2009) Evaluation of the cost-effectiveness of root canal treatment using conventional approaches versus replacement with an implant. *International Endodontic Journal*, 42, 874–883.

Petersen, P.E., Bourgeois, D., Ogawa, H., et al. (2005) Point of care. *Journal of the Canadian Dental Association*, 71, 267–272.

Porter, M. and O'Brien, M. (1994) The "Buy-Max" mouthguard: oral, perioral and cerebral protection for contact sports. *Journal of the Irish Dental Association*, 40, 98–101.

Ramos-Jorge, M.L., Bosco, V.L., Peres, M.A., *et al.* (2007) The impact of treatment of dental trauma on the quality of life of adolescents: a case-control study in southern Brazil. *Dental Traumatology*, 23, 114–119.

Ranalli, D.N. (2000) Sports dentistry in general practice. *General Dentistry*, 48, 158–164.

Rodd, H.D. and Chesham, D.J. (1997) Sports-related oral injury and mouthguard use among Sheffield school children. *Community Dental Health*, 14, 25–30.

Soporowski, N.J., Tesini, D.A., Weiss, A.I. (1994) Survey of orofacial sports-related injuries. *Journal of the Massachusetts Dental Society*, 43, 16–20.

Stenger, J.M., Lawson, E.A., Wright, J.M., *et al.* (1964) Mouthguards: protection against shock to head, neck and teeth. *Journal of the American Dental Association*, 69, 273–281.

Takeda, T., Ishigami, K., Hoshina, S., *et al.* (2005) Can mouthguards prevent mandibular bone fractures and concussions? A laboratory study with an artificial skull model. *Dental Traumatology*, 21, 134–140.

Truman, B.I., Gooch, B.F., Sulemana, I., *et al.* (2002) Task Force on Community Preventive Services. Reviews of evidence on interventions to prevent dental caries, oral and pharyngeal cancers, and sports-related craniofacial injuries. *America Journal of Preventive Medicine*, 23(1 Suppl), 21–54.

Vanet R. (1951) Gridiron challenge. *Dental Survey*, 27, 1258–1259.

Vastardis, P.D. (2005) Athletic mouthguards: indications, types, and benefits. *Dentistry Today*, 24, 52–55.

von Arx, T., Flury, R., Tschan, J., *et al.* (2008) Exercise capacity in athletes with mouthguards. *International Journal of Sports Medicine*, 29, 435–438.

Wisniewski, J.F., Guskiewicz, K., Trope, M., *et al.* (2004) Incidence of cerebral concussions associated with type of mouthguard used in college football. *Dental Traumatology*, 20, 143–149.

13

Tooth erosion

W. Peter Holbrook

Introduction

Tooth erosion is the term used to describe tooth wear caused by acid that is not of bacterial origin. A search of the dental research literature clearly illustrates the increasing awareness of this phenomenon in recent years (Lussi 2006). This type of tooth wear has an etiology distinct from other forms of tooth wear such as attrition and abrasion, but frequently the clinical manifestations of observed tooth wear can be attributed to a mix of etiological factors that can sometimes make an accurate diagnosis difficult (Addy and Shellis 2006; Holbrook 2009).

Prevalence of the condition

The prevalence of tooth erosion, at least in European studies, would appear to be increasing (Nunn *et al.* 2003; Lussi 2006) especially among young adults and adolescents with a higher prevalence usually found in males (Nunn *et al.* 2003; Arnadottir *et al.* 2010). Few longitudinal studies of tooth erosion have been reported in the literature (Dugmore and Rock 2003; El Aidi *et al.* 2008), and this may be related in part to the lack of a suitable index for scoring erosion in individuals and groups similar to the permanent dentition's decayed, missing, and filled (DMF) and primary dentition's decayed, missing, and filled (dmf) indices used for recording caries. The Basic Erosive Wear Examination (BEWE) index (Bartlett *et al.* 2008) has attempted to remove this barrier to scoring erosion. This index would appear to have several advantages over other popular scoring methods for tooth wear such as that of Smith and Knight (1984) or Lussi (1996) that are more adapted to recording the epidemiology of tooth wear. Preliminary investigations of the use

of the BEWE index on studies of erosion in Iceland have proved to be helpful (Holbrook et al. 2010).

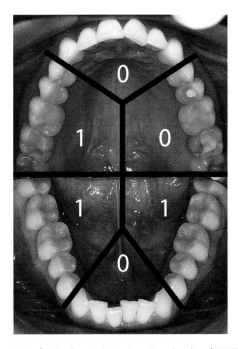

Figure 13-1 The Basic Erosive Wear Examination (BEWE) index for a case with mild erosion. The maxillary and mandibular dentitions are divided into six 'sextants' (right and left posterior, upper and lower segments that include the premolars and molars, plus the upper and lower anterior segments, that include the canines and incisors). Scores are assigned as follows: 0 = no erosive wear, 1 = initial loss of surface texture, 2 = distinct defect, hard tissue loss <50%, 3 = hard tissue loss >50% of surface area. Only three sextants in this case showed erosion, and the risk level for this dentition was rated mild (cumulative BEWE score of 3 for all sextants). Photograph courtesy of Sverrir Hlödversson.

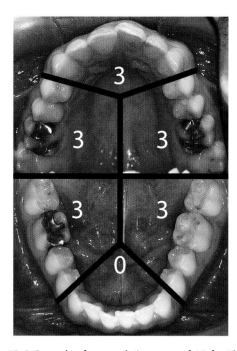

Figure 13-2 Example of a cumulative score of 15 for The Basic Erosive Wear Examination (BEWE), indicating a high risk level of continued erosive wear (Bartlett *et al.* 2008; Holbrook *et al.* 2010). Photograph courtesy of Sverrir Hlödversson.

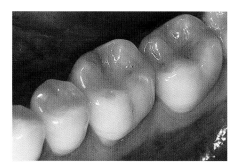

Figure 13-3 Typical 'cupping' of the cusp tip from erosion. The mesio-buccal cusp tip of the lower left first permanent molar in this photograph shows the typical cusp-tip wear that is often observed in people with early erosion in their dentitions.

In these studies erosive wear scores were calculated for subgroups within a large sample of referred patients (Holbrook *et al.* 2010) and for groups within a national survey of erosion in children and adolescents in Iceland. With the adoption of a reliable scoring index for erosion there opens up the possibility of assessing changes in the degree of erosion with time and the results of measures to prevent the onset of erosion or the continuation of the disease.

Etiology of tooth erosion

The etiology of tooth erosion is relatively straightforward. The causative agents are acids that can be extrinsic in the form of acidic foods and drinks. Environmental acids causing erosion may be linked to uncontrolled industrial environments such as battery manufacture (Wiegand and Attin 2007; Suyama *et al.* 2010). Intrinsic acids that cause erosion are gastric acid that is refluxed in patients with such conditions as bulimia, anorexia, hiatus hernia, and gastroesophageal reflux disease (GERD) (Holbrook *et al.* 2009). Acid attack on dental hard tissues leads to a softening of the tissue that is, consequently, liable to have further tooth wear from the other forces known to cause tooth wear such as attrition and abrasion. Thus, the etiology behind any observed case of tooth wear may result from a combination of several factors, and this can affect the measures taken to prevent further advance of any observed tooth wear.

Early detection of erosion

Diagnosis, early detection, scoring of severity, and monitoring progress of erosion are important parameters that are all less well developed than their counterparts for dental caries. For many years, dental caries has been scored for individuals and populations using well-tried methods largely related to the score of permanent decayed, missing, and filled teeth (DMFT) or surfaces (DMFS) and primary decayed, missing, and filled teeth (dmft) and surfaces (dmfs). The sensitivity of the diagnostic method behind such a caries score was for many years a visual-tactile examination. Greater sensitivity could be obtained by using radiographs. Later, diagnostic criteria were altered, such as the introduction of ICDAS, and diagnostic devices were developed, such as Diagnodent, QLF, and DiFOTI (Fejerskov and Kidd 2008), and used to increase the ability of the clinician to diagnose caries at as early a stage as possible. This could give an opportunity to introduce effective caries-preventive measures that could even include recalcification of initial lesions so that the observed degree of caries could actually reduce. Unfortunately no accepted method of detecting erosion at an initial stage has yet gained clinical acceptance. Some preliminary studies including fluorescent and optical methods, profilometry, and assessments of surface hardness (Schlueter *et al.* 2005; Attin 2006; Chew *et al.* 2010) have suggested that early detection of enamel erosion might become a reality, but no reliable and sensitive methods for the grading and monitoring erosion *in vivo* are yet available. Such a development would offer an opportunity for adopting specific preventive measures for individual patients or possibly particular teeth in the mouth of an individual. Currently neither the diagnostic techniques nor the preventive measures developed for erosion have yet reached the level of usefulness available for caries detection, monitoring of progression, and prevention.

Table 13-1 Comparison of the results of routine tests of salivary parameters in three groups of patients: those referred for testing because of (i) xerostomia, (ii) tooth erosion, and (iii) dental caries

Patient group	Stimulated flow/min mean (s.d.)	Buffer capacity (Dentobuff® test kit pH) Mean (s.d.)	pH mean (s.d.)	Streptococcus mutans count mean (s.d.)	Lactobacillus count mean (s.d.)
Xerostomia (n=90)	0.9 mL (0.7)	4.7 (0.8)	6.6 (0.8)	10^5/mL [1.6]	$10^{3.4}$/mL [2.0]
Erosion (n=88)	1.7 mL (0.8)	5.4 (0.7)	7.5 (0.7)	$10^{4.8}$/mL [1.6]	$10^{2.3}$/mL [2.2]
Caries (n=45)	1.5 mL (0.9)	5.2 (0.8)	7.0 (0.9)	10^5/mL [1.8]	$10^{3.6}$/mL [1.9]

Protection against erosion: the effects of saliva

The protective effect of saliva against erosion is important because it provides virtually the only inherent protection against erosion in the oral cavity. Acid in the mouth is diluted by the flow of saliva, and the buffering action of saliva neutralizes acid retained in the mouth. Furthermore, the deposition of salivary glycoprotein on to the enamel, or dentine, surface protects hydroxyapatite crystals and reduces their decalcification in the low pH environment at which erosion occurs. Salivary calcium is also potentially important in promoting some recalcification of a decalcified tooth surface following acid challenges (Dawes 2008). The association of some easily measurable salivary parameters with caries, erosion, and xerostomia is shown in Table 13.1 where the study group consisted of patients referred for salivary testing (Holbrook and Sæmundsson 2006).

The interplay of causative and protective factors for erosion in the mouth may seem relatively simple when compared with the more complex factors associated with dental caries. Low salivary flow rates and a low salivary buffer capacity are associated with tooth erosion and also with caries. The use by patients suffering from dry mouth of acidic products to stimulate their salivary flow can result in tooth erosion (Lajer *et al.* 2009). However, it has been shown that the explanatory value of factors associated with tooth erosion explained only a very small part of the observed degree of erosion in one study of patients referred for investigation (Holbrook *et al.* 2009).

Prevention of erosion

Prevention of erosion can be divided into two main areas: prevention for the individual and prevention for a population or subgroups of a given population. For the individual the main aim at present is to stop the progress of erosion that has been diagnosed whereas for populations, the aim is largely to try and reduce the erosive effects of various lifestyle factors that could otherwise lead to the onset of erosion and in addition to slow down the progress of any erosion that could have started.

Prevention for the individual

As was noted by Holbrook *et al.* (2003), it is first necessary to diagnose the observed tooth wear as being erosive in nature, to grade its severity, and monitor its progression. Diagnosis also requires determination of the likely causative factors of the observed erosion and the possible combination of different types of tooth wear to give the observed clinical picture. Although some aspects of diagnosis and grading erosion have advanced in recent years, there still remains the problem of monitoring progress of erosion to determine the effects of preventive measures employed to stop erosion continuing in an individual. Equally it is important to develop a diagnostic method suitable for clinical use to determine if erosion has commenced in an individual previously free of this problem.

Erosion due to intrinsic factors

A careful case history including medical, dental, and lifestyle factors should be taken whenever a patient presents with tooth wear, to determine the likely causes. If the medical history indicates the possible presence of a gastric reflux disease such as GERD, bulimia, or anorexia then this usually will require referral to a gastroenterologist or other medical specialist for further investigation. Confirmed cases of these reflux diseases are usually treated, and this may remove the cause of the erosion. However, it should not be assumed that systemic treatment of the underlying condition is sufficient, and some local preventive measures against erosion are usually helpful. Dissolving an antacid tablet in the mouth has been shown to raise the intra-oral pH quickly; these tablets should be taken immediately following symptoms of reflux (Meurman *et al.* 1988).

Patients with symptoms of dry mouth (xerostomia) often turn to acidic drinks to stimulate their salivary flow. If the dry mouth is a chronic problem due, for example, to the side effects of medication, radiotherapy, or Sjögrens syndrome then the long-term use of acidic drinks could lead to tooth erosion. Non-erosive products should be recommended for these patients, and an increasing range of salivary-stimulating lozenges and mouth rinses together with saliva-replacement mouth rinses and gels that do not cause tooth erosion are now available. It is often helpful for patients experiencing xerostomia to have printed information on suitable products and instructions on their use. The dentist should then complement this with advice on products that help counterbalance the erosive potential of xerostomia.

Erosion due to extrinsic factors

Acidic drinks

Much of the tooth erosion seen today by dental professionals and increasingly reported in the dental literature is not caused by underlying factors such as reflux disease or xerostomia but by significant changes in lifestyle particularly seen in the increasing consumption of acidic drinks by adolescents and young adults (Arnadóttir *et al.* 2003; Jensdottir *et al.* 2004). These drinks contain citric, ascorbic, phosphoric, or even lactic acids. Their erosive effects are caused by the low pH that decalcifies the apatite crystals of the teeth and also the chelating effect of the relatively weak organic acids. This reduces the possibilities for recalcification of the teeth from saliva, which is normally supersaturated with respect to calcium ions (Dawes 2008). Soft drinks are consumed not only to quench thirst but also with meals, socially, and as sports/energy drinks to provide carbohydrate and thirst quenching in relation to physical activity (Rytömaa *et al.* 1988). Even bottled carbonated waters sometimes contain citric acid and have an erosive potential similar to cola drinks (Þorvaldsdóttir *et al.* 2008). There is clear evidence of the erosive nature of several sports drinks, but the risk of erosion also comes from the pattern of drinking, especially swishing the drink around the mouth before swallowing. This is a habit among consumers of soft drinks (Johansson *et al.* 2004) as well as wine tasters, among whom the erosive effect, particularly of white wine, is well known (Gray *et al.* 1998).

Preventing erosion in an individual case where the cause is thought to be a high consumption of acidic drinks is not easy. The level of risk may be as low as 0.5 L of acidic drink per day (Holbrook *et al.* 2009). Getting patients who present with erosion to chart their consumption of acidic drinks for a week might help the dentist give them pertinent advice. The following factors are known to increase erosion: (1) frequent consumption of acidic drinks, (2) swishing the drink before swallowing, (3) consuming acidic drinks just before sleep, when the protective benefits of saliva are reduced, and (4) brushing

teeth immediately following the acid challenge, which increases the wear of the enamel due to the abrasive action of toothpaste on the still softened tooth surface. Switching to a less abrasive toothpaste might be helpful in reducing the overall tooth wear in patients with erosion (Wiegand *et al.* 2008); this probably applies to patients with erosion due to intrinsic as well as extrinsic factors.

Changing the lifestyle factors of adolescents and young adults is particularly difficult and measures, such as drinking acidic beverages through a straw, chewing a piece of cheese, or drinking milk immediately following consumption of cola beverages are unlikely to appeal to this age group. However, severe cases of erosion cause considerable dental discomfort or even pain, and patients experiencing this are more likely to cooperate.

Other extrinsic causes of erosion

Erosion due to extrinsic factors is overwhelmingly caused by acidic drinks (Jensdottir *et al.* 2006), but other causes do exist. Vegetarians and vegans are particularly at risk of tooth erosion if they consume acidic fruits and vegetables, especially raw when the constituent acids in these foods are active (Linkosalo and Markkanen 1985). Some medications are also known to be erosive, and the low pH of steroids used in inhalers, for example for treating asthma, may contribute to erosion (Al-Dlaigan *et al.* 2002; O'Sullivan *et al.* 1998). Acidic sweets and lozenges may also have an erosive potential not realized by those prescribing, selling, or using them (Nunn *et al.* 2001). Health professionals prescribing or advising the use of acidic preparations in the mouth should advise patients of the potential risk. The formulation of some medications has indeed considered the erosive potential of the preparation, and modifications have been made to minimize any erosive effect (Lajer *et al.* 2009; Jensdottir *et al.* 2010).

Industrial causes of erosion are no longer common in developed countries although they do sometimes occur (Westergaard *et al.* 2001; Suyama *et al.* 2010). Regulations to cover the working environment are likely to be the most successful preventive measure.

Preparations to prevent erosion

Although fluoride is the mainstay of preventive measures against dental caries, its effectiveness against tooth erosion, however, is less clear. This is partly due to the problems in grading erosion and monitoring the disease accurately enough to obtain suitable data for statistical analysis, particularly in longitudinal clinical studies. Many studies of products aimed at preventing tooth erosion were conducted *in vitro* using enamel slabs and testing microhardness as a means of assessing the protective effect. *In situ* models have also been used for testing the effect of potential protective products on tooth pieces inserted into the mouths of volunteer subjects for periods of time, followed by their removal and testing with methods including microhardness (Lussi 1996; West *et al.* 1998) and profilometry (Lussi 1996; Hooper 2005).

Given the limitations of the studies reported so far, there is an increasing interest in chemical methods for preventing both the initiation and progress of tooth erosion. Double-blind or placebo-controlled trials of products used by subjects with erosion or at risk of developing erosion have yet to be conducted. A lot of research on erosion prevention has involved the use of preparations containing fluoride, but the results have been variable (Sorvari *et al.* 1988; Bartlett *et al.* 1994; Grenby 1996; Attin *et al.* 1998; Attin *et al.* 1999; Ganss *et al.* 2001; Larsen 2001). There is little doubt, however, that a fluoride-rich enamel surface created through mouth rinsing, varnish, or toothpaste containing fluoride would produce an apatite structure that would be less easily dissolved than a fluoride-free enamel. The low pH of many acidic drinks and foods is, however, sufficient to cause dissolution even of hydroxyfluorapatite and fluorapatite. Furthermore, the abrasivity of toothpaste can add to the observed tooth wear following acid challenge that will soften the enamel (Attin *et al.* 1998; Attin *et al.* 1999; Attin *et al.* 2001). This is the reason why many protocols for preventing tooth wear emphasize the need to not brush teeth immediately after consuming acidic foods or beverages or following an episode of heartburn, reflux, or vomiting (Attin *et al.* 2001). Fluoride preparations are not all equivalent, and there are some reliable studies reporting an increased resistance to erosion when the tooth surface enamel or dentine has been treated with tin, titanium, fluoride, or with dilute hydrofluoric acid (Ganss *et al.* 2010a, 2010b). Fluoride-containing preparations that have shown some protective effect against erosive forces include pastes containing casein phosphopeptide-amorphous calcium phosphate (Poggio *et al.* 2009; Ranjitkar *et al.* 2009; Cochrane *et al.* 2010), and this has been effective in reducing erosion *in vitro* (Ranjitkar *et al.* 2009) indicating possible new modalities for treatment and prevention of erosion. Numerous other fluoride preparations have been tested for their protective effect against erosion. These include hydrofluoric acid (Hjortsjö *et al.* 2009), amine fluoride, and fluoride salts of sodium, cerium, titanium, tin, and zirconium (Wiegand *et al.* 2010; Wegehaupt 2010).

Reduction in the erosive effects of acidic drinks is clearly possible (Grenby 1996), and modification of soft drinks and indeed other acidic food products is a potentially useful development that has not yet been appreciated by the food manufacturing industry. One modified fruit drink was developed for children and shown to have reduced erosive potential (Ribena tooth kind, Hughes *et al.* 1999a, 1999b; West *et al.* 1999). This modified drink contained calcium as did a modified orange drink tested in *in vitro* studies (Jensdottir *et al.* 2005). Unfortunately, both of these products have failed to gain significant acceptance in the market.

Saliva-stimulating products are useful for treating xerostomia related to Sjögrens or sicca syndrome, the side effects of medication or radiotherapy. Fluoride-containing Xerodent lozenges and calcium-modified acidic candies (Jensdottir *et al.* 2009; Lajer *et al.* 2010) are examples of products intended to reduce dry mouth symptoms while not causing erosion. Similarly, fluoride-containing chewing gum (Sjögren *et al.* 1997) could have a beneficial effect against erosion although this requires further clinical investigation. The stimulation of saliva with these products leads to dilution of acid in the mouth as well as increasing the amount of salivary pellicle on teeth that will contribute to protecting the tooth surface against acid attack. The known protective effect of pellicle coating the tooth surface has lead to investigation of the potential benefits of coating the tooth surface with casein in various topical preparations. Indeed a study by Gedlaia in 1992 (Gedalia *et al.* 1992) showed the benefit of eating cheese at the end of a meal as a means of preventing acid erosion of teeth. Patients with gastroesophageal reflux and those with bulimia need advice and medication to reduce the effect of regular sever acid attack on their teeth. Regular use of antacids following reflux symptoms has been proposed (Meurman *et al.* 1988; Sunram and Bartlett 2001).

The increasing awareness of tooth erosion has lead to an increase in research and to several reports of unusual products and treatments that may have a protective effect for the tooth surface against erosion. These include green tea (Kato *et al.* 2009), and recently the use of the matrix-metalloproteinase inhibitor epigallocatechin gallate that together with chlorhexidine prevented erosion induced using Coca-Cola® in an *in situ* bovine enamel model in volunteers (Kato *et al.* 2010). As with other approaches to erosion prevention such as use of fluoride and drink modification, properly structured clinical trials with relevant monitoring of the erosion are needed for these new approaches.

References

Addy, M. and Shellis, R.P. (2006) Interaction between attrition, abrasion and erosion in tooth wear. In: *Dental Erosion* (Ed. A. Lussi), pp. 17–31, Monographs in Oral Science, Karger, Basel Switzerland.

Al-Dlaigan, Y.H., Shaw, L., Smith, A.J. (2002) Is there a relationship between asthma and dental erosion? A case control study. *International Journal of Paediatric Dentistry*, 12, 189–200.

Arnadóttir, I.B., Holbrook, W.P., Eggertsson, H., *et al.* (2010) Prevalence of dental erosion in children: a national survey. *Community Dentistry and Oral Epidemiology*, 38, 521–526.

Arnadóttir, I.B., Saemundsson, S.R., Holbrook, W.P. (2003) Dental erosion in Icelandic teenagers in relation to dietary and lifestyle factors. *Acta Odontologica Scandinavica*, 61, 25–28.

Attin, T., Deifuss, H., Hellwig, E. (1999) Influence of acidified fluoride gel on abrasion resistance of eroded enamel. *Caries Research*, 33, 135–139.

Attin, T., Knofel, S., Buchalla, W., et al. (2001) In situ evaluation of different remineralization periods to decrease brushing abrasion of demineralised enamel. *Caries Research*, 35, 216–222.

Attin, T., Zirkel, C., Hellwig, E. (1998) Brushing abrasion of eroded dentin after application of sodium fluoride solutions. *Caries Research*, 32, 344–350.

Attin, T. (2006) Methods for assessment of dental erosion In: *Dental Erosion* (Ed. A. Lussi), pp. 152–172, Monographs in Oral Science 20, Karger, Basel Switzerland.

Bartlett, D.W., Smith, B.G., Wilson, R.F. (1994) Comparison of the effect of fluoride and non-fluoride toothpaste on tooth wear in vitro and the influence of enamel fluoride concentration and hardness of enamel. *British Dental Journal*, 176, 346–348.

Bartlett, D.W., Ganss, C., Lussi, A. (2008) Basic Erosive Wear Examination (BEWE): a new scoring system for scientific and clinical needs. *Clinical Oral Investigation*, 12 Suppl 1, S65–S68.

Chew, H.P., Zakian, C.M., Pretty, I.A. (2010) Measurement of dental erosion with two optical methods. *Journal of Dental Research*, 89 Special Issue B: abstract 3132.

Cochrane, N.J., Cai, F., Huq, N.L., et al. (2010) New approaches to enhanced remineralization of tooth enamel. *Journal of Dental Research*, 89, 1187–1197.

Dawes, C. (2008) Salivary flow patterns and the health of hard and soft oral tissues. *Journal of the American Dental Association*, 139 Suppl, 18S–24S.

Dugmore, C.R. and Rock, W.P. (2003) The progression of tooth erosion in a cohort of adolescents of mixed ethnicity. *International Journal of Paediatric Dentistry*, 13, 295–303.

El Aidi, H., Bronkhorst, E.M., Truin, G.J. (2008) A longitudinal study of tooth erosion in adolescents. *Journal of Dental Research*, 8, 731–735.

Fejerskov, O. and Kidd, E. (2008) *Dental Caries: the disease and its clinical management* 2nd ed., Blackwell Munksgaard, Oxford, UK.

Ganss, C., Hardt, M., Lussi, A., et al. (2010) Mechanism of action of tin-containing fluoride solutions as anti-erosive agents in dentine—an in vitro tin-uptake, tissue loss, and scanning electron microscopy study. *European Journal of Oral Science*, 118, 376–384.

Ganss, C., Klimek, J., Schaffer, U., et al. (2001) Effectiveness of two fluoridation measures on erosion progression in human enamel and dentine in vitro. *Caries Research*, 35, 325–330.

Ganss, C., Neutard, L., von Hinckeldey, J., et al. (2010) Efficacy of a tin/fluoride rinse: a randomized in situ trial on erosion. *Journal of Dental Research*, 89, 1214–1218.

Gedalia, I., Davidov, I., Lewinstein, I., et al. (1992) Effect of hard cheese exposure with and without fluoride prerinse on the rehardening of softened human enamel. *Caries Research*, 26, 290–292.

Gray, A., Ferguson, M.M., Wall, J.G. (1998) Wine tasting and dental erosion. Case report. *Australia Dental Journal*, 43, 32–34.

Grenby, T.H. (1996) Lessening dental erosive potential by product modification. *European Journal of Oral Science*, 104, 221–228.

Hjortsjö, C., Jonski, G., Thrane, P.S., et al. (2009) Effect of stannous fluoride and dilute hydrofluoric acid on early enamel erosion over time in vivo. *Caries Research*, 43, 449–454.

Holbrook, W.P., Hlödversson, S.Ö., Arnarsdottir, E.K., et al. (2010) Assessing tooth erosion using the BEWE index. *Journal of Dental Research*, 89 Special Issue B: abstract 1995.

Holbrook, W.P, Arnadöttir, I.B., Kay, E.J. (2003) Prevention. Part 3: Prevention of tooth wear. *British Dental Journal*, 26, 75–81.

Holbrook, W.P., Furuholm, J., Gudmundsson, K., et al. (2009) Gastric reflux is a significant causative factor of tooth erosion. *Journal of Dental Research*, 88, 422–426.

Holbrook, W.P. and Sæmundsson, S.R. (2006) Analysis of saliva from patients with caries, erosion and xerostomia. *Journal of Dental Research*, 85 Special Issue B, abstract 2449.

Hooper, S.M., Hughes, J.A., et al. (2005) A methodology for testing the erosive potential of sports drinks. *Journal of Dentistry*, 33, 343–348.

Hughes, J.A., West, N.X., Parker, D.M. (1999a) Development and evaluation of a low erosive blackcurrant juice drink in vitro and in situ. 1. Comparison with orange juice. *Journal of Dentistry*, 27, 285–289.

Hughes, J.A., West, N.X., Parker, D.M. (1999b) Development and evaluation of a low erosive blackcurrant juice drink. 3. Final drink and concentrate, formulae comparisons in situ and overview of the concept. *Journal of Dentistry*, 27, 354–350.

Jensdottir, T., Arnadottir, I.B., Thorsdottir, I., et al. (2004) Relationship between dental erosion, soft drink consumption, and gastroesophageal reflux among Icelanders. *Clinical Oral Investigation*, 8, 91–96.

Jensdottir, T., Bardow, A., Holbrook, P. (2005) Properties and modification of soft drinks in relation to their erosive potential in vitro. *Journal of Dentistry*, 33, 569–575.

Jensdottir, T., Buchwald, C., Nauntofte, B., et al. (2009) Erosive potential of calcium-modified acidic candies in irradiated dry mouth patients. *Radiotherapy and Oncology*, 93, 534–538.

Jensdottir, T., Buchwald, C., Nauntofte, B., et al. (2010) Erosive potential of calcium-modified acidic candies in irradiated dry mouth patients. *Oral Health and Preventive Dentistry*, 8, 173–178.

Jensdottir, T., Holbrook, P., Nauntofte, B., et al. (2006) Immediate erosive potential of cola drinks and orange juices. *Journal of Dental Research*, 85, 226–230.

Johansson, A.K., Lingström, P., Imfeld, T., et al. (2004) Influence of drinking method on tooth-surface pH in relation to dental erosion. *European Journal of Oral Science*, 112, 484–489.

Kato, M.T., Leite, A.L., Hannas, A.R., et al. (2010) Gels containing MMP inhibitors prevent dental erosion in situ. *Journal of Dental Research*, 89, 468–472.

Kato, M.T., Magalhães, A.C., Rios, D., et al. (2009) Protective effect of green tea on dentin erosion and abrasion. *Journal of Applied Oral Science*, 17, 560–564.

Lajer, C., Buchwald, C., Nauntofte, B., et al. (2009) Erosive potential of saliva stimulating tablets with and without fluoride in irradiated head and neck cancer patients. *Radiotherapy and Oncology*, 93, 534–538.

Lajer, C., Buchwald, C., Nauntofte, B., et al. (2010) Erosive potential of saliva stimulating tablets with and without fluoride in irradiated head and neck cancer patients. *Oral Health and Preventive Dentistry*, 8, 173–178.

Larsen, M.J. (2001) Prevention by means of fluoride of enamel erosions as caused by soft drinks and orange juice. *Caries Research*, 35, 229–234.

Linkosalo, E. and Markkanen, H. (1985) Dental erosions in relation to lactovegetarian diet. *Scandanavian Journal of Dental Research*, 93, 436–441.

Lussi, A. (1996) Dental erosion clinical diagnosis and case history taking. *European Journal of Oral Science*, 104, 191–198.

Lussi, A. (2006) Erosive tooth wear—a multifactorial condition of growing concern and increasing knowledge. In: *Dental Erosion* (Ed. A. Lussi), pp. 1–8, Monographs in Oral Science 20, Karger, Basel, Switzerland.

Meurman, J.H., Kuittinen, T., Kangas, M., et al. (1998) Buffering effect of antacids in the mouth—a new treatment of dental erosion? *Scandinavian Journal of Dental Research*, 96, 412–417.

Nunn, J.H., Gordon, P.H., Morris, A.J., *et al.* (2003) Dental erosion-changing prevalence? A review of British national childrens' surveys. *International Journal of Paediatric Dentistry*, 13, 98–115.

Nunn, J.H., Ng, S.K., Sharkey, I., *et al.* (2001) The dental implications of chronic use of acidic medicines in medically compromised children. *Pharmacy World and Science*, 23, 118–119.

O'Sullivan, E.A. and Curzon, M.E. (1998) Drug treatments for asthma may cause erosive tooth damage. *British Medical Journal*, 317, 820.

Poggio, C., Lombardini, M., Dagna, A., *et al.* (2009) Protective effect on enamel demineralization of a CCP-ACP paste: an AFM in vitro study. *Journal of Dentistry*, 37, 949–954.

Ranjitkar, S., Kaidonis, J.A., Richards, L.C., *et al.* (2009) The effect of CPP-ACP on enamel wear under severe erosive conditions. *Archives of Oral Biology*, 54, 527–532.

Rytömaa, I., Meurman, J.H., Koskinen, J., *et al.* (1988) In vitro erosion of bovine enamel caused by acidic drinks and other foodstuffs. *Scandinavian Journal of Dental Research*, 96, 324–333.

Schlueter, N., Ganss, C., De Sanctis, S., *et al.* (2005) Evaluation of a profilometrical method for monitoring erosive tooth wear. *European Journal of Oral Science*, 113, 505–511.

Sjögren, K., Lingström, P., Lundberg, A.B. (1997) Salivary fluoride concentration and plaque pH after using a fluoride-containing chewing gum. *Caries Research*, 31, 366–372.

Smith, B.G. and Knight, J.K. (1984) An index for measuring the wear of teeth. *British Dental Journal*, 156, 435–438.

Sorvari, R., Kiviranta, I., Luoma H. (1988) Erosive effect of a sport drink mixture with and without addition of fluoride and magnesium on the molar teeth of rats. *Scandinavian Journal of Dental Research*, 96, 226–231.

Sorvari, R., Meurman, J.H., Alakuijala, P. (1994) Effect of fluoride varnish and solution on enamel erosion in vitro. *Caries Research*, 28, 227–232.

Sundram, G. and Bartlett, D. (2001) Preventive measures for bulimic patients with dental erosion. *European Journal of Prosthodontics and Restorative Dentistry*, 9, 25–29.

Suyama, Y., Takaku, S., Okawa, Y., *et al.* (2010) Dental erosion in workers exposed to sulfuric acid in lead storage battery manufacturing facility. *Bulletin of the Tokyo Dental College*, 51, 77–83.

Þorvaldsdóttir, S.A., Sigurjónsson, J.H., Halldórsdóttir, H., *et al.* (2008) Erosion and soft drinks. *The Icelandic Dental Journal*, 26, 22–24.

Wegehaupt, F.J., Sener, B., Attin, T., *et al.* (2010) Application of cerium chloride to improve the acid resistance of dentine. *Archives of Oral Biology*, 55, 441–446.

West, N.X., Hughes, J.A., Parker, D.M., *et al.* (1999) Development and evaluation of a low erosive blackcurrant juice drink. 2. Comparison with a conventional blackcurrant juice drink and orange juice. *Journal of Dentistry*, 27, 341–344.

West, N.X., Maxwell, A., Hughes, J.A., *et al.* (1998) A method to measure clinical erosion: the effect of orange juice consumption on erosion of enamel. *Journal of Dentistry*, 26, 329–335.

Westergaard, J., Larsen, I.B., Holmen, L., *et al.* (2001) Occupational exposure to airborne proteolytic enzymes and lifestyle risk factors for dental erosion—a cross-sectional study. *Occupational Medicine* (London), 51, 189–197.

Wiegand, A. and Attin, T. (2007) Occupational dental erosion from exposure to acids: a review. *Occupational Medicine*, 57, 169–176.

Wiegand, A., Egert, S., Attin, T. (2008) Toothbrushing before or after an acidic challenge to minimize tooth wear? An in situ/ex vivo study. *American Journal of Dentistry*, 21, 13–6.

Wiegand, A., Hiestand, B., Sener, B., *et al.* (2010) Effect of TiF4, ZrF4, HfF4 and AmF on erosion and erosion/abrasion of enamel and dentin in situ. *Archives of Oral Biology*, 55, 223–228.

14

The etiology, diagnosis, and management of dentin hypersensitivity

Hardy Limeback

Introduction

One of the most common reasons for a patient to complain to the dentist or dental hygienist these days, outside of dissatisfaction with the cosmetic appearance of the teeth, is sensitivity to hot or cold stimuli. The literature describing techniques to reduce tooth sensitivity resulting from the placement of the ever-evolving posterior composite, a porcelain inlay, and a full coverage restoration is vast and will not be discussed in this chapter. The main focus of this chapter is a different kind of dentin sensitivity, most commonly referred to as 'dentin hypersensitivity.' This kind of tooth sensitivity is usually the result of dentin losing the connective tissue layers and surface mineralized tissues that protect it from the oral environment. These protective tissues are enamel, cementum, and the periodontal ligament and attached gingiva. The most common area of the tooth affected is the cervical margin at the cemento-enamel junction (CEJ). This chapter will review in detail what dentin hypersensitivity is, how prevalent it is, what causes it, and what the dental team can do to provide immediate pain relief, long-term pain relief (a 'cure'), and then prevent it from happening again or prevent it from happening in patients at risk.

A tooth that is sensitive to cold stimulus at the gingival margin is an extremely common complaint by patients, particularly after a recent dental procedure such as a dental scaling appointment. Dentin hypersensitivity results primarily from the exposure of opened dentinal tubules on the root surface to the oral environment. By definition, hypersensitivity implies that the tooth is experiencing sensitivity that is greater than the usual sensitivity to various stimuli.

Review articles on dentin hypersensitivity have appeared during the last 2 decades on a regular basis in the dental literature (Cox 1994; Ciancio 1995; Ling and Gillam 1996; Wichgers and Emert 1997; Bartlett and Ide 1999; Bal and Kundalgurki 1999; Orchardson and Gillam 2006). One thorough review examined the efficacy of potassium-containing toothpaste (Poulsen 2009).

Some of these reviews provide a cursory update of the current literature on dentin hypersensitivity. Most provide only a brief overview of the causes and certain treatment protocols for dentin hypersensitivity. This chapter is designed to summarize and expand on these reviews and provide the reader with a more comprehensive, up-to-date analysis of the subject of dentin hypersensitivity.

It is essential to mention that the literature cited in this chapter represents a variety of different levels of evidence. The best evidence that a particular treatment is likely to be effective is from a double-blinded, randomized, placebo-controlled clinical trial that is preferably a prospective and intervention type study. (See Chapter 5 on evidence-based dentistry.)

Prevalence of dentin hypersensitivity

Chabanski and Gillam (1997) summarized the studies where the prevalence, etiology, and oral distribution of dentin hypersensitivity were examined. Dentin hypersensitivity occurred in 8–35% of the population, depending on the population studied and methodology used to evaluate the condition. About 40 million adults in the United States at one time or another and 10 million consider themselves chronically affected, according to

Comprehensive Preventive Dentistry, First Edition. Edited by Hardy Limeback.
© 2012 John Wiley & Sons, Ltd. Published 2012 by John Wiley & Sons, Ltd.

one market survey (Kanapka 1990). In Ireland clinicians studying dentin hypersensitivity examined 250 subjects who reported a sensitivity rate of 57.2%. It occurred most frequently in the 30- to 39-year-old age group (Irwin and McCusker 1997). This was a high prevalence rate compared to previous studies, suggesting that an increase in the levels of sensitivity within the general population had occurred. However, more than half of patients attending general dental practices complained of dentin hypersensitivity at one time or another, usually in the third and fourth decades of life (Gillam et al. 1999). A group in Taiwan found that out of 780 patients exactly half had a history of dentin sensitivity or were experiencing the problem (Liu et al. 1998). Premolars and molars were the most common teeth sensitive to the stimuli; the incisors were the least sensitive.

The highest prevalence of dentin hypersensitivity was reported in a group of periodontal patients. Chabinski et al. (1996) assessed 507 patients attending a periodontal clinic. Eighty-four percent complained of dentin hypersensitivity. This suggests that periodontal disease and/or its treatment plays a significant role in the etiology of dentin hypersensitivity. It seems intuitive that any time a new root surface is exposed through periodontal surgery, one can expect dentin sensitivity to occur, but there are not a lot of studies to show that this is indeed the case. Perhaps simply burnishing the exposed root surface (see below) is enough to avoid acute sensitivity until the root surface builds up permanent resistance to hot or cold stimuli. One should use caution when using the results of just one periodontal practice for extrapolation to the general population. The questionnaire study conducted by Gillam et al. (1999) of general practice patients, for example, showed that about half of the patients complain about dentin hypersensitivity, but it is not a serious concern for them, even for those who had periodontal therapy. For those patients receiving periodontal care, the post-operative hypersensitivity did not last longer than a week. Dentin hypersensitivity seems to be more common in females, but this difference does not reach statistical significance (Addy 1992; Gillam et al. 1999; Rees and Addy 2002). It affects mostly those people in the 3 decades between 20 and 50 years of age (Bissada 1994; Gillam et al. 2002). Addy (1992) reports that people complain about dentin sensitivity more in the winter, and this makes obvious sense since cold air is one of tests for dentin sensitivity (see below). The most common sites of dentin hypersensitivity are the buccal surfaces of the canines and premolars (Addy 1992; Brännström 1992; Hefti and Stone 2000). More than two-thirds of the teeth with reported dentin hypersensitivity have gingival recession, but only 25% have evidence of abrasion, attrition, or erosion (Orchardson and Collins 1987).

Differential diagnosis

Any time dentin is newly exposed, patients with responsive pulp tissues and active afferent nerve endings in the odontoblast layer will complain of sensitivity to cold stimuli (mostly cold liquids). Clinicians can easily find areas of dentin exposed when restorations fail and dislodge. A margin that has lost its bond to the dentin, or a hairline crack in the restoration, may also illicit new sensitivity in a tooth. To distinguish this from dentin hypersensitivity at the cervical margin, one needs only to cover the crack or margin with a cotton roll and use a quick, short blast of compressed air from the air-water syringe directed to the gingival margin. Tooth sensitivity from hyper-occlusion, caries, or periapical osteitis tends to be more of a throbbing, dull ache, instead of an acute, sharp pain. Some patients describe the pain of dentin hypersensitivity as an excruciatingly sharp pain, others, simply an annoyance.

Patients who have recently had amalgam restorations placed may complain of tooth sensitivity, which may subside as metal oxides eventually occlude the narrow metal-to-tooth spaces. The sensitivity may persist in the case of composite resin restorations. The placement of restorations may even make exposed cervical root surfaces more sensitive to air. Bruxism or clenching could confound cervical hypersensitivity as well. One of the most difficult clinical presentations to diagnose is tooth sensitivity from a hairline fracture, or cracked tooth syndrome (Seltzer and Boston 1997). In this situation, a hairline fracture has recently formed and the patient seeks immediate relief from the pain on occlusion. It is fairly simple to pinpoint which cusp is fractured on the molars using a 'tooth sleuth.' When these hairline fractures do not remineralize, the cusp will eventually be lost.

As has already been mentioned, periodontal patients frequently complain of dentin hypersensitivity. The degree to which their dentin is exposed after periodontal therapy will likely determine the degree of discomfort. Older patients usually do not present with dentin hypersensitivity because their dentin tubules have occluded, and the pulp chambers have decreased in size resulting in decreased vascularity, loss of afferent nerve endings, and dentin sclerosis (Dai et al. 1991).

Several other conditions may cause teeth to feel sensitive. These include myofascial pain or temporomandibular disorders, chronic sinusitis, otitis media, and other chronic facial pain syndromes (Sessle 1987). After the clinician has eliminated other sources of sensitivity as the cause of tooth sensitivity, a simple blast of cold air from the air/water syringe will pinpoint the offending root surface.

A summary flow chart (Figure 14-1) on how to diagnose and manage dentin hypersensitivity was

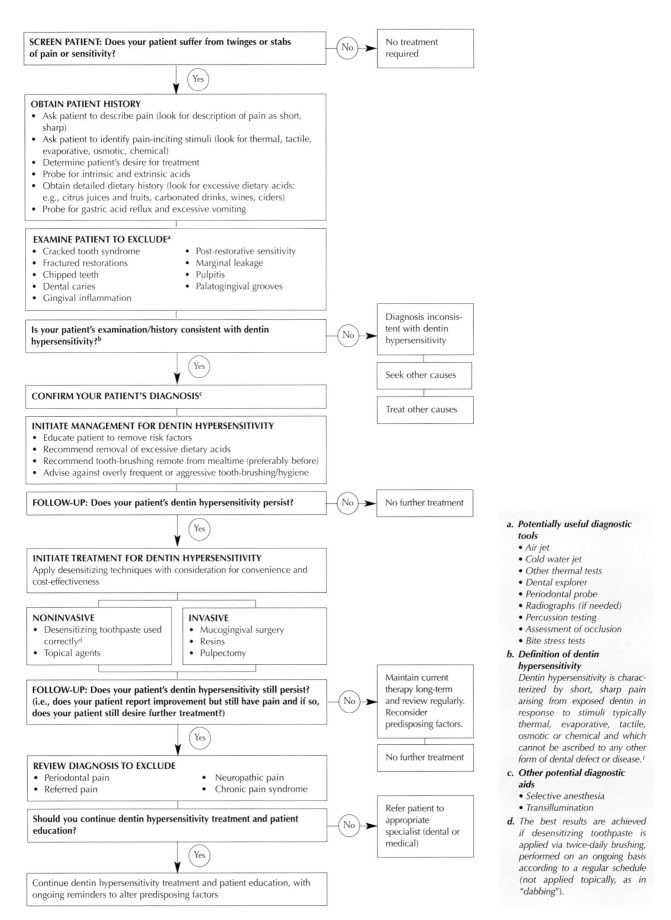

Figure 14-1 Flow chart of Differential Diagnosis of Dentin Hypersensitivity and Management Strategies. Reprinted from Canadian Advisory Board on Dentin Hypersensitivity, 2003, with permission from the Canadian Dental Association.

provided by the Canadian Advisory Board on Dentin Hypersensitivity (2003), and this flow chart was cited in the Journal of the American Dental Association (JADA) article by Orchardson and Gillam (2006).

Assessing the degree of response to stimuli that cause dentin hypersensitivity

Patients will have different responses to mechanical (tactile), chemical, thermal, cold air, cold liquid, thermo-electric, and electric stimuli (reviewed by Gillam and Newman 1993). Researchers in the field have attempted to quantify these responses by means of various pain-response questionnaires, which may include the verbal rating scale, the visual analogue scale, the verbal descriptor checklist, and the McGill pain questionnaire. For the purpose of the differential diagnosis in the practice setting, a simple blast of cold air directed only at the cervical margin where the root surfaces are exposed, and then inquiring about the intensity of the pain, is probably the most common way that a dentist or dental hygienist screens for dentin hypersensitivity. Visual analogue scales or pain questionnaires have not yet been adapted from the clinical research setting to the every day practice setting.

Summary of quick chairside diagnosis

To determine the history of pain, look for the following symptoms:

- Complaints of hot and cold sensitivity (air, beverages, certain foods)
- May be generalized (patient cannot localize)
- Not constant, not 'throbbing,' may even disappear for days or weeks
- Patient may use fingernail to pinpoint area of sensitivity

The clinical examination includes the following:

- Gingival recession
  - May present with abfraction lesion
  - Usually area not covered by plaque or calculus
- Use of an explorer can uncover exposed dentin versus open margins around fillings

The differential examination includes the following:

- Test for cracked tooth syndrome with tooth sleuth, transillumination
- Check hyper-occlusion trauma with articulating paper, percussion
- Check for caries with bitewing radiographs, caries detectors
- Check for periapical inflammation or infection with periapical radiographic views, percussion, pulp testers

The diagnostic strategy includes the following:

- Cover gingival recession with cotton rolls.
- Apply air jet to the occlusal on fillings and interproximally to rule out microleakage of fillings, cracked tooth syndrome.
- Allow the patient to rehydrate the teeth.
- Apply air jet to the gingival margin, 3–5 mm from the surface.
- Move from tooth to tooth to pinpoint the sensitive tooth.
- Repeated stimuli will dampen the response.

Etiology of dentin hypersensitivity

Gingival recession and toothbrush/paste abrasion

The primary consideration to determine the cause of dentin hypersensitivity is to first assess gingival recession and any exposure of the root surface. The most obvious reason for gingival recession is excessive force applied during oral hygiene, but it may also be the result of defective gingival anatomy such as an area of minimal attached gingiva. In one study by Khocht et al. (1993), it was the increasing hardness of the toothbrush bristles that was blamed for excessive gingival recession. In this study, patients who reported hard toothbrush use at home had twice the percentage of surfaces with recession. Nearly one-tenth of gingival surfaces showed signs of recession. The abrasiveness of the dentifrice and the oral hygiene technique used are also likely contributors of gingival recession as well as the use of various oral hygiene aids (West et al. 1998). An exposed root surface in patients with dentin hypersensitivity usually is not covered by plaque; thick plaque would cover the dentinal tubules and prevent an irritating stimulus such as air from disturbing the dentin. See Figure 14-2.

Automatic, electronic toothbrushes have been tested for their propensity to cause gingival abrasion (Van Der Weijden et al. 2001). One study showed that the pressures applied to the gingival, and the amount of toothpaste used, are related to the size of the head of the toothbrush (Boyd et al. 1997). Thus, Rota-Dent seemed to apply the least amount of pressure and toothpaste to oral tissues compared with Oral B and Interplak mechanical toothbrushes and manual toothbrushes. The question of whether hard bristles are more damaging than soft bristles has not been fully established since some studies show that softer brushes with higher density bristles retain more toothpaste. It is, perhaps, the increase in abrasive toothpaste that causes more dentin abrasion (Dyer et al. 2000; Dyer et al. 2001).

If the results of the study by Boyd et al. (1997) are corroborated in other clinical trials, then it would mean that electric toothbrushes would pose less of a risk for

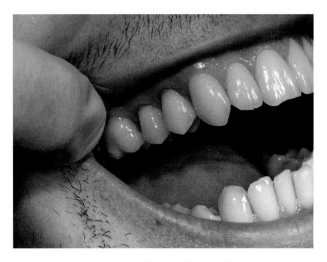

Figure 14-2 A patient complaining of gingival hypersensitivity on the first and second maxillary premolars. This patient was disclosed with Redcote disclosing dye to reveal plaque deposits. Note that the hygiene on the facial surfaces of the premolars is relatively good and that there is interproximal plaque. The dye clearly shows the outline of the cervical root surface that is exposed. (Photo courtesy of Dr. Amir Azarpazhooh)

gingival recession and dentin abrasion than manual toothbrushes, especially if they have smaller heads than regular manual toothbrushes. Electric toothbrushes provide about 7,000 strokes per minute and the sonic brushes about 30,000 strokes per minute of toothbrushing (Engel *et al.* 1993). If gingival recession and dentin abrasion were related to the number of brush strokes performed each day, one would assume that electric brushes provide a higher risk for damage to soft and hard tissues than manual toothbrushes, which would lead to increased dentin hypersensitivity. However, Hefti *et al.* (2000) showed that the Sonicare electric toothbrush was as effective in reducing dentin hypersensitivity as the conventional electric toothbrush. In this study, the overall brushing area covered in each stroke was not compared, and it is not clear why powered toothbrushes would reduce dentin hypersensitivity in the first place. Perhaps the key factor is the delivery of fluoride to the exposed dentin to encourage remineralization of the dentin tubules. More studies will be required to clearly establish whether electric toothbrushes should be used by patients at risk for dentin hypersensitivity.

Oral acid erosion of exposed root surfaces

Progressive erosion of exposed root surfaces by means of intra-oral acids will also result in dentin hypersensitivity. Two main sources of oral acids are gastric acids and acids that are purposely introduced into the oral cavity. Gastric acid may enter the oral cavity as a result of an eating disorder or as a result of an underlying

pathological disorder. Rytomaa *et al.* (2000) found that bulimics had increased tooth sensitivity to cold and touch. Dental erosion was found to be common when there is gastric reflux disease (Lasarchik and Filler 2000), but the authors did not determine how common dentin hypersensitivity was in these patients.

Under normal conditions, dietary acids do not present a problem in terms of causing dental erosion. However, excessive ingestion of citrus fruits or fruit juices, or carbonated soft drinks containing phosphoric acid, has been shown to cause dental erosion (Zero 1996; O'Sullivan and Curzon 2000). Cases of dental erosion have even been documented in wine tasters (Gray *et al.* 1998) and competitive swimmers (Guersten 2000). The effects of these sources of acids are made worse if the patient has an underlying disorder affecting salivary gland function. For example, dental erosion is common in patients with Sjogren's syndrome (Atkinson and Fox 1993).

Vital bleaching and dentin hypersensitivity

Another source of intra-oral acid is carbamide peroxide. Peroxide in aqueous solution will lower the pH when it is chemically activated. In addition to the direct affect on neuronal responses in the pulp (Nathanson 1997), peroxides used for vital tooth bleaching also cause dentin hypersensitivity by demineralizing peritubular dentin and allowing the transport of fluids through the tubules. (See mechanism in the next section.) Price *et al.* (2000) determined the pH produced by various vital bleaching agents, and some of them would obviously demineralize dentin if they were allowed to come in contact with the surface for extended periods of time. However, adding potassium nitrate and fluoride to the vital bleaching gel lessens dentin hypersensitivity (Tam 2001). Fluoride likely minimizes demineralization of the dentin tubules, and potassium nitrate may dampen pulp tissue nerve impulses.

The mechanism involved in the etiology of dentin hypersensitivity

When there is hypersensitivity of the dentin, it could be caused by either inflammatory changes in the pulp or mechanical changes in the patency of dentinal tubules. The most widely accepted mechanism of dentin hypersensitivity is the hydrodynamic theory, first proposed by Gysi in 1900.

The evidence to support this hypothesis was presented by Brännström in 1963. Basically, the mechanism is as follows. Any fluid flow in the dentin tubules, whether to the surface or to the pulp side, that extends throughout the length of the tubules will be registered by the odontoblasts that are closely associated pulp tissue

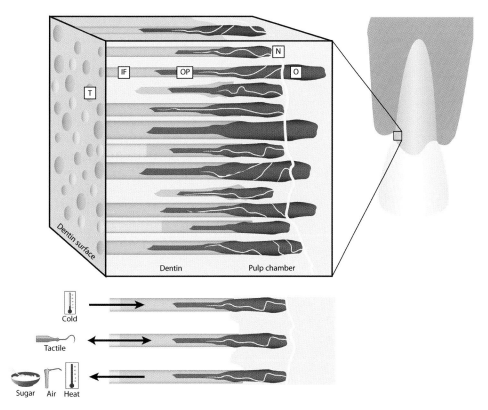

Figure 14-3 Schematic of the mechanism of the hydrodynamic theory. The tooth on the right has dentin exposed. The left diagram shows a schematic magnification of this area showing open dentin tubules (T) on the root surface. Any stimulus that causes movement (depicted by the black arrows) of the intratubular fluid (IF) within the tubule is detected by the odontoblast process (OP), which is in contact with mechanoreceptors of the A-delta nerves (N), which are in intimate contact with the odontoblast layer (O). Hot and cold, tactile, air, and sugar all affect fluid movement.

mechanoreceptor nerves. Any noxious stimulus that can make the intratubular fluid move, such as thermal, tactile, or chemical stimuli near the exposed surface of the tubules, will elicit a response. Where tubules are closed on the surface, these stimuli do not register. Sclerotic dentin is not sensitive; however, it is usually when the dentin tubules are exposed.

A hydrostatic pressure gradient usually occurs from the pulp to the surface, that is, the pulpal pressure is higher than the oral pressure (Pashley 1992). As a result, there is a spontaneous outward flow of dentinal fluid due to the filtration of fluid. However, this spontaneous outward flow is 50 times less than the lowest thresholds for activating mechanoreceptors, initiating action potentials, and causing pain. On the other hand, the dehydrating effect of a blast of air from an air syringe could desiccate the dentin, resulting in a rapid outward movement of fluid in the tubule because of capillary forces at a rate of 2 to 3 mm/sec (Brännström 1992). The rapid outward movements of flow during a 4-minute evaporation application with the air syringe can result in the aspiration of odontoblasts into the dentinal tubules (Brännström 1992). Any time there is a stimulus on the

exposed root surface that can cause fluid movement, mechanoreceptors in the pulp respond. Thus, friction from a bur, or mechanical deformation from the application of an explorer, can make intratubular fluid flow. Solvents, acids, and chemicals dissolve water and 'pull' the intratubular fluid toward the surface. Hygroscopic chemicals such as sucrose and hyperosmotic solutions will also cause fluid movement because they dissolve more water. The sharp pain associated with dentin hypersensitivity occurs when the movement of fluids affects the A-delta nerve fiber endings, which are interwoven with the cells of the odontoblast cell layers (Alquist and Franzen 1999).

When mechanoreceptors detect the movements of dentinal fluid, pressure is transduced by the opening of ion channels, leading to an increase in the flow of sodium ions, thus initiating generator action potentials leading to the perception of pain (Rossman *et al.* 2005).

A summary of the various stimuli and their effects is shown in Figure 14-3.

Since A-delta nerve fibers are myelinated, they are fast conducting nerve fibers. Thus, the typical response to stimulation of the fibers is a sharp and immediate painful response. Changes in the anatomy of the pulp at the odontoblast cell layer, or alterations to tubule morphology, have been studied in an attempt to determine how these changes may affect the response of the pulp to stimuli.

Treatment strategies to manage dentin hypersensitivity

There are several approaches to managing dentin hypersensitivity. Treating the acute pain is the first objective. This is followed up with preventive strategies in an attempt to provide permanent relief to dentin hypersensitivity. Orchardson and Gillam (2006) boil down their recommendations to manage dentin hypersensitivity to three main recommended strategies in their JADA paper.

1. Avoid the painful stimulus.
2. Occlude the dentin tubules in the following ways:
   o plugging the tubule openings
   o increasing the intra-tubular dentin mineralization
   o inducing tertiary dentin formation
3. Decrease intradental nerve excitability.

An understanding of the biology of dentin and the effects of various treatments on the response of the pulp to external stimuli will aid in the treatment of dentin sensitivity. The long-range goal of the dental practitioner is to, of course, encourage permanent relief from dentin hypersensitivity. Apart from taking last resort and aggressive steps such as root canal therapy or extraction, long-term results will be attained if the tooth is allowed to 'heal' naturally. This is achieved by permanently occluding the surface's opening of the dentin tubules and by reducing the size of the dentin tubules so that fluid movement is limited in the future. This will reduce the dependency on agents that simply mask the symptoms of dentin hypersensitivity. It is important, however, to provide immediate relief to patients when their chief complaint is pain from dentin hypersensitivity. While the acute pain is being managed, the dentist can also work to prove long-term, more permanent solutions to the problem.

Providing immediate relief in the dental office

The primary goal of treating patients with acute dentin hypersensitivity is to immediately relieve their discomfort. This is particularly true for patients who specifically seek dental treatment on an emergency basis for dentin hypersensitivity. The health care professional has several options including procedures that occlude the openings of the exposed dentin tubules or procedures that cover the dentin tubules and protect the exposed surfaces from further stimuli. Ideally, treatment of acute dentin hypersensitivity should be with a procedure that is easy to apply, rapid in its effectiveness, non-invasive, and provides permanent relief. Patients lose confidence in the practitioner who continues to apply a therapy that does not prove to be effective. As a last resort, of course, drastic measures that include restorations, periodontal surgery, root canal therapy, and even extraction of the offending tooth have all been carried out in an attempt to find immediate relief to the dentin hypersensitivity. It is obviously in the dental practitioner's best interest to use the most effective, non-invasive technique to manage acute pain from dentin hypersensitivity before these last resort measures are undertaken.

Burnishing the root surface

Although long-term relief from dentin sensitivity involving abrasives in toothpaste and mechanical burnishing of the dentin tubules may to be important, attempting to burnish the dentin tubules with a blunt periodontal scaler or a ball burnisher will likely be ineffective as an 'emergency' procedure in the dental office setting.

Occluding dentin tubules with chemical precipitates

Several chemical combinations have been used in an attempt to immediately seal the dentin tubules in patients suffering from acute dentin hypersensitivity. These include calcium phosphates, strontium chloride, potassium oxalate, and ferric oxalate. In the dental office, the practitioner usually applies the solution directly to the exposed surface. In a split-mouth placebo-controlled trial, calcium phosphates had mixed results and may not be any more effective than placebo (Yates et al. 1998).

Strontium chloride has been tested with success for immediate treatment of dentin sensitivity (Kishore et al. 2002). Strontium has an affinity for mineralized tissues, and its chloride salt tends to precipitate on the surface of dentin tubules to occlude the openings (Pearce et al. 1994). Strontium has been an active ingredient in the original Sensodyne dentifrice formulation for some time.

The oxalates have been extensively tested and have been shown to provide immediate relief. There is a concern, however, that abrasion will remove the precipitates in a short time following application, resulting in a return to hypersensitivity when the tubules become unblocked. In one study (Ling et al. 1997), investigators showed that ferric oxalate (Sensodyne Sealant) penetrates deeper into dentin tubules than potassium oxalate (Butler Protect) and may, therefore, provide longer-lasting relief from dentin hypersensitivity. The effect of these precipitates on the retention of restorations bonded directly to the treated dentin was studied, and it was found that the oxalate precipitates reduced the bond strength of glass ionomer restorations (Haveman and Charlton 1994).

This is important to note especially when a restoration becomes the treatment option after more conservative approaches have failed. There are no studies to determine how long after these treatments that restorations can be placed without affecting the retention negatively.

In a recent review, Cunha-Cruz et al. (2011) concluded that only monohydrogen monopotassium oxalate showed any significant reduction in dentin hypersensitivity.

Lasers

The use of lasers in treating dentin hypersensitivity is a novel approach. The concept is a simple one. The laser is used to thermally decompose the surface mineral, denature the protein, vaporize the water, and release carbonate. Re-deposition of mineral will not only ablate the dentin tubules, but the mineral will be more resistant to further erosion. There have been some properly conducted clinical trials to test the effectiveness of various lasers for the treatment of dentin hypersensitivity. For example, Gerschman et al. (1994) reduced dentin sensitivity with the Galium/Aluminum/Arsenide laser in a double-blind study. Lan and Lui (1996) and Yonaga et al. (1999) used the Nd:YAG laser and Moritz et al. (1996) used the CO_2 laser to effectively reduce dentin hypersensitivity. The same group assessed neodymium: yttrium-aluminum-garnet lasers for dentin desensitization (Gutknecht et al. 1997). Because lasers effectively alter dentin surface mineral at very high temperatures (500–1,300°C), there is a concern that despite the extremely brief pulses and minimal penetration into dentin, the laser may injure the pulp (Zhang et al. 1998). Some studies have already demonstrated that the laser induces micro-cracks on the mineral surface, which may contribute to further microleakage and sensitivity (Fried et al. 1997; Kimura et al. 2000).

This has yet to be addressed in careful clinical studies. There is also a concern about the reproducibility in dentin hypersensitivity clinical studies, which would make testing of the efficacy of this modality and a comparison to standard technique more difficult (Ide et al. 2001). This is perhaps why the laser is being tested in conjunction with conventional chemical therapy to see if the laser can improve the effectiveness of the chemical treatments (Moritz et al. 1998; Lan et al. 1999).

Bonding agents

Ever since bonding agents were used to decrease dentin sensitivity under restorations, they have become more popular in the treatment of cervical hypersensitivity. The strategy with these agents is to provide a long-term blockage of the surface dentin tubules and protect the dentin surface from further erosion. Thus, products that achieve effective bonding to dentin under restorations should all be effective in providing immediate relief to dentin hypersensitivity. Davidson and Suzuki (1997) and Schupbach et al. (1997) discussed the usefulness of the Gluma bonding system for treating dentin hypersensitivity, particularly since it was designed to replace the desensitizing agents that contained the toxin glutaraldehyde. Gillam et al. (1997) compared the effectiveness of All-Bond with Butler Protect and found little difference between the two because of the placebo effect. Browning et al. (1997) was unable to show that Amalgabond Plus was better than Copalite varnish at reducing sensitivity to cold air 1 week after treatment. Zhang et al. (1999) were able to show that Pain-Free¯ Desensitizer effectively blocked dentin permeability. Morris et al. (1999), however, were unable to show that this agent worked any better at reducing dentin hypersensitivity than a 0.7% fluoride solution (DentinBloc) or the placebo. Other dentin bonding agents have been tested (Ide et al. 1998; Dondi dall'Orologio et al. 1999; Ferrari et al. 1999) to varying degrees of success.

A meta-analysis will not be able to make sense of the variety of results from these studies. The placebo effect is so strong that it is impossible at this stage to place any value for one particular treatment over the other until head-to-head studies of various bonding agents, fluoride therapies, or topical solutions are carried out relative to a placebo treatment. There is no one bonding agent that stands out in terms of its effectiveness against dentin hypersensitivity.

Iontophoresis

Parkell used to distribute the 'Desensitron' for reducing dentin hypersensitivity. This instrument is not well known to North American dentists but was popular in some other countries. When contacted, the manufacturer responded with the following: "Unfortunately, the Desensitron has been discontinued. It was a battery-powered, iontophoretic device that drove the (fluoride) ions from a 2% NaFl solution onto a tooth's surface. The device did not utilize potassium nitrate. The device became unpopular in the marketplace since desensitization may be accomplished by what are perceived to be simpler means."

Long-term therapy and home care

Potassium nitrate

One of the most popular ways to treat dentin hypersensitivity on an ongoing basis is for the patient to switch their regular toothpaste to one that contains 5% potassium nitrate. (See Figure 14-4.)

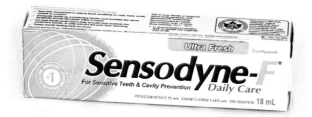

Figure 14-4 The current Sensodyne formulation sold in Canada. This product has been awarded the Canadian Dental Association (CDA) Seal of Recognition for sensitivity protection. The CDA Seal of Recognition is based on the same criteria as the ADA Seal of Acceptance.

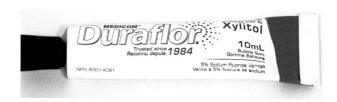

Figure 14-5 Duraflor Varnish (a product available in Canada and the US). This varnish can be dispensed on a pad and applied directly to the cervical margins with a brush or cotton tip applicator. Individual doses are now available. There are many fluoride varnishes on the market today. The FDA has approved them for the treatment of dentin sensitivity but not for caries control (see the chapter on fluorides).

Several clinical trials have been conducted using this formulation to determine if toothpastes with potassium nitrate are more effective than placebo in reducing dentin hypersensitivity, but a recent meta-analysis of eight clinical trials failed to show that there was any efficacy of this active ingredient (Poulsen *et al.* 2001). This contrasts the conclusion made by Orchardson and Gillam (2000), who did not do a meta-analysis. No one yet has any proof that potassium affects dentin hypersensitivity; however, McCormack and Davies (1996) proposed a 'nitric oxide second messenger' mechanism as to how potassium ions might attenuate the response of the A-delta fibers in pulp. Peacock and Orchardson (1999) found that potassium citrate and nitrates work equally well to attenuate nerve impulses, but oxalate lowers the ability of potassium to reduced nerve conductance. Given that there is biological evidence that potassium salts attenuate pulp nerve impulses, the Cochrane meta-analysis likely points out just how difficult it is to 'prove' clinically that a desensitizing agent is effective, rather than offering an 'in-depth' analysis as to whether it is actually no better than placebo. As with many other medicinal treatments, investigators studying active ingredients in toothpaste have not yet been able to reduce the placebo effect to a level that allows proper investigation of the effect of potassium nitrate on dentin hypersensitivity. There are so many variables affecting clinical trials that the Cochrane analysis should be interpreted 'with a grain of (potassium) salt.' Nevertheless, the advantage of using potassium salts in toothpastes or mouth rinses on a daily basis is that mild relief is likely attained, and in the presence of topical fluoride sources and salivary mineral, the dentin tubules eventually mineralize naturally resulting in long-term relief. The only way to determine this, however, is to return to the use of regular toothpaste without potassium nitrate using properly conducted cross-over and split-mouth studies to see if symptoms return. These kinds of studies have not been done carefully.

Slow-release fluoride

Since the main goal of long-term therapy is to encourage the natural mineralization of the dentin tubules, several attempts have been made to introduce slow-release agents or devices into the oral cavity to manage dentin hypersensitivity. These include, of course, the various fluoride-fortified resins materials (Tavares *et al.* 1994), glass-ionomer cements (Hansen 1992), and fluoride varnishes (Hansen 1992; Gaffar *et al.* 1999; Kielbassa *et al.* 2001). Figure 14-5 shows a product that is commonly sold directly to dentists through dental supply companies.

In a well-conducted clinical trial, an acrylic device designed to release fluoride at 0.04 mg/day, successfully reduced dentin hypersensitivity in periodontal patients after surgery compared with patients who wore the placebo device (Marini *et al.* 2000).

Successful application of the bonding agents, glass ionomer cements, and other sealing agents may require isolation of the area that is sensitive. Often the area of the root just apical to the cemento-enamel junctions may not be exposed to the environment, and yet it is still exquisitely sensitive. Retraction chord can be used to maximize the application of the sealant to the exposed root. See Figure 14-6.

Additional home care products designed to treat dentin hypersensitivity

Many formulations of toothpastes have been developed to treat dentin hypersensitivity. Sensodyne's strontium chloride formulation was designed to block dentin tubules and seemed to perform as well as the other desensitizing toothpastes in a double-blind study (Collins *et al.* 1984). Since it does not contain fluoride, this toothpaste may not provide a long-term solution to the problem. Strontium acetate has also been tested and compared with other formulations, and it did not perform any better (West *et al.* 1997). A 0.4% concentration of stannous fluoride as an active ingredient in toothpaste

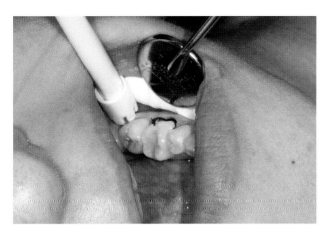

Figure 14-6 Retraction chord in place prior to administering a sealant to the exposed root surface of a mandibular molar.

and brush-on gels (for example, GelKam) can provide both dentin tubule-occluding effects for immediate relief and long-term effectiveness because of the fluoride content (Miller *et al.* 1994; Thrash *et al.* 1994; Luchese *et al.* 1997). A toothpaste (Enamelon), specifically designed to combine fluoride and calcium at the tooth surface to treat caries, has also been tested for its effectiveness in treating dentin hypersensitivity and showed promise (Kaufman *et al.* 1999).

Recently a new system of professional and home application has been introduced in North America called 'ProArgin' (Colgate Oral Pharmaceuticals) (Figure 14-7). Pro-ArginTM/MC Technology, contains calcium carbonate and arginine, an amino acid naturally found in saliva that provides protective oral health benefits. Arginine and calcium carbonate in the Pro-Argin[TM/MC] Technology bind to the dentin surface. This helps attract a calcium-rich layer into the dentin tubules to effectively plug and seal them. The layer resists acids, such as low pH beverages. There appears to be immediate relief with statistically better results than the placebo abrasive toothpaste containing 1,450 ppm fluoride (Fu *et al.* 2010).

Eventual success in managing dentin hypersensitivity will, of course, depend on how to control destructive behavior leading to gingival recession. Some authors believe that changing tooth brushing habits rather than the toothpaste will be more likely to help control dentin hypersensitivity (Bergstrom and Lavstedt 1979); however, the accumulated evidence in the laboratory suggests that the more abrasive the toothpaste, the more likely it will cause gingival recession and exposure of the dentin tubules on the root surfaces (Desautels and Labreche 1988; Addy *et al.* 1991). Unfortunately, there are not very many studies that clinically assess the abrasivity of dentifrices; most of the studies so far have been conducted in the laboratory on acrylic blocks or

dentin slices under controlled laboratory conditions. Nevertheless, these laboratory studies suggest that silica-base gel toothpastes are less abrasive than regular toothpastes, but they are more abrasive than carbonate-based toothpastes.

The main problem in determining the long-term efficacy of a dentifrice in the treatment of dentin hypersensitivity is being able to document how effective the product really is and whether it can be compared to other effective means of treating dentin hypersensitivity. There are now guidelines on how to properly conduct a clinical trial on dentin hypersensitivity (Gillam 1997; Holland *et al.* 1997; FDI Commission 1997).

The application of ozone in the management of dentin hypersensitivity

The application of ozone in the treatment of DH was described more than 50 years ago (Ciriello 1955). There have been some anecdotal reports from the KaVo Company (the manufacturer of HealOzone technology) that HealOzone can be used to manage DH, but it wasn't until this century that ozone was investigated for its effectiveness in treating dentin hypersensitivity. In his groundbreaking book, Bocci (2005) suggests that ozone not only prevents infection but also stimulates the synthesis of fibronectin, collagen, hyaluranic acid, and chondroitin sulphate (all important organic molecules in the formation of tertiary dentin).

In a recent study using a crossover prospective design that evaluated the efficacy of HealOzone at 1,600 ppm for 60 seconds in the treatment of DH, the subjects' pain levels were reduced by about half immediately after the ozone treatment; however, over time, there was no statistically significant difference in pain reduction between the ozone-treated teeth and non-treated teeth (Millar and Hodson 2007). In a randomized triple-blinded clinical trial (the examiners, patients, and statistician were blinded to the test versus control until after the trial). Azarpazhooh and Limeback (2009) failed to show that ozone achieved a higher degree of desensitization than air. Nevertheless, all subjects, both test and control, reported improvements of up to 50% in dentin hypersensitivity, confirming once again how difficult dentin desensitization trials can be in separating real effects from powerful placebo effects.

Additional therapies not yet fully explored

An area that has not been investigated for the long-term therapy of dentin hypersensitivity is the use of professional topical fluorides used by the patient on a daily basis for home use. Also, the use of custom trays in which 1.0% neutral sodium fluoride is applied (for example,

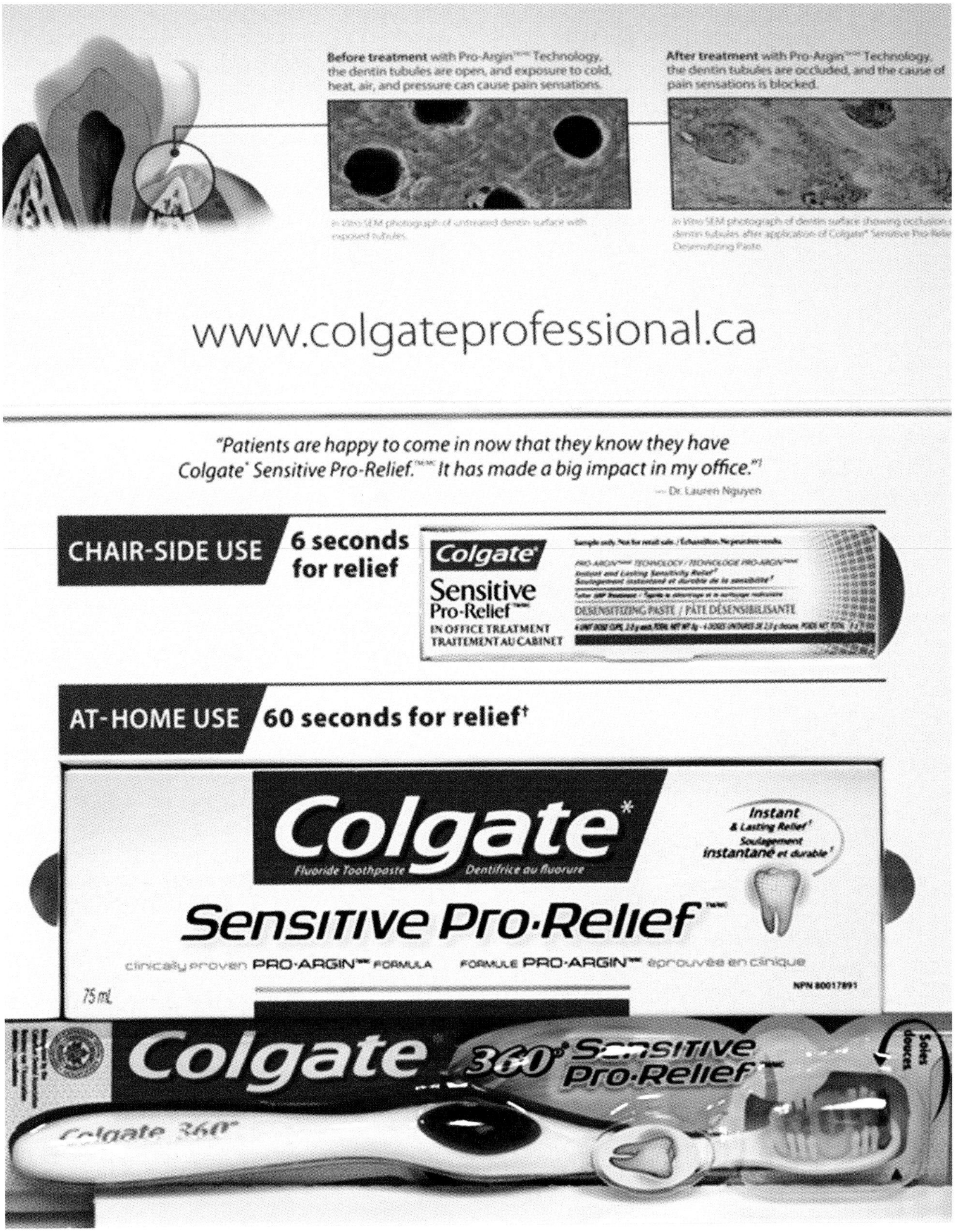

Figure 14-7 A new system for managing dentin hypersensitivity: Colgate Sensitive Pro-Relief with ProArgin technology. Used with permission from Colgate Oral Pharmaceuticals.

Prevident) may be an alternative approach in treating those patients who simply do not respond to conventional therapies. Combination therapies should also be considered and will likely be more successful than single procedures. For example, a new product, Fluoridex (Discus Dental), contains 1.1% neutral NaF (5,000 ppm) and 5% potassium nitrate. Additionally, clinicians should consider doing everything possible. For example, start by using a non-invasive bonding agent to seal the tubules. This should be accompanied by an alteration in the destructive oral hygiene habits (for example, changing to an electric toothbrush with a small head, using less abrasive toothpaste). Finally, patients may be placed on repeated topical fluoride regimens for application at home. If these combination approaches fail, the dentist may be facing a pulpitis that may not be reversible.

When all else fails...

For those patients where there is irreversible loss of attached gingiva at the cervical margin, consideration should be made placing a free gingival graft over the exposed area. There have not been any good clinical trials to demonstrate how effective this technique is in treating dentin hypersensitivity in comparison to conventional techniques. When cervical dentin hypersensitivity results in irreversible pulpitis, the dentist must obviously consider the ultimate solution to the problem, which may involve large restorations, root canal therapy, or even extraction. These are, unfortunately, very invasive solutions to what may seem to be a simple problem, but patients who are unable to tolerate the pain from hypersensitive teeth may be ready for this therapy when all else has failed.

The most common treatments used in clinical practice

Cunha-Cruz *et al.* (2010) published a study where she and her cohorts surveyed dentists to find out what they considered the most effective treatments of dentin hypersensitivity. Dentists found fluoride products such as fluoride varnishes to be the group of products most successful. Second was the use of bonging agents in general and products such as Gluma desensitizing agent (Heraeus Kulser). Gluma's patented Glutaraldehyde/HEMA formula seals dentinal tubules, and also inhibits the growth of bacteria. Third, MI Paste and MI Paste Plus were being used as a successful treatment of dentin hypersensitivity.

Why it is so difficult to prove interventions can be successful?

Currently no single technique uniformly and reliably measures pain from dentin hypersensitivity in a clinical trial. Visual Analogue Scales (VAS) can be useful in measuring relief after therapy. They are objective, easy to use, sensitive to treatment effects, and sufficiently reproducible to indicate that dentin hypersensitivity has been reduced. There are no ordinal scores. The data derived from VAS tests are continuous and can be analyzed by using parametric statistical techniques.

Several factors in DH clinical trials might compound the study outcomes and obscure any particular effect of the testing product on tooth hypersensitivity. The following factors are included:

- A strong placebo effect
- Spontaneous 'healing' during the clinical trial
- Large variations of symptoms
- Hawthorne Effect (The behavior of the subjects change because they are involved in a clinical trial and are under observation.)
- Experimental Subordination (Subjects want to do well in a trial and report improvement even when there is none; this contributes to the placebo effect.)

Prevention strategies in avoiding dentin hypersensitivity

This area of clinical practice has not received much attention in terms of experimental studies. There are obviously things that a clinician can do to reduce the prevalence of dentin hypersensitivity by managing the causes of the problem. For example, where there is heavy occlusion or bruxism, adjusting the bite and relieving the tooth under heavy occlusion will lessen the progression of the problem, and potentially relieve the symptoms. Changing oral hygiene habits from aggressive anterior-posterior scrubbing with a firm toothbrush to a gentle roll technique with a soft toothbrush is another approach. Reducing dietary acid exposure (Chapter 13 on erosion) is something that is also under the control of the patient. For example, avoiding acidic fruit drinks such as apple and grapefruit drinks, or substituting them with calcium fortified, high pH drinks (such as milk) will go a long way to reduce loss of mineral from the surface of the dentinal tubules. Referring patients to a specialist to cope with eating disorders could help much more than simply applying fluorides to treat the symptoms. Finally, good oral hygiene with a low-abrasive fluoridated toothpaste is a good strategy to avoid ending up with dentin hypersensitivity in the first place.

Conclusion

The dental practitioner has many effective therapies from which to choose in managing the often-frustrating condition known as 'dentin hypersensitivity.' An attempt should be made to treat acute pain in the dental office and then seek a long-term solution to this problem. Intervention strategies should be initiated in an attempt to prevent further exposure of cervical root structures and further abrasion of already exposed root structures. Very often, in the presence of ongoing gingival recession, dentin abrasion or erosion or parafunction that cannot be eliminated, long-term fluoride therapy will help in promoting a permanent cure that, ultimately, involves encouraging the natural mineralization of the dentin tubules.

Disclaimer and conflict of interest statement

The author's interest in dentin hypersensitivity stems from his experience in his own private dental practice. The author has no financial interest in any of the products mentioned in this chapter. In 2005 he and his graduate student (A. Azarpazhooh) were provided by CurOzone with the funds to test the HealOzone unit and its proposed effectiveness in reducing dentin hypersensitivity. This study certainly is not the last word on the use of ozone to treat dentin hypersensitivity: other studies are needed and will provide clinicians with more guidance as to whether this modality is safe and effective in the management of dentin hypersensitivity.

References

Addy, M. (1992) Clinical aspects of dentine hypersensitivity. *Proceedings of the Finnish Dental Society*, 88(Suppl I), 23–30.

Addy, M., Goodfield, S., Harrison, A. (1991) The use of acrylic to compare the abrasivity and stain removal properties of toothpastes. *Clinical Materials*, 7, 219–225.

Ahlquist, M. and Franzen, O. (1999) Pulpal ischemia in man: effects on detection threshold, A-delta neural response and sharp dental pain. *Endodontics and Dental Traumatology*, 15, 6–16.

Atkinson, J.C. and Fox, P.C. (1993) Sjogren's syndrome: oral and dental considerations. *Journal of the American Dental Association*, 124, 74–86, 78–82, 84–86.

Azarpazhooh, A., Limeback, H., Lawrence, H.P., et al. (2009) Evaluating the effect of an ozone delivery system on the reversal of dentin hypersensitivity: a randomized, double-blinded clinical trial. *Journal of Endodontics*, 35, 1–9.

Bal, J. and Kundalgurki, S. (1999) Tooth sensitivity prevention and treatment. Oral Health, 89, 33–34, 37–38, 41.

Bartlett, D.W. and Ide, M. (1999) Dealing with sensitive teeth. *Primary Dental Care*, 6, 25–27.

Bergstrom, J. and Lavstedt, S. (1979) An epidemiologic approach to toothbrushing and dental abrasion. *Community Dentistry and Oral Epidemiology*, 7, 57–64.

Bissada, N.F. (1994) Symptomatology and clinical features of hypersensitive teeth. Archives of Oral Biology, 39, 31S–32S.

Bocci, V. (2005) *Ozone. A new Medical Drug.* p. 34. Springer, Dordrecht, The Netherlands.

Boyd, R.L., McLey, L., Zahradnik, R. (1997) Clinical and laboratory evaluation of powered electric toothbrushes: in vivo determination of average force for use of manual and powered toothbrushes. *Journal of Clinical Dentistry*, 8(3 Spec No), 72–75.

Brännström, M. (1992) Etiology of dentin hypersensitivity. *Proceedings of the Finnish Dental Society*, 88(Suppl I), 7–13.

Brännström, M. (1963) Dentin sensitivity and aspiration of odontoblasts. *Journal of the American Dental Association*, 66, 366–370.

Browning, W.D., Johnson, W.W., Gregory, P.N. (1997) Reduction of postoperative pain: a double-blind, randomized clinical trial. *Journal of the American Dental Association*, 128, 1661–1667.

Canadian Advisory Board on Dentin Hypersensitivity. (2003) Consensus based recommendations for the diagnosis and management of dentin hypersensitivity. *Journal of the Canadian Dental Association*, 69, 221–226.

Chabanski, M.B. and Gillam, D.G. (1997) Aetiology, prevalence and clinical features of cervical dentine sensitivity. *Journal of Oral Rehabilitation*, 24, 15–19.

Chabanski, M.B., Gillam, D.G., Bulman, J.S. et al. (1996) Prevalence of cervical dentine sensitivity in a population of patients referred to a specialist Periodontology Department. *Journal of Clinical Periodontology*, 23, 989–992.

Ciancio, S.G. (1995) Chemical agents: plaque control, calculus reduction and treatment of dentinal hypersensitivity. *Periodontology 2000*, 8, 75–86.

Ciriello, G. (1955) Ozone and dentinal sensitivity. *Rivista Italiano Stomatologica*, 10, 159–164.

Collins, J.F. and Perkins, L. (1984) Clinical evaluation of the effectiveness of three dentifrices in relieving dentin sensitivity. *Journal of Periodontology*, 55, 720–725.

Cox, C.F. (1994) Etiology and treatment of root hypersensitivity. *American Journal of Dentistry*, 7, 266–270.

Cunha-Cruz, J., Stout, J.R., Heaton, L.J., et al. (2011) Dentin hypersensitivity and oxalates: a systematic review. *Journal of Dental Research*, 90, 304–310.

Cunha-Cruz, J., Wataha, J.C., Zhou, L., et al. (2010) Treating dentin hypersensitivity: therapeutic choices made by dentists of the northwest PRECEDENT network. *Journal of the American Dental Association*, 141, 1097–1105.

Dai, X.F., Ten Cate, A.R., Limeback, H. (1991) The extent and distribution of intratubular collagen fibrils in human dentine. *Archives Oral Biology*, 36, 775–778.

Davidson, D.F. and Suzuki, M. (1997) The Gluma bonding system: a clinical evaluation of its various components for the treatment of hypersensitive root dentin *Journal of the Canadian Dental Association*, 63, 38–41.

Desautels, P. and Labreche, H. (1988) Abrasion relative des dentrifices—un dentifrice pour chacun. *Le Journale Dentaire du Quebec*, 25, 65–74.

Dondi dall'Orologio, G., Lorenzi, R., Anselmi, M., et al. (1999) Dentin desensitizing effects of Gluma Alternate, Health-Dent Desensitizer and Scotchbond Multi-Purpose. *American Journal of Dentistry*, 12, 103–106.

Dyer, D., Addy, M., Newcombe, R.G. (2000) Studies in vitro of abrasion by different manual toothbrush heads and a standard toothpaste. *Journal of Clinical Periodontology*, 27, 99–103.

Dyer, D., MacDonald, E., Newcombe, R.G., et al. (2001) Abrasion and stain removal by different manual toothbrushes and brush actions: studies in vitro. *Journal of Clinical Periodontlogy*, 2, 121–127.

Engel, D., Nessly, M., Morton, T., et al. (1993) Safety testing of a new electronic toothbrush. *Journal of Periodontology*, 64, 941–946.

FDI Commission (1999) Guidance on the assessment of the efficacy of toothpastes. Work Project (8–95). *International Dental Journal*, 49, 311–316.

Ferrari, M., Cagidiaco, M.C., Kugel, G., *et al.* (1999) Clinical evaluation of a one-bottle bonding system for desensitizing exposed roots. *American Journal of Dentistry*, 12, 243–249.

Fried, D., Glena, R.E., Featherstone, J.D.B., *et al.* (1997) Permanent and transient changes in the reflectance of CO_2 laser irradiated dental hard tissues at lambda = 9.3, 9.6, 10.3, and 10.6 microns and at fluences of $1–20 J/cm^2$. *Lasers in Surgery and Medicine*, 20, 22–31.

Fu, Y., Li, X., Que, K., *et al.* (2010) Instant dentin hypersensitivity relief of a new desensitizing dentifrice containing 8.0% arginine, a high cleaning calcium carbonate system and 1450 ppm fluoride: a 3-day clinical study in Chengdu, China. *America Journal of Dentistry*, 20A–26A.

Gaffar, A. (1999) Treating hypersensitivity with fluoride varnish. *Compendium of Continuing Education in Dentistry*, 20 (1 Spec No), 27–33.

Gerschman, J.A., Ruben, J., Gebart-Eaglemont, J. (1994) Low level laser therapy for dentinal tooth hypersensitivity. *Australian Dental Journal*, 39, 353–357.

Gillam, D.G., Aris, A., Bulman, J.S. (2002) Dentine hypersensitivity in subjects recruited for clinical trials: clinical evaluation, prevalence and intra-oral distribution. *Journal of Oral Rehabilitation*, 29, 226–231.

Gillam, D.G., Coventry, J.F., Manning, R.H., *et al.* (1997) Comparison of two desensitizing agents for the treatment of cervical dentine sensitivity. *Endodontics and Dental Traumatology*, 13, 36–39.

Gillam, D.G. and Newman, H.N. (1993) Assessment of pain in cervical dentinal sensitivity studies. A review. *Journal of Clinical Periodontology*, 20, 383–394.

Gillam, D.G., Seo, H.S., Bulman, J.S., *et al.* (1999) Perceptions of dentine hypersensitivity in a general practice population. *Journal of Oral Rehabilitation*, 26, 710–714.

Gray, A., Ferguson, M.M., Wall, J.G. (1998) Wine tasting and dental erosion. Case report. *Australian Dental Journal*, 43, 32–34.

Guersten, W. (2000) Rapid general dental erosion by gas-chlorinated swimming pool water. Review of the literature and case report. *American Journal of Dentistry*, 13, 291–293.

Gutknecht, N., Moritz, A., Dercks, H.W., *et al.* (1997) Treatment of hypersensitive teeth using neodymium:yttrium-aluminum-garnet lasers: a comparison of the use of various settings in an in vivo study. *Journal of Clinical Laser Medicine and Surgery*, 15, 171–174.

Gysi, A. (1900) An attempt to explain the sensitiveness of dentine. *British Journal of Science*, 43, 865–868.

Hansen, E.K. (1992) Dentin hypersensitivity treated with a fluoride-containing varnish or a light-cured glass-ionomer liner. *Scandinavian Journal of Dental Research*, 100, 305–309.

Haveman, C.W. and Charlton, D.G. (1994) Dentin treatment with an oxalate solution and glass ionomer bond strength. *America Journal of Dentistry*, 7, 247–251.

Hefti, A.F. and Stone, C. (2000) Power toothbrushes, gender, and dentin hypersensitivity. *Clinical Oral Investigation*, 4, 91–97.

Holland, G.R., Narhi, M.N., Addy, M., *et al.* (1997) Guidelines for the design and conduct of clinical trials on dentine hypersensitivity. *Journal of Clinical Periodontology*, 24, 808–813.

Ide, M., Morel, A.D., Wilson, R.F., *et al.* (1998) The role of a dentine-bonding agent in reducing cervical dentine sensitivity. *Journal of Clinical Periodontology*, 25, 286–290.

Ide, M., Wilson, R.F., Ashley, F.P. (2001) The reproducibility of methods of assessment for cervical dentine hypersensitivity. *Journal of Clinical Periodontology*, 28, 16–22.

Irwin, C.R. and McCusker, P. (1997) Prevalence of dentine hypersensitivity in a general dental population. *Journal of the Irish Dental Association*, 43, 7–9.

Kanapka, J.A. (1990) Over-the-counter dentifrices in the treatment of tooth hypersensitivity. Review of clinical studies. *Dental Clinics of North America*, 34, 545–560.

Kaufman, H.W., Wolff, M.S., Winston, A.E., *et al.* (1999) Clinical evaluation of the effect of a remineralizing toothpaste on dentinal sensitivity. *Journal of Clinical Dentistry*, 10(1 Spec No), 50–54.

Khocht, A., Simon, G., Person, P. (1993) Gingival recession in relation to history of hard toothbrush use. *Journal of Periodontology*, 9, 900–905.

Kielbassa, A.M., Attin, T., Hellwig, E., *et al.* (2001) In vivo study on the effectiveness of a lacquer containing CaF2/NaF in treating dentine hypersensitivity. *Clinical Periodontology*, 28, 121–127.

Kimura, Y., Wilder-Smith, P., Yonaga, K. (2000) Treatment of dentine hypersensitivity by lasers: a review. *Journal of Periodontology*, 10, 715–721.

Kishore, A., Mehrotra, K.K., Saimbi, C.S. (2002) Effectiveness of desensitizing agents. *Journal of Endodontics*, 28, 34–35.

Lan, W.H. and Liu, H.C. (1996) Treatment of dentin hypersensitivity by Nd:YAG laser. *Journal of Clinical Laser Medicine and Surgery*, 14, 89–92.

Lan, W.H., Liu, H.C., Lin, C.P. (1999) The combined occluding effect of sodium fluoride varnish and Nd:YAG laser irradiation on human dentinal tubules. *Journal of Endodontics*, 25, 424–426.

Lazarchik, D.A. and Filler, S.J. (2000) Dental erosion: predominant oral lesion in gastroesophageal reflux disease. *American Journal of Gastroenterology*, 95(8 Suppl), S33–S38.

Ling, T.Y. and Gillam, D.G. (1996) The effectiveness of desensitizing agents for the treatment of cervical dentine sensitivity (CDS)—a review. *Journal of the Western Society of Periodontology/Periodontal Abstracts*, 44, 5–12.

Ling, T.Y., Gillam, D.G., Barber, P.M., *et al.* (1997) An investigation of potential desensitizing agents in the dentine disc model: a scanning electron microscopy study. *Journal of Oral Rehabilitation*, 24, 191–203.

Liu, H.C., Lan, W.H., Hsieh, C.C. (1998) Prevalence and distribution of cervical dentin hypersensitivity in a population in Taipei, Taiwan. *Journal of Endodontics*, 24, 45–47.

Lucchese, A., Mongiorgi, R., Prati, C., *et al.* (1997) Treatment of dentin sensitivity with stannous fluoride gel. Electron microscopic study and evaluation of dentin permeability. *Minerva Stomatologica*, 46, 659–663.

Marini, I., Checchi, L., Vecchiet, F., *et al.* (2000) Intraoral fluoride releasing device: a new clinical therapy for dentine sensitivity. *Journal of Periodontology*, 71, 90–95.

McCormack, K. and Davies, R. (1996) The enigma of potassium ion in the management of dentine hypersensitivity: is nitric oxide the elusive second messenger? *Pain*, 68, 5–11.

Millar, B.J. and Hodson, N. (2007) Assessment of the safety of two ozone delivery devices. *Journal of Dentistry*, 35, 195–200.

Miller, S., Truong, T., Heu, R., *et al.* (1994) Recent advances in stannous fluoride technology: antibacterial efficacy and mechanism of action towards hypersensitivity. *International Dental Journal*, 44(1 Suppl 1), 83–98.

Moritz, A., Gutknecht, N., Schoop, U., *et al.* (1996) The advantage of CO2-treated dental necks, in comparison with a standard method: results of an in vivo study. *Journal of Clinical Laser Medicine and Surgery*, 14, 27–32.

Moritz, A., Schoop, U., Goharkhay, K., *et al.* (1998) Long-term effects of CO_2 laser irradiation on treatment of hypersensitive dental necks: results of an in Vivo study. *Journal of Clinical Laser Medicine and Surgery*, 16, 211–215.

Morris, M.F., Davis, R.D., Richardson, B.W. (1999) Clinical efficacy of two dentin desensitizing agents. *American Journal of Dentistry*, 12, 72–76.

Nathanson, D. (1997) Vital tooth bleaching: sensitivity and pulpal considerations. *Journal of the America Dental Association*, 128 (Suppl), 41S–44S.

O'Sullivan, E.A. and Curzon, M.E. (2000) A comparison of acidic dietary factors in children with and without dental erosion. *ASDC Journal of Dentistry for Children 2000*, 67, 186–192, 160.

Orchardson, R. and Collins, W.J. (1987) Clinical features of hypersensitive teeth. *British Dental Journal*, 162, 253–256.

Orchardson, R. and Gillam, D.G. (2000) The efficacy of potassium salts as agents for treating dentin hypersensitivity. *Journal of Orofacial Pain*, 14, 9–19.

Orchardson, R. and Gillam, D.G. (2006) Managing dentin hypersensitivity. *Journal of the American Dental Association*, 137, 990–998.

Pashley, D.H. (1992) Dentin permeability and dentin sensitivity. *Proceedings of the Finnish Dental Society*, 88 Suppl 1, 31–37.

Peacock, J.M. and Orchardson, R. (1999) Action potential conduction block of nerves in vitro by potassium citrate, potassium tartrate and potassium oxalate. *Journal of Clinical Periodontology*, 26, 33–37.

Pearce, N.X., Addy, M., Newcombe, R.G. (1994) Dentine hypersensitivity: a clinical trial to compare 2 strontium densensitizing toothpastes with a conventional fluoride toothpaste. *Journal of Periodontology*, 65, 113–119.

Poulsen, S., Errboe, M., Lescay Mevil, Y., *et al.* (2006) Potassium containing toothpastes for dentine hypersensitivity. *Cochrane Database of Systematic Reviews* 2006 (3), CD001476.

Price, R.B., Sedarous, M., Hiltz, G.S. 2000 The pH of tooth-whitening products. *Journal of the Canadian Dental Association*, 66, 421–426.

Rees, J. and Addy, M. (2002) A cross sectional study of dentin hypersensitivity. *Journal of Clinical Periodontology*, 29, 997–1003.

Rossman, L.E., Hasselgren, G., *et al.* (2005) Diagnosis and Management of Orofacial Dental Pain Emergencies. In: *Pathways of the Pulp.* (Eds. S. Cohen and K. Hargreaves) 9th edn. pp. 31–77, Elsevier Health Sciences, Amsterdam, Netherlands.

Rytomaa, I., Jarvinen, V., Kanerva, R., *et al.* (1998) Bulimia and tooth erosion. *Acta Odontologica Scandinavica*, 56, 36–40.

Schupbach, P., Lutz, F., Finger, W.J. (1997) Closing of dentinal tubules by Gluma desensitizer. *European Journal of Oral Sciences*, 105, 414–421.

Seltzer, S. and Boston, D. (1997) Hypersensitivity and pain induced by operative procedures and the "cracked tooth" syndrome. *General Dentistry*, 45, 148–159.

Sessle, B.J. (1987) The Neurobiology of facial and dental pain. Present Knowledge, future direction. *Journal of Dental Research*, 66, 962–981.

Tam, L. (2001) Effect of potassium nitrate and fluoride on carbamide peroxide bleaching. *Quintessence International*, 32, 766–770.

Tavares, M., DePaola, P.F., Soparkar, P. (1994) Using a fluoride-releasing resin to reduce cervical sensitivity. *Journal of the American Dental Association*, 125, 1337–1342.

Thrash, W.J., Dodds, M.W., Jones, D.L. (1994) The effect of stannous fluoride on dentinal hypersensitivity. *International Dental Journal*, 44(1 Suppl 1), 107–118.

Van Der Weijden, G.A., Timmerman, M.F., Piscaer, M., *et al.* (2001) Oscillating/rotating electric toothbrushes compared: plaque removal and gingival abrasion. *Journal of Clinical Periodontology*, 28, 536–543.

West, N., Addy, M., Hughes, J. (1998) Dentine hypersensitivity: the effects of brushing desensitizing toothpastes, their solid and liquid phases, and detergents on dentine and acrylic: studies in vitro. *Journal of Oral Rehabilitation*, 25, 885–895.

West, N.X., Addy, M., Jackson, R.J., *et al.* (1997) Dentine hypersensitivity and the placebo response. A comparison of the effect of strontium acetate, potassium nitrate and fluoride toothpastes. *Journal of Clinical Periodontology*, 24, 209–215.

Wichgers, T.G. and Emert, R.L. (1997) Dentin hypersensitivity. *Oral Health*, 87, 51–53, 55–56, 59, quiz 61.

Yates, R., Owens, J., Jackson, R., *et al.* (1998) A split mouth placebo-controlled study to determine the effect of amorphous calcium phosphate in the treatment of dentine hypersensitivity. *Journal of Clinical Periodontology*, 25, 687–692.

Yonaga, K., Kimura, Y., Matsumoto, K. (1999) Treatment of cervical dentin hypersensitivity by various methods using pulsed Nd:YAG laser. *Journal of Clinical Laser Medicine and Surgery*, 17, 205–210.

Zero, D.T. (1996) Etiology of dental erosion—extrinsic factors. *European Journal of Oral Science*, 104, 162–177.

Zhang, Y., Agee, K., Pashley, D.H., *et al.* (1999) The effects of Pain-Free Desensitizer on dentine permeability and tubule occlusion over time, in vitro. *Journal of Clinical Periodontology*, 25, 884–891.

Zhang, C., Matsumoto, K., Kimura, Y., *et al.* (1998) Effects of CO_2 laser in treatment of cervical dentinal hypersensitivity. *Journal of Endodontics*, 24, 595–597.

15

Caries risk assessment

Ferne Kraglund and Hardy Limeback

Introduction

The concept of caries resistance was introduced in the first chapter. Some people just don't seem to get dental caries despite poor oral hygiene and/or poor dietary habits. Then some people, despite meticulous oral hygiene and a conscientious effort to avoid cariogenic diets, somehow always manage to get new decay. The caries process has not been controlled in this latter group, and it is these patients where all the tools of preventing dental decay become essential. But how do we determine whether one person is more at risk than the other? In this chapter the concept of risk assessment will be explored.

Dental caries—who is at risk?

As discussed in the introduction chapter, dental caries is a chronic, transmissible disease of multifactorial etiology. The specific manner in which etiological factors influence the disease process is complex, including host and pathogen adaptations, and is not completely understood. It is especially difficult to predict with accuracy which patient will develop dental decay (Brown 1995).

Dental caries is a slowly progressive disease; it is not the consequence of a singular event but rather a sequel of processes occurring over a time (Angmar-Månsson and Al-Khateeb 1998). Not everyone has the same oral flora. Bacterial biofilms are sophisticated ecosystems that respond to different oral environments. They can shift from normal healthy microflora to the acidogenic (acid-forming) and acidoduric (tolerate living in acidic environments) microorganisms that are associated with dental caries. Bacteria in biofilms, such as dental plaque, are better able to survive and exhibit stronger resistance to various environmental factors because they are 1,000

times more resistant to antibodies, antibiotics, and antimicrobial products. These attributes lead to persistent bacterial infections in some people that will undoubtedly represent a new challenge in the treatment of dental caries (Kutsch and Kutsch 2006).

Caries distribution

The prevalence of dental caries among children and adolescents living in industrialized nations declined in the 1970s and 1980s (Marthaler et al. 1996; Fontana and Zero 2006). It was suggested by most experts that regular exposure to fluoride was the most significant contribution to this decline in caries (Petersson and Bratthall 1996; Burt 1998). The decline has since stabilized in many countries; however, in some areas, there are reports that the prevalence of caries is again on the rise (Dye et al. 2007). It was reported in Oral Health in America: A Report of the Surgeon General that dental caries is the single most common chronic disease of childhood, with a prevalence rate five times greater than that of asthma (US NIDCR 2000). Due to the universal nature of this disease, management of dental caries, typically in the form of operative procedures, remains the most routine practice in the dental office (Tranæus et al. 2005; Evans et al. 2008). The diminished pervasiveness and severity of dental caries in many developed countries, along with an increasing number of dentate elderly retaining their teeth longer, have brought about a noticeably skewed distribution of disease in the population (Pitts 1998; Hausen et al. 2000). From the North Carolina risk assessment studies, it was shown that the pattern of dental caries has changed in such a way that the high caries minority is suffering very different patterns of caries prevalence, risk, and activity than the low caries

Comprehensive Preventive Dentistry, First Edition. Edited by Hardy Limeback.
© 2012 John Wiley & Sons, Ltd. Published 2012 by John Wiley & Sons, Ltd.

majority that have no or few cavitated lesions (Stamm *et al.* 1988; Stamm *et al.* 1991; Leverett *et al.* 1993). It has been estimated that approximately 60–75% of the caries occurs in only 20–25% of the population. In addition, findings from the National Preventive Dentistry Demonstration Program showed that most severe disease was limited to only 5% of the children (Disney *et al.* 1992). With the earlier high prevalence of dental caries observed in western civilization between the 1950s and 1980s, most of society was categorized as having the disease (Moss and Zero 1995). This led health professionals to use a population-based approach in which its goal was to alter the distribution of disease by controlling the underlying determinants of dental caries in the entire population (Beck 1998; Rose 2001; Hänsel Petersson 2003). Fluoridation of public water systems is an example of a population-based strategy that was intended to be a preventive treatment for all members of society. Whereas water fluoridation in the early days was shown to be a successful and cost-effective population-wide strategy, the appropriateness of providing costly preventive measures (for example, sealants) to whole populations has been questioned (Burt 1998).

Consequently, the low prevalence and skewed distribution of disease have led some investigators to argue for a high-risk targeted approach to diagnosing and treating dental caries (FDI Working Group 1988; Disney *et al.* 1992). Using the high-risk approach, the goal would be to identify highly susceptible persons and to use efficacious individual-based preventive measures to diminish their risk (Moss and Zero 1995). This method operates to decrease the risk of a small number of highly vulnerable individuals to include them into the majority of the population with no or few caries (Stamm *et al.* 1991; Pitts 1997). In order to use a high-risk approach, one must have accurate and feasible measures for identifying those individuals that are exceedingly prone to dental caries (Hausen 1997). A caries risk assessment may aid in the identification of etiological factors so that suitable preventive treatment may be rendered for that particular individual (Hänsel Petersson 2003). There is still much debate in the scientific community as to the appropriate way to approach the diagnosis and treatment of dental caries. Batchelor and Sheiham (2002) have argued in favor of a population approach as opposed to a high-risk approach because the latter would fail to deal with the majority of new carious lesions in the population. On the contrary, Axelsson *et al.* (1991; 1993) have had much success using targeted approaches for prevention of dental diseases. Using a high-risk strategy does not imply that the general population does not require preventive dental care, but rather

that the intensity of treatment should vary depending on the need. A joint approach for caries prevention in which both strategies are used may maximize the advantages of both methods by addressing those most in need, while acquiring smaller, but still significant, changes in the population's distribution of disease (Pitts 1998).

Treatment of dental caries

Historically, it was thought that dental caries was a progressive disease that inevitably led to the eventual loss of a tooth unless a dentist intervened surgically. The conventional method of dealing with dental decay involved detection of the carious lesions, followed by drilling and filling (Fontana and Zero 2006; Doméjean-Orliaguet *et al.* 2006; Evans *et al.* 2008). Although treating dental caries by restorative means will offer relief from pain and restore function to the tooth, it will likely not prevent the lifelong continuation of the disease process and will undoubtedly allow recurrent decay necessitating further surgical interventions (Kutsch *et al.* 2007). Restoration of the carious lesions removes areas of cariogenic microorganisms, but it does not alter the risk level of the patient. Research demonstrates that placing dental restorations contributes very little to the management of the caries disease process because there is no measurable effect on the cariogenic bacterial load in the mouth when restorative procedures are completed (Wright *et al.* 1992; Featherstone 2003; Jensen *et al.* 2007).

A great deal of dental work is focused on treating the symptoms of this bacterial infection rather than focusing on the causative factors. Restorations, by themselves, are incapable of modifying the etiological factors of dental caries in order to eradicate caries-forming bacteria (Young *et al.* 2007). When health professionals are dealing with other systemic diseases, measures to eradicate the causes of the disease are used, such as immunizations and antibiotics. Dental professionals need to consider dental caries in the same manner and treat the disease rather than just the clinical manifestations of the disease. It is believed that our current understanding of the caries disease process is strong enough to accomplish this (Featherstone *et al.* 2003).

Numerous dental researchers have advocated following the medical model for dental caries. This approach entails regarding dental caries as a disease process, to manage its etiological factors, and to employ prevention strategies rather than simply repairing the damage caused by the disease (Newbrun 1992; Anderson *et al.* 1993; Edelstein 1994; Limeback 1996). Medical management of dental caries is not only possible, but it has been shown to provide superior outcomes as compared to surgical intervention alone. It was demonstrated that patients treated via a caries risk assessment and medical model approach had developed significantly fewer new carious lesions than patients being treated solely with the conventional surgical approach (that is, drill and fill) (Kutsch and Kutsch 2006).

Modern caries management

Modern caries management is based on evidence-based dentistry, with a more intense focus on prevention. Comprehensive caries control involves focusing on the whole patient to manage the individual risk factors of the patient to promote and maintain optimum oral health (Young et al. 2007a). Preventive dentistry is thus characterized by risk factor management in which we hope to maximize the protective factors while minimizing the pathological factors (Young et al. 2007b). Modern management of dental caries includes the following sequence of treatment:

1. Detection of carious lesions at an earlier stage (incipient lesions, non-cavitated lesions).
2. Diagnosis of the caries disease process.
3. Identification of the patient's caries risk factors.
4. Treatment planning, including tooth restoration, risk factor modification/elimination, arresting active lesions, and preventing future lesions.
5. Altering the caries risk status of the patient.

Measures of caries control involve identifying the disease process and the risk factors; this is achieved by first performing a caries risk assessment for the patient to identify his/her risk factors for caries development. When the risk factors have been detected, the dental professional provides preventive measures aimed at remineralizing incipient lesions, suppressing microbial levels, and preventing the appearance of new lesions. The clinician uses a variety of behavioral, chemical, and minimally invasive surgical techniques to bring back a positive balance between the pathologic and protective factors that favor a healthy oral environment (Hildebrandt 1995; Young et al. 2007b). Caries control measures may include restorative treatment (with or without fluoride releasing materials), sealants, oral hygiene instruction, patient education, dietary analysis and modification, fluoride treatments (for example, gel, varnish), xylitol chewing gum, and antimicrobial therapies (for example, chlorhexidine gluconate). With a better understanding of the caries process, there comes a change in operative dentistry philosophy. Although there is considerable variability between dentists, there is more emphasis on preventive dentistry than ever before (Doméjean-Orliaguet 2006). The shift in emphasis appears to be occurring in dental schools in which curriculum and practical skills are focused more on caries risk assessment, modern management of the caries disease (including minimally inva-

sive dentistry), and delayed restoration of teeth until the surfaces have become cavitated (or are likely to become cavitated). Restorations are only placed after all practical efforts of prevention and remineralization have been attempted (Hildebrandt 1995; Anusavice 2005).

Caries risk assessment

Caries risk assessment (CRA) is the process of collecting data regarding various factors (for example, bacterial levels) and indicators (for example, previous caries experience) to predict caries activity in the immediate future (Hänsel Petersson et al. 2003).

Formal CRA has been described as a four-step process:

1. Identification of measurable risk factors.
2. Development of a multifactorial tool.
3. Risk assessment to determine a patient's risk profile.
4. Application of preventive measures tailored to the risk profile (Moss and Zero 1995).

For the past 30 years, researchers have focused on developing an instrument that is easy to administer, simple, quick, and accurate. The risk assessment tool should estimate caries risk, identify the primary etiological factors, provide an inventory of the patient's current preventive practices, and serve as a guide for selecting specialized preventive care tailored to that individual's needs (Tinanoff 1995a; Tinanoff 1995b; Reich et al. 1999). It is likely that most dentists incorporate some informal CRA into their practice based on their overall impression of the patient and previous caries experience (Fontana and Zero 2006).

Research has shown that experienced clinicians are often able to assess caries risk very quickly and accurately (Carvalho et al. 1992; Isokangas et al. 1993). Although determination of the overall risk level may be relatively easy, pinpointing the specific factors associated with the disease process often proves to be more difficult. For that reason, it is worthwhile for dental practitioners to conduct a formal CRA to determine the precise factors involved in the patient's disease progression (Kidd 1999).

Performing a CRA assists practitioners to provide their patients appropriate levels of preventive care and to eliminate wasteful use of resources (Abernathy et al. 1987; Powell 1998). By matching the person's risk level to his/her proposed preventive therapy, the profession stands a greater chance of positively impacting a patients' oral health. If dental professionals were able to identify, in advance, individuals at the greatest risk of developing dental caries, the cost of caries prevention procedures could be markedly reduced and their efficiency greatly increased (Stamm et al. 1991).

Dental caries management by formal risk assessment represents a significant change in the mindset of the profession and should be incorporated into daily practice as dictated by practices of evidence-based standards of care. CRA should be routinely built into preliminary and recall examinations as the findings help to guide the patient's designated course of treatment. This is especially important before extensive prosthodontic, restorative, and orthodontic treatment is undertaken to ensure a favorable prognosis (Angmar-Månsson *et al.* 1998; Jenson *et al.* 2007).

CRA may be valuable in the clinical management of caries by helping dental clinicians in the following ways:

1. Categorize the level of the patient's risk of developing caries to control the intensity of treatment rendered.
2. Pinpoint main etiological factors that contribute to the development of decay and thus determine appropriate form of therapy (Zero *et al.* 2001; Fontana and Zero 2006).
3. Assist in restorative treatment decisions (for example, choice of restorative material) (Zero *et al.* 2001; Fontana and Zero 2006).
4. Improve prognosis of planned therapeutic care (Zero *et al.* 2001; Douglass 1998).
5. Provide information on what additional diagnostic tests and screening are required (Douglass 1998; Zero *et al.* 2001; Fontana and Zero 2006).
6. Educate and motivate patients to improve and maintain optimum oral health (Kidd 1999; Fontana and Zero 2006; Jenson *et al.* 2007).
7. Guide timing of subsequent recall appointments (Kidd 1999; Kidd 2001).

CRA tools screen people based on risk factors and predictors and classify patients into one of three risk categories: low, moderate, or high (Burgess 1995; Ngo and Gaffney 2005). Ordinarily, if new caries have developed since the last examination, the patient is categorized as either moderate or high risk depending on the interval since the last examination, and the number and severity of carious lesions. If, however, the patient is caries-free since the last examination, his/her risk level would be designated as low or moderate risk depending on his/her oral hygiene status, fluoride exposure, and microbiological count (Reich *et al.* 1999).

Reaching a consensus on the moderate risk group represents the greatest diagnostic challenge. It can be rather simple to identify low risk-low caries and high risk-high caries patients. However, it is much more complicated to recognize moderate risk individuals that may have exhibited little or no disease for long periods followed by a sudden development of carious lesions. It is for these patients, along with people who are at risk without any apparent signs or symptoms of disease, that

benefit the most from identification from CRA (Kutsch *et al.* 2007; Jenson *et al.* 2007).

Although dental caries has long been established to be a disease of multifactorial etiology, many of the traditional caries prediction models have focused on individual factors associated with high caries activity (Disney *et al.* 1992). More recently, the multifactorial etiology of caries points in the direction of constructing a more promising risk assessment model that includes the various factors that contribute to the development of caries as no single test can simultaneously measure the three principal components of dental caries: host resistance, cariogenicity of the diet, and microbial pathogens (Hänsel Petersson 2002).

Risk assessment models

Two types of variables can be used in the development of multivariable caries risk models: risk factors and risk indicators or sometimes called etiologic and non-etiologic factors, respectively (Powell 1998). A risk factor is an environmental, behavioral, biologic, or lifestyle exposure or characteristic that increases the probability of a disease occurring (Beck 1998). They are part of the causal chain of disease development because they satisfy the conditions of causality, such as strength of association, temporal relationship, consistency of association, dose-response relationship, and biological plausibility. (See Chapter 5 on evidence-based dentistry.) Collection of information regarding true risk factors, such as *Streptococcus mutans*, during risk assessment may help clinicians plan preventive therapy (Powell 1998).

A risk predictor, on the other hand, is normally a biologic marker that is indicative of the disease process, but is not thought to be etiological for that disease. It is often used synonymously with risk marker in the literature (Beck *et al.* 1992). Some risk indicators for caries, such a previous caries experience, can be powerful predictors for future lesion development without being a direct cause of the disease but offer little direction in prescribing preventive measures. Risk factors and indicators are most commonly pathological in nature (that is, associated with disease occurrence); however, they may also be protective if they decrease an individual's probability of developing the disease (for example, fluoride exposure) (Douglass 1998).

There are two frameworks that can be used for the development of CRA instruments: the risk model and the prediction model. The risk model, or sometimes called the etiologic model, is employed when you want to identify the risk factors for the disease to implement the most effective prevention and treatment interventions.

It contains only true risk factors and is typically simple to use, but it is not intended to predict future caries risk. Because of its simplicity and stability across different subgroups of the population, it is often used for screening in public health domains (Beck *et al.* 1992; Beck *et al.* 1998). In contrast, a prediction model uses both risk factors and risk predictors to maximize its ability to identify low- and high-risk individuals (that is, maximize sensitivity and specificity). Although risk predictors (such as baseline caries) will not influence the incidence of disease, they can be strong predictors that are inexpensively and easily obtained. Risk factors (such as *Streptococcus mutans* counts) are often more costly to measure; however, they tend to be more reliable in caries prediction (Beck *et al.* 1992; Beck *et al.* 1998). Often investigators want to use a combination risk and prediction model that encompasses both risk factors and risk indicators. The variables directly involved in the caries process either as a protective or risk factor include, but are not limited to, specific microorganisms, dental plaque, type and frequency of carbohydrates and sugars in the diet, and fluoride exposure. Conversely, risk indicators, such as previous dental experience, are often included in CRA tools because they are indirectly related to the occurrence of dental caries without participating in the actual development of carious lesions (Beck *et al.* 1992; Beck *et al.* 1998). There are some CRA instruments that support both types of models. The Cariogram (Bratthall *et al.* 2004) and the CRA form developed at the University of Toronto (Burgess 1995) do just that; they act as prediction models in that they can identify those who are high risk, and they are also risk models because they can identify the risk factors involved in order to facilitate appropriate intervention planning. Bratthall and Hänsel Petersson (2004) conducted an internet-based search for risk models. Although they found numerous reports dealing with caries prediction-based models using one or a few risk factors, there have been few attempts made in cariology to construct any practical and comprehensive risk assessment instruments. It was concluded at the 2001 National Institutes of Health conference that "caries is an etiologically complex disease process. It is likely that numerous microbial, genetic, immunological, behavioural, and environmental contributors to risk are at play in determining the occurrence and severity of clinical disease. Assessment tools based on a single risk indicator are therefore unlikely to accurately discriminate between those at high and low risk. Multiple indicators combined on an appropriate scale and accounting for possible interactions, will certainly be required" (NIH Consensus Development Conference 2001).

Caries risk analyses using a combination of variables have shown superior results than single factors (Disney *et al.* 1992) Beck *et al.* 1992; Tinanoff 1995a; Tinanoff 1995b).

Selection of risk assessment instrument

The underlying principle of risk assessments is that individuals with elevated levels of risk factors will receive more aggressive preventive interventions. Because of this, examiners must be cautious in how they categorize patients in the various risk levels. One must decide at what stage a risk factor changes from low to moderate to high-risk categorization (Douglass 1998). This can prove to be a difficult task as many etiological factors do not have a clear demarcation between absence and presence, but normally range from excellent to poor (for example, oral hygiene) or from low to high (such as lactobacilli counts). Regrettably, no perfect risk factors are available for caries risk assessment; clinicians must be willing to accept a certain proportion of errors in the prediction of future caries activity. This remains true for medical conditions as well. For example, Hausen (1997) used data from the Kuopio Ischaemic Heart Disease Risk Factor Study to construct a logistic risk function. He discovered from the Receiver Operating Characteristic (ROC) curves, a summary of the predictive power of a multiple level risk factor, that the individual risk assessments of acute myocardial infarction and dental caries are equally inaccurate.

In creating a CRA tool, a trade-off between sensitivity (percentage of truly diseased persons who test positively) and specificity (percentage of persons without the disease who test negatively) must be made (Fletcher and Fletcher 2005). In doing so, a balance is struck between the number of false positives (that is, patients assumed to be high risk but do not develop caries) and false negatives (that is, patients assumed to be low risk but develop caries) (Hausen 1997). It is imperative that the values of sensitivity and specificity remain high to ensure that a patient labelled as high risk truly has the disease, and the threat of identifying low risk individuals as diseased should be minimal (Angmar-Månsson and Al-Khateeb 1998).

Because it is impractical to believe that a diagnostic test would have sensitivity (Se) and specificity (Sp) values of 100%, different criteria and cut-off points have been established by researchers investigating caries risk. Wilson and Ashley (1989) suggested that Se and Sp values each be set at 80% to be considered an acceptable test for caries risk. Alternatively, it has been recommended by Fleiss and Kingman (1990) that the combined Se and Sp of a risk model should be at least 160%, which has become the gold standard among many researchers (Hausen 1997; Zero *et al.* 2001). Unfortunately, this benchmark value has only been achieved by a small number of caries prediction instruments (Streiner *et al.* 1992; Scheinin *et al.* 1992; Leverett *et al.* 1993).

Caries risk prediction remains an inexact science despite the sizeable amount of research devoted to the topic. Examiners must appreciate that a certain proportion of errors will be made, and risk misclassification may result in providing inappropriate management, including elements of overtreatment and undertreatment (Pitts 1998). When considering the cut-off points of Se and Sp and the trade-off between them, one must weigh the consequences of having too many false positives or false negatives (Hausen 1997).

If the CRA tool is to be used at the public health level for mass screenings, it may be advantageous to have a higher specificity. Public health administrators would want to avoid false positives and as a result the overtreatment of individuals that do not necessarily require the preventive services. This is especially crucial in environments where resources are scarce. Avoiding false positives would also be desirable in situations where the recommended disease management is invasive or costly to the patient (Zero *et al.* 2001). On the contrary, it may be more advantageous from an ethical and economical standpoint to increase the sensitivity of the test to avoid false negatives. Failure to identify those at risk for caries development may result in unnecessary treatment in the future that may be more costly and painful to the patient due to the progression of undiagnosed disease. By raising the sensitivity of the risk model, the number of false positives would increase. Although it may result in overtreatment of some patients, if the clinician uses an appropriate preventive strategy, this would result in little to no harm to the patient in that dental caries would not be permitted to start or progress. The patient would, however, experience some economical loss for the cost of the preventive therapy.

Risk factors

A multitude of caries risk factors and indicators have been identified over decades of research. For example, in a systematic review of risk factors for dental caries in young children, Harris *et al.* (2004) found that 106 risk factors were significantly related to the prevalence of dental caries.

With so many factors, it can seem daunting to decide which variables should be chosen for inclusion in the CRA instrument. The risk factors selected for research are typically dictated by the purpose of the study because there are very few standardized CRA instruments available (Powell 1998). The few CRA models currently in use are recent additions to the discipline and tend to focus on the principal factors associated with caries development, namely diet, microbial pathogens, and

host susceptibility factors. The University of Toronto's CRA model is congruent with these instruments (for example, Cariogram, CAMBRA [Caries Management by Risk Assessment], Featherstone *et al.* 2007) in that it maintains its focus on the basic caries risk elements that can easily be identified in the dental clinic and modified through preventive care practices. The most commonly used caries risk factors and indicators in multifactorial CRA models include levels of cariogenic bacteria (that is, *Streptococcus mutans* and lactobacilli), salivary factors (such as flow rate and buffering capacity), carbohydrate intake, oral hygiene, fluoride exposure, previous caries experience, and socioeconomic characteristics Eriksen and Bjertness 1991; Tinanoff 1995a; Tinanoff 1995b: Bratthall *et al.* 2005). Each of these caries risk predictors will be discussed in the following sections.

Streptococcus mutans and lactobacilli

As was discussed in the introduction chapter, dental caries is an infectious disease of microbial origin; the etiologic agents are regular inhabitants of the oral cavity that cause demineralization of dental hard tissue when their pathogenicity and proportions are altered in response to environmental conditions. Microorganisms such as *Streptococcus mutans* (SM) and *Lactobacillus* sp. (LB) have acquired a significant advantage over other oral acidogenic bacteria due to their acidoduric nature. Not only are SM able to survive in an acidic environment, but they have also adapted the ability to increase their rate of acid production, thus driving the pH in the oral cavity lower and forming a cariogenic plaque (Moss and Zero 1995).

Whereas SM are the primary initiators of the formation of carious lesions (Loesche 1986), LB contribute substantially to the propagation of the lesion due to their ability to survive at a lower pH than SM. In addition, SM have evolved the capacity to store energy for occasions when fermentable carbohydrates are scarce in the oral cavity. This incredible adaptation allows oral SM levels to remain relatively constant regardless of dietary modifications. LB have yet to develop this ability, and thus LB counts are often used to determine a patient's compliance to dietary changes (Hildebrandt 1995).

Traditionally, SM and LB counts have been the principal biological indicators used for prediction of future caries experience (Pienihäkkinen 1987; Krasse 1988; Demers *et al.* 1990; Disney *et al.* 1992; Beck *et al.* 1992; Scheinen *et al.* 1992; Drake *et al.* 1994; Hänsel Petersson *et al.* 2003).

Studies have shown that not only are these microorganisms related to the incidence of dental caries but that children with high levels of these pathogens develop a significantly greater number of carious lesions than children with low levels (Zickert *et al.* 1982). Nevertheless, salivary levels of SM and LB have been more successful in identifying low-risk children than those at an elevated risk for developing dental caries (van Houte 1993).

These salivary tests aid dental professionals in identifying the two extremes in a disease susceptible population but are less effective in predicting caries in moderate risk groups. The accuracy of tests for SM in predicting future caries in the whole population is less than 50%. Unfortunately, despite their prevalent use in CRA, the predictive power of microbiologic tests remains uncertain at the individual level as well (Eriksen *et al.* 1991; van Houte 1993). With the exception of findings in young children, salivary levels of SM have been disappointing with regard to risk assessment (Tinanoff 1995a; Tinanoff 1995b). Salivary tests for LB are even less sensitive than tests for caries prediction than SM. This is to be expected as LB are not primarily responsible for the initiation of dental caries, but they are found in large quantities when a considerable amount of carbohydrates have been consumed (Fontana and Zero 2006).

LB counts are commonly analyzed to reflect dietary changes, and the test results can be useful to motivate patients and to monitor changes in oral hygiene, diet, and microbial therapies (Hänsel Petersson *et al.* 2003).

Some dental offices use SM and LB counts to not only estimate caries risk but to monitor improvement in oral hygiene and diets for educating the patient regarding their own oral health. There are kits available for conveniently culturing saliva and determining bacterial counts. In Europe, Orion Diagnostica sells kits for estimating *Streptococcus mutans* counts (Dentocult SM Strip Mutans) in both saliva and plaque samples, as well as Dentocult LB for estimating lactobacilli counts in saliva. In North America Ivoclar-Vivadent sells the CRT test kit, which also estimates salivary SM and LB levels. In both of these cases, agar plates or strips immersed in nutrient broth have to be incubated for 2 days to encourage growth of the bacteria. Patients return in 2 days to view their results.

A new system has been developed, where the SM counts can be estimated by measuring the bioluminescence produced by plaque bacteria metabolizing adenosine triphosphate (ATP). Preliminary studies (Fazilat *et al.* 2010) indicate that the CariScreen Caries Susceptibility Test (CariFree), which is a simple 1-minute chairside bacterial test for estimating patients' caries risk through the direct measurement of biological activity of the plaque, to be a useful tool for measuring SM levels in plaque (Figure 15-1).

Patients are offered immediate feedback in terms of the cariogenic potential of their plaque.

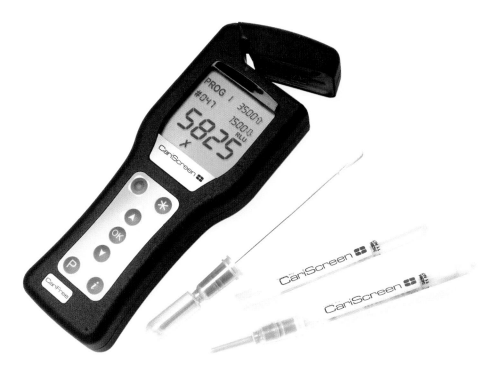

Figure 15-1 Photograph of the CarieScreen (Oral Biotech Inc.) caries susceptibility tester. A plaque sample is obtained using the swab that comes with the kit (shown), mixed with bioluminescent reagents, and inserted into the tester that measures Adenosine Triphosphate (ATP) production by means of a bioluminescence reaction. A score under 1,500 is considered to be relatively healthy; a score above 1,500 shows risk for decay. Reprinted with permission from Oral Biotech, Inc.

Other salivary factors

Saliva serves multiple protective functions against the initiation and progression of dental caries. It assists to clear food particles and bacteria from the oral cavity, and it buffers the acids produced by microorganisms in dental plaque. The number of individuals suffering from a reduced salivary flow rate is increasing, especially in the elderly population. Xerostomia (dry mouth) may be the consequence of a variety of conditions including radiation therapy to the head and neck region and medical ailments such as Sjögren's syndrome, Parkinson's disease, and uncontrolled diabetes mellitus (Hunter 1988).

Xerostomia, however, is most commonly attributed to the side effects of many frequently prescribed medications including antihistamines, anticholinergics, and tricyclic antidepressants.

Although xerostomia has long been known to be a risk factor for individuals of any age, the elderly are especially susceptible to salivary changes due to the large number of medications they are often required to take. This can be especially problematic for this cohort as they are generally retaining more teeth than they have previously but suffer from unfavorable salivary conditions, which puts them at an even higher risk of developing dental caries (Fure 1998; Petersen 2005).

Individuals with chronically reduced salivary function have been found to have a significant increase in caries activity. Many dentists rely on the patient's complaint of xerostomia to diagnose hyposalivation; however, this subjective complaint often does not correlate with objective findings of reduced salivary flow. Testing an individual's unstimulated salivary flow rate can be accomplished easily in clinical practice, and it has a strong predictive validity for assessing caries risk. GC America provides a complete salivary test kit with instructions on how to measure saliva flow (Figure 15-2).

The stimulated flow rate, using paraffin wax, is also customarily measured to conclude if preventive strategies based on salivary stimulation (for example, chewing sugarless gum) will benefit the patient. Low un-stimulated salivary flow rates increase the risk for caries in adults (Flink 2007), and stimulated salivary flow low rates under 0.3 mL/min are considered to be low and associated with caries, but one reviewer suggests that other factors may be more important than low stimulated saliva (Billings 1993).

Salivary buffering capacity appears to be another risk factor for caries (Pienihäkkinen 1988; Wilson and Ashley 1989). This can be measured easily using the Ivoclar-Vivadent CRT test kit (Dentobuff) or the GC America buffering capacity test (Figure 15-3).

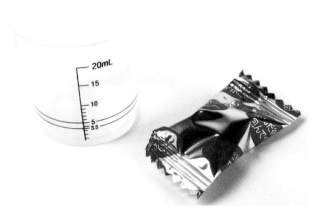

Figure 15-2 Stimulated salivary flow test kit. These two items, offered by GC America in their saliva test kits, are used to measure stimulated saliva flow. The patient chews on a piece of paraffin wax provided in the sealed pouch, and collects ALL of the saliva in the dispensing cup. Ideally, collection should be supervised so no swallowing occurs. After 5 minutes, the volume of the saliva is measured from the markings on the cup. The stimulated salivary flow rate is expressed as mL/min. Rates less than 0.3 mL/min are considered to be low and associated with caries.

Fluoride exposure

Topical fluoride exposure, oral hygiene habits, and diet are often not strong predictive factors for caries development, but they are often still included in CRA instruments because they may be prescriptive for the preventive actions recommended. Determining a problem in one or more of these areas will aid the dentist and patient to customize a care plan using these elements to alter other caries risk variables, such as bacterial and salivary factors (Tinanoff 1995a; Tinanoff 1995b). In order to prevent dental caries, it has been recommended that a constant, low ambient level of fluoride should be maintained in the oral environment. (See Chapter 16 on fluorides.)

Caries have been on the decline worldwide, and experts surveyed felt that the main reason was the widespread use of fluoridated toothpaste (Bratthall *et al.* 1996). When completing a CRA, the various sources of fluoride must be taken into account such as fluoridated drinking water, food and drinks, fluoridated toothpaste and mouth rinse, as well professionally applied topical fluoride. Since there may be more than one source of fluoride, all contributing at the so-called optimum exposure, patients may or may not be at risk. A patient living a lifetime in a non-fluoridated region, consuming foods made with non-fluoridated water, and not using fluoridated toothpaste will likely have a higher risk for caries. (See Chapter 16 on fluorides.)

(a)

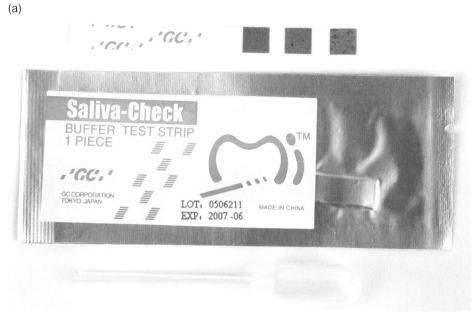

(b)

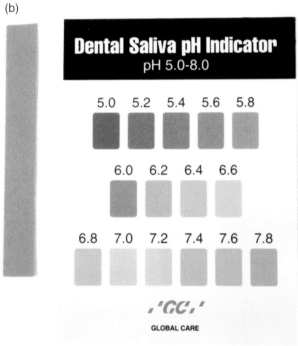

Figure 15-3 The Salivary Buffer Capacity test (GC America). (a) A sealed pouch containing a pH indicator paper strip and a plastic pipette. The pipette is used to transfer a drop of saliva collected during the salivary flow test (Figure 15-2) onto the pH indicator paper strip. After 30 seconds, the color is compared to the colors in the pH Indicator Chart. (b) for color comparison. Red colors indicate higher risk for caries. The pH of resting and stimulated saliva can also be measured directly using the other pH test paper provided in the kit (not shown), but this is not as important as measuring buffer capacity.

Plaque

Because dental caries is a microbiological disease, a prerequisite for caries development is the presence of dental plaque on the teeth, and unless this biofilm is present caries will not occur, regardless of any other risk factors. Researchers have failed to demonstrate a consistent relationship between dental plaque scores and caries (Hunter 1988). Not all patients with poor plaque control inevitably develop caries; however, those who clean their teeth infrequently or ineffectively may be at higher risk for developing carious lesions (Kidd 1999). Furthermore, conditions that hinder long-term maintenance of good oral hygiene, such as mental and physical disabilities and oral appliances, are positively associated with a higher caries risk (NIH Consensus Development Conference 2001). An inconsistent relationship between oral hygiene and dental caries prevalence may be due to the manner in which data are collected. Many risk assessment models use plaque indices that were developed for the study of periodontal disease to record the oral hygiene status of patients. This can be an inaccurate means of recording because they are often based on smooth surface scores, whereas the majority of caries occurs in the pits and fissures or the interproximal surfaces of teeth (Tinanoff 1995a; Tinanoff 1995).

However, when patients present with teeth that are covered with plaque, where oral hygiene is absent, there is no doubt that the dentition is at risk (Figure 15-4a and 15-4b).

(a)

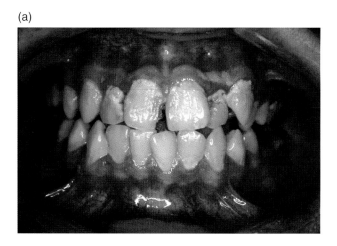

(b)

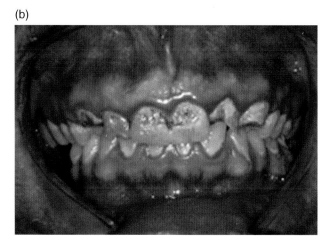

Figure 15-4 (a) There is abundant plaque visible, even on the gingiva of the maxilla. The caries can be clearly seen at the cervical margins of the lateral teeth and one obvious carious lesion on the right central incisor. This patient is at high risk for caries. (b) A photograph of an adult patient who is clearly at risk for losing a few teeth from dental decay. Most gingival margins have decayed. Courtesy of Dr. Kim Kutsch of Oral Biotech, Albany OR, USA.

Patients can be shown where the plaque resides with disclosing solutions. (See Chapter 1.) In some cases the caries risk has been increased by dental treatment. Orthodontics can result in widespread white spot lesions because plaque is not removed at the gingival margins and the teenager has increased sugar consumption. This is illustrated in Figure 15-5.

Fermentable carbohydrates

Consumption of sugar and carbohydrates is considered an important etiological factor in the development of dental caries (Zero 2004). The role of diet is primarily local in nature rather than systemic as bacteria metabolize carbohydrates and sugar, producing acidic by-products that cause the demineralization of the enamel surface. Whether this disease activity proceeds to a carious lesion depends on various dietary elements, as well as the patient's oral hygiene, exposure to fluoride, and the ability of the saliva to neutralize plaque acids (Burt and Pai 2001).

Several dietary elements need to be addressed when assessing a patient's caries risk level. Whether or not a food is cariogenic depends on a number of factors specific to the individual who eats it, namely the predominant oral bacteria in plaque, salivary flow rate, and buffering capacity, and fluoride availability in the oral cavity. The clinician must also take into account the retentiveness of the food, protective elements in food (such as fluoride, calcium, phosphate), the frequency of meals and snacks, sugar-containing non-foods (such as lozenges, gum, medications), and patterns of consumption (for example, sipping sugared drinks over a long period of time). Patients are typically asked to fill out a 24-hour diet diary and may be requested to complete an

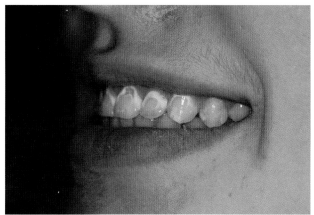

Figure 15-5 This photograph of a patient after orthodontic treatment was completed shows the new caries that developed between the brackets and the gingival margins. Courtesy of Dr. David Boag, DDS, Peach Tree, Georgia, USA.

additional dietary record of up to a week if the practitioner believes the patient to be at high risk for dental caries.

Assessing diet alone is usually inadequate at predicting caries. Studies in humans have not found a consistent relationship between consumption of cariogenic foods and dental caries experience. In a longitudinal study by Burt *et al.* (1988), the between meal sugar consumption was found to be only marginally related to interproximal caries increment but not at all related to caries in the pits and fissures. Dental caries is a multifactorial disease, and thus caries risk is not always directly correlated to fermentable carbohydrate consumption. For example, it was found that children developed very few caries if they had good oral hygiene irrespective of their dietary intake, but if oral hygiene was poor, a high sugar intake revealed an increase in caries prevalence (van Houte 1994). It is thus more prudent to consider dietary factors in association with other caries factors such as oral hygiene practices and fluoride exposure.

Previous caries experience

Without a doubt, previous caries experience remains the most powerful single predictor of future caries development (Hausen 1997; Pitts 1998; Powell 1998). It is the most common risk indicator used by dentists in both clinical practice and in CRA research because it provides the strongest predictive ability (Abernathy *et al.* 1987; Pienihäkkinen 1987; Beck *et al.* 1992). Studies of children and adolescents show that individuals developing carious lesions early in life tend to develop more caries in the coming years (Helfenstein *et al.* 1991; Li and Wang 2002). This tendency has also been demonstrated with an increase in caries risk among children whose mothers have caries, and adults are more likely to develop root caries if they have existing coronal caries (Locker *et al.* 1989).

Previous caries experience is often used in prediction models because it is fast, simple, and inexpensive to record. However, it cannot specify the particular risk factors that are causing the dental caries and, therefore, it cannot be used alone to specify appropriate preventive strategies directed at eliminating or modifying the patient's risk for caries development (Bratthall *et al.* 2005). Documenting caries experience over the past 1 to 2 years, and current disease activity, tends to be more indicative of the patient's true caries risk level. It has been shown that short-term predictions (that is, less than 2 years) are more reliable than long-term predictions of risk (more than 5 years). Dental caries develop under precise oral conditions, and these circumstances are more likely to change during studies of longer duration due to lifestyle or behavioral modifications (Powell 1998).

Sociodemographic indicators

Some researchers take the patient's age into account when assessing caries risk because teeth are exposed to different levels of the oral environment at various stages throughout life.

Dental caries used to be considered a disease of childhood. This belief arose when the prevalence of caries was much higher and when few children reached adulthood caries-free. This is no longer the case, and the caries disease process is spread out more throughout life (Burt and Eklund 1999). Adults of all ages still develop coronal caries and thus dental caries must now be considered a lifetime disease. Currently age, as a risk indicator, is considered to be less critical in the prediction of caries. The interaction of the principal risk factors (diet, bacteria, and host factors) takes precedence over an individual's age for appropriately categorizing caries risk level (Powell 1988).

Some investigators use other demographic risk indicators in their caries risk models, such as gender. Women, in both childhood and adulthood, tend to present with higher DMF (Decayed, Missing, Filled) scores than men. However, females generally tend to have superior oral hygiene and fewer missing teeth than males. Therefore, it is unlikely that women have higher caries susceptibility than men, but rather it is a combination of seeking out more dental care and/or earlier tooth eruption in the case of children and adolescents (Burt and Eklund 1999). A person's medical status is an indicator that incorporates some of the same elements as a few other risk factors, such as bacterial load and salivary characteristics. Xerostomia and lack of physical or cognitive abilities will alter the saliva and bacterial counts in an individual's oral cavity, especially in the elderly and special needs patients, and thus resulting in a higher risk for caries activity. Medical status is not often formally assessed because it is indirectly considered by its effect on stronger predicting etiologic risk factors such as salivary flow rate (Fure 1998). Socioeconomic status (SES) is a broad measure of individual or family's relative economic and social ranking with regards to factors such as income, education, and occupation. A large number of reports over the past few decades have demonstrated that social and behavioral factors are associated with dental caries, and some studies have specifically indicated that dental caries can now be regarded as a disease of poverty (Graves *et al.* 1986; Palmer and Pitter 1988; Petersen 2005). The sharpest decline in caries prevalence has been in the upper SES groups, while reductions in disease rates in lower SES groups have been much more modest (Tinanoff 1995a; Tinanoff 1995b).

There is much discussion on whether or not to include socioeconomic variables in CRA instruments. Certainly these indicators will often select for high-risk individuals because they will be more inclined to develop higher levels of tooth decay than people living under less extreme conditions (Hobdell *et al.* 2003). But much like medical status, they do not indicate which risk factors are responsible for the development of disease, and they are often indirectly considered with stronger etiological factors (Bratthall *et al.* 2005). There is little doubt that dietary and health practices are affected by education, income, and environment; however, bacterial levels and cariogenic diet are normally already considered to be direct causes of caries and are regularly assessed. It, therefore, may be redundant to assess both socioeconomic variables and biological factors in the same CRA model.

Overall

It was concluded at the risk assessment conference at the University of North Carolina that clinical variables were stronger predictors of dental caries than non-clinical variables. Past experience of caries activity was the most significant indicator of future caries development, along with fluoride exposure, microbial agents, tooth morphology, and socioeconomic status (Powell 1998). Given that dental caries is a multifactorial disease, it only makes sense to use multiple predictors in order to accurately predict risk for the disease. It has been established that analyses applying a combination of biological and social factors have shown better results than any single risk factor studies. Work must be continued in this area to determine which caries risk factors and indicators are most effective for defined populations.

In practice, the idea of caries risk assessment is catching on. Recent dental school graduates are more likely to assess caries risk. Oral hygiene, salivary flow, and the presence of active caries were considered to be the most important risk factors (Riley *et al.* 2010; Yorty *et al.* 2011).

Multifactorial caries risk assessment models

It has been noted by a couple of researchers that the majority of CRA studies have been conducted in children and adolescent populations (Eriksen and Bjertness 1991; Powell 1998). There are relatively few studies involving adult subjects, and those that do exist focus mainly on older adults (aged 50+ years) and the development of root caries (Beck *et al.* 1988; Powell *et al.* 1991; Ravald and Birkhed 1992; Rivald *et al.* 1993; Joshi *et al.* 1993; Locker 1996). We are only just beginning to see studies that investigate general caries activity in populations that include younger adults (Bader *et al.* 2005; Ruiz Miravet *et al.* 2007; Sonbul *et al.* 2008). This is promising because the younger adult population may express different disease factors due to lifestyle changes that they encounter early into adulthood, such as living away from home for the first time, changes in dental care utilization, and access to dental care in rural settings (Skillman *et al.* 2010).

The following two examples are of multifactorial caries risk assessment instruments. Firstly, the Cariogram is a widely available tool that has been validated and has received much attention in the discipline of cariology.

It has been used extensively to identify caries risk factors for a variety of populations globally (Twetman *et al.* 2005; Ruiz Miravet *et al.* 2007; Al Mulla *et al.* 2009; Holgerson *et al.* 2009). This program is still freely available from the University of Malmo in Sweden in several languages, the software is compatible with Windows 7. Unfortunately, the creator of this very useful and validated CRA tool, Professor Bratthall, passed away in 2006, and the Cariogram has not been updated. Nevertheless, it can still be used in dental offices that use Windows. Secondly, the caries risk assessment form (Caries Risk and Preventive Needs Assessment) from the Faculty of Dentistry at the University of Toronto (Figure 15-1) is a university-developed model used by the students in the dental school clinic.

Cariogram

The Cariogram, developed in 1996, was originally conceived as an educational model aiming to demonstrate the multifactorial etiology of dental caries in a simple manner. It is a graphical picture illustrating the interactions of caries-related factors and the overall risk profile of the patient. In the beginning, the pie chart presentation included three components: diet, bacteria, and susceptibility. Based on this model, an interactive computer program was developed in 1997. Changes made to the program included the addition of two more sections to the pie chart—'circumstances' and 'chance of avoiding caries.' The circumstances sector included factors that did not participate directly in the development of caries but were risk predictors of dental caries, such as past caries experience and systemic diseases (Bratthall *et al.* 2005). An example of a pie-chart result after entering various caries risk scores is shown in Figure 15-6.

The program prompts the clinician to enter a weight (0 to 3, with '0' representing a low risk and '3' representing a high risk) for nine risk factors (caries experience, related general diseases, dietary contents, dietary frequency, plaque amount, *Streptococcus mutans*, fluoride, saliva secretion, and saliva buffering capacity) and a clinical judgment score. An algorithm was constructed

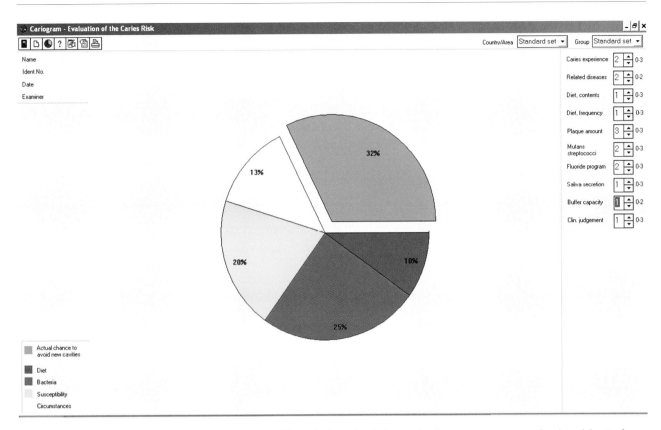

Figure 15-6 A sample result of a Cariogram Caries Risk analysis. This 'Cariogram' software program was developed by Professor Douglass Bratthall from the Dental School in Malmö, Sweden and is now available for download from that dental school for Window versions up to Windows 7, even though Dr. Bratthall is now deceased. By entering values of caries risk factors in the right-hand column, a pie chart is generated showing estimates of the chances of avoiding new caries (green).

so that all the factors entered into the model could be weighed and the patient's chance of avoiding caries could be calculated. This was represented as the final pie piece in the diagram. With this interactive program, it is possible to demonstrate to the patient how their caries risk can change as a result of various actions. Additionally, the patient's risk profile can be saved or printed, and the program offers recommendations for preventive measures that should be adopted to avoid new caries activity.

'Caries risk and preventive needs assessment' instrument

The Faculty of Dentistry at the University of Toronto developed its own caries risk assessment instrument (Caries Risk and Preventive Needs Assessment) and implemented it into their school-based dental clinic in 1996 (Figure 15-7).

It was introduced to the undergraduate students as a preventive dentistry assignment to help students focus their attention on their patients' caries preventive needs. The CRA form was intended to provide a guide for students to consider the various factors that may influence caries risk, as well as the preventive measures available to reduce the risk of disease (Burgess 1995).

There are five sections of the form:

1. Basic patient data: includes information regarding medical conditions, disabilities, and oral appliances that may influence the patient's overall caries risk.
2. Basic caries risk factors: 11 factors (for example, past caries and oral hygiene) are assessed and given a score ('0' for low, '1' for moderate, or '2' for high risk). A total risk score is calculated by summing the scores of the 11 risk factors.
3. Caries preventive factors: provides an inventory of the preventive practices routinely used by the patient.
4. Supplementary caries susceptibility tests: provides suggestions for additional diagnostic tests and procedures that could be used to investigate the patient's caries risk level.
5. Assessment summary: provides space to summarize the patient's risk factors and to propose preventive treatment.

Caries Risk and Preventive Needs Assessment

Student_____   Date_____

Patient_____   Age_____ Chart#_____

Conditions that will likely increase caries risk   Detailed explanation of how caries is affected

Conditions that will likely increase caries risk	Detailed explanation of how caries is affected
Medical condition summary	
Physical disability? Low dental IQ?	
Major lifestyle change? Negative attitude?	
Workplace/home environment	
Intra-oral appliance planned	

Rating of the Basic Caries Risk Factors

	Rating			PATIENT SCORE	COMMENTS
	=2	=1	=0		
Caries Activity coronal/root/incipient clinical/radiographic	≥two	one	none		
Past Caries coronal/smooth surface (DMFS)	free, smooth surface, or lower anterior	proximal	none or pit and fissure only		
Root caries index[a]	≥0.3	<0.3 to >0	0		
Usual Fluoride Exposure	<1/day	1/day	≥2/day		
Carbohydrate between meal frequency	>3/day	2/day	<1/day		
Oral Hygiene	Poor	Fair	Good		
Modified Gingival Bleeding Index (MGBI)[b]	>9	5–8	0–4		
Salivary Tests – stimulated *flow* (SSF) ml/min	≤0.5	<0.5 to >0.7	≥0.7		
– resting *flow* (if SSF <0.7) ml/min	≤0.1	<0.1 to >0.3	≥0.3		
Mutans streptococci CFU/ml	≥1,000,000	intermediate	≤10,000		
Lactobacilli CFU/ml	≥100,000	intermediate	≤1,000		
	Total Risk Score →				**Patient Caries Risk** High (≥7) Medium (4–6) Low (0–3)

[a]RCI: # teeth with carious roots (decayed or filled)/total # of teeth with exposed roots
[b]MGBI: use Stimudent test numbers collected from all facial-interproximal locations: (0 = no symptoms, 1 = inflammation/no bleeding, 2 = inflammation/slight bleeding, 3 = inflammation + bleeding)

Figure 15-7 Caries risk and preventive needs assessment.

The risk factors selected for assessment in this instrument were obtained from the literature. Although this CRA tool has been used for more than a decade, it has now been evaluated (Kraglund 2009). This tool was able to accurately categorize an individual's risk for future caries development, as demonstrated by two trends that emerged from the data. Firstly, as the caries risk elevated, the number of teeth affected by caries also increased. The number of carious teeth rose proportionately across the risk groups (0.20 for low, 1.13 for moderate, and 2.09 for high-risk groups). Secondly, as the caries risk rose, the number of individuals displaying caries at the follow-up exam also increased. Approximately 9% of the low-risk subjects presented with caries at the recall exam, while nearly 70% of the high-risk group exhibited new carious lesions. Predicting caries in the moderate risk group proved to be more challenging; just over half of the moderate risk group presented with dental decay at the follow-up appointment. Defining the appropriate criteria to select moderate risk individuals represents the utmost diagnostic challenge because it is difficult to know where to set the cut-off point between risk categorizations. Often it can be rather straightforward to identify low-risk and high-risk individuals; however, it is much more complicated to recognize moderate risk individuals that may have exhibited little or no dental disease for long periods of time followed by a sudden burst of caries activity.

With the University of Toronto CRA tool, all of the risk factors, except the usual fluoride exposure, were found to be significantly associated with caries increment in the bivariate analysis. This was not surprising because dental caries is a disease of multifactorial etiology and thus there were many elements related to the development of caries in this population. It should be noted, however, that the majority of the differences were found solely between the high- and low-risk groups. Again, this demonstrates the ease in identifying low risk, low caries and high risk, high caries patients, while detecting a moderate risk for caries development proves to be a more complex task.

Fluoride exposure was the only variable that was not significantly associated with dental caries in this study. Typically, exposure to various sources of fluoride has been shown to be a protective factor and helps to prevent the formation or progression of caries development (Marinho *et al.* 2003). However, it is becoming increasingly difficult to determine differences in fluoride exposure if there are several sources. One might be able to determine that extremely low fluoride exposure was a significant risk factor, but the patient would have to be from area with no exposure to professional fluorides, fluoridated products, and foods processed with fluoridated water.

The overall risk score from the CRA instrument, which is the summation of multiple risk factors, was by far the strongest predictor of future caries activity. This supports the current literature, which suggests that due to the multifactorial etiology of dental caries, the identification of several risk factors would increase the probability of formulating an accurate risk profile for our patients. Multifactorial CRA tools are becoming more popular and their use more prevalent as they present an overall picture of the interaction of the multitude of caries risk factors.

Summary

Table 15-1 summarizes various risk factors associated with caries. The statistical significance of the risk factors in predicting future decay are offered only as an estimate, since many studies have assigned different predictive values for these factors.

The dated method of relying on a single factor to dictate the development of a multifactorial disease often would lead to inaccurate predictions. For example, although consumption of fermentable sugars certainly plays a key role in the development of caries, reliance on

Table 15-1 Summary from the literature-predictors of caries

	P<0.01	P<0.05	P<0.05	NS
Primary teeth	SES, Existing caries	Sugared beverage and candy use	SM, plaque	Diet, Poor OH
Mixed dentition	Plaque on primary teeth Existing caries	DMFS at baseline	SM, LB, low F	Diet, Poor OH
Permanent teeth	Baseline DMFS Existing caries	Low saliva Ca, PO_4, F	SM, LB	Diet, Poor OH
Root caries	History of caries Existing root caries	LB, yeast		SM

this single factor as a predictor for future development of caries would often be misleading. Many individuals remain caries-free despite a high intake of sugar (high-risk behavior), likely due to the interaction of several low-risk behaviors. When all variables (except overall risk score) are considered in logistic regression analyses, individual risk factors such as caries experience (past and present), carbohydrate frequency, plaque and gingivitis scores, and stimulated salivary flow are, usually, significantly associated with caries activity. From the literature, it is clear that past caries experience remains the most powerful single predictor of future caries development. It is the most common risk indicator used in clinical practice and in research due to its strong predictive value. Although caries experience is a powerful indicator of caries activity, it cannot specify the particular risk factors that are causing the dental caries and, therefore, it cannot be used alone to specify appropriate preventive strategies directed at eliminating or modifying the patient's risk for caries development. Dental caries occurs as a result of the interaction of a dietary substrate, microbial pathogens, and host factors.

Dental decay does not occur in the absence of bacteria or in the absence of fermentable carbohydrates. However, bacterial counts alone cannot predict future caries experience very accurately and thus we must rely on the overall risk score (that is, the interaction of multiple factors) to assess risk level. Additionally, some researchers have suggested that microbial tests are not cost-effective and contribute only marginally to the prediction of future dental caries development if other clinical and sociodemographic data are available (Alanen *et al.* 1994). Given that the majority of caries occurs in a minority of the population, it is worthwhile to identify those patients at high risk for caries so that more aggressive preventive measures can be initiated. The multifactorial CRA tools described in this chapter are useful for that purpose.

References

Abernathy, J.R., Graves, R.C., Bohannan, H.M., *et al.* (1987) Development and application of a prediction model for dental caries. *Community Dentistry and Oral Epidemiology*, 15, 24–28.

Al Mulla, A.H., Kharsa, S.A., Kjellberg, H., *et al.* (2009) Caries risk profiles in orthodontic patients at follow-up using cariogram. *Angle Orthodontics*, 79, 323–330.

Alanen, P., Hurskainen, K. Isokangas P., *et al.* (1994) Clinician's ability to identify caries risk subjects. *Community Dentistry and Oral Epidemiology*, 22, 86–89.

Anderson, M.H., Bales, D.J., Omnell, K.A. (1993) Modern management of dental caries: the cutting edge is not the dental bur. *Journal of the American Dental Association*, 124, 37–44.

Angmar-Månsson, B.E. and Al-Khateeb, S. (1998) Caries diagnosis. *Journal of Dental Education*, 62, 771–780.

Anusavice, K.J. (2005) Present and future approaches for the control of caries. *Journal of Dental Education*, 69, 538–554.

Axelsson, P., Lindhe, J., Nystrom, B. (1991) On the prevention of caries and periodontal disease. Results of a 15-year longitudinal study in adults. *Journal of Clinical Periodontology*, 18, 182–189.

Axelsson, P., Paulander, J., Svardstrom, G., *et al.* (1993) Integrated caries prevention: effect of a needs-related preventive program on dental caries in children. County of Värmland, Sweden: results after 12 years. *Caries Research*, 27 (Suppl 1), 83–94.

Bader, J.D., Perrin, N.A., Maupomé, G., *et al.* (2005) Validation of a simple approach to caries risk assessment. *Journal of Public Health Dentistry*, 65, 76–81.

Batchelor, B. and Sheiham, A. (2002) The limitations of a 'high-risk' approach for the prevention of dental caries. *Community Dentistry and Oral Epidemiology*, 30, 302–312.

Beck, J.D. (1998) Risk revisited. *Community Dentistry and Oral Epidemiology*, 26, 220–225.

Beck, J.D., Kohout, F., Hunt, R.J. (1988) Identification of high caries in adults: attitudes, social factors and diseases. *International Dental Journal*, 38, 231–238.

Beck, J.D., Weintraub, J.A., Disney, J.A., *et al.* (1992) University of North Carolina Caries Risk Assessment Study: comparisons of high risk prediction, any risk prediction, and any risk etiologic models. *Community Dentistry and Oral Epidemiology*, 20, 313–321.

Billings, R.J. (1993) An epidemiologic perspective of saliva flow rates as indicators of susceptibility to oral disease. *Critical Reviews in Oral Biology and Medicine*, 4, 351–356.

Bratthall, D. and Hänsel Petersson, G. (2005) Cariogram—a multifactorial risk assessment model for a multifactorial disease. *Community Dentistry and Oral Epidemiology*, 33, 256–264.

Bratthall, D., Hänsel Petersson, G., Stjernswärd, J.R. (2004) Cariogram manual, Internet version 2.01. April 2, 2004.

Bratthall, D., Hänsel Petersson, G., Sundberg, H. (1996) Reasons for the caries decline: what do the experts believe? *European Journal of Oral Science*, 104, 416–422; discussion 423–425, 430–432.

Brown, J.P. (1995) Developing clinical teaching methods for caries risk assessment: introduction to the topic and its history. *Journal of Dental Education*, 59, 928–931.

Burgess, R.C. (1995) Assessment of caries risk factors and preventive practices. *Journal of Dental Education*, 59, 962–971.

Burt, B.A. (1998) Prevention policies in the light of the changed distribution of dental caries. *Acta Odontologica Scandinavica*, 56, 179–186.

Burt, B.A., Eklund, S.A., Morgan, K.L., *et al.* (1988) The effects of sugar intake and frequency of ingestion on dental caries increment in a three-year longitudinal study. *Journal of Dental Research*, 67, 1422–1429.

Burt, B.A. and Pai, S. (2001) Sugar Consumption and caries risk: a systematic review. *Journal of Dental Education*, 65, 1017–1023.

Campus, G., Cagetti, M.G., Senna, A., *et al.* (2009) Caries risk profiles in Sardinian schoolchildren using Cariogram. *Acta Odontologica Scandinavica*, 67, 146–152.

Carvalho, J.C, Thylstrup, A., Ekstrand, K. (1992) Results after 3 years non-operative occlusal caries treatment of erupting permanent molars. *Community Dentistry and Oral Epidemiology*, 20, 187–192.

Demers, M., Brodeur, J-M., Mouton, C., *et al.* (1990) Caries predictors suitable for mass-screenings in children: a literature review. *Community Dental Health*, 7, 11–21.

Disney, J.A., Graves, R.C., Stamm, J.W., *et al.* (1992) The University of North Carolina Caries Risk Assessment study: further developments in caries risk prediction. *Community Dentistry and Oral Epidemiology*, 20, 64–75.

Doméjean-Orliaguet, S., Gansky, S.A., Featherstone, J.D. (2006) Caries risk assessment in an educational environment. *Journal of Dental Education*, 70, 1346–1354.

Douglass, C.W. (1998) Risk assessment in dentistry. *Journal of Dental Education*, 62, 756–761.

Drake, C.W., Hunt, R.J., Beck, J.D., *et al.* (1994) Eighteen-month coronal caries incidence in North Carolina older adults. *Journal of Public Health Dentistry*, 54, 24–30.

Dye, B.A., Tan, S., Smith, V., *et al.* (2007) Trends in oral health status: United States, 1988–1994 and 1999–2004. *Vital Health Statistics*, 11, 248, 1–92.

Edelstein, B.L. (1994) The medical management of dental caries. *Journal of the American Dental Association*, 125 (Suppl), 31S–39S.

Eriksen, H.M. and Bjertness, E. (1991) Concepts of health and disease and caries prediction: a literature review. *Scandinavian Journal of Dental Research*, 99, 476 483.

Evans, R.W., Pakdaman, A., Dennison, P.J., *et al.* (2008) The caries management system: an evidence-based preventive strategy for dental practitioners. Application for adults. *Australian Dental Journal*, 53, 83–92.

Fazilat, S., Sauerwein, R., McLeod, J., *et al.* (2010) Application of adenosine triphosphate-driven bioluminescence for quantification of plaque bacteria and assessment of oral hygiene in children. *Pediatric Dentistry*, 32, 195–204.

FDI Working Group. (1988) Review of methods of identification of high caries risk groups and individuals. Fédération Dentaire Internationale Technical Report No. 31. *International Dental Journal*, 38, 177–189.

Featherstone, J.D. (2003) The caries balance: contributing factors and early detection. *Journal of the California Dental Association*, 31, 129–133.

Featherstone, J.D.B., Adair, S.M., Anderson, M.H., *et al.* (2003) Caries management by risk assessment: consensus statement, April 2002. *Journal of the California Dental Association*, 31, 257–69.

Featherstone, J.D.B., Doméjean-Orliaguet, S., Jenson, L. (2007) Caries risk assessment in practice for age 6 through adult. *Journal of the California Dental Association*, 35, 703–707, 710–713.

Fleiss, J.L. and Kingman, A. (1990) Statistical management of data in clinical research. *Critical Reviews in Oral Biology and Medicine*, 1, 55–66.

Fletcher, R.W. and Fletcher, S.W. Diagnosis. In: *Clinical Epidemiology: the Essentials*. (Eds. R.W. Fletcher and S.W. Fletcher) pp. 35–58, 4th edn. *Lippincott Williams and Wilkins Baltimore*.

Flink, H. (2007) Studies on the prevalence of reduced salivary flow rate in relation to general health and dental caries, and effect of iron supplementation. *Swedish Dental Journal. Supplement*, 192, 3–50.

Fontana, M. and Zero, D.T. (2006) Assessing patients' caries risk. *Journal of the American Dental Association*, 137, 1231–1239.

Fure, S. (1998) Five-year incidence of caries, salivary and microbial conditions in 60-, 70- and 80-year-old Swedish individuals. *Caries Research*, 32, 166–174.

Graves, R.C., Bohannan, H.M., Disney, J.A., *et al.* (1986) Recent dental caries and treatment dental patterns in US children. *Journal of Public Health Dentistry*, 46, 23–29.

Hänsel Petersson, G., Fure, S., Bratthall, D. (2003) Evaluation of a computer-based caries risk assessment program in an elderly group of individuals. *Acta Odontologica Scandinavica*, 61, 164–171.

Hänsel Petersson, G., Twetman, S., Bratthall, D. (2002) Evaluation of a computer program for caries risk assessment in schoolchildren, *Caries Research*, 36, 327–340.

Hänsel Petersson, G. (2003) Assessing caries risk-using the Cariogram model. *Swedish Dental Journal*. Supplement, 158, 1–65.

Harris, R., Nicoll, A.D., Adair, P.M., *et al.* (2004) Risk factors for dental caries in young children: a systematic review of the literature. *Community Dental Health*, 21(1 Suppl), 71–85.

Hausen, H., Kärkkäinen, S., Seppä, L. (2000) Application of the high-risk strategy to control dental caries. *Community Dentistry and Oral Epidemiology*, 28, 26–34.

Hausen, H. (1997) Caries prediction-state of the art. *Community Dentistry and Oral Epidemiology*, 25, 87–96.

Helfenstein, U., Steiner, M., Marthaler, T.M. (1991) Caries prediction on the basis of past caries including precavity lesions. *Caries Research*, 25, 372–326.

Hildebrandt, G.H. (1995) Caries risk assessment and prevention for adults. *Journal of Dental Education*, 59, 972–979.

Hobdell, M.H., Oliveira, E.R, Bautista, R., *et al.* (2003) Oral diseases and socio-economic status (SES). *British Dental Journal*, 194, 91–96.

Holgerson, P.L., Twetman, S., Stecksèn-Blicks, C. (2009) Validation of an age-modified caries risk assessment program (Cariogram) in preschool children. *Acta Odontologica Scandinavica*, 67, 106–112.

Hunter, P.B. (1988) Risk factors in dental caries. *International Dental Journal*, 38, 211–217.

Isokangas, P., Alanen, P., Tiekso, J. (1993) The clinician's ability to identify caries risk subjects without saliva tests—a pilot study. *Community Dentistry and Oral Epidemiology*, 21, 8–10.

Jenson, L., Budenz, A.W., Featherstone, J.D.B., *et al.* (2007) Clinical protocols for caries management by risk assessment. *Journal California Dental Association*, 35, 714–723.

Joshi, A., Papas, A.S., Giunta, J. (1993) Root caries incidence and associated risk factors in middle aged and older adults. *Gerondotology*, 10, 83–89.

Kidd, E.A. (1999) Caries management. *Dental Clinics of North America*, 43, 743–764.

Kraglund, F. (2009) Evaluation of a caries risk assessment model in an adult population. M.Sc. Thesis, University of Toronto, Canada.

Krasse, B. (1988) Biological factors as indicators of future caries. *International Dental Journal*, 38, 219–225.

Kutsch, V.K. and Kutsch, C.L. (2006) Disease prevention: caries risk assessment. *Dentistry Today*, 25, 86, 88–9.

Kutsch, V.K., Milicich, G., Domb, W., *et al.* (2007) How to integrate CAMBRA into private practice. *Journal of the California Dental Association*, 35, 778–785.

Leverett, D.H., Proskin, H.M., Featherstone, J.D., *et al.* (1993) Caries risk assessment in a longitudinal discrimination study. *Journal of Dental Research*, 72, 538–543.

Li, Y. and Wang, W. (2002) Predicting caries in permanent teeth from caries in primary teeth: an eight year cohort study. *Journal of Dental Research*, 81, 561–566.

Limeback, H. (1996) Treating dental caries as an infectious disease. Applying the medical model in practice to prevent dental caries. *Ontario Dentist*, 73, 23–25.

Locker, D., Slade, G.D., Leake, J.L. (1989) Prevalence of and factors associated with root decay in older adults in Canada. *Journal of Dental Research*, 69, 768–772.

Locker, D. (1996) Incidence of root caries in an older Canadian population. *Community Dentistry and Oral Epidemiology*, 24, 403–407.

Loesche, W.J. (1986) Role of Streptococcus mutans in human dental decay. *Microbiological Reviews*, 50, 353–380.

Marinho, V.C., Higgins, J.P., Logan, S., *et al.* (2003) Topical fluoride (toothpastes, mouthrinses, gels or varnishes) for preventing dental caries in children and adolescents. *Cochrane Database Systematic Reviews*, 4, CD002782.

Marthaler, T.M., O'Mullane, D.M., Vrbic, V. (1995) The prevalence of dental caries in Europe 1990–1995. ORCA Saturday afternoon symposium 1995. *Caries Research*, 30, 237–255.

Moss, M.E. and Zero, D.T. (1995) An overview of caries risk assessment and its potential utility. *Journal of Dental Education*, 59, 932–940.

Newbrun, E. (1992) Preventing dental caries: breaking the chain of transmission. *Journal of the American Dental Association*. 123, 55–59.

Ngo, H. and Gaffney, S. (2005) Risk Assessment in the Diagnosis and Management of Caries. In: *Preservation and Restoration of Tooth Structure* (Eds. G.J. Mount and W.R. Hume), 2nd edn pp. 61–82. Knowledge Books and Software, Brighton, Queensland, Australia.

NIH Consensus Development Conference on Diagnosis and Management of Dental Caries Throughout Life. Bethesda, MD, March 26–28, 2001. Conference Papers. *Journal of Dental Education*, 65, 935–1179.

Palmer, J.D. and Pitter, A.F. (1988) Differences in dental caries levels between 8-year-old children in Bath from different socio-economic groups. *Community Dental Health*, 4, 363–367.

Petersen, P.E. and Yamamoto, T. (2005) Improving the oral health of older people: the approach of the WHO Global Oral Health Programme. *Community Dentistry and Oral Epidemiology*, 33, 81–92.

Petersen, P.E. (2005) Sociobehavioural risk factors in dental caries—international perspectives. *Community Dentistry and Oral Epidemiology*, 33, 274–249.

Petersson, G.H. and Bratthall, D. (1996) The caries decline: a review of reviews. *European Journal of Oral Science*, 104, 436–443.

Pienihäkkinen, K. (1987) Caries prediction through combined use of incipient caries lesions, salivary buffering capacity, lactobacilli and yeasts in Finland. *Community Dentistry and Oral Epidemiology*, 15, 325–328.

Pitts, N.B. (1997) Diagnostic tools and measurements—impact on appropriate care. *Community Dentistry and Oral Epidemiology*, 25, 24–35.

Pitts, N.B. (1998) Risk assessment and caries prediction. *Journal of Dental Education*, 62, 762–770.

Powell, L.V., Mancl, L.A., Senft, G.D. (1991) Exploration of prediction models for caries risk assessment of the geriatric population. *Community Dentistry and Oral Epidemiology*, 19, 291–295.

Powell, L.V. (1998) Caries prediction: a review of the literature. *Community Dentistry and Oral Epidemiology*, 26, 361–371.

Powell, L.V. (1998) Caries risk assessment: relevance to the practitioner. *Journal of the America Dental Association*, 129, 349–353.

Ravald, N., Birkhed, D., Hamp, S.E. (1993) Root caries susceptibility in periodontally treated patients. Results after 12 years. *Journal of Clinical Periodontology*, 20, 124–129.

Ravald, N. and Birkhed, D. (1992) Prediction of root caries in periodontally treated patients maintained with different fluoride programmes. *Caries Research*, 26, 450–458.

Reich, E., Lussi, A., Newbrun, E. (1999) Caries-risk assessment. *International Dental Journal*, 49, 15–26.

Riley, J.L. 3rd, Qvist, V., Fellows, J.L., et al. (2010) Dentists' use of caries risk assessment in children: findings from the Dental Practice-Based Research Network. *General Dentistry*, 58, 230–234.

Rose, G. (2001) Sick individuals and sick populations. International *Journal of Epidemiology*, 30, 427–432.

Ruiz Miravet, A., Montiel Company, J.M., Almerich Silla, J.M. (2007) Evaluation of caries risk in a young adult population. *Medicina Oral, Patologia Oral, y Cirugia Bucal*, 12, E412–418.

Scheinin, A., Pienihäkkinen, K., Tiesko, J. et al. (1992) Multifactorial modeling for root caries prediction. *Community Dentistry and Oral Epidemiology*, 20, 35–37.

Skillman, S.M., Doescher, M.P., Mouradian, W.E. et al. (2010) The challenge to delivering oral health services in rural America. *Journal of Public Health Dentistry*, 70 (Suppl 1), S49–57.

Sonbul, H., Al-Otaibi, M., Birkhed, D. (2008) Risk profile of adults with several dental restorations using the Cariogram model. *Acta Odontologica Scandinavica*, 66, 351–357.

Stamm, J.W., Disney, J.A., Graves, R.C., et al. (1988) The University of North Carolina caries risk assessment study, I: rationale and content. *Journal of Public Health Dentistry*, 48, 225–232.

Stamm, J.W., Stewart, P.W., Bohannan, H.M., et al. (1991) Risk assessment for oral diseases. *Advances in Dental Research*, 5, 4–17.

Stecksén-Blicks, C., Holgerson, P.L., Twetman, S. (2007) Caries risk profiles in two-year-old children from northern Sweden. *Oral Health and Preventive Dentistry*, 5, 215–21.

Steiner, M., Helfenstein, U., Marthaler, T.M. (1992) Dental predictors of high caries increment in children. *Journal of Dental Research*, 71, 1926–1933.

Tayanin, G.L., Petersson, G.H., Bratthall, D. (2005) Caries risk profiles of 12–13-year-old children in Laos and Sweden. *Oral Health and Preventive Dentistry*, 3, 15–23.

Tinanoff, N. (1995a) Critique of evolving methods for caries risk assessment. *Journal of Dental Education*, 59, 980–985.

Tinanoff, N. (1995b) Dental caries risk assessment and prevention. *Dental Clinics of North America*, 39, 709–719.

Tranæus, S., Shi, X-Q., Angmar-Månsson, B. (2005) Caries risk assessment: methods available to clinicians for caries detection. *Community Dentistry and Oral Epidemiology*, 33, 265–273.

Twetman, S., Petersson, G.H., Bratthall, D. (2005) Caries risk assessment as a predictor of metabolic control in young Type 1 diabetics. *Diabetes Medicine*, 22, 312–315.

U.S. National Institute of Dental and Craniofacial Research. 2000. Oral health in America: a report of the surgeon general, executive summary. Rockville, Md.: U.S. National Institute of Dental and Craniofacial Research.

van Houte, J. (1993) Microbiological predictors of caries risk. *Advances in Dental Research*, 7, 87–96.

van Houte, J. (1994) Role of micro-organisms in caries etiology. *Journal of Dental Research*, 73, 672–681.

Wilson, R.F. and Ashley, P.P. (1989) Identification of caries risk in schoolchildren: salivary buffering capacity and bacterial counts, sugar intake and caries experience as predictors of 2-year and 3-year caries increment. *British Dental Journal*, 167, 99–102.

Wright, J.T., Cutter, G.R., Dasanayake, A.P., et al. (1992) Effect of conventional dental restorative treatment on bacteria in saliva. *Community Dentistry and Oral Epidemiology*, 20, 138–143.

Yorty, J.S., Walls, A.T., Wearden, S. (2011) Caries risk assessment/treatment programs in U.S. dental schools: an eleven-year follow-up. *Journal of Dental Education*, 75, 62–67.

Young, D.A., Featherstone, J.D.B., Roth, J.R., et al. (2007a) Caries management by risk assessment: implementation guidelines. *Journal of the California Dental Association*, 35, 799–805.

Young, D.A., Featherstone, J.D.B., Roth, J.R. (2007b) Curing the silent epidemic: caries management in the 21st century and beyond. *Journal of the California Dental Association*, 35, 681–685.

Zero, D. (2004) Sugars: the arch criminal? *Caries Research*, 38, 277–285.

Zero, D.T., Fontana, M., Lennon, Á.M. (2001) Clinical applications and outcomes using indicators of risk in caries management. *Journal of Dental Education*, 65, 1126–1132.

Zickert, I., Emilson, C.G., Krasse B. (1982) Streptococcus mutans, lactobacilli and dental health in 13–14 year-old Swedish children. *Community Dentistry and Oral Epidemiology*, 10, 77–81.

16

Fluoride therapy

Hardy Limeback and Colin Robinson

Introduction

For over 60 years, dental professionals have been attempting to control caries with fluoride and its various inorganic and organic compounds (Ripa 1993). For most of this time, the build up of fluoride in the mineralized tooth tissues during tooth development was thought to render them more resistant to the effects of plaque acids. More recently, however, there has been a paradigm shift in terms of our understanding of how fluoride works (Fejerskov 2004; National Research Council 2006). It is now well established that fluoride has a direct topical influence on the dynamic mineralization-remineralization process that occurs under the plaque biofilm that adheres to tooth enamel (crown portion of the tooth) as well as cementum and dentin (exposed surfaces of the root). The idea that fluoride pills taken daily during tooth development, or the consumption of fluoridated water, will make teeth 'stronger' and more resistant to decay has been largely abandoned in many countries. (See the section below on fluoride supplements.)

Fluoride appears to provide its benefit when present in the oral cavity. Its effectiveness depends on how frequently it is administered in the mouth, and the mechanism of fluoride's topical anti-caries effect will depend on the mode of application, its chemical formulation and, especially its concentration. The beneficial effects of topical fluoride application were first seen as a result of daily exposure to very low concentrations of fluoride by means of the drinking water or diets enriched in fluoride. Subsequent trials using various means of topical fluoride administration showed significant reductions in caries. This culminated in the addition of fluoride to toothpastes and mouth rinses with concentrations of fluoride 1,000-fold higher than fluoridated water. These became quite popular, and indeed became the gold standard, especially after the endorsement of the professional dental organizations.

Before discussing various fluoride therapies, dental professionals should be able to feel comfortable in dealing with different concentrations and modes of expression used in the literature. Some fluoride levels are extremely low (for example, the fluoride concentration in serum, 0.01 parts per million [ppm]), and others are extremely high (topical fluoride varnish ~20,000 ppm).

The following table shows various fluoride levels, which the reader can use as a resource in this context, and some sample calculations relating a number of ways of expressing fluoride concentration (Table 16-1).

Sample calculations:
Converting 1.0 ppm F to micromolar

$1.0\,ppm = 1\,mg/L$
$= 0.001\,gm/L$
$= 0.001\,gm/L \times mole/19\,gm\,F$
$= 0.00005263\,moles/L$
$= 0.05263\,mM = 52.63\,\mu M$
Therefore, multiply ppm by 52.63 to get μM
(for example, $1,000\,ppm = 52,630\,\mu M$)

Converting toothpaste concentrations to ppm F

$5\%\,NaF = 5\,gm\,NaF/100\,mL$
$= 5 \times 19/42\,gm\,F/100\,cc$
$= 2.26\,gm\,F/100\,mL$

Comprehensive Preventive Dentistry, First Edition. Edited by Hardy Limeback.
© 2012 John Wiley & Sons, Ltd. Published 2012 by John Wiley & Sons, Ltd.

Table 16-1 Conversion of fluoride concentrations

Fluoride concentration	ppm	μM	mM
5% NaF fluoride varnish	22,620	1,180,000	1,183.00
1.23% F in 'APF' topical fluoride gel	12,300	647,000	647.35
0.8% MFP = 0.8 gm	1,060	55,800	55.8
0.4% SnF$_2$ gel	970	51,100	51.1
0.05% NaF daily mouth rinse	226	11,800	11.84
1 mg/mL fluoridated water	1.0	52.63	0.05263
Salivary fluoride levels (fluoridated areas)	0.019–0.038	1–2	0.001–0.002
Baseline fluoride in saliva	0.0056	0.3	0.0003

= 22,600 mg F/L

= 22,600 ppm F

0.0219% SnF$_2$ = 0.0219 gm SnF$_2$/100 cc × 38/156.7

= 0.00531 gm F/100 mL

= 53.1 mg F/L

= 53.1 ppm F

0.4% SnF$_2$ = 0.4 gm SnF$_2$/100 cc × 38/156.7 gm F/ SnF$_2$

= 0.097 gm/100 mL

= 970 mg/L

= 970 ppm

0.8% MFP = 0.8 gm Na$_2$PO$_3$F/100 mL

= 0.8 gm × 19/144 F/100 mL

= 0.1055 gm F/100 mL

= 1,055 mg F/L

= 1,055 ppm F

Converting fluoride levels in plaque

0.3 mmol F/gm plaque weight = 0.0003 moles F/gm plaque

= 0.0003 × 19 gm F/gm plaque

= 0.0057 gm F/gm plaque

= 5.7 mg × 1,000 F/kg plaque

= 5,700 ppm F

1 μM/mL = 19 micrograms/mL

= 19,000 μg/L

= 19 mg/L

= 19 ppm F

How fluoride works

Fluoride's effect on tooth mineral

Our current understanding of how fluoride affects tooth mineral to reduce dental caries has been reviewed extensively (ten Cate 1999; Robinson *et al.* 2000; Aoba 2004; Robinson 2009). Enamel is composed primarily (~95%) of hydroxyapatite (HA) crystals in which are substituted a number of other ions including fluoride. Well-formed HA crystals have a hexagonal configuration of phosphate and calcium ions with a central hydroxyl ion (Figure 16-1).

The incorporation of magnesium and carbonate because of a poor fit in the crystal (schematically shown in Figure 16-1b) tends to destabilize the crystal, making it more susceptible to acid dissolution. In developing enamel, carbonate will substitute for phosphate ions and if the concentration is high enough for hydroxyl ions. Magnesium can substitute to a limited extent for calcium but often resides at the crystal surfaces. There are reports that a very small amount of separate phases, for example, whitlockite (calcium magnesium phosphate) might be present. Carbonated apatite (and some reports of magnesium whitlockite) occur in developing enamel.

Fluoride, however, substituting for the hydroxyl group fits extremely well and stabilizes the HA molecule forming fluoridated apatite. If all of the hydroxyl ions are substituted fluorapatite (FA) forms. The fluoride ion is extremely electronegative and forms very strong hydrogen bonds with hydroxyl and acid phosphate groups in the HA crystal rendering the enamel surface more difficult to protonate. Essentially this makes the enamel more difficult to demineralize, and it also favors the remineralization process. This is the primary chemical mechanism of fluoride's action to protect the tooth against acids produced by plaque metabolism, as follows:

$Ca_{10}(PO_4)_6(OH)_2 + Mg^{++}$ = magnesium whitlockite

$Ca_{10}(PO_4)_6(OH)_2 + CO_3^-$ = carbonated apatite

$Ca_{10}(PO_4)_6(OH)_2 + 2F^-$ = $Ca_{10}(PO_4)_6(F)_2$ (fluorapatite) + 2(OH$^-$)

Fluoridated apatite and/or fluorapatite are generally found in the surface layers of enamel that contains high fluoride concentrations of fluoride. This can arise both during development and from topical exposure (see below).

Changes in the chemistry of enamel during carious attack

The acidogenic plaque bacteria, primarily *S. mutans*, produce mainly lactic acid, which dissociates into lactate and protons. The lower pH encourages apatite crystal

(a)

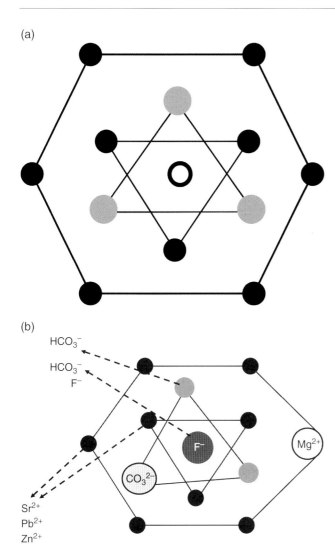

(b)

HCO_3^-

HCO_3^-

F^-

Sr^{2+}
Pb^{2+}
Zn^{2+}

CO_3^{2-}

F^-

Mg^{2+}

Figure 16-1 (a, b) The crystal chemistry of apatite. Reprinted from Robinson 2009, with permission from the European Academy of Paediatric Dentistry. (a) Unit cell of hydroxyapatite showing central hydroxyl ion surrounded by triangles of calcium and phosphate, the whole surrounded by a hexagon of calcium ions. (b) Unit cell of hydroxyapatite showing the central ion (the hydroxyl ion has been replaced with a fluoride ion.) and possible location of other substituent ions notably carbonate and magnesium. ● = Calcium ion, ● = phosphate ion, O = hydroxyl ion.

dissolution into component ions (Ca^{++}, PO_4^{---}, OH^-, Mg^{++}, CO_3^{--}). When the acid is neutralized, the Mg^{++}, CO_3^- are lost, the fluoride (F^-) ion enters the remineralizing crystal and replaces the hydroxyl group (OH^-) resulting in a crystal that is enriched in fluorapatite (FA) (Figure 16-2).

The carious lesion begins with demineralization of the enamel surface. However, only soluble components (carbonate and magnesium rich) are likely to be removed. This allows acid to pass into the subsurface regions with minimal damage to the fluoride-rich and therefore acid-resistant surface. This relatively intact surface layer also acts as a barrier to dissolved calcium and phosphate. The exit of these ions is slowed down resulting in a buildup of calcium-phosphate ions. This together with the high fluoride tends to favor reprecipitation preserving the apparent integrity of the surface layer. This feature of an incipient lesion is extremely important. Without an intact surface layer, plaque would get trapped in the early cavitations and undoubtedly speed the progress of the carious lesion. The fluoride composition of a typical white spot lesion on the surface of enamel is shown in Figure 16-3.

After the formation of the surface zone, subsurface enamel is progressively demineralized, and more distinct zones can be seen based on their pore structure. During this process some crystals become enriched with fluoride, making them more resistant to future acid dissolution. In addition, as fluoride ions accumulate in remineralizing apatite crystals, there is a net loss of magnesium and carbonate (Figure 16-4).

In short, the removal of destabilizing carbonate and magnesium and accumulation of fluoride by the lesion renders it less acid soluble. Since the surface layer stays relatively intact, reactions occur in the subsurface layers increasing the fluoride content even at the earliest stages of the incipient lesions. The balance between demineralization and remineralization ("demin-remin" cycles) is determined by the amount of acid produced by the plaque biofilm and how quickly the acid is either washed away by saliva or neutralized by salivary buffers.

Fluoride encourages remineralization for two reasons. First, the solubility products of fluoride-enriched minerals are lowered. Secondly, as fluoride is incorporated into recrystallizing apatite crystals, hydroxyl groups are released, which neutralize some of the protons produced by the bacteria (the hydroxyl groups 'mop up' some protons and combine with them to form water). The removal of protons increases the pH, and this will further drive the solubility reaction toward the precipitation of apatite. This process follows:

1. Solubility equilibrium:

$$2(H_2O) = 2H^+ + 2(OH^-)$$
$$10\ Ca^{++} + 6\ PO_4^{---} + 2H_2O = Ca_{10}(PO_4)_6(OH)_2 + 2H^+$$

Conversely as hydroxyapatite crystals grow, hydroxyl ions are accumulated and the pH will therefore drop, inhibiting further remineralization.

2. Fluoride substitution reaction:

$$Ca_{10}(PO_4)_6(OH)_2 + 2F^- = Ca_{10}(PO_4)_6(F)_2 + 2(OH^-)$$
$$2H^+ + 2(OH^-) = 2(H_2O)$$

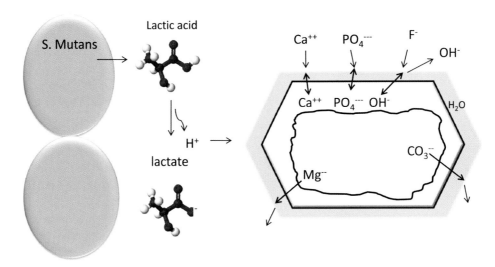

Figure 16-2 Changes in composition of the apatite crystals during acid demineralization and neutral remineralization.

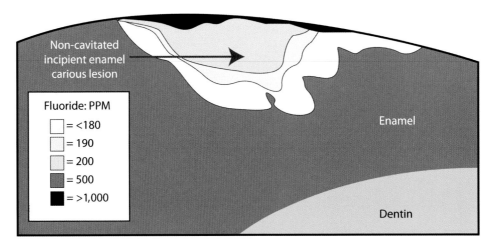

Figure 16-3 An illustration of an incipient enamel carious lesion. The table (*inset*) indicates the level of fluoride in the lesion. Note that the surface layer is enriched in fluoride. This is one of the reasons the surface layer stays intact and the integrity of the enamel is preserved allowing for potential remineralization and 'healing' of the lesion. Adapted from Weatherell *et al.* 1977.

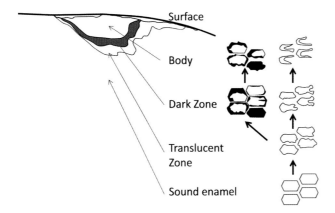

Figure 16-4 An illustration of a carious lesion showing various stages of demineralized enamel crystals (*right*) and remineralized crystals (*left*), that are enriched in fluoride (*black coloring*). Created from Robinson *et al.* 2000 and Robinson 2009.

As indicated above, however, if fluoride is added to the environment, re-precipitation will release hydroxyl groups and raise the pH encouraging precipitation of more crystals.

Therefore, when bacterial acids are produced, fluoride, through the formation of fluoridated apatite and fluorapatite, not only encourages remineralization but can also help to control low pH levels. Clearly, the reservoir of fluoride in the enamel is limited for this purpose if the production of acid is great and the severity of the pH gradient will determine if there is a net loss of mineral components. If the conditions intraorally are such that remineralization is favored, such as during good salivary buffering, then the 'demin-remin' cycle will favor remineralization. The 'demin-remin process is repeated numerous times as soon as the tooth erupts into the mouth and continues during the following months and years. As long as there is no cavitation, or excessive loss of subsurface mineral, there is the potential for a

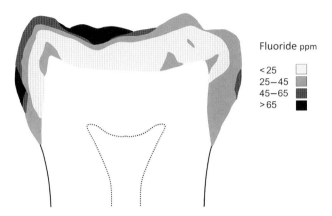

Figure 16-5 Cross-sectional analysis of a human molar showing fluoride distribution. The legend indicates fluoride concentration in various regions of human enamel. Note that the enamel is enriched in fluoride in the pits and fissures as well as in the proximal contact areas. This is the result of many 'demin-remin' cycles that encourage fluoride build up in those areas under daily 'acid attack.' Adapted from Robinson and Weatherell (1995) with permission.

complete reversal of the lesion. Essentially, the enamel lesion is arrested, or 'healed' and even more resistant to decay than when the incipient lesion initially formed.

Analysis of mature teeth after years of fluoride exposure (Figure 16-5) indicates that the fluoride incorporation occurs where there are plaque deposits that are not usually removed with toothbrushing, that is, in the pits and fissures of the occlusal surfaces and in the approximal contact areas.

Fluoride profiles have been mapped (Figure 16-6) showing that the fluoride concentration at the extreme surface starts out at about 1,000 ppm and drop precipitously toward the dentin, where it increases slightly and then drops again (Weatherell *et al.* 1974; Weatherell *et al.* 1977; Nakagaki *et al.* 1987; Thuy *et al.* 2003).

Even when fluoridated toothpaste is used, these levels diminish with age presumably due to wear and/or erosion. However, on surfaces where plaque collects, the fluoride content may vary but does not seem to decrease. This also depends on the morphological characteristics of the tooth (Figure 16-7).

If fluoride in enamel is enriched where plaque is not removed regularly, one can conclude that the presence of plaque, and the 'demin-remin' cycles produced by plaque,

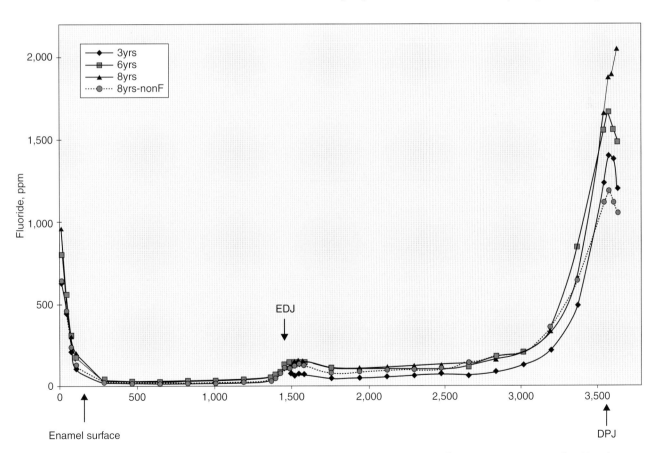

Figure 16-6 Fluoride content of the teeth from the enamel surface to the pulp as a result of increasing exposure to fluoridated water. The enamel has more fluoride near the surface as a result of years of fluoride exposure, but the levels are not much higher statistically. Adapted from Thuy *et al.* 2003.

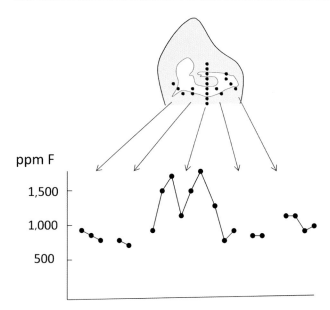

Figure 16-7 Analysis of the fluoride in the approximal contact area of a premolar. The illustration is of a white spot lesion (*white area*) in the proximal zone of a premolar. The dots represent the areas of the tooth in the region of the contact zone that were analyzed for fluoride content. Clearly the central region of the white spot, the area that was likely covered by plaque the longest (that is, when flossing is absent), had more fluoride content. This was the result of frequent 'demin-remin' cycles in the presence of fluoride. Adapted from Robinson 2009, with permission from the European Academy of Paediatric Dentistry.

helps to deposit fluoride where it is needed most—under plaque biofilm. This apparent paradox makes perfect sense. Fluoride accumulation in enamel is aided by plaque, which itself accumulates fluoride that is applied topically. However, the architecture of the plaque has been shown to be complex. The surface area to mass ratios of plaque biomass mirrored the fluoride distribution. Interaction with plaque biomass components would seem to restrict diffusion of fluoride through the plaque layers (Watson *et al.* 2005).

Thus, while fluoridated toothpaste (1,000 ppm) can significantly increase the fluoride content of plaque, very little of the fluoride appears to make it to the enamel surface (Figure 16-8) Fluoride accumulation in the underlying enamel must therefore be relatively slow, and this implies that the concentrations active at the tooth surface must be many times lower than the amounts applied via toothpaste, for example. It seems likely that what little fluoride is present may be released at low pH and diffuses into the incipient lesion where it is needed during the 'demin-remin' cycles.

Fluoridated water does not, on the other hand, increase the fluoride of enamel significantly (Figure 16-8c). It is possible that stagnation areas under plaque in people living in fluoridated areas may contain enough fluoride to provide a measure of protection from caries. The mechanism of action of fluoride as delivered by fluoridated water is still unclear. (See also the section on water fluoridation.)

Overall, the data, however, point convincingly to the fact that fluoride's action is primarily at the level of the incipient lesion, and plaque may actually aid in providing the fluoride.

Topical fluorides

Thus far we have introduced the concept of 'demin-remin' (demineralization-remineralization) and how topical fluoride plays a role in building resistant incipient lesions that may become arrested and may even remineralize. Topical fluorides are now available in a variety of different formulations and concentrations. The most obvious topical source is, of course, saliva, and it is important to consider this first.

Salivary fluoride

Salivary fluoride contributes very little in terms of topical fluoride when there are other sources of fluoride available (Limeback 1999; Cury 2008). For example, salivary fluoride levels can be as low as 0.006 ppm (Oliveby 1990). Foods and beverages (including fluoridated water), with fluoride levels 100 times that level, are consumed several times a day. Add to this the fluoridated consumer products that contain typically 1,000–1,100 ppm fluoride that are used two to three times a day. Following such exposures, salivary levels seldom return to baseline resting/fasting levels. Such elevated salivary fluoride can therefore be a source of extra topical fluoride during 'demin-remin' cycles. A summary of salivary fluoride levels compared to other sources on a daily basis is presented in Figure 16-9.

Fluoridated toothpaste

The evidence that fluoridated toothpastes work better than their non-fluoridated vehicle controls in reducing caries is quite extensive. There are several thorough reviews (Rolla 1991; Marinho *et al.* 2003b; Marinho 2009; Walsh *et al.* 2010). Although there is a dose response with fluoridated toothpaste, it is not clear from the many clinical trials carried out whether there is an optimal dose. The vast majority of clinical studies were carried out with toothpaste containing 1,000 ppm and compared to vehicle controls (minus fluoride). Some studies showed increased protection with moderately elevated concentrations (1,500 and 2,500 ppm), but none have looked at concentrations higher than that (Hausen 2004). Thus, we still don't know, for example, if high-risk

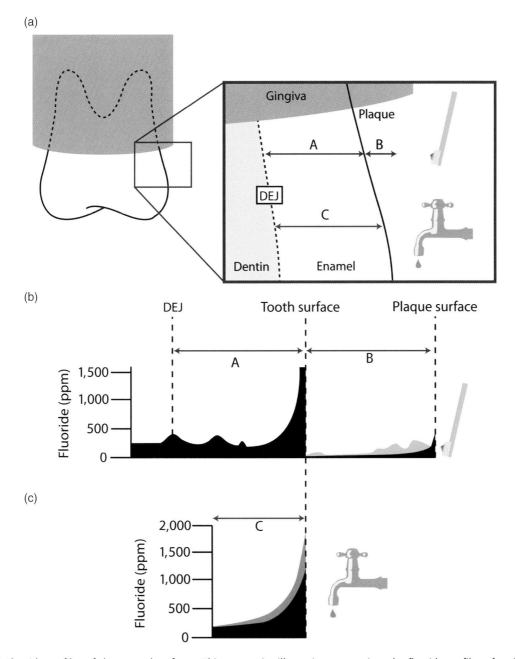

Figure 16-8 Fluoride profiles of the enamel surfaces. This composite illustration summarizes the fluoride profiles of various regions associated with the development of an incipient enamel carious lesion. The box at the top shows the areas from which these profiles were obtained. (a) The region of the enamel from tooth surface to the Dento-enamel junction (DEJ) underlying areas of frequent plaque deposits. (b) The region of the surface of the plaque to the layer immediately adjacent the surface of the enamel. (c) The region of smooth surface enamel exposed to fluoridated water. Representative profiles are presented in black. In B the green profile represents that increase in fluoride in plaque that is achieved with toothpaste containing 1,000 ppm fluoride. Note that very little of the fluoride enters the layers of plaque immediately adjacent the enamel surface. In C the fluoride content from fluoridation (*blue*) is only slightly elevated relative to the non-fluoridated tooth.

patients benefit from ever-increasing concentrations of fluoride in toothpaste.

Because of the risk of dental fluorosis from swallowing fluoridated toothpaste, toothpastes with fluoride at levels typically around the 1,000 ppm are sold over the counter. Each gm of toothpaste contains 1 mg fluoride at this level. The CONCENTRATION available in the mouth would, however, depend upon the amount placed on the toothbrush. Also since young children tend to swallow a significant amount of toothpaste, there is an increased risk for dental fluorosis by early use of fluorides at these concentrations. So called 'pea-sized'

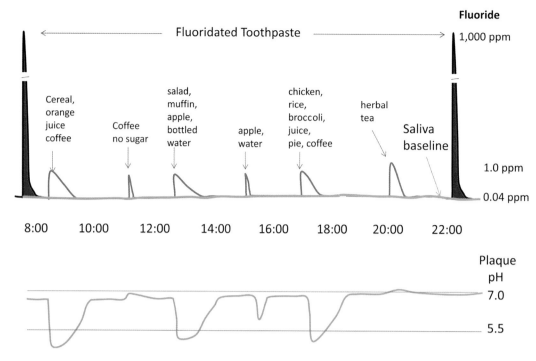

Figure 16-9 Hypothetical 1-day fluoride profile of saliva. The top profile shows what oral fluoride levels can be achieved in the saliva in a typical day of a person who brushes twice a day with 1,000 ppm fluoride, eats three meals, and has three snacks. This person might by living in a fluoridated area and consuming foods (*blue profile*) that were prepared with fluoridated water (1 ppm). The baseline salivary levels would be higher than normal (*green profile*) but may seldom exceed 0.04 ppm. It is important to have fluoride present when plaque forms acid. The plaque pH profile is shown in the graph at the bottom. Notice that the 'apple and water' snack did not approach critical pH. Similarly, the unsweetened coffee and herbal tea did not cause the plaque pH to decrease at all. Those, therefore, were all 'safe' snacks. The three meals produced a pH drop that could potentially contribute to caries but enough time (in the presence of fluoride) was available for the enamel to remineralize.

amounts of toothpaste were therefore recommended (ADA 1991; Pendrys 2000).

Since 1991 the American Dental Association (ADA) has placed the following labeling requirements on the fluoridated toothpastes that were awarded their 'Seal of Acceptance':

"Do not swallow. Use only a pea-sized amount for children under six. To prevent swallowing, children under six years of age should be supervised in the use of toothpaste."

Subsequently, the Canadian Dental Association sponsored two conferences to develop appropriate recommendations for fluoride (Canadian Dental Association 1993; Limeback *et al.* 1999), but it wasn't until 2003 that it followed the ADA's lead to recommend a pea-sized amount of fluoride (Canadian Dental Association 2010). DenBesten *et al.* (1996) measured how much fluoride was retained in small children when a pea-sized amount of fluoridated toothpaste was used (0.25 gm) instead of a large strip (1.0 gm) to confirm that the ADA recommendations would reduce fluoride retention (Figure 16-10). The salivary fluoride levels were less than half of the salivary fluoride concentrations when

1.0 gm of toothpaste was used, and levels returned to baseline more rapidly.

Using an alternative approach in Europe and Australia, toothpastes were made available for children at half the normal concentration (500 ppm fluoride) although there is some evidence that this lower concentration is not very effective (Walsh *et al.* 2010). Some toothpastes with a very high fluoride content (5,000 ppm) are supplied by dentists or are available over the counter in drug stores. Based on the fact that such concentrations can even harm adults when excess amounts are swallowed (Eichmillar *et al.* 2005), toothpastes with 5,000 ppm fluoride should be used with extreme caution. Table 16-2 lists some currently available fluoridated toothpastes.

It is worth noting that given the almost ubiquitous availability of fluoride toothpastes, many have not actually been tested clinically (Zero 2006). According to Dr. Zero, very few of the currently marketed dentifrice products have ever been tested in clinical caries trial. Toothpastes have increasingly been used over the last 20 years for other additives, including anti-calculus agents (tartar control), anti-plaque/anti-gingivitis agents, tooth-

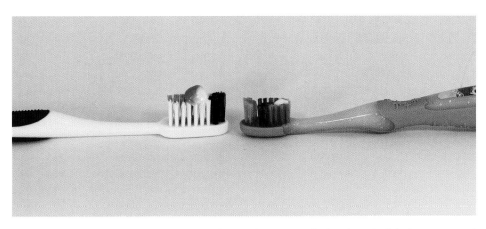

Figure 16-10 Pea-size amount of toothpaste as recommended in North America. The brush on the left shows a typical 'pea-size' amount on toothbrush intended for children. The toothbrush on the right has a very small 'smear' or 'rice-sized' amount of toothpaste on a toddler's toothbrush.

Table 16-2 Common fluoridated toothpastes

Toothpaste type and fluoride content	Example brand	Fluoride level (ppm)	Target population
Amine fluoride	Elmex (GABA-Colgate), Europe	1,250	General population
Sodium fluoride	Crest Cavity Protection (Proctor & Gamble)	1,100	General population
MFP	Colgate Cavity Protection (Colgate Oral Pharmaceuticals)	1,100	General population
Stannous fluoride	GelKam (Colgate Oral Pharmaceuticals)	970	General population and root caries
Sodium fluoride	Prevident (Colgate Oral Pharmaceuticals)	5,000	High risk patient (adult)
Sodium fluoride	Little Kids (Preventive Dental Care Systems), Australia	500	Children age 1–5 years

desensitizing agents, breath-freshening agents, whitening/stain removal formulations, and remineralizing agents. According to Dr. Zero, the only claim that has been associated with a long-term health benefit is the anti-caries effects of fluoride, and thus this claim must be given precedence above all others.

Perhaps toothpastes and mouthwashes should be tested in well-conducted clinical trials to measure better outcomes such as lowered rates of caries and periodontal disease. Claims like "removes 25% more plaque than brushing alone" or "40% less tartar build-up" may have no clinical relevance unless they can be shown to have positive outcomes in terms of reduced caries or improved periodontal health.

Particularly important would be to show that the fluoride in these new toothpaste formulations still has the same bio-availability, and that none of the other ingredients interfere with the ability of fluoride to promote remineralization. Some abrasives are known to be incompatible with fluoride. Abrasives containing calcium, for example, interfere with fluoride because the fluoride can react with calcium and precipitate as calcium fluoride in the toothpaste tube and render the fluoride less active. When Proctor and Gamble switched from its first formulation containing stannous fluoride to sodium fluoride, it had to find an abrasive that would not interfere with fluoride. Silica gel was used for that purpose. Similarly Colgate Oral Pharmaceuticals developed a form of fluoride called Sodium Monofluorophosphate (MFP), which did not precipitate with calcium-containing abrasives but released its fluoride in plaque through the action of salivary and bacterial pyrophosphatases. Studies showed that some MFP remains undissociated in the oral cavity and that more fluoride is taken up when NaF rinses are administered (Vogel *et al.* 2000). One would suspect, then, that NaF would 'outperform' MFP. Proctor and Gamble sponsored a meta-analysis of the literature and claimed to show that NaF was superior to MFP by about 6%. Colgate responded with its own meta-analysis to contradict this finding and claimed that both formulations worked equally well (Proskin 1993; Volpe *et al.* 1993).

Fluoridated mouth rinses

Mouth rinses can also deliver significant fluoride to the oral cavity. There is in fact evidence that fluoridated mouth rinses are effective even when there is regular use of fluoridated toothpastes and the drinking water is optimally fluoridated (Adair 1998; Marinho *et al.* 2003a; Marinho *et al.* 2004).

Fluoride rinses have been tested at two main concentrations of fluoride: 0.05% NaF (225 ppm fluoride, which is recommended for daily use), and 0.2% NaF (900 ppm fluoride, which is recommended for weekly rinse). There are other concentrations on the market, and these generally have much lower levels of fluoride to reduce the risk of excess fluoride ingestion and dental fluorosis in children who still have growing teeth (Table 16-3).

How fluoride rinses work

We have already established that topical application of fluoride at the 1,000-ppm level (applied as a slurry) does not penetrate well through the plaque biofilm. However, the rapid movement of mouthwash in the oral cavity may result in better access of fluoride to stagnation areas, together with the fact that better penetration of biofilms is thought to occur in a non-stagnant system. At least one study (Vogel *et al.* 2010) has ruled out that fluoride rinses contribute to the formation of calcium fluoride (as discussed in the next sections). Therefore, one has to conclude that the added fluoride present in the saliva and released from oral reservoirs (plaque, enamel, mucosa) within an hour after rinsing, contributes to the formation of fluoridated apatite/fluorapatite during the frequent daily exposures to sugar and the pH drop in the incipient lesion underneath plaque biofilms.

An interesting experiment was carried out to examine the benefits of 0.2% fluoride rinsing (Ogaard *et al.* 1988; Ogaard *et al.* 1991). Shark enameloid slabs, which contain nearly 100% fluorapatite, were mounted in Hawley retainers worn by volunteer subjects. This model system allowed the formation of protected plaque biofilms on the shark enameloid (Ogaard *et al.* 1988). Under ordinary cariogenic challenges, test subjects were asked to rinse with 0.2% neutral NaF 1 minute each day after brushing with non-fluoridated toothpaste. It was clear from the experiments that even enamel-like tissue with 100% fluorapatite was not protected against demineralization. What did inhibit mineral loss, though, was bathing the enamel slabs in 0.2% NaF rinse. This inhibition was through saturation of the saliva and plaque with fluoride, not through the formation of calcium fluoride. (See the next section.) A summary of the results of this study is shown in Figure 16-11.

Professional fluoride gels

Fluoride gels have been used for many years in the dental office to reduce the risk of caries. In the last 10 years there have been several reviews (meta-analyses and systematic reviews) of clinical trials showing that professional fluorides are effective in reducing caries (Seppä 2004; Petersson *et al.* 2004; Azarpazhooh and Main 2008; Milgrom *et al.* 2009; Poulsen 2009; Marinho 2009). However, there is also good evidence that professional topical fluoride application is not very effective for populations that are at low risk for caries (Rozier 2001; Marinho 2002; American Dental Association Council on Scientific Affairs 2006).

The American Dental Association Council on Scientific Affairs (2006) developed guidelines, based on the strength of the evidence, for the use of professional fluoride gels. The recommendations can be summed as follows:

1. Low risk groups for caries should not receive professional fluorides.
2. Moderate risk patients should receive professional fluorides every 6 months.
3. High-risk patients should receive professional fluorides at 3- to 6-month intervals.

Additional comments were made in relation to these recommendations:

1. Varnishes have been shown to work as well as gels, and the varnishes are preferred because less fluoride is ingested.
2. Fluoride foams have only been tested in two clinical trials and percent uptake of fluoride in enamel *in vitro* is not a substitute for clinical trials.
3. One-minute applications have not been endorsed; a full 4-minute application of the gels or foams is required. Rinses are not endorsed either.

Table 16-3 Common fluoridated mouth rinses

Fluoride concentration in the mouth rinse	PPM F (recommended doses)	Examples
0.63% SnF$_2$ or 0.153% F 0.2% NaF or 0.09% F	1528 (use daily as prescribed) 900 (use as a weekly rinse as directed by the manufacturer)	Rx: GelKam (Colgate Oral Pharmaceutricals, Inc.) OTC: Oral-B Fluorinse Proctor and Gamble (Canada) Rx: Prevident Dental Rinse
0.05% NaF or 0.0225% F	225 (use once daily as directed by the manufacturer)	OTC Brand names*: Act, CVS, Duane Reade, H.E. Buddy, Hannaford, Tom's of Maine, Swan, Shop Rite, Equate, Sunmark, Meijer, The Natural Dentist Healthy Teeth, Hello!, Publix, Weis, Western
0.44 NaF mg/mL or 0.2 mg F/mL	200 Acidulated to pH 4 (5 mL/day)	Rx: Phos-Flur Anti-Cavity Rinse* (Colgate Oral Pharmaceuticals, Inc.)
0.0221% NaF or 0.001% F	100 (use once daily as directed by the manufacturer)	Listerine Smart Rinse (Johnson and Johnson, Inc) Crest ProHealth Complete (Proctor and Gamble, Inc.)
0.00219% SnF$_2$ or 0.00531% F	53.1 (use once daily as directed by the manufacturer)	Crest ProHealth For Me (Proctor and Gamble, Inc.)

* Accepted by the ADA as of December 2010

(a)

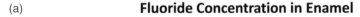

Fluoride Concentration in Enamel

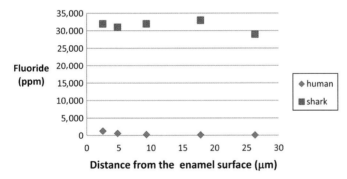

Ogaard B, Rolla C, Ruben J, Dijkman T, Arends J: Microradiographic study of demineralization of shark enamel in a human caries model. Scand J Dent Res 1988; 96: 209–11.

(b)

Demineralization in vivo-high caries risk

Figure 16-11 Effect of 0.2% NaF rinse on dissolution of shark enamel in a cariogenic human caries model. (a) Results of the analysis of fluoride in the shark enameloid block (*red*) and human enamel blocks (*blue*). Shark enamel contains nearly 100% fluorapatite. These were attached to an orthodontic appliance and subjected to the usually human cariogenic challenges. In (b) it is evidence that under demineralizing conditions *in situ*, enamel blocks from human teeth demineralize, but so do shark enameloid blocks. Pre-rinsing with fluoridated mouthwash reduces the extent of the demineralization in the human blocks.

With these recommendations in mind, one clearly can see that professional fluoride therapy should be geared to individual needs and not be administered to every patient. It has to be kept in mind that fluoride varnish therapy is gaining acceptance in the US in clinical practice, but the products that are sold to dental professionals are being used off-label, since no FDA fluoride varnish has been approved for its anti-caries benefit.

How professionally applied fluorides work

It may strike the average practitioner odd that it only takes two applications per year for professional fluoride to have a significant effect on caries rates. It is now believed that the mechanism involved depends on the formation of calcium fluoride. When acidic fluoride at high concentrations is applied to the tooth, surface calcium is 'etched' from the surface of the tooth. The free calcium that is released, and calcium that is present in saliva, react with the fluoride ions present in the topical fluoride to form calcium fluoride. When the saliva returns the plaque pH to neutral, the calcium fluoride precipitates and deposits as tiny granules of insoluble fluoride that occupy the etched areas. Later, when a cariogenic food is consumed and lactic acid is produced by plaque, the pH drops and the calcium fluoride 'spheres' dissolve, releasing fluoride ions locally. These fluoride ions participate during the 'acid attack' in much the same

way that fluoride from other daily sources participate. (See the previous section.) Saliva stimulated by the ingestion of the food then neutralizes the acid, and the calcium fluoride re-precipitates, acting as a reservoir ready to respond to future acid attacks (Figure 16-12).

It turns out that the presence of plaque does not interfere with the benefit that professional topical fluoride therapy can provide (Johnson and Lewis 1995). In other words, there is no clinical advantage to removing all of the plaque before a professional topical fluoride application. The surface CaF_2 layer may not even be the reason for prolonged protection by professional fluorides from future 'acid attacks' since it has been shown by Cherisoni et al. (2011) that the surface layers are lost soon after the professional fluoride application. These workers hypothesize that the calcium fluoride molecules that remain between apatite crystal rods effectively decrease enamel permeability.

Slow release fluoride strategies

There have been numerous studies to examine the potential for attaching slow-release devices (plastic or glass beads containing fluoride) to teeth in order to raise the salivary fluoride levels over a long period of time, which in turn, lowers caries risk. (See Toumba et al. [2009] for a review.) They have potential and there is some evidence for caries effectiveness, but the evidence is not yet strong enough to support their widespread use (Marinho 2009).

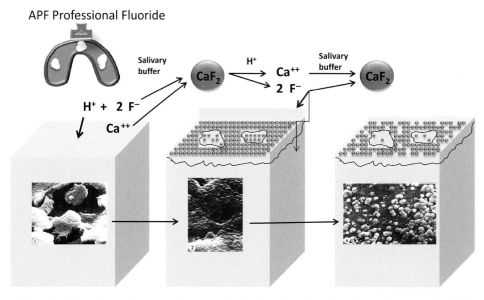

Figure 16-12 Fluoride administered as a high concentration topical gel at low pH etches the surface enamel. Calcium is released and combines with fluoride to form CaF_2 'spheres' on the surface. When plaque acids are produced, these spherical deposits are depleted, releasing fluoride locally to take part in remineralization. A return to neutral pH by saliva reforms the CaF_2 spheres. The insert images in the block are actual scanning electron microscope (SEM) images of the enamel surface immediately after applying acidulated phosphate fluoride, or APF (left). The middle block shows an SEM close-up of the CaF_2 spheres. The right block shows the SEM picture of the CaF_2 layer that has been partially depleted. SEM images adapted from Larsen and Fejerskov (1978) with permission.

Glass ionomer sealants and restorations are known to provide a long-term release of fluoride, and these materials can even be recharged with fluoride, but whether they significantly lower caries incidence has yet to be shown (Wiegand *et al.* 2007). The reader is also referred to the chapter on sealants in this text for a discussion of glass ionomer sealants and their effectiveness.

Summary of how fluorides work

There is a common thread in terms of how all fluoride therapies work. During repeated demineralization-remineralization cycles, fluoride is incorporated into the incipient white spot lesion. This not only makes that area of the tooth more resistant to acid than other areas of the enamel smooth surface but is also a result of enhanced remineralization of fluoride-enriched mineral. This is shown in Figure 16-13.

Does fluoride affect the growth or metabolism of plaque bacteria?

In a previous chapter we presented evidence to show that plaque bacteria are affected by the diet. Fluoride exists in several mineral forms in the diet and cannot be avoided. It is the thirteenth most common element on earth. It occurs naturally in many areas in the drinking water and in plant foods that are able to sequester fluoride from the soil. Tea, for example, is rich in fluoride (Whyte *et al.* 2005). There are numerous anthropogenic sources of fluoride as well, including pollution, artificial fluoridation, fluoridated salt, fluoride supplements, fluoridated dentifrices, fluoride mouth rinses, and, of course, professional fluorides. With so many sources of fluoride, one would assume that the oral flora has adapted to the fluoride exposures experienced on a day-to-day basis. Nevertheless, it has always been assumed that one of the ways that fluoride works is through its inhibition of the metabolism and growth of cariogenic bacteria.

Cariogenic bacteria have to thrive in an episodic low pH environment. Some are aciduric (able to grow at low pH), others are acidogenic (produce organic acids from sugar substrates). The bacteria that produce the low pH environment in the first place are primarily the mutans streptococci (MS). The *Lactobacillus* (LB) species, which can survive at low pH, find protected niches to grow, such as in enamel or dentin cavitations, or next to overhanging amalgams. Both bacterial species are believed to be the primary infective microorganisms that cause dental caries (Van Houte 1994), and yet when quantified clinically, they do make good predictors of future decay (Van Houte 1993). A significantly broader range of bacterial species can cause root caries. (For review, see Bowden [1990] and Jordan [1986].)

SUMMARY OF HOW FLUORIDE WORKS

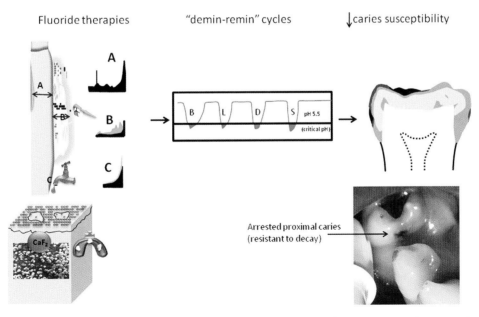

Figure 16-13 How all fluoride therapies work to increase caries resistance. All fluoride therapies can now be assumed to provide protection against caries through the same mechanism. The therapies (fluoridated toothpaste and mouth rinses, fluoridated water, and professional topical fluorides) provide the fluoride that is required during the daily 'demin-remin' cycles. The result is a stable, fluoride-enriched remineralized incipient lesion that can be considered to be arrested or 'healed.' The figure also shows a clinical image of a brown-stained arrested incipient lesion in the proximal zone.

Along with LB, these bacteria have great tolerance for acidic conditions. MS can also synthesize extracellular glucans from dietary sucrose, which not only acts as an energy source when food is scarce, but the glucans are 'sticky' and help the bacterial cells cling to each other, to the plaque biofilm, and to the tooth surface. The metabolism of the extracellular bacterial starch when dietary sugars are scarce is believed to lower the resting pH of the saliva in patients at high risk for caries. This extracellular glycan is a virulence factor that must be taken into account. As more sucrose is consumed, more MS grows and it becomes harder to remove.

Half of the plaque biofilm is primarily composed of the acidogenic MS and LB species, and the other half contains other microorganisms, such as non-mutans streptococci, actinomyces, and veillonellae (van Houte 1980). Small numbers of strains of Neisseria, Bacteroides, Bifidobacterium, Clostridium, Eubacterium, Propionibacterium, or Rothia all have acidogenic potential. Caries can occur without MS (deStoppelaar *et al.* 1969; Boyar et al. 1989; Marshet al. 1989; Macpherson *et al.* 1990) especially on the root surfaces, where *A. viscosus* is the prime etiologic microorganism (Jordan 1986; Bowden *et al.* 1990; Nyvad and Kilian 1990).

In the introduction we showed how fluoride disrupted the growth of some bacteria in culture but not others. Fluoride has been extensively tested in bacterial cultures *in vitro* for its ability to inhibit the metabolism of cariogenic microorganisms. (See Hamilton [1990].) At mM concentrations, fluoride inhibits the glycolytic enzyme, enolase, which converts 2-P-glycerate to P-enolpyruvate.

Enolase
$$2\text{-PG} \rightleftharpoons \text{PEP}$$

This results in the inhibition of sugar transport via the PEP phosphotransferase system (PTS). Acidic conditions outside of the cell wall of the bacteria (for example, when APF fluoride is applied) convert fluoride ions to hydrogen fluoride (HF), which is able to diffuse into the bacteria. Inside the cell, where the cytoplasm is alkaline, HF disassociates into fluoride ions and protons. The fluoride ions inhibit metabolic enzymes and the added protons acidify the cytoplasm, causing a reduction in both the proton gradient and enzyme activity.

When fluoride inhibits the membrane-bound, proton-pumping H⁺/ATPase, the cell's ability to expel protons to the environment at the expense of ATP is inhibited.

$$HF \rightleftharpoons H^+ + F^-$$

ATPase
$$ATP \rightleftharpoons ADP + HPO_4^-$$

The levels that are required to inhibit cell growth and metabolism *in vitro*, however, far exceed those that are normally found *in vivo* (Maltz and Emilson 1982; ten Cate 2001).

The minimal dose of fluoride required to reduce the prevalence of caries by means of an anti-bacterial effect is not known. One study showed that *in vitro* the pH decline could be inhibited in MS with fluoride as low as 10 ppm NaF (Bradshaw *et al.* 2002; Pandit *et al.* 2011). However, generally, much higher levels of fluoride are required, notably those found only in toothpastes, rinses, and professional fluorides.

Watson *et al.* (2005) measured how far fluoride from toothpaste penetrates into plaque that was generated on enamel surfaces. In fairly thick plaques of the sort resident in fissures and in interproximal regions, very little of the fluoride was found to reach the inner layers of the plaque biofilm. It has been difficult to show that the more fluoride you deposit in the plaque, the less acid it produces (Balzar Ekenbäck *et al.* 2001; ten Cate 2001; Marquis *et al.* 2003).

Experiments to measure plaque inhibition *in vivo* after fluoride exposure suggest that plaque regrows quickly following removal by fluoridated toothpaste. In one study (Brailsforth *et al.* 2005) interproximal plaque levels, including acidogenic MS and LB, were back to baseline levels within 6 hours after using fluoride-containing toothpaste. Van der Mei *et al.* (2006) found the same result.

Slurries of toothpaste containing the most amount of fluoride available over the counter (5,000 ppm) reduced plaque growth on smooth surfaces after 4 days of no brushing, compared to rinsing with water, but rinsing with slurries made with toothpaste containing 1,500 ppm did not inhibit plaque accumulation on the teeth. Continuous use of 5,000 ppm toothpaste can, however, reduce plaque over a period of 3 and 6 months (Baysan *et al.* 2001). It appears possible that *S. mutans* can adapt to high concentrations of fluoride (Van Loveren *et al.* 1990). In one experiment MS exposed to Duraflor varnish at 0.1% fluoride (1,000 ppm F), resistant strains of MS were isolated. In another study (Ostela *et al.* 1991), professional stannous fluoride/amine fluoride was applied three times during the first week of the study. Fluoride had no effect on LB counts, and MS counts were inhibited only 2 to 3 weeks following the intensive professional fluoride therapy. Chlorhexidine in these experiments was more effective in controlling bacterial levels.

Thus, it seems that extremely high levels of fluoride and repeated exposures are required to significantly affect MS and LB metabolism and growth. The role that plaque plays in caries prevention, therefore, seems to be to concentrate fluoride and provide a reservoir of fluoride during the early 'demin-remin' cycles. In fact one might even go as far to propose that the presence of plaque is essential during these early stages of building resistance to net demineralization. Obviously if acid is produced several times during the day, say in patients who frequently consume sugary snacks or drinks, the fluoride protective mechanism will be overwhelmed and the plaque will play a destructive role rather than facilitate the buildup of fluoride-rich crystals in white spot incipient lesions.

Systemic fluoride

Fluoride metabolism

Fluoride from systemic administration (supplements, milk, water, and salt) enters the oral cavity where it provides topical benefits before it is swallowed. It then enters the GI system where it is absorbed and metabolized Figure 16-14.

Because fluoride has a dissociation constant (Ka) of -3.189 (Vanderborgh 1968), 99.9% of the fluoride ions will be protonated by the HCl acid in the stomach to produce hydrogen fluoride (HF). HF being neutral can readily penetrate gut epithelial cell walls and enter the cell cytoplasm. In the neutral pH environment of the cytoplasm, the HF dissociates into protons and fluoride ions. Any increase of fluoride in the cell can cause interference with cellular function. Approximately 90% of the absorbed fluoride then passes into the serum where it is quickly distributed and diluted. The clearance of fluoride depends greatly on the pH balance (Whitford 1990). Serum fluoride levels seldom exceed 0.06 ppm but are more typically in the 0.01-ppm range (Sowers *et al.* 2005). The fluoride concentration of saliva (Oliveby *et al.* 1989; Oliveby *et al.* 1990; Whitford *et al.* 1990), sweat (WHO Expert Committee on Oral Health Status and Fluoride Use 1994) and breast milk (Ekstrand *et al.* 1981) is less than the serum, which means that these biological fluids would not be

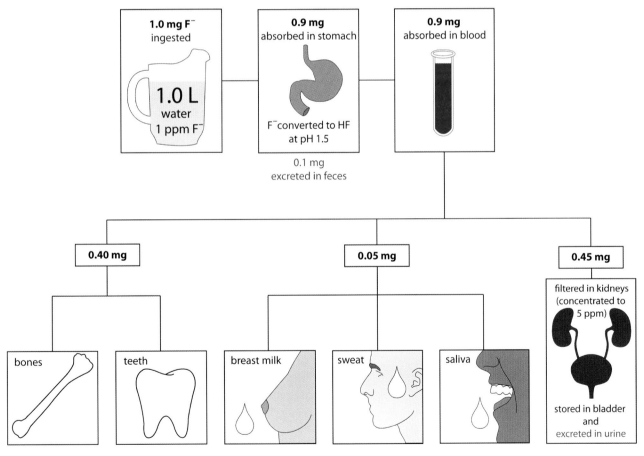

Figure 16-14 The fate of 1 mg of fluoride that is ingested by humans. This illustration shows how fluoride is handled by the human body. When 1 mg of fluoride is ingested, 90% of it is absorbed into the blood stream (10% is excreted in the feces). Nearly half of the absorbed fluoride is quickly taken up by bone and growing teeth. About 0.45 mg of fluoride in the blood is filtered in the kidneys, stored in the bladder, and eventually excreted. Only a small amount of fluoride (0.05 mg) is excreted in other bodily fluids (breast milk, sweat, saliva).

efficient for eliminating fluoride (besides, nearly all of the saliva is re-ingested). As the serum circulates, about 50% is sequestered into the mineral phases of developing teeth and areas where there is bone growth. The remaining fluoride is freely filtered in the kidneys, stored in the bladder, and excreted. A small amount of fluoride is excreted in the feces (Whitford 1990). Thus, at any given time each tissue contains fluoride. The kidneys and bladder may contain up to 5 ppm of fluoride, but bone can accumulate fluoride throughout life where levels under normal conditions can exceed 1,000 ppm primarily in tissue surfaces.

The systemic side effects of fluoride stem from these ingested amounts of fluoride. In addition to ingestion of foods, beverages, and consumer products, people might also accumulate fluoride from breathing fluoride-polluted air or absorbing fluoride from fluorinated drugs such as general anesthetics. (See the NRC Report [2006] for a review.)

As discussed previously, it has long been assumed that fluoride can benefit teeth through ingestion (systemic route) by increasing the fluoride content on the surface enamel prior to eruption of the teeth. Now researchers have concluded that fluoride's effect in reducing caries is primarily a topical effect (Limeback 1999; Featherstone 2000; Centers for Disease Control and Prevention 2001; Fejerskov 2004; Hellwig 2004; Cheng *et al.* 2007). Some of the fluoride derived from systemic fluoride finds its way to the saliva (via the blood stream), but those levels are so small as to be insignificant during demineralization-remineralization cycles, where fluoride benefits the most (Figure 16-9).

Water fluoridation

A discussion in this section on the benefits (and risks) of fluoridation will be limited to a review of the literature of what the clinician in private practice should know in order to determine the risks for future caries in patients and whether there is also need for additional fluoride therapy. For example, do children living in non-fluoridated areas still need fluoride supplements? What are the risks for children living in fluoridated areas to develop dental fluorosis? Do adults benefit from water fluoridation? The literature on water fluoridation is vast. In this chapter, we do not attempt to address every social, scientific, and public health issue related to water fluoridation, a practice that has been in effect for over 65 years. Instead, the reader will find this section relevant to private practice in that it will help the practitioner make important decisions on caries risk assessment.

The declining benefit of water fluoridation

The dental decay rates in the 1950s and 1960s were considerably high and a major health problem. Using decayed, missing, and filled teeth (DMFT) as the accepted measure of disease incidence, water fluoridation trials showed that adding fluoride to the drinking water at about 1.0 ppm lowered decay rates by as much as 50% to 60% (McDonagh *et al.* 2000; Young 2008). The magnitude of the benefit of fluoridated water declined in the 1970s and 1980s (reviewed by Ripa [1993]). This was to be expected since a worldwide trend to declining dental decay rates, even in non-fluoridated areas, had occurred (Diesendorf 1986; Brathall *et al.* 1996; de Liefde 1998), making it difficult to measure the efficacy of water fluoridation. (See also Chapter 1.) The general, widespread use of fluoridated toothpaste was rated as the most important factor responsible for the worldwide decline in dental caries (Brathall *et al.* 1996), but other factors that were cited as contributing factors included improved diets, changes in oral flora, improved dental materials and therapies, and improved dental hygiene.

Does water fluoridation simply delay dental decay?

Diesendorf (1986) first pointed out that there may simply be a delay in caries increment in fluoridated areas. Prior to the introduction of fluorides for caries prevention, the mean age of tooth eruption rates have been remarkably constant (Limeback 1999), but since the introduction of fluorides, estimates for the delay in tooth eruption range from 0.7 years (Virtanen *et al.* 1994) to as much as 2 years (Campagna *et al.* 1995). Fluoride incorporation in the primary dentition and in the alveolar bone, which must be resorbed prior to the eruption of the permanent teeth is believed to be the cause of this generalized delay in tooth eruption. Using existing data it is possible to estimate the effects on dental decay rates of a delay of tooth eruption of 1.0 year or 1.5 years. These delays, as Figure 16-15 shows, could account for a 20% or 33.3% apparent difference in dental decay rates, respectively.

In a study where the emergence time was factored into the analysis, a Belgian group of researchers could not find a benefit of lower caries prevalence (Komárek *et al.* 2005). Thus, in modern times where there is fluoride ingestion from many sources, it is difficult to demonstrate the benefit from fluoridated water.

There have been studies to show that fluoridated water could reduce coronal caries in adults and reduce root caries (Hunt *et al.* 1989; Yeung 2007; Griffin 2007; Rihs *et al.* 2008). These benefits are topical and likely cumulative, but researchers continue to search for a 'pre-eruptive' or systemic benefit. Some would argue that the pre-eruptive benefit still has not been demonstrated (Mascarenhas and Scott 2008). Despite all the fluoride sources to which people are exposed, children who are life-long residents in a fluoridated area might still benefit from pre-eruptive exposure to fluoride according to some researchers (Singh *et al.* 2007), but the benefit is likely very small when corrections for a delay in tooth eruption are taken into account. The most recent studies

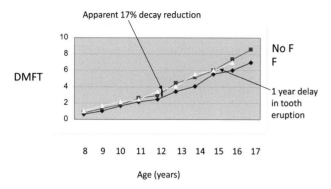

Figure 16-15 The effect of 1-year delay in tooth eruption on the caries prevalence. The data of Brunelle and Carlos (1990) is plotted here showing caries prevalence (as measured by decayed, missing, and filled teeth, or DMFT) in fluoridated (F) and non-fluoridated (no F) areas. There is an approximate 17% difference in caries rates in 12-year-old children, which disappears when a 1-year delay in tooth eruption is taken into account (*yellow line*). No statistical analysis was provided by the authors.

published comparing fluoridated and non-fluoridated communities have required large sample sizes to find statistically significant differences in dental decay rates, and when these were found, they were clinically quite small (Table 16-4).

These more modern studies indicate that the number of tooth surfaces saved is clinically small. It is not surprising then that recent cost-benefit analyses do not show a large savings in restorative costs (Maupomé *et al.* 2007). The studies listed in Table 16-4 are ecological studies comparing disease rates in communities. It is difficult to draw clear cause and effect conclusions from such studies unless several confounders are taken into account. This was not done in the US, but it was done to a certain extent in Australia and in Denmark. When several communities are compared, regression analysis permits the influence of confounding factors (Ekstrand *et al.* 2010), but only cross-sectional studies using individual data will permit conclusions to be made concerning the benefit of fluoride added to the drinking water. Randomized, double-blinded clinical trials to test the benefit of fluoridated drinking water, where all the important confounders have been accounted for in the regression analysis, are lacking. As mentioned previously, only the Komárek study corrected for a delay in tooth eruption. The claims, therefore, that the evidence for water fluoridation's benefit is overwhelming must now be re-evaluated as a result of so many other

Table 16-4 A summary of recent publications on surveys of the dental decay rates in children

Study author	Country	Number of subjects	Age of subjects (years)	Surfaces saved with optimum fluoridation
Heller *et al.* 1997	US	18,755	12	0.5*
Brunelle and Carlos 1990	US	16,498	12	0.5*
Angelillo *et al.* 1990	Italy	643	12	0.6
Selwitz *et al.* 1998	US	495	8–16	1.2
Ismail 1991	Canada	219	10–12	0.7
Clark 1991	Canada	1131	6–14	0.8
Slade *et al.* 1995	Australia	9,690 vs 10,195	5–15	0.2
				1.1
Jackson *et al.* 1995	US	243	7–14	1.2*
Kumar *et al.* 1998	US	1,493	7–14	−0.2
Armfield and Spencer 2004	Australia	5129	4–9	1.5
		4803	10–15	NS
Komarek *et al.* 2005	Belgium	4468	7–12	NS
Spencer *et al.* 2008	Australia	8183 (SA)	5–15	NS
Nyvad *et al.* 2009	Lithuania	300	12–15	NS
Ekstrand 2010	Denmark	191 municipalities	15	1.0–2.0
Armfield 2010	Australia	128,990	5–15	0.5

* Difference was statistically significant.

sources of fluoride masking any real benefit that water fluoridation might have.

Expert panels that reviewed the literature averaged old with new studies (conditions changed considerably over the years), and did not correct for confounders such as variation in diet, exposure to sunshine (vitamin D levels), nutrition (although, in many cases, low socioeconomic status [SES] accounts for poor nutrition), other factors in the drinking water such as calcium, strontium, and magnesium and, lastly, delayed tooth eruption.

Will decay rates rise if fluoridation is halted?

The studies in Table 16-4 indicate that if water fluoridation were halted in these communities, decay rates would climb marginally, and they would not even be detectable without large sample sizes. A study done in the 1980s in Wick, Scotland (Stephen *et al.* 1987) showed that there would be an increase in dental decay, but another study in the Netherlands (Kalsbeek *et al.* 1993) showed that the difference disappeared after a few years. A close examination of the results of the Dutch experiments comparing Culemborg and Tiel after cessation of fluoridation suggested that fluoridation reduced the progression of caries. Other studies have failed to find a lasting difference in dental decay rates when fluoridation is halted (Kobayashi *et al.* 1992; Seppä *et al.* 1998; Künzel and Fischer 2000). Durham, North Carolina experienced an inadvertent cessation of fluoridation, but there was no measurable increase in the dental decay rates up to 5 years after the event (Burt *et al.* 2000). Maupomé *et al.* (2001) showed that caries rates declined faster in two communities that stopped fluoridation, compared to one in the same province of Canada that continued to fluoridate.

Fluoridated water is used in the manufacturing of beverages and foods that are consumed in non-fluoridated areas (the 'halo' effect). This, in part, explains why it is so difficult to show a difference in caries prevalence rates between fluoridated and non-fluoridated communities. This has often been cited as one of the reasons for the decline of caries in non-fluoridated communities (Ripa 1993; Lewis and Banting 1994). Because most of Europe does not use fluoridated water, this 'halo' effect from the diet is not an important factor in the general decline of caries worldwide (Brathall *et al.* 1996). However, ingestion of foods and beverages made with fluoridated water, especially by children (Rojas-Sanchez *et al.* 1999) contributes significantly to the daily intake of fluoride in non-fluoridated communities, which means that the daily ingestion of fluoride cannot be monitored or controlled.

In determining fluorosis risk, total intake of fluoride from all sources should be considered. One cannot avoid the ingestion of fluoride when it is added to the drinking water. Excess fluoride intake is common and can lead to side effects that have to be taken into account. The benefits of water fluoridation, which are less and less clinically significant these days, have to be weighed against these side effects (see below).

Fluoride supplements

Where drinking water low in fluoride cannot be fluoridated, fluoride tablets were introduced. Fluoride supplements were originally designed to provide the systemic fluoride that a child would not consume living in a non-fluoridated area. At the time studies to distinguish the topical effects from the systemic effects of fluoridated water were rare. There was one early attempts to distinguish the systemic from the topical effects. In a 1-year caries trial with 242 children comparing fluoride lozenges that were sucked and swallowed with fluoride 'pills' that were swallowed right away, Bibby *et al.* (1955) found only four new caries in the children who consumed the lozenges versus 6.6 new caries in the children who swallowed the pills.

Feltman and Kosel (1961) showed in a placebo-controlled trial that systemic fluoride ingested in tablet form by pregnant mothers enters the placenta and reaches the developing fetus. Their study showed that the offspring benefited in terms of caries, but they also found that 1% of their subjects developed gastric problems. Feltman and Kosal (1961) also recognized that fluoride delays tooth eruption, which could account for some of the benefit.

Generally fluoride supplements were provided as fluoride tablets, but in some cases, clinicians attempted to provide prescriptions of liquid fluoride that the parents would add to drinking water in the refrigerator at home to simulate fluoridated drinking water. The problem with the fluoride drop prescription was that instructions were often incorrectly followed leading to incorrect dosages, and the schedules were complicated, especially when there were children of different ages in the household. This also resulted in poor compliance. Fluoride tablets became the method of choice for fluoride supplementation.

Although some countries (Canada and the UK, for example) have abandoned fluoride supplements for preventing caries, the US still favors the use of fluoride supplements. In 1994 a fluoride supplement schedule was modified from older versions in the US for the purpose of guiding clinicians on appropriate supplement doses for children that live in areas low in fluoride in the drinking water. Since then, the evidence of the effectiveness of fluoride supplements was further reviewed, as was the

Table 16-5 The American Dental Association (ADA) Recommended Fluoride Supplementation Schedule (Compiled from information found in Rozier *et al.* 2010)

Age	Fluoride supplement dosage according to fluoride in the drinking water (parts per million)		
	<0.3	0.3–0.6	>0.6
Birth to 6 months	None	none	none
6 months to 3 years	0.25 mg/day	none	none
3 to 6 years	0.5 mg/day	0.25 mg/day	none
6 to 16 years	1.0 mg/day	0.5 mg/day	none

risk for dental fluorosis from fluoride supplements, especially when prescribed by physicians instead of dentists, who are the only ones who can really assess caries risk (Ismail and Bandekar 1999; Bader *et al.* 2004; Sohn *et al.* 2007; Ismail and Hasson 2008).

Some dental researchers in the US have doubts whether the US should continue to recommend fluoride supplements for children in low fluoride areas. Burt (1999) recommended abandoning their use over a decade ago, and Levy (2003) reviewed the various problems associated with continued use of fluoride supplements and stated:

> There continues to be controversy concerning the use of dietary fluoride supplements, and now they are not generally recommended.

Nevertheless, the American Dental Association convened another panel of experts and in 2010 published their latest recommendations. The 1994 fluoride supplement schedule remained unchanged (Table 16-5), despite some additional reviews of the literature that were published. The levels of evidence and strength of recommendations were this time published with the schedule (Rozier *et al.* 2010). The strength of recommendation for avoiding fluoride altogether is based on expert opinion, not clinical evidence, and these recommendations were therefore given a "strength of recommendation = D." The quality of the evidence for this dosage schedule was given a fair rating (category B recommendation) because of methodological weaknesses in the few clinical studies that met the criteria for the review by the panel of experts.

Fluoride tablets are available in the US for sale, but they are not FDA approved. Some manufacturers have voluntarily removed fluoride supplements from the market, especially those that were combined with vitamins. Fluoride supplements should only be prescribed by dentists where there is clear evidence for high risk of caries and non-compliance with using other fluoridated products.

Fluoridated salt

Where water fluoridation could not be initiated, some countries have introduced salt fluoridation. Caries remain a significant problem in some Latin America countries, as well as some countries in the Caribbean, and some of these countries have converted their salt supplies to fluoridated salt. The countries that have embarked on salt fluoridation programs include Bolivia, Equador, Columbia, Peru, Jamaica, Costa Rica, Mexico, Uruguay, and Venezuela. Switzerland, Germany, and France now sell fluoridated salt, and Switzerland started the practice in 1955 (Marthaler 2005).

Salt is usually fluoridated at 250 ppm (which is 250 mg F/kg salt, or 0.25 mg/gm salt). Table salt in the kitchen can contribute 1 to 4 g of the daily salt intake. Thus, a person could potentially ingest 1 mg of fluoride a day at a salt intake of 4 grams a day. Some restrictions remain in effect in Europe, however, in that fluoridated salt cannot be added to commercial products or to food at restaurants.

The evidence that fluoridated salt is actually effective is weak. The main evidence provided has been an observation of before and after caries rates in countries where fluoridated salt was introduced. One fairly well-conducted study showed that 350 mg fluoride/kg salt did not produce dental fluorosis but failed to show significant reduction in caries after 11.5 years (Stephen *et al.* 1999). Nevertheless, on a theoretical basis, fluoridated salt should provide some protection against caries because it increases salivary fluoride levels when the meals prepared with fluoridated salt are ingested (Hedman *et al.* 2006).

Fluoridated milk

In a recent Cochrane collaboration review Yeung *et al.* 2005, 144 articles were found that reported effects of fluoridated milk on caries. There were really only two intervention studies with sufficient quality that could be used to assess whether fluoride in milk can actually reduce caries. Some studies could not show any benefit of fluoridated milk, but these did not meet the criteria of quality set out by the reviewers. The two studies that met the inclusion criteria showed a reduction in dental decay when milk was fortified with fluoride and fed to children on a daily basis. Maslak *et al.* (2004) used 2.5 ppm fluoride and Stephen (1984) used 6 ppm. The children generally consumed one typical serving (200 mL) of the beverage (test and control milk). In the trial by Stephen it took about 5 years to achieve a 31.2% reduction in DMFT. No correction was made for delay in tooth eruption. A high concentration of fluoride is needed for two reasons: (1) the children did not drink the beverage throughout the day and (2) calcium in the milk complexes with fluoride, which would reduce its availability for topical benefits.

Excess fluoride intake and dental fluorosis

The first noticeable sign to the clinician that there has been too much fluoride intake is dental fluorosis. The relationship between the prevalence/severity of dental fluorosis and fluoride ingestion is dose dependent (Fejerskov *et al.* 1990). When dental decay rates were high, a certain amount of dental fluorosis was considered an acceptable 'trade off' of providing an 'optimum' dose of 1.0 ppm fluoride in the water. However, recent studies have shown that fluorosis has increased dramatically in North America (Clark 1994; Beltrán-Aguilar *et al.* 2005; Beltrán-Aguilar *et al.* 2010), and that the optimum fluoride in drinking water has been more difficult to determine (Warren *et al.* 2009; Ekstrand *et al.* 2010). Infants and toddlers are especially at risk for dental fluorosis of the anterior teeth since it is during the first 3 years of life that the permanent front teeth are the most sensitive to the effects of fluoride. Fluoride accumulates at the transition/maturation stage of tooth development so that the entire tooth surface can be affected. Children fed formula made with fluoridated water are at higher risk to develop dental fluorosis (Hujoel *et al.* 2009; Levy *et al.* 2010). The CDC and ADA issued warnings (as soon as the NRC Report was published) that parents should consider using non-fluoridated water to reconstitute infant formula. Children affected with dental fluorosis usually have mild fluorosis that is considered simply a 'cosmetic side effect' of fluoride ingestion. However, a larger proportion of children suffer from the more objectionable fluorosis (moderate to severe), the kind that requires extensive cosmetic treatment or restorative dental work. Estimates of the prevalence of objectionable fluorosis

ranges from 1% to as much as 12.5 %. Sometimes parents and patients are more concerned about the yellow discoloration of fluorotic teeth than the minor white spots (Shulman *et al.* 2004). Where there is an increase in severe fluorosis in the population, those teeth are actually more susceptible to decay (NRC report 2006; Waidyasekera *et al.* 2010).

Diagnosis of dental fluorosis

Fluoride exposure from birth to age 3 years only affects the anterior incisors and first molars (Table 16-6, Figure 16-16).

Dental fluorosis is a symmetrical condition, occurring on pairs of teeth that are undergoing enamel maturation (final mineralization) at the same time (Limeback 2007). An astute clinician can deduce from the fluorosis pattern when most of the excess fluoride intake had taken place (Figure 16-17). For example, exposure during the first year of life would result in fluorosis on the incisal third of the central incisors and the cusp tips of the first molars (Ishii and Suckling 1991). Excess exposure to fluoride occurring later in life, from age 3 to 6 years, results in dental fluorosis on the cervical edges of the central and lateral incisors but might involve all of the canines, premolars, and second molars starting at the incisal. Excess fluoride intake continuously from birth results in fluorosis in all of the teeth and on all of the surfaces. Severe fluorosis, characterized by deep pitting and major loss of enamel tissue, is not common but can occur in 1–4% of North American children. It can also be present in immigrants who grew up in countries where endemic fluorosis is prevalent (India, Africa, China, Middle East).

Several indices of dental fluorosis have been developed for the purpose of measuring fluorosis severity in dental health surveys and epidemiological studies (Thylstrup and Fejerskov 1978; Horowitz *et al.* 1984; Rozier 1994). All of them are improvements of the original Dean's index (Dean 1934). Vieira *et al.* (2005) even developed and validated a visual analogue scale. But essentially, dental fluorosis is still compartmentalized into these categories: very mild, mild, moderate, and severe.

Teeth with very mild fluorosis sometimes demonstrate developmental striae, which appear as slightly white, opaque lines. Faint white spots or lines are only found on less than 25% of the enamel surface.

Teeth with mild fluorosis have more distinct chalky white areas covering up to half of the tooth surface.

Teeth with moderate fluorosis have more than half of their tooth surfaces covered with very distinct white opaque areas. There may be some structural loss of surface enamel where thin layers of surface enamel 'flakes' off. Some teeth can have intrinsic orange to brown staining.

Table 16-6 Timing of chronic daily fluoride ingestion and the corresponding dental fluorosis pattern that can be expected

Fluoride intake (mg/kg/day)	When exposed	Probable sources of excess fluoride	Permanent teeth affected	Dental fluorosis severity
<0.05	Birth to 3 years	– Fluoridated tap water used for infant formula	Incisors, first molars	Mild
0.10–0.15		– Early toothpaste use – General anesthetics – Fluoride supplements – Fluoridated water	Incisors, first molars plus tips of canines and premolars	Moderate
>0.15		– Any combination of the above plus excess swallowing of fluoridated toothpaste – Pollution (or drinking water >4 ppm fluoride)	All teeth	Severe
<0.05	3–6 years	– Fluoridated tap water used for infant formula – Early fluoridated toothpaste use	Premolars, canines, second molars	Mild
0.10–0.15		– Fluoridated water – Fluoride supplements – Swallowing fluoridated toothpaste – Pollution – Multiple exposures to general anesthetics	Premolars, canines, second molars	Moderate
>0.15		– Excess intake from combinations of the above	All teeth	Severe
<0.05	0–6 yrs	– Fluoridated water – Early fluoridated toothpaste use	All teeth	Mild
0.10–0.15		– Fluoridated water – Fluoride supplements – Swallowing fluoridated toothpaste – Pollution – Multiple exposures to general anesthetics	All teeth	Moderate
>0.15		– May also be increased retention in addition to the above intakes (such as kidney problems)	All teeth	Severe

More severe forms of fluorosis are demonstrated by enamel that has pitting and brown staining on all of the surfaces of the teeth (Figure 16-18). Often the surface enamel appears to be properly mineralized, but there is usually extensive wear of the surface enamel. The characteristic brown stain was originally described by Dr. Frederick McKay, which would eventually lead to the discovery of the association between fluoride ingestion and low caries rates (Peterson 1997). Brown staining is very common in endemic fluorosis areas but occurs much less frequently in the US, Canada, Australia, New Zealand, and the UK.

Prevalence of dental fluorosis

The overall prevalence of dental fluorosis increases as the concentration of fluoride in the drinking water increases. Dental and skeletal fluorosis is a major health problem in area of endemic fluorosis (World Health Organization Expert Committee on Oral Health Status and Fluoride Use 1994). In countries where fluoride levels are low naturally, or where fluoridation is common, the majority of fluorosis is of the mild category (National Research Council 2006). However, overall dental fluorosis prevalence is at a high level and steadily

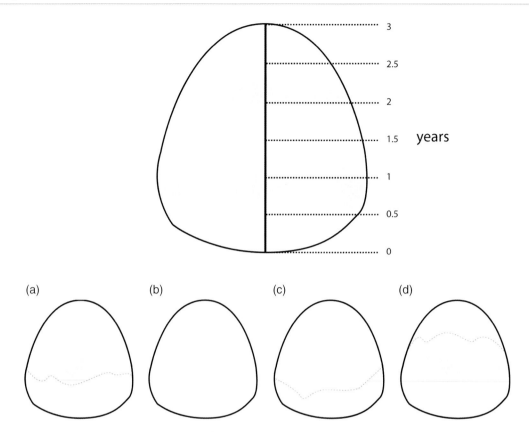

Figure 16-16 Dental fluorosis in relation to the stage of tooth development and exposure to fluoride. The central incisor takes approximately 3 years to go through complete enamel mineralization (*top*). (a) Exposure during the first year of mineralization may only affect the incisal third of the tooth. (b) Exposure to fluoride throughout the entire mineralization period will affect the entire tooth surface. (c) Exposure to fluoride in the second and third year of mineralization will leave the incisal third of the tooth unaffected. (d) Exposure during the last year of mineralization will affect the cervical third of the tooth surface.

increasing in countries that fluoridate their water supplies (Aoba and Fejerskov 2002; Whelton *et al*. 2004). The York reviewers found that, overall, there was a significant proportion of children with objectionable fluorosis in fluoridate communities (McDonagh *et al*. 2000). Efforts to reduce the exposure to excess fluoride are under way in some countries (Leake *et al*. 2002; Spencer and Lo 2008).

The mechanism of the formation of dental fluorosis

It has long been assumed that fluoride interferes with the enzymes that are responsible for the removable of enamel proteins (Whitford 1997; DenBesten *et al*. 2002). Now it appears that fluoride causes dental fluorosis by interfering with proper crystal formation and ameloblast cell function (Bronckers *et al*. 2009; Sharma *et al*. 2010). Fluoride that enters the ameloblast cause endoplasmic reticulum (ER) stress resulting in the reduction of the extracellular production of the enzymes that break down the enamel matrix enamel proteins (Sharma *et al*. 2010). Additionally, accelerating crystal growth

extracellularly the same way that fluoride helps to remineralize incipient carious lesions, there is an enhanced proton production. Since fluoride also interferes with ameloblast cell function in terms of pH regulation, neutralization of the lower acidic environment, which is crucial for continued crystal growth, is also inhibited. The subsurface enamel becomes hypocalcified with disoriented crystals, and it is this poorly formed enamel that reflects light differently causing an appearance of opaque white lines or spots.

The treatment of dental fluorosis

Mild fluorosis that is considered objectionable is usually treated with bleaching or microabrasion (Figure 16-19) or removal of the maturation enamel with fine polishing burs alone or in combination with a strong acid (Wong and Winter 2002; Price *et al*. 2003; Limeback *et al*. 2006).

In the more severe cases, simple microabrasion may not be adequate to remove the fluorotic enamel. Dentists generally provide more extensive treatment (such as,

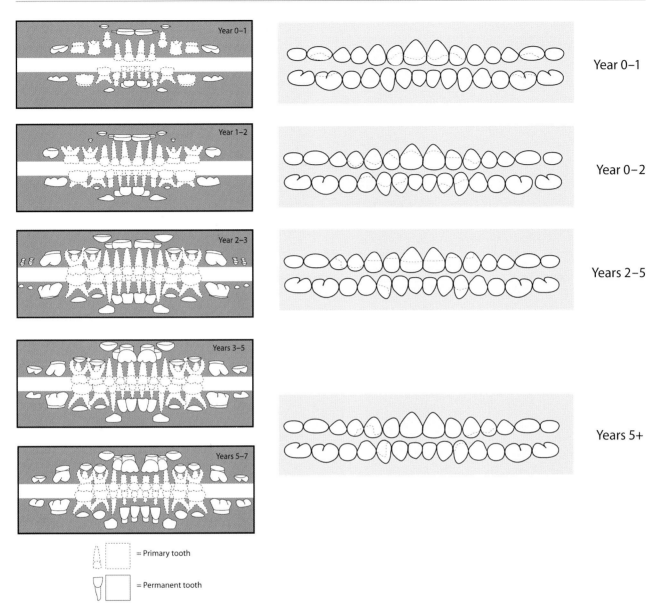

Figure 16-17 Identification of exposure periods to excess fluoride intake based on fluorosis patterns observed. The left panel indicates the stages of tooth permanent tooth development in the human dentition. The right panel shows the pattern of fluorosis that one can expect with the exposure periods indicated on the right (white areas = fluorosis). This is based on observations by the author (*see text*) and in part from the data of Ishii and Suckling (1991). Note that fluorosis can still occur after the age of 5 years, but only the posterior teeth, which develop later than the incisors, are affected.

composite resins, porcelain veneers, and sometimes full coverage restorations). The actual cost of treating dental fluorosis caused by water fluoridation has never been estimated.

Sources of excess systemic fluoride

Water, beverages, and food

Fluoride is the thirteenth most abundance element in the earth's crust (Krebs 2006) and occurs naturally in ocean water at levels of about 1.3 ppm (Warrington 1990), up to

15 ppm in groundwater, and up to 2,000 ppm in soil (Natural Resources Canada 2004). Certain foods contain more fluoride than others. Dark tea, for example, is enriched in fluoride (Whyte *et al.* 2005) and can range between 3 and 6 ppm. Accidental fluoridation overfeeds have resulted in entire communities suffering acute fluoride poisoning, one resulting in death (Gessner *et al.* 1994), and there have been accidental exposures of the concentrated fluoridation chemicals that have resulted in severe acute fluoride chemical burns and life-threatening sequelae (Bjornhagen *et al.* 2003).

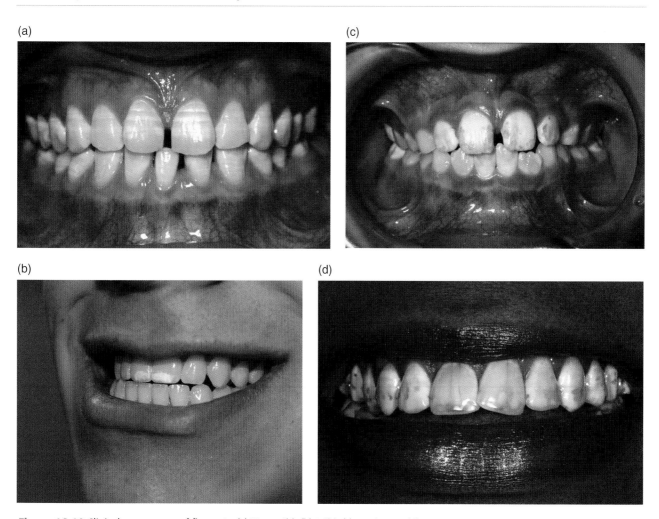

Figure 16-18 Clinical appearance of fluorosis. (a) Very mild. (b) Mild. (c) Moderate. (d) Severe.

Medicines

In addition to fluoride supplements already discussed, many common pharmaceuticals used in medicine are fluorinated. The list of fluorinated drugs number in the hundreds, but the more common ones include Celebrex, Cipro, Diflucan, Prozac, Dalmane, Lipitor, and nearly all of the halogenated general anesthetics. Depending on the molecular formula, these drugs contain from 3–17% fluorine by weight. Some have been shown to lose free fluoride from defluorination by cytochrome P450 enzymes (Pradhan *et al.* 1995; Martinez *et al.* 1997). Most fluorinated general anesthetics elevate serum fluoride but some to levels that pose risks to kidney function, at least during the fluoride exposure (Nishiyama *et al.* 1998).

Pollution

Increased fluoride intake can occur from inhaling fluoride-polluted air. In Canada the mean concentration of fluoride in ambient air is generally low ($<0.05\,\mu g/m^3$), but samples were much higher near steel plants in Hamilton ($0.2\,\mu g/m^3$), within $0.5\,km$ of a phosphate fertilizer plant in BC ($0.5\,\mu g/m^3$), within $1\,km$ of a brick manufacturing plant in Brampton ($0.7\,\mu g/m^3$), and on Cornwall Island ($0.43\,\mu g/m^3$) within $4\,km$ of an aluminum plant (Government of Canada 1993). The highest fluoride levels found in air have been documented in China where coal is burned extensively for industrial power generation. In some areas, where dental fluorosis has been documented to be quite severe and skeletal fluorosis has been observed, the concentration of fluoride in ambient can be as high as $11\,\mu g/m^3$ (Feng *et al.* 2003).

Is dental fluorosis predictive of bone fluorosis?

Generalized dental fluorosis of all the permanent teeth indicates that the bone is potentially a major source of the excess fluoride that causes dental fluorosis in children. This possibility has been conclusively demonstrated in animal models (Angmar-Månsson *et al.* 1990). The

(a)   (b)

(c)   (d)

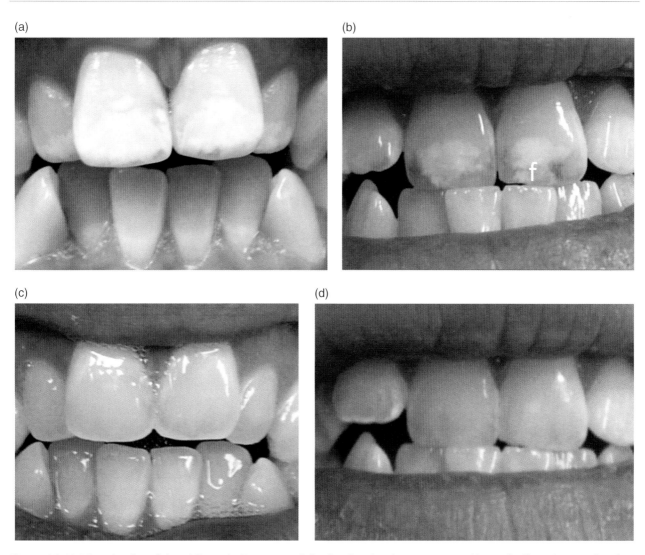

Figure 16-19 Microabrasion of dental fluorosis. Two cases of simple microabrasion are presented here. The fluorotic enamel surfaces (a) and (b) were abraded with a fine diamond bur to expose normal enamel (c) and (d) without significantly changing the dimensions of the teeth.

excess fluoride will have the effect of delaying tooth eruption and possibly contributing to malocclusion (Sutton 1988). There is no reason to believe that fluoride preferentially accumulates in alveolar bone. People ingesting fluoridated water for many years have higher levels of fluoride in their entire skeletal systems (NRC Report 2006). Several ecological studies have been published suggesting that there is an increased risk in hip fractures when dental fluorosis is endemic (NRC 2006). However, relating to fluoridation, so far the consensus is that despite causing mostly mild fluorosis, fluoridated water at 1 ppm or less is not associated with significant bone fractures (McDonagh *et al.* 2000). Even so, one would have to be cautious about a lifetime of excess chronic intake of fluoride because even very low daily fluoride intake associated with mild fluorosis has been

seen to be associated with changes in bone density (Kroger *et al.* 1994; Arnold *et al.* 1997; Levy *et al.* 2009; Chachra *et al.* 2010).

Acute toxicity—clinical signs, diagnosis, treatment

Most accidental fluoride poisonings in the US have occurred in children younger than 6 years. Several hundred of these acute poisonings occur annually, some resulting in death (Shulman and Wells 1997). Most of the fluoride sources are oral care products. Whitford defines the probably toxic dose (PTD) as:

> the minimum dose that could cause toxic signs and symptoms, including death, and that should trigger immediate therapeutic intervention and hospitalization

Table 16-7 Some sources of fluoride poisoning—A guide to probable toxic doses for a small toddler

Fluoride source	Concentration	Amount usually used	Amount containing a probable toxic dose* for a 10-kg toddler (=50 mg)
Fluoride supplements	0.25 mg F	1 tab/day (toddler)	200 tablets
	0.5 mg F	1 tab/day (3–6 years)	100 tablets
	1.0 mg F	1 tab/day >6 years	50 tablets
Fluoridated toothpaste	NaF 0.22%	Pea-size amount per brushing (0.5 cc)	50 cc
	MFP 0.76%	Pea-size amount per brushing (0.5 cc)	50 cc
	SnF$_2$ 0.4%	Pea-size amount per brushing (0.5 cc)	50 cc
Accidental overfeed of fluoridated water	For example, 0.1 mg fluoride/ml (100 ppm)	1 L/ day	Two cups
Fluoridated mouth rinse	NaF 0.05% (226 ppm)	Mouthful/day (not recommended for toddlers)	One cup
	NaF 0.2% (904 ppm)	Mouthful/week (not recommended for toddlers)	Approximately one capful
Professional fluoride gel	2.2% NaF gel 10,000 ppm	5 ml every 6 months	5 ml
	APF 1.23% F (12,300 ppm)	5 ml every 6 months	4 ml
High fluoride toothpaste	1.1% NaF (5,000 ppm)	Pea-size amount on toothbrush or as directed	10 cc
Household glass etcher/cleaner	3% HF (28,500 ppm)	Accidental ingestion?	1.7 ml

*Probable toxic dose is 5 mg/kg body weight, requiring emergency care or hospitalization.

and that dose has generally been accepted to be 5 mg F/km body weight. The sources of a probably toxic dose in low weight 28-month toddler weighing 10 km (22 pounds) are listed in Table 16-7.

This table can be used for quickly judging whether or not toddlers or children weighing more than 10 kg have consumed a toxic dose of fluoride. Acute doses of fluoride usually result in immediate gastric distress because the fluoride is converted to HF, which enters the epithelium lining of the stomach (Spak *et al.* 1990; NRC Report 2006, p. 270).

The clinical signs and symptoms of acute fluoride toxicity are shown in Table 16-8.

Every parent (and health care professional) should be aware of the potential emergency that could result from an ingestion of a sizable amount of fluoride. When the fluoride source is known and severe symptoms develop, emergency care, including a visit to the local hospital, should be considered.

Chronic fluoride toxicity—non-dental clinical signs, diagnosis, and treatment

Excess fluoride ingestion can lead to joint pain and bone problems. This is a major problem in areas of endemic fluorosis. Dentists should be aware that administration of too much fluoride for home use may put the patient at risk for joint pain or bone problems (Eichmiller *et al.* 2005). If a dentist suspects excess chronic fluoride intake, it would be prudent to refer to a physician with some knowledge in fluoride toxicity. Fluoride tests are not routine in family practice, and referral to a physician or hospital with experience in dealing with fluoride poisoning should be considered.

Medical management of fluoride toxicity

The average medical doctor may not be prepared to deal with fluoride poisoning. Hospital emergency physicians and most poison control centers may know what to do about acute fluoride intoxication, however, chronic fluoride poisoning is more difficult to recognize and manage. When everyone in an entire community appears to have symptoms of nausea and vomiting, fluoridation overfeed, especially in small communities, should be considered as a potential cause, and the public health department should be alerted. Bottle-fed infants that do not tolerate formula may improve with straight formula or formula reconstituted with distilled water or water

Table 16-8 Symptoms and treatment of acute fluoride poisoning

Acute symptoms	Excess salivation, tremors, weakness, convulsions, shallow breathing, nausea, vomiting, abdominal pain, diarrhea, and eventually shock
Emergency home treatment for a probable toxic dose (5 mg fluoride/kg) See Table 16-7 for estimates of amounts and potential sources	1. Contact Poison Control Center and provide the following: • Patient's age, weight, and condition • Name of the product (ingredients and strengths if known) • Time swallowed • Amount swallowed 2. Follow instructions of the hospital emergency department or the poison control center. 3. Give milk every 4 hours.
If symptoms worsen, go immediately to hospital emergency department—take the product container along.	Expect: • Gastric lavage • IV calcium • Supportive therapy
Prognosis	Depends on dose: if patient survives 48 hours, recovery is likely

that has been treated by reverse osmosis (RO). Patients who consume large quantities of water or who have renal problems should avoid fluoridated water altogether. Physicians should at least consider that some joint pain complaints may simply be the result of exposure to too much fluoride and develop a strategy to reduce the fluoride intake. Finally, patients should be reminded to inform their dentists if they want to avoid fluorides so that alternative therapies to prevent dental decay can be initiated.

Conclusion

For more than 6 decades, fluoride has been the first line of defense against caries. After years of laboratory research, animal experiments, and clinical trials, researchers now have a good idea how fluoride works to prevent tooth decay. They have also learned more about how fluoride interferes with a number of host biological processes. Dental fluorosis is an increasing problem in North America, and clinicians should be aware of the total daily fluoride intake to which their patients are exposed. Once the background exposure is known, side effects can be minimized while ensuring maximum anticaries benefit is attained.

References

Adair, S.M. (1998) The role of fluoride mouthrinses in the control of dental caries: a brief review. *Pediatric Dentistry*, 20, 101–104.

Alarcán-Herrera, M.T., Martín-Domínguez, I.R., Trejo-Vázquez, R. et al. (2001) Well water fluoride, dental fluorosis and bone fractures in the Guadiana Valley of Mexico. *Fluoride*, 34, 139–149.

American Dental Association. (2011) Statement on FDA toothpaste warning labels. [online] Available at the ADA website http://www.ada.org/1761.aspx.

American Dental Association, Council on Access Prevention and Interprofessional Relations (1995) Caries diagnosis and risk assessment: a review of preventive strategies and management. *Journal of the American Dental Association*, 126 (Suppl).

American Dental Association, Council on Scientific Affairs (2006) Professionally applied topical fluoride. Evidence-based clinical recommendations. *Journal of the American Dental Association*, 137, 1151–1159.

Angelillo, I.F., Romano, F., Fortunato, L., et al. (1990) Prevalence of dental caries and enamel defects in children living in areas with different water fluoride concentrations. *Community Dental Health*, 7, 229–236.

Angmar-Månsson, B., Lindh, U., Whitford, G.M. (1990) Enamel and dentin fluoride levels and fluorosis following single fluoride doses: a nuclear microprobe study. *Caries Research*, 24, 258–262.

Aoba, T. (2004) Solubility properties of human tooth mineral and pathogenesis of dental caries. *Oral Diseases*, 10, 249–257.

Aoba, T. and Fejerskov, O. (2002) Dental fluorosis: chemistry and biology. *Critical Reviews in Oral Biology and Medicine*, 13, 155–170.

Armfield, J.M. (2010) Community effectiveness of public water fluoridation in reducing children's dental disease. *Public Health Reports*, 125, 655–664.

Armfield, J.M. and Spencer, A.J. (2004) Consumption of nonpublic water: implications for children's caries experience. *Community Dentistry and Oral Epidemiology*, 32, 283–296.

Azarpazhooh, A. and Main, P.A. (2008) Fluoride varnish in the prevention of dental caries in children and adolescents: a systematic review. *Journal of the Canadian Dental Association*, 74, 73–79.

Bader, J.D., Rozier, R.G., Lohr, K.N., et al. (2004) Physicians' roles in preventing dental caries in preschool children: a summary of the evidence for the U.S. Preventive Services Task Force. *American Journal of Preventive Medicine*, 26, 315–325.

Balzar Ekenbäck, S., Linder, L.E., Sund, M.L., et al. (2001) Effect of fluoride on glucose incorporation and metabolism in biofilm cells of Streptococcus mutans. *European Journal of Oral Science*, 109, 182–186.

Baysan, A., Lynch, E., Ellwood, R., et al. (2001) Reversal of primary root caries using dentifrices containing 5000 and 1100 ppm fluoride. *Caries Research*, 35, 41–46.

Beltrán-Aguilar, E.D., Barker, L., Canto, M.T., et al. (2005) Surveillance for dental caries, dental sealants, tooth retention, edentulism, and enamel fluorosis—United States, 1988–1994 and 1999–2002. *Morbidity and Mortality Weekly Reports: Surveillance Summary*, 54, 1–43.

Beltrán-Aguilar, E.D., Barker, L., Dye, B.A. (2010) Prevalence and severity of dental fluorosis in the United States, 1999–2004. *NCHS Data Brief*, no 53. National Center for Health Statistics, Hyattsville, MD.

Bibby, B.G., Wilkins, E., Witol, E. (1955) A preliminary study of the effects of fluoride lozenges and pills on dental caries. *Oral Surgery, Oral Medicine and Oral Pathology*, 8, 213–216.

Bjornhagen, V., Hojer, J., Karlson-Stiber, C. (2003) Hydrofluoric acid-induced burns and life-threatening systemic poisoning-favorable outcome after hemodialysis. Journal of Toxicology. *Clinical Toxicology*, 41, 855–860.

Bohannan, H.M., Stamm, J.W., Graves, R.C. (1985) Fluoride mouthrinse programs in fluoridated communities. *Journal of the American Dental Association*, 111, 783–789.

Bowden, G.H. (1990) Microbiology of root surface caries in humans. *Journal of Dental Research*, 69, 1205–1210.

Boyar, R.M., Thylstrup, A., Holmen, L., *et al.* (1989) The microflora associated with the development of initial enamel decalcification below orthodontic bands in vivo in children living in a fluoridated-water area. *Journal of Dental Research*, 68, 1734–1738.

Boyle, D.R. and Chagnon, M. (1995) An incidence of skeletal fluorosis associated with groundwaters of the maritime carboniferous basin, Gaspé region, Quebec, Canada. *Environmental Geochemistry and Health*, 17, 5–12.

Bradshaw, D.J., P.D. Marsha, P.P., Hodgson, R.J., *et al.* (2002) Effects of Glucose and Fluoride on Competition and Metabolism within in vitro Dental Bacterial Communities and Biofilms. *Caries Research*, 36, 81–86.

Brailsford, S.R., Kidd, E.A., Gilbert, S.C., *et al.* (2005) Effect of withdrawal of fluoride-containing toothpaste on the interproximal plaque microflora. *Caries Research*, 39, 231–235.

Bratthall, D., Hänsel-Petersson, G., Sundberg, H. (1996) Reasons for the caries decline: what do the experts believe? *European Journal of Oral Science*, 104 (Pt 2), 416–22; discussion 423–5, 430–2.

Briggs, D. (2003) Environmental pollution and the global burden of disease. *British Medical Bulletin*, 68, 1–24.

Bronckers, A.L., Lyaruu DM, DenBesten, P.K. (2009) The impact of fluoride on ameloblasts and the mechanisms of enamel fluorosis. *Journal of Dental Research*, 88, 877–893.

Brown, H.K. and Poplove, M. (1963) The Brantford-Sarnia-Stratford fluoridation caries study: final survey. *Canadian Journal of Public Health*, 56, 319–324.

Brunelle, J.A. and Carlos, J.P. (1990) Recent trends in dental caries in U.S. children and the effect of water fluoridation. *Journal of Dental Research*, 69 (Spec No), 723–7; discussion 820–3.

Burt, B.A. (1999) The case for eliminating the use of dietary fluoride supplements for young children. *Journal of Public Health Dentistry*, 59, 269–274.

Burt, B.A., Keels, M.A., Heller, K.E. (2000) The effects of a break in water fluoridation on the development of dental caries and fluorosis. *Journal of Dental Research*, 79, 761–769.

Campagna, L., Tsamtsouris, A., Kavadia, K. (1995) Fluoridated drinking water and maturation of permanent teeth at age 12. *Journal of Clinical Pediatric Dentistry*, 19, 225–228.

Canadian Dental Association. (2010) CDA Position on Use of Fluorides in Caries Prevention. Available at http://www.cda-adc.ca/_files/position_statements/fluorides.pdf.

Canadian Dental Association. (1993) Fluoride recommendations released. Canadian Conference on the Evaluation of Current Recommendations Concerning Fluorides, April 9–11, 1992. *Journal of the Canadian Dental Association*, 59, 330, 334–6.

Centers for Disease Control and Prevention (2001) Recommendations for Using Fluoride to Prevent and Control Dental Caries in the United States. *Morbidity and Mortality Weekly Report*, 50(RR14), 1–42.

Cheng, K.K., Chalmers, I., Sheldon, T.A. (2007) Adding fluoride to water supplies. *British Medical Journal*, 335(7622), 699–702.

Chersoni, S., Bertacci, A., Pashley, D.H. *et al.* (2011) In vivo effects of fluoride on enamel permeability. *Clinical and Oral Investigations*, 15, 443–449.

Clark, D.C. (1994) Trends in prevalence of dental fluorosis in North America. *Community Dentistry and Oral Epidemiology*, 22, 148–152.

Clark, D.C., Hann, H.J., Williamson, M.F., *et al.* (1995) Effects of lifelong consumption of fluoridated water or use of fluoride supplements on dental caries prevalence. *Community Dentistry and Oral Epidemiology*, 23, 20–24.

Council on Scientific Affairs (2010) *Journal of the American Dental Association*, 114, 1480–1489.

Cury, J.A. and Tenuta, L.M. (2008) How to maintain a cariostatic fluoride concentration in the oral environment. *Advances in Dental Research*, 20, 13–6.

Danielson, C., Lyon, J.L., Egger, M. (1992) Hip fractures and fluoridation in Utah's elderly population. *Journal of the American Medical Association*, 268, 746–748.

de Liefde, B. (1998) The decline of caries in New Zealand over the past 40 years. *New Zealand Dental Journal*, 94, 109–113.

De Stoppelaar, J.D., Van Houte, J., Backer Dirks, O. (1969) The relationship between extracellular polysaccharide-producing streptococci and smooth surface caries in 13-year-old children. *Caries Research*, 3, 190–199.

Dean, H.T. (1934) Classification of mottled enamel diagnosis. *Journal of the American Dental Association*, 21, 1421–1426.

DenBesten, P., Ko, H.S. (1996) Fluoride levels in whole saliva of preschool children after brushing with 0.25 g (pea-sized) as compared to 1.0 g (full-brush) of a fluoride dentifrice. *Pediatric Dentistry*, 18, 277–280.

DenBesten, P.K., Yan, Y., Featherstone, J.D., *et al.* (2002) Effects of fluoride on rat dental enamel matrix proteinases. *Archives of Oral Biology*, 47, 763–770.

Department of Health and Human Services (1991) Review of fluoride: benefits and risks. Report of the Ad Hoc Subcommittee on Fluoride, p. 46, Department of Health and Human Services Washington, DC.

Diesendorf, M. (1986) The mystery of declining tooth decay. *Nature*, 322(6075), 125–129.

Eichmiller, F.C., Eidelman, N., Carey, C.M. (2005) Controlling the fluoride dosage in a patient with compromised salivary function. *Journal of the American Dental Association*, 136, 67–70.

Ekstrand, J., Boreus, L.O., de Chateau, P. (1981) No evidence of transfer of fluoride from plasma to breast milk. *British Medical Journal (Clinical Research Edition)*, 283(6294), 761–762.

Ekstrand, K.R., Christiansen, M.E.C., Qvist, V., *et al.* (2010) Factors associated with inter-municipality differences in dental caries experience among Danish adolescents. An ecological study. *Community Dentistry and Oral Epidemiology*, 38, 29–42.

Environment Canada (1976) National inventory of sources and emissions of fluoride (1972). *Environmental Protection Service. Internal Report APCD 75-7*. Environment Canada, Air Pollution Directorate.

Erdal, S. and Buchanan, S.N. (2005) A quantitative look at fluorosis, fluoride exposure, and intake in children using a health risk assessment approach. *Environmental Health Perspectives*, 113, 111–117.

Featherstone, J.D.B. (2000) The Science and Practice of Caries Prevention. *Journal of the American Dental Association*, 131, 887–899.

Fejerskov, O. (2004) Changing paradigms in concepts on dental caries: consequences for oral health care. *Caries Research*, 38, 182–191.

Fejerskov, O., Larsen, M.J., Richards, A., *et al.* (1994) Dental tissue effects of fluoride. *Advances in Dental Research*, 8, 15–31.

Fejerskov, O., Manji, F., Baelum, V. (1990) The nature and mechanisms of dental fluorosis in man. *Journal of Dental Research*, 69 (Spec No), 692–700; discussion 721.

Felsenfeld, A.J. and Roberts, M.A. (1991) A report of fluorosis in the United States secondary to drinking well water. *Journal of the American Medical Association*, 265, 486–488.

Feltman, R. and Kosel, G. (1961) Prenatal and postnatal ingestion of fluorides-fourteen years of investigation-Final report. *Journal of Dental Medicine*, 16, 190–198.

Feng, Y.W., Ogura, N., Feng, Z.W. (2003) The Concentrations and Sources of Fluoride in Atmospheric Depositions in Beijing, China. *Water Air and Soil Pollution*, 145, 95–107.

Fomon, S.J. and Ekstrand, J. (1999) Fluoride intake by infants. *Journal of Public Health Dentistry*, 59, 229–234.

Fomon, S.J., Ekstrand, J., Ziegler, E.E. (2000) Fluoride intake and prevalence of dental fluorosis: trends in fluoride intake with special attention to infants. *Journal of Public Health Dentistry*, 60, 131–139.

Gessner, B.D., Beller, M., Middaugh, J.P., *et al.* (1994) Acute fluoride poisoning from a public water system. *New England Journal of Medicine*, 330, 95–99.

Government of Canada (Environment Canada, Health Canada) (1993) *Inorganic Fluorides. Priority Substance List Assessment Report.* Pp.13, Government of Canada.

Griffin, S.O., Regnier, E., Griffin, P.M., *et al.* (2007) Effectiveness of fluoride in preventing caries in adults. *Journal of Dent Research*, 86, 410–415.

Hamilton, I.R. (1990) Biochemical effects of fluoride on oral bacteria. *Journal of Dent Research*, 69 Spec No, 660–667; discussion 682–683.

Hausen, H. (2004) Benefits of topical fluorides firmly established. *Evidence Based Dentistry*, 5, 36–37.

Hedman, J., Sjöman, R., Sjöström, I., *et al.* (2006) Fluoride concentration in saliva after consumption of a dinner meal prepared with fluoridated salt. *Caries Research*, 40, 158–162.

Heller, K.E., Eklund, S.A., Burt, B.A. (1997) Dental caries and dental fluorosis at varying water fluoride concentrations. *Journal of Public Health Dentistry*, 57, 136–143.

Hellwig, E. and Lennon, A.M. (2004) Systemic versus topical fluoride. *Caries Research*, 38, 258–262.

Horowitz, H.S., Driscoll, W.S., Meyers, R.J., *et al.* (1984) A new method for assessing the prevalence of dental fluorosis: The Tooth Surface Index of Fluorosis. *Journal of the American Dental Association*, 109, 37–41.

Hujoel, P.P., Zina, L.G., Moimaz, S.A. (2009) Infant formula and enamel fluorosis: a systematic review. *Journal of the American Dental Association*, 140, 841–854.

Hunt, R.J., Eldredge, J.B., Beck, J.D. (1989) Effect of residence in a fluoridated community on the incidence of coronal and root caries in an older adult population. *Journal of Public Health Dentistry*, 49, 138–141.

Ishii, T. and Suckling, G. (1991) The severity of dental fluorosis in children exposed to water with a high fluoride content for various periods of time. *Journal of Dental Research*, 70, 952–956.

Ismail, A.I. and Bandekar, R.R. (1999) Fluoride supplements and fluorosis: a meta-analysis. *Community Dentistry and Oral Epidemiology*, 27, 48–56.

Ismail, A.I. and Hasson, H. (2008) Fluoride supplements, dental caries and fluorosis: a systematic review. *Journal of the American Dental Association*, 139, 1457–1468.

Ismail, A.I., Shoveller, J., Langille, D., *et al.* (1993) McNally Should the drinking water of Truro, Nova Scotia, be fluoridated? *Water fluoridation in the 1990s. Community Dentistry and Oral Epidemiology*, 21, 118–125.

Jackson, R.D., Kelly, S.A., Katz, B.P., *et al.* (1995) Dental fluorosis and caries prevalence in children residing in communities with different levels of fluoride in the water. *Journal of Public Health Dentistry*, 55, 79–84.

Johnston, D.W. and Lewis, D.W. (1995) Three-year randomized trial of professionally applied topical fluoride gel comparing annual and biannual applications with/without prior prophylaxis. *Caries Research*, 29, 331–336.

Jordan, H.V. (1986) Cultural methods for the identification and quantitation of Streptococcus mutans and lactobacilli in oral samples. *Oral Microbiology and Immunology*, 1, 23–27.

Jordan, H.V. (1986) Microbial etiology of root surface caries. *Gerodontology*, 5, 13–20.

Kalsbeek, H., Kwant, G.W., Groeneveld, A., *et al.* (1993) Caries experience of 15-year-old children in The Netherlands after discontinuation of water fluoridation. *Caries Research*, 27, 201–205.

Kobayashi, S., Kawasaki, K., Takagi, O., *et al.* (1992) Caries experience in subjects 18–22 years of age after 13 years' discontinued water fluoridation in Okinawa. *Community Dentistry and Oral Epidemiology*, 20, 81–83.

Komárek, A., Lesaffre, E., Härkänen, T., *et al.* (2005) A Bayesian analysis of multivariate doubly-interval-censored dental data. *Biostatistics*, 6, 145–155.

Krebs, R. (2006) *The History and Use of Our Earth's Chemical Elements. A reference Guide*, (Ed. R. Krebs) 2nd edn. Pp 246. Greenwood Publishing Group, Westport CT.

Känzel, W., Fischer, T., Lorenz, R., *et al.* (2000) Decline of caries prevalence after the cessation of water fluoridation in the former East Germany. *Community Dentistry and Oral Epidemiology*, 28, 382–389.

Larsen, M.J. and Fejerskov, O. (1978) Structural studies on calcium fluoride formation and uptake of fluoride in surface enamel in vitro. *Scandinavian Journal of Dental Research*, 86, 337–345.

Leake, J., Goettler, F., Stahl-Quinlan, B., *et al.* (2002) Has the level of dental fluorosis among Toronto children changed? *Journal of the Canadian Dental Association*, 68, 21–25.

Levy, S.M., Eichenberger-Gilmore, J., Warren, J.J., *et al.* (2009) Associations of fluoride intake with children's bone measures at age 11. *Community Dentistry and Oral Epidemiology*, 37, 416–426.

Levy, S.M. (2003) An update on fluorides and fluorosis. *Journal of the Canadian Dental Association*, 69, 286–291.

Levy, S.M., Broffitt, B., Marshall, T.A., *et al.* (2010) Associations between fluorosis of permanent incisors and fluoride intake from infant formula, other dietary sources and dentifrice during early childhood. *Journal of the American Dental Association*, 141, 1190–1201.

Lewis, D.W. and Banting, D.W. (1994) Water fluoridation: current effectiveness and dental fluorosis. *Community Dentistry and Oral Epidemiology*, 22, 153–158.

Li, J., Nakagaki, H., Tsuboi, S., *et al.* (1994) Fluoride profiles in different surfaces of human permanent molar enamels from a naturally fluoridated and a non-fluoridated area. *Archives of Oral Biology*, 39, 727–731.

Limeback, H. (1999) A re-examination of the pre-eruptive and post-eruptive mechanism of the anti-caries effects of fluoride: is there any anti-caries benefit from swallowing fluoride? *Community Dentistry and Oral Epidemiology*, 27, 62–71.

Limeback, H. (2007) Point of Care. How do I diagnose fluorosis? *Journal of the Canadian Dental Association*, 73, 809–812.

Limeback, H., Ismail, A., Banting, D., *et al.* (1998) Canadian Consensus Conference on the appropriate use of fluoride supplements for the prevention of dental caries in children. *Journal of the Canadian Dental Association*, 64, 636–639.

Limeback, H., Vieira, A.P., Lawrence, H. (2006) Improving esthetically objectionable human enamel fluorosis with a simple microabrasion technique. *European Journal of Oral Science*, 114 (Suppl 1), 123–126, discussion 127–129, 380.

Macpherson, L.M., MacFarlane, T.W, Stephen, K.W. (1990) An intra-oral appliance study of the plaque microflora associated with early enamel demineralization. *Journal of Dental Research*, 69, 1712–1716.

Maltz, M. and Emilson, C.G. (1982) Susceptibility of Oral Bacteria to Various Fluoride Salts. Journal of Dental Research, 61, 786–790.

Marinho, V.C. (2009) Cochrane reviews of randomized trials of fluoride therapies for preventing dental caries. *European Archives of Paediatric Dentistry*, 10, 183–191.

Marinho, V.C., Higgins, J.P., Logan, S., *et al.* (2002) Fluoride gels for preventing dental caries in children and adolescents. *Cochrane Database of Systematic Reviews*, 2002 (2), CD002280.

Marinho, V.C., Higgins, J.P., Logan, S., *et al.* (2003a) Fluoride mouthrinses for preventing dental caries in children and adolescents. *Cochrane Database of Systematic Reviews*, 2003(3), CD002284.

Marinho, V.C., Higgins, J.P., Logan, S., *et al.* (2003b) Fluoride toothpastes for preventing dental caries in children and adolescents. *Cochrane Database of Systematic Reviews*, 2003(1), CD002278.

Marinho, V.C., Higgins, J.P., Sheiham, A., *et al.* (2004) One topical fluoride (toothpastes, or mouthrinses, or gels, or varnishes) versus another for preventing dental caries in children and adolescents. *Cochrane Database of Systematic Reviews*, 2004(1), CD002780.

Marquis, R.E., Clock, S.A., Mota-Meira, M. (2003) Fluoride and organic weak acids as modulators of microbial physiology. *FEMS Microbiology Reviews*, 26, 493–510.

Marsh, P.D., Featherstone, A., McKee, A.S, *et al.* (1989) A microbiological study of early caries of approximal surfaces in schoolchildren. *Journal of Dental Research*, 68, 1151–1154.

Marthaler, T.M. and Petersen, P.E. (2005) Salt fluoridation—an alternative in automatic prevention of dental caries. *International Dental Journal*, 55, 351–358.

Martinez, L.J., Li, G., Chignell, C.F. (1997) Photogeneration of fluoride by the fluoroquinolone antimicrobial agents lomefloxacin and fleroxacin. *Photochemistry and Photobiology*, 65, 599–602.

Mascarenhas, A.K. and Scott, T. (2008) Does exposure to fluoridated water during crown completion and maturation phases of permanent first molars decrease pit and fissure caries? *Journal of Evidence Based Dental Practice*, 8, 17–18.

Maslak, E.E., Afonina, I.V., Kchmizova, T.G. (2004) The effect of a milk fluoridation project in Volgograd. *Caries Research* 38, 377 (abstract 60).

Matsuo, S., Kiyomiya, K., Kurebe, M. (1998) Mechanism of toxic action of fluoride in dental fluorosis: whether trimeric G proteins participate in the disturbance of intracellular transport of secretory ameloblast exposed to fluoride. *Archives of Toxicology*, 72, 798–806.

Maupomé, G., Clark, D.C., Levy, S.M., *et al.* (2001) Patterns of dental caries following the cessation of water fluoridation. *Community Dentistry and Oral Epidemiology*, 29, 37–47.

Maupomé, G., Gullion, C.M., Peters, D., *et al.* (2007) A comparison of dental treatment utilization and costs by HMO members living in fluoridated and nonfluoridated areas. *Journal of Public Health Dentistry*, 67, 224–233.

McDonagh, M.S., Whiting, P.F., Wilson, P.M., *et al.* (2000) Systematic review of water fluoridation. *British Medical Journal*, 321, 855–859.

McKnight-Hanes, M.C., Leverett, D.H., Adair, S.M., *et al.* (1988) Fluoride content of infant formulas: soy-based formulas as a potential factor in dental fluorosis. *Pediatric Dentistry*, 10, 189–194.

Milgrom, P., Zero, D.T., Tanzer, J.M. (2009) An examination of the advances in science and technology of prevention of tooth decay in young children since the Surgeon General's Report on Oral Health. *Academy of Pediatrics*, 9, 404–409.

Nakagaki, H., Koyama, Y., Sakakibara, Y., *et al.* (1987) Distribution of fluoride across human dental enamel, dentine and cementum. *Archives Oral Biology*, 32, 651–654.

National Research Council. (2006) Fluoride in Drinking Water. A Scientific Review of EPA's Standards. National Research Council: The National Academies Press.

Natural Resources Canada. (2004) *Geological Survey of Canada Open File Report 4703*. Soil and Till Geochemical Metadata for Canada.

Nishiyama, T. and Hanaoka, K. (1998) Inorganic fluoride kinetics and renal and hepatic function after repeated sevoflurane anesthesia. *Anesthesia and Analgesia*, 87, 468–473.

National Research Council (NRC). (2006) *Fluoride in Drinking-Water, A scientific Review of EPA's Standards*, NRC, p. 123, Washington, DC.

Nyvad, B. and Kilian, M. (1990) Microflora associated with experimental root surface caries in humans. *Infection and Immunity*, 58, 1628–1633.

Ogaard, B., Rölla, G., Dijkman, T., *et al.* (1991) Effect of fluoride mouthrinsing on caries lesion development in shark enamel: an in situ caries model study. *Scandinavian Journal of Dental Research*, 99, 372–377.

Ogaard, B., Rölla, G., Ruben, J., *et al.* (1998) Microradiographic study of demineralization of shark enamel in a human caries model. *Scandinavian Journal of Dental Research*, 96, 209–211.

Oliveby, A., Lagerlöf, F., Ekstrand, J., *et al.* (1989) Studies on fluoride excretion in human whole saliva and its relation to flow rate and plasma fluoride levels. *Caries Research*, 23, 243–246.

Oliveby, A., Twetman, S., Ekstrand, J. (1990) Diurnal fluoride concentration in whole saliva in children living in a high- and a low-fluoride area. *Caries Research*, 24, 44–47.

Ostela, I., Karhuvaara, L., Tenovua, J. (1991) Comparative antibacterial effects of chlorhexidine and stannous fluoride-amine fluoride containing dental gels against salivary mutans streptococci. *Scandinavian Journal of Dental Research*, 99, 378–383.

Pandit, S., Kim, J.E., Jung, K.H., *et al.* (2011) Effect of sodium fluoride on the virulence factors and composition of Streptococcus mutans biofilms. *Archives of Oral Biology*, 56, 643–649.

Pendrys, D.G. (2000) Risk of enamel fluorosis in nonfluoridated and optimally fluoridated populations: considerations for the dental professional. *Journal of the America Dental Association*, 131, 746–755.

Peterson, J. (1997) Solving the mystery of the Colorado Brown Stain. *Journal of the History of Dentistry*, 45, 57–61.

Petersson, L.G., Twetman, S., Dahlgren, H., *et al.* (2004) Professional fluoride varnish treatment for caries control: a systematic review of clinical trials. *Acta Odontologica Scandinavica*, 62, 170–176.

Poulsen, S. (2009) Fluoride-containing gels, mouth rinses and varnishes: an update of evidence of efficacy. *European Archives of Paediatric Dentistry*, 10, 157–161.

Pradhan, K.M., Arora, N.K., Jena, A., *et al.* (1995) Safety of ciprofloxacin therapy in children: magnetic resonance images, body fluid levels of fluoride and linear growth. *Acta Paediatrics*, 84, 555–560.

Proskin, H.M. (1993) Statistical considerations related to a meta-analytic evaluation of published caries clinical studies comparing the anticaries efficacy of dentifrices containing sodium fluoride and sodium monofluorophosphate. *American Journal of Dentistry*, 6 Spec No., S43–S49.

Riggs, B.L., Baylink, D.J., Kleerekoper, M., *et al.* (1987) Incidence of hip fractures in osteoporotic women treated with sodium fluoride. *Journal of Bone and Mineral Research*, 2, 123–126.

Rihs, L.B., de Sousa Mda, L., Wada, R.S. (2008) Root caries in areas with and without fluoridated water at the Southeast region of São Paulo State, Brazil. *Journal of Applied Oral Science*, 16, 70–74.

Riordan, P.J. (1993) Perceptions of dental fluorosis. *Journal of Dental Research*, 72, 1268–1274.

Ripa, L.W. (1993) A half-century of community water fluoridation in the United States: review and commentary. *Journal of Public Health Dentistry*, 53, 17–44.

Robinson, C. and Weatherell, J.A. (1995) The Chemistry of Mature Enamel in: *Dental Enamel Formation to Destruction* 1995 (Eds. Robinson, C., Shore, R.C, and Kirkham, J.) CRC Press, Boca Raton.

Robinson, C. (2009) Fluoride and the caries lesion: interactions and mechanism of action. *European Archives of Paediatric Dentistry*, 10, 136–140.

Robinson, C., Shore, R.C., Brookes, S.J., *et al.* (2000) The chemistry of enamel caries. *Critical Reviews in Oral Biology and Medicine*, 11, 481–495.

Rojas-Sanchez, F., Kelly, S.A., Drake, K.M., *et al.* (1999) Fluoride intake from foods, beverages and dentifrice by young children in communities with negligibly and optimally fluoridated water: a pilot study. *Community Dentistry and Oral Epidemiology*, 27, 288–297.

Rølla, G., Ogaard, B., Cruz Rde, A. (1991) Clinical effect and mechanism of cariostatic action of fluoride-containing toothpastes: a review. *International Dental Journal*, 41, 171–174.

Rozier, R.G., Adair, S., Graham, F., *et al.* (2010) Evidence-based clinical recommendations on the prescription of dietary fluoride supplements for caries prevention: a report of the American Dental Association. *Journal of the American Dental Association*, 141, 1480–1489.

Rozier, R.G. (1984) Epidemiologic indices for measuring the clinical manifestations of dental fluorosis: overview and critique. *Advances in Dental Research*, 8, 39–55.

Rozier, R.G. (1999) The prevalence and severity of enamel fluorosis in North American children. *Journal of Public Health Dentistry*, 59, 239–246.

Rozier, R.G. (2001) Effectiveness of methods used by dental professionals for the primary prevention of dental caries. *Journal of Dental Education*, 65, 1063–1072.

Selwitz, R.H., Nowjack-Raymer, R.E., Kingman, A., *et al.* (1998) Dental caries and dental fluorosis among schoolchildren who were lifelong residents of communities having either low or optimal levels of fluoride in drinking water. *Journal of Public Health Dentistry*, 58, 28–35.

Seppä, L. (2004) Fluoride varnishes in caries prevention. *Medical Principles and Practice*, 13, 307–311.

Seppä, L., Kärkkäinen, S., Hausen, H. (1998) Caries frequency in permanent teeth before and after discontinuation of water fluoridation in Kuopio, Finland. *Community Dentistry and Oral Epidemiology*, 26, 256–262.

Sharma, R., Tsuchiya, M., Skobe, Z., *et al.* (2010) The acid test of fluoride: how pH modulates toxicity. PLoS One, 5, e10895.

Shulman, J.D., Maupome, G., Clark, D.C., *et al.* (2004) Perceptions of desirable tooth color among parents, dentists and children. *Journal of the American Dental Association*, 135, 595–604, quiz 654–655.

Silva, M. and Reynolds EC. (1996) Fluoride content of infant formulae in Australia. *Australia Dental Journal*, 41, 37–42.

Singh, K.A., Spencer, A.J., Brennan, D.S. (2007) Effects of water fluoride exposure at crown completion and maturation on caries of permanent first molars. *Caries Research*, 41, 34–42.

Sohn, W., Ismail, A.I., Taichman, L.S. (2007) Caries risk-based fluoride supplementation for children. *Pediatric Dentistry*, 2, 23–31.

Sowers, M., Whitford, G.M., Clark, M.K (2005). Elevated serum fluoride concentrations in women are not related to fractures and bone mineral density. *Journal of Nutrition*, 135, 2247–2252.

Spak, C.J., Sjöstedt, S., Eleborg, L., *et al.* (1990) Studies of human gastric mucosa after application of 0.42% fluoride gel. *Journal of Dental Research*, 69, 426–429.

Spencer, A.J. and Do, L.G. (2008) Changing risk factors for fluorosis among South Australian children. *Community Dentistry and Oral Epidemiology*, 36, 210–218.

Stephen, K.W., Boyle, I.T., Campbell, D., *et al.* (1984) Five-year double-blind fluoridated milk study in Scotland. *Community Dentistry and Oral Epidemiology*, 12, 223–229.

Stephen, K.W., McCall, D.R., Tullis, J.I. (1987) Caries prevalence in northern Scotland before, and 5 years after, water defluoridation. *British Dent Journal*, 163, 324–326.

Stephen, K.W., Macpherson, L.M.D., Gorzo, I., *et al.* (1999) Effect of fluoridated salt intake in infancy: a blind caries and fluorosis study in 8th grade Hungarian pupils. *Community Dentistry and Oral Epidemiology*, 27, 210–215.

Susa, M. (1999) Heterotrimeric G proteins as fluoride targets in bone (review). *International Journal of Molecular Medicine*, 3, 115–126.

Sutton, P.R. (1988) Can water fluoridation increase orthodontic problems? *Medical Hypotheses*, 26, 63–64.

Swan, E. (2000) Dietary fluoride supplement protocol for the new millennium. *Journal of the Canadian Dental Association*, 66, 362–363.

ten Cate, J.M. (1999) Current concepts on the theories of the mechanism of action of fluoride. *Acta Odontologica Scandinavica*, 57, 325–329.

ten Cate, J.M. (2001) 2001 Consensus statements on fluoride usage and associated research questions. *Caries Research*, 35(S1), 71–73.

ten Cate, J.M. (2004) Fluorides in caries prevention and control: empiricism or science. *Caries Research*, 38, 254–257.

Thuy, T.T., Nakagaki, H., Ha, N.T., *et al.* (2003) Fluoride profiles in premolars after different durations of water fluoridation in Ho Chi Minh City, Vietnam. *Archives of Oral Biology*, 48, 369–376.

Thylstrup, A. and Fejerskov, O. (1978) Clinical appearance of dental fluorosis in permanent teeth in relation to histologic changes. *Community Dentistry and Oral Epidemiology*, 6, 315–328.

Toumba, K.J., Al-Ibrahim, N.S., Curzon, M.E. (2009) A review of slow-release fluoride devices. *European Archives of Paediatric Dentistry*, 10, 175–182.

van der Mei, H.C, White, D.J, Atema-Smit, J., *et al.* (2006) A method to study sustained antimicrobial activity of rinse and dentifrice components on biofilm viability in vivo. *Journal of Clinical Periodontology*, 33, 14–20.

van Houte, J. (1980) Bacterial specificity in the etiology of dental caries. *International Dental Journal*, 30, 305–326.

Van Houte, J. (1993) Microbiological Predictors of Caries Risk *Advances in Dental Research*, 7, 87–96.

Van Houte, J. (1994) Role of Micro-organisms in Caries Etiology. *Journal of Dental Research*, 73, 672–681.

van Loveren, C., Lammens, A.J., ten Cate, J.M. (1990) Development and establishment of fluoride-resistant strains of Streptococcus mutans in rats. *Caries Research*, 24, 337–343.

Van Loveren, C., Van de Plassche-Simons, Y.M., De Soet, J.J., *et al.* (1991) Acidogenesis in relation to fluoride resistance of Streptococcus mutans. *Oral Microbiology and Immunology*, 6, 288–291.

Vanderborgh, N.E. (1968) Evaluation of the lanthanum fluoride membrane electrode response in acidic solutions: the determination of the pka of hydrofluoric acid. *Talanta*, 10, 1009–1013.

Vieira, A.P., Lawrence, H.P., Limeback, H., *et al.* (2005) A visual analog scale for measuring dental fluorosis severity. *Journal of the American Dental Association*, 136, 895–901.

Virtanen, J.I., Bloigu, R.S., Larmas, M.A. (1994) Timing of eruption of permanent teeth: standard Finnish patient documents. *Community Dentistry and Oral Epidemiology*, 22, 286–288.

Vogel, G.L., Mao, Y., Chow, L.C., *et al.* (2000) Fluoride in plaque fluid, plaque, and saliva measured for 2 hours after a sodium fluoride monofluorophosphate rinse. *Caries Research*, 34, 404–411.

Vogel, G.L., Tenuta, L.M., Schumacher, G.E., *et al.* (2010) No calcium-fluoride-like deposits detected in plaque shortly after a sodium fluoride mouthrinse. *Caries Research*, 44, 108–115.

Volpe, A.R., Petrone, M.E., Davies, R.M. (1993) A critical review of the 10 pivotal caries clinical studies used in a recent meta-analysis comparing the anticaries efficacy of sodium fluoride and sodium monofluorophosphate dentifrices. *American Journal of Dentistry*, 6 Spec No:S13–42.

Waidyasekera, K., Nikaido, T., Weerasinghe, D., *et al.* (2010) Why does fluorosed dentine show a higher susceptibility for caries: an ultra-morphological explanation. *Journal of Medical and Dental Science*, 57, 17–23.

Walsh, T., Worthington, H.V., Glenny, A.M., *et al.* (2010) Fluoride toothpastes of different concentrations for preventing dental caries in children and adolescents. *Cochrane Database Systematic Reviews*, 2010(1), CD007868.

Warren, J.J., Levy, S.M., Broffitt, B., *et al.* (2009) Considerations on optimal fluoride intake using dental fluorosis and dental caries outcomes—a longitudinal study. *Journal of Public Health Dentistry*, 69, 111–115.

Warren, J.J. and Levy, S.M. (2003) Current and future role of fluoride in nutrition. *Dental Clinics of North America*, 47, 225–243.

Warrington, P.D. (1990) *Ambient water quality criteria for fluoride. Technical Appendix*. British Columbia Ministry of the Environment, Victoria, BC.

Watson, P.S., Pontefract, H.A., Devine, D.A., *et al.* (2005) Penetration of fluoride into natural plaque biofilm. *Journal of Dental Research*, 84, 451–455.

Weatherell, I.A., Deutsch, D., Robinson, C., *et al.* (1977) Assimilation of fluoride by enamel through the life of the tooth. *Caries Research*, 1 (Suppl 1), 85–115.

Weatherell, J.A., Robinson, C., Hallsworth, A.S. (1974) Variations in the chemical composition of human enamel. *Journal of Dental Research*, 53, 180–192.

Whelton, H.P., Ketley, C.E., McSweeney, F., *et al.* (2004) A review of fluorosis in the European Union: prevalence, risk factors and aesthetic issues. *Community Dentistry and Oral Epidemiology*, 32 (Suppl 1), 9–18.

Whitford, G.M. (1997) Determinants and mechanisms of enamel fluorosis. *Ciba Foundation Symposium*, 205, 226–241, discussion 241–245.

Whitford, G.M. (1990) The physiological and toxicological characteristics of fluoride. *Journal of Dental Research*, 69 (Spec No), 539–549, discussion 556–557.

Whitford, G.M. (1999) Fluoride metabolism and excretion in children. *Journal of Public Health Dentistry*, 59, 224–228.

World Health Organisation Expert Committee on Oral Health Status and Fluoride Use (1994) Fluorides and oral health. WHO Technical Report Series No. 846, pp. 6, World Health Organisation, Geneva.

Whyte, M.P., Essmyer, K., Gannon, F.H, *et al.* (2005) Skeletal fluorosis and instant tea. *American Journal of Medicine*, 118, 78–82.

Wiegand, A., Buchalla, W., Attin, T. (2007) Review on fluoride-releasing restorative materials—fluoride release and uptake characteristics, antibacterial activity and influence on caries formation. *Dental Materials*, 23, 343–362.

Wong, F.S. and Winter, G.B. (2002) Effectiveness of microabrasion technique for improvement of dental aesthetics. *British Dental Journal*, 193, 155–158.

Yeung, A., Hitchings, J.L., Macfarlane, T.V., *et al.* (2005) Fluoridated milk for preventing dental caries. *Cochrane Database of Systematic Reviews*, 2005(3), CD003876.

Yeung, C.A. (2007) Fluoride prevents caries among adults of all ages. *Evidence Based Dentistry*, 8, 72–73.

Young, C.E. (2008) A systematic review of the efficacy and safety of fluoridation. *Evidence Based Dentistry*, 9, 39–43.

Zero, D. (2006) Proceedings: Dentifrices, mouthwashes, and remineralization/caries arrestment Strategies. *BMC Oral Health*, 6 (Suppl 1), S9.

17

Dental sealants

Hien Ngo and W. Kim Seow

Introduction

A definition of pit and fissure sealant was proposed by Simonsen in 1978. He defined it as "a material that is introduced into the occlusal pits and fissures of caries susceptible teeth, thus forming a micro-mechanically bonded, protective layer cutting access of caries-producing bacteria from their source of nutrients." This definition leaves out glass-ionomer and resin-modified glass-ionomer sealants because these are chemically bonded to enamel; therefore, it is important to modify the above definition to read "..., thus forming a micromechanically or chemically bonded, ...". Pit and fissure sealant has been used both as primary and secondary preventive measures against occlusal caries. After nearly 4 decades of clinical use, the pit and fissure sealant is now recognized as one of the most effective methods for preventing occlusal caries in children. Their cost effectiveness has been demonstrated in school-based preventive programs especially among high-risk groups, such as children with disabilities or from low social economic backgrounds.

Reporting on the prevalence and distribution of caries in developed countries, Burt made the following three observations: (1) there is an overall decline in prevalence and severity in child populations, (2) there is a skewed distribution with a small number of children carrying a larger burden of the disease, and (3) most of carious lesions are found in pits and fissures (Burt 1998). More recent epidemiological data suggest that dental caries of the pit and fissure system is a major issue in school-aged children, with evidence showing that, in the US, 90% of carious lesions occur in the pits and fissures of permanent molars (Brown and Selwitz 1995; Beltran-Aguilar et al. 2005).

However older children and young adults present different patterns of caries compared to younger children. Longitudinal data indicate that proximal surfaces are more susceptible to caries in older children. At the age of 13 years, proximal caries contributes approximately 30% to the caries increment with the majority of lesions still located in the pits and fissures. This percentage increases steadily to over 40 and 50% at 19 and 27 years of age, respectively (Mejare et al. 2004). It is also well known that the development of caries on proximal surfaces can lead to the breakdown of marginal ridges and reduced physical integrity of the tooth. This is the start of a vicious cycle of restoration and breakdown, which often eventually ends with loss of the tooth. It is therefore equally justified to protect proximal surfaces, in a similar way with the occlusal surfaces, with sealants to reduce the risk of caries.

Recently, advances in adhesive materials have facilitated the use of sealants to be extended to therapeutic uses such as managing incipient lesions by infiltrating these with low viscosity resin (Meyer-Lueckel and Paris 2008; Ekstrand et al. 2010). This is a relatively new concept and still lacks evidence to support its routine use.

This chapter critically reviews the clinical use of pit and fissure sealants and discusses the concept of protecting the occlusal surface of erupting molars. In addition, a novel concept of preventing proximal caries is proposed.

Comprehensive Preventive Dentistry, First Edition. Edited by Hardy Limeback.
© 2012 John Wiley & Sons, Ltd. Published 2012 by John Wiley & Sons, Ltd.

Oral biofilm

The topic of caries as a disease is addressed in other chapters. In this chapter, we revisit some of the key concepts of caries that are relevant to the rationale behind the use of sealants as a protective coating and also when it is used to infiltrate the enamel in the treatment of incipient lesions.

Dental caries is a chronic, lifestyle associated, dieto-microbial, and site-specific disease that can affect dental hard tissue, through a localized and excessive demineralization of tooth structures (Zero *et al.* 2009). There is a dynamic interaction between the fluid phase of oral biofilms and the mineral contents of enamel, dentin, and cementum. These interactions are mostly governed by the bacterial metabolic activity and the resulting fluctuation in the pH of plaque fluid. The presence of bacteria in the oral cavity is essential because the resident microflora inside the oral biofilm contributes to the well being of the host in general and more specifically to the underlying tooth structure. A healthy pellicle layer and biofilm are protective against erosion, can store fluoride and minerals to facilitate remineralization, and delay cavitation (Marsh 1994; Ngo and Gaffney 2005). The challenge for the clinician is to select treatment strategies, which modulate the pH fluctuation in favor of remineralization without disrupting the beneficial behavior of the resident microflora (Marsh 1994).

On the crown of a tooth, carious lesions usually start in enamel and because this tissue is acellular, the living reparative events that are generally triggered by an infectious process in soft tissues cannot occur. Furthermore, the stability of enamel is entirely dependent on the chemical balance of its immediate surrounding environment. The breakdown of enamel is gradual and will eventually expose the pulpo-dentinal organ to bacterial metabolic products long before any bacteria can be detected at the dentino-enamel junction (Thylstrup and Qvist 1987).

The concepts, described above, underpin the rationale for sealants in general. They prevent the growth of biofilms in hard to reach areas on a tooth and therefore have the ability to disrupt bacterial physiology and prevent the initiation and progression of lesions (Oong *et al.* 2008).

Site specificity

Caries susceptibility is site specific, and these sites can be roughly divided into the following segments:

1. Exposed smooth surfaces: Because demineralization is associated with stagnant accumulation of oral biofilms, these exposed smooth surfaces are considered to be the least susceptible because they are subjected to good mechanical cleansing and salivary flow. It is important to point out that in some situations, the "exposed" status of a surface can change. For example, the distal and mesial surfaces of a first permanent

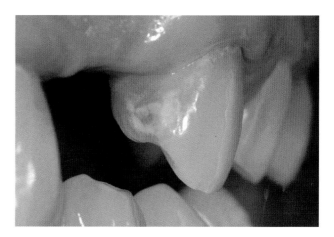

Figure 17-1 A non-cavitated carious lesion was formed on the mesial surface of the maxillary left canine during the time this surface was "hidden." It is likely that, when it became "exposed," the lesion became arrested.

molar can be classified as "exposed" toward the end of the mixed dentition stage, when the second primary molar exfoliates and the second permanent molar is still unerupted. The authors propose that in high-risk children, these surfaces can be protected from future proximal caries prior to their returning to a "hidden" status upon the eruption of the second permanent molar and premolar. These surfaces should be sealed, with a thin and hard-wearing sealant, while they are still "exposed," therefore having easy access. This principle should be extended to any smooth surfaces deemed to be at risk.

2. Hidden smooth surfaces: Smooth surfaces with well-established contacts are considered to be "hidden" because they are less accessible to mechanical cleansing and chemical protection from saliva and fluoride and are more susceptible to caries. Common examples of "hidden" sites are the interproximal surfaces, however, the same surface can change its risk status over time (Figure 17-1). For example, a large carious white spot lesion that was formed on the proximal surface of a tooth when it was "hidden" could become "exposed" with the removal of an adjacent tooth. Another example is the occlusal surface of an erupting tooth can be classified as "hidden" while it is covered by an operculum and inaccessible to a toothbrush. It becomes "exposed" after eruption and benefits from the self-cleansing effect of a functional occlusion.

A slowly erupting permanent molar usually has problems of plaque accumulating under the operculum and requires professional preventive care throughout the erupting phase (Carvalho *et al.* 1992).

The prolonged period of eruption results in large areas of plaque stagnation under the operculum so

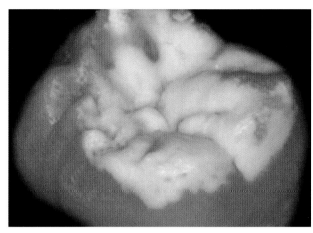

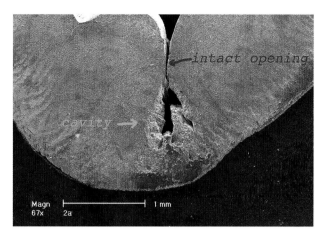

Figure 17-3 Cross section of a pit showing the restricted opening that is surrounded by bulbous cusps with steep inclines and an advanced lesion at the base.

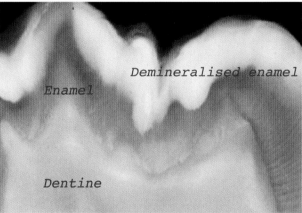

Figure 17-2 The pattern of demineralization follows the pattern of plaque accumulation under the operculum. On an erupting tooth, it is possible for the entire occlusal surface to be demineralized.

that the area of demineralization would not be limited to the pits and fissures but usually extends to an extensive area of enamel under an operculum, as shown in Figure 17-2.

Later in this chapter we will describe a method that will temporarily protect the occlusal surfaces of erupting teeth from caries during the eruption period.

3. Pits and fissures: These are found on the occlusal surface of posterior teeth and on buccal and palatal surfaces of molars. Epidemiological and clinical data consistently show that the pit and fissure systems of molars are the most vulnerable to caries; this is supported anecdotally by clinicians. The risk status of the occlusal surface and external opening of the pits and fissures will be lowered when they become "exposed," after full eruption to the oral environment and mechanical cleansing. However, the risk status at the base of pits and fissures does not usually change because their morphological features tend to harbor undisturbed microflora and restrict access to the remineralization properties of healthy saliva.

Development of occlusal caries

Caries affecting pit and fissures are the first types of lesions encountered in children. In addition to general risk factors, the following three site-specific risk factors are associated with the development and progression of occlusal caries (Carvalho *et al.* 1989):

1. Morphology of pit and fissure systems
2. Eruption stage
3. Functional use

Even in populations with low caries prevalence, the occlusal surfaces of permanent molars are more often affected by caries than the proximal surfaces. The fact that occlusal caries is usually attributed to the plaque retentive nature of pit and fissure systems, provides the rationale for preventing caries by fissure widening, prophylactic odontomy, or sealing with adhesive materials. It is fortunate that the invasive prophylactic odontomy approach has not gained much acceptance since it was suggested in the 1920s.

The pit and fissure system of the occlusal surface is composed of shallow fissures with occasional deep pits. The high risk for caries is associated in particular with those pits that have narrow openings and a bulbous widening at the base, which is close to the dentino-enamel junction (DEJ) and provides a very short route for a lesions to penetrate into dentine (Figure 17-3).

Because these features tend to be associated with bulbous cusps with steep inclines, they can be employed as risk features. These types of pits and fissures should be sealed when possible (Figure 17-4).

The risk status of a pit can be assessed individually, because it is possible to have both low- and high-risk pits

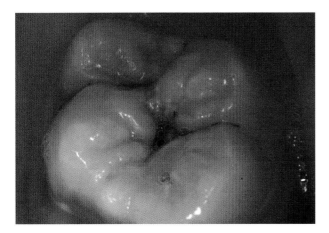

Figure 17-4 Clinical appearance of a high-risk pits and fissures.

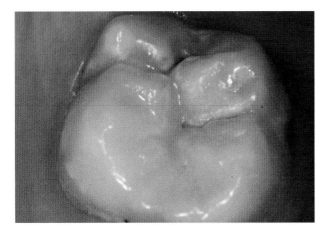

Figure 17-5 This pit and fissure system presents a shallow pit on the mesial section and a deep pit on the distal part.

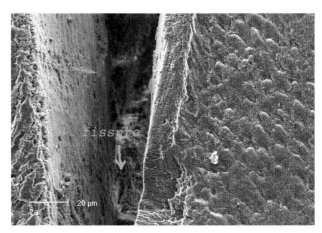

Figure 17-6 The walls of pit and fissure systems are lined with aprismatic enamel.

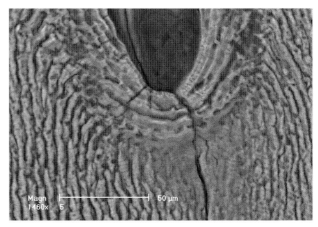

Figure 17-7 A back-scattered electron view reveals the layers in the aprismatic enamel that run perpendicular to the direction of enamel rods. The crack in the middle is an artefact.

on the same occlusal surface. The pit and fissure system illustrated in Figure 17-5 is complex; it contains a low-risk shallow pit on the mesial section, and a high-risk deep pit in the distal fissure, which shows early signs of demineralization. The clinical management in this case should be placement of a pit and fissure sealant, which will play a dual role. It will be preventive in the mesial section and therapeutic in the distal pit.

At a microscopic level, an important feature of the enamel lining the pits and fissures is the presence of a layer of aprismatic enamel (Figure 17-6). This layer exists both in permanent and deciduous teeth, and it may require longer etching time before an adequate seal can be achieved with resin sealants (Eccles 1989).

This aprismatic layer reduces the permeability of enamel by sealing the ends of enamel rods (Figure 17-7). The space between the enamel rods forms a major diffusion pathway for acid and bacterial products. It can be hypothesized that the aprismatic layer protects the underlying prismatic enamel by the combination of

having more tightly packed apatite crystals and lack of the inter-prismatic space (Figure 17-8).

There is a considerable difference in plaque accumulation on the occlusal surface of erupting and fully erupted molars, due to the lack of functional usage (Ekstrand *et al.* 1993) and the presence of an operculum, which covers an erupting or partially erupted tooth. There is also the risk of food debris impacted in the space between the enamel and the soft tissue (Figure 17-9).

The duration of the eruption period is a further risk factor because teeth with longer eruption time tend to have more occlusal caries. For example, occlusal caries is much more prevalent in molars, which have a relatively long eruption time of 12 to 18 months, compared to premolars, with an eruption time of only a few months. Occlusal caries in molars is usually initiated during the eruption period due to conditions conducive for plaque accumulation. In a study where children with erupting molars were provided

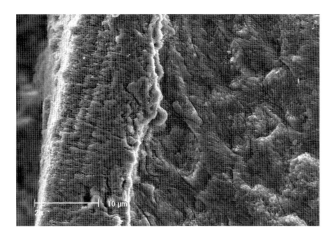

Figure 17-8 The aprismatic layer, on the left, is around 10 micron thick and is composed of tightly packed hydroxyapatite (HAP) crystals.

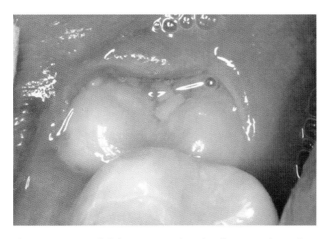

Figure 17-9 Food debris impacted under the operculum of an erupting molar, presenting a site-specific risk of caries.

with intensive education and professional cleaning over a period of 3 years, there was a significantly lower rate of teeth requiring restoration. The authors concluded that "our data indicate that professional care for erupting teeth on an individual basis has long term effect on occlusal surfaces" (Carvalho *et al.* 1992). These results suggest that certain erupting teeth would benefit from temporary protection of the partially exposed surfaces.

Pit and fissure sealant: historical perspective

Due to the high prevalence and early onset of occlusal caries, its prevention has been one of the major quests in dentistry since GV Black. As early as the 1920s, it was suggested that enamel fissures should be converted into nonretentive depressions on the occlusal surface to decrease plaque retention (Hyatt 1923). In the 1940s it was suggested that occlusal surfaces should be treated with strong antibacterial agents such as ammonical silver

nitrate (Klein and Knutsan 1942), followed by zinc chloride and potassium ferrocyanide (Ast *et al.* 1950) to prevent occlusal caries. However, the efficacy of these methods has never been established.

The major event that made resin pit and fissure sealants possible came from the early work of Buonocore (1955) who earned the title of being the "Father of Adhesive Dentistry" by introducing the acid etch and bonding technique for resin-based materials. The purpose of his original research was the development of a sealant to prevent occlusal caries on posterior teeth. However, the impact of his work revolutionized operative dentistry and allowed the development of current minimally invasive techniques that are based on resin-based technologies (Handelman and Shey 1996). The first group to be developed was the unfilled resins that were introduced in the late 1940s. These had a short existence because their clinical performance was very poor. In the 1960s, Bowen converted them to an entirely acceptable restorative group by introducing bis-GMA and including a variety of fillers for physical reinforcement and control of setting shrinkage (Bowen 1963; Bowen 1970).

In the same time period, Smith recognized the biological benefits of the polyalkenoic acid group and combined these with zinc oxide to develop the polycarboxylate cements, which was the first group of materials to have both self-adhesion and fluoride-releasing capabilities (Smith 1967). Wilson and others (1985) modified this through the use of a powdered glass instead of zinc oxide and thus introduced glass-ionomer cements, which exists today as both restorative and preventive materials.

Effectiveness of fissure sealants

Pit and fissure sealing is strongly recommended in protecting permanent molars against the initiation of occlusal caries. The protective effect of a sealant is even more important in a high caries risk population (Simonsen 2002; Beiruti *et al.* 2006; Ahovuo-Saloranta *et al.* 2010). As recommended by several authors, pit and fissure sealants can be applied to arrest the progression of an early non-cavitated carious lesion (Simonsen 2002; Locker *et al.* 2003; Beauchamp *et al.* 2008).

Eruption status greatly influences the retreatment rate of resin-based sealants. In one study, at a review period of 36 months, the retreatment rate was 54% when the operculum was over the distal margin ridge at baseline, 25.8% when it was level with the distal margin, and nil required retreatment when the soft tissue was below the marginal ridge (Figure 17-10). This case will be later used in the demonstration of placement steps. This trend in retreatment rates is likely to be related to effective moisture control. When a tooth is partially erupted and deemed to be at high risk, the use of fluoride varnish or glass-ionomer

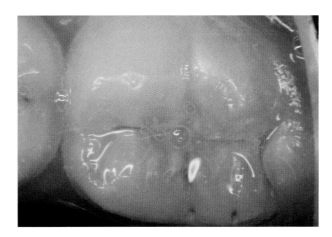

Figure 17-10 The tooth is not fully erupted so moisture control is difficult. It is recommended that glass-ionomer sealant be used if an occlusal protection is required immediately due to its high risk.

sealant would be good provisional alternatives to protect the tooth until adequate moisture control can be achieved for the placement of a resin sealant.

Who should place pit and fissure sealants?

In many countries the rate of utilization of pit and fissure sealants is still as low as 10%. It is disappointing for a treatment modality that has proven efficacy and long track records, so if delegating is part of the answer then this should be encouraged. However, it is essential that it be delegated to a person with the appropriate training. When children are seen in a school dental service system, most fissure sealants are placed by trained oral therapists. The efficacy and cost effectiveness of this approach is well proven when it is a part of an overall preventive program. The types of auxiliary team members that have been studied include dental assistants, hygienists, and therapists, and there are variations in the third-party insurance system and legislation that govern the scope of work of these professions. Stiles reported that there is no difference in the retention rates of pit and fissure sealants, which were placed by a dentist or a trained auxiliary (Stiles *et al.* 1976). This was later reconfirmed in a 5-year clinical trial using dental assistants (Holst *et al.* 1998).

Retention

For resin sealants, retention rates of over 90% are commonly reported in the first year. Even after 15 years, approximately 28% of sealed permanent first molar teeth showed complete sealant retention and 35% partial retention. Only approximately 30% of sealed surfaces had become carious or restored compared to 80% in the unsealed group (Simonsen 1991). However, it should be remembered that these high retention rates can only be achieved under optimal conditions.

It should be emphasized that isolation is the key to the success of resin pit and fissure sealants because saliva contamination can decrease the bond strength of sealant to etched enamel by 40%. Even when the contaminated enamel is washed thoroughly, there is still a 4% decrease (Thomson et al. 1981). It has been suggested that using a dentin-bonding agent on etched enamel before placing the resin sealant (Hitt and Feigal 1992) can enhance the penetration of the sealant. It was found that the bonding agent increased bond strength, reduced microleakage and enhanced the wetting of the resin sealant (Borem and Feigal 1994; Choi *et al.* 1997). The results of a 5-year clinical trial confirmed that the application of a dentin-bonding agent can reduce the risk of failure by 50% (Feigal *et al.* 2000; Hebling and Feigal 2000). However a 2-year clinical trial comparing the performance of pit and fissure sealant with and without a bonding agent concluded that there is no significant advantage in using a bonding agent (Boksman *et al.* 1993).

It is suggested that the use of a dentin-bonding agent would tend to increase the time, cost, and complexity of the procedure without the certainty of improving performance. In a compromised situation, it may be more beneficial to choose a more technique-tolerant material like glass-ionomer cement.

Introduction of resin-based pit and fissure sealants

The first reported clinical trial on a pit and fissure sealant showed 87% caries reduction after 12 months (Cueto and Buonocore 1967). A filled enamel adhesive, a mixture of methyl-2-cyanoacrylate monomer with the powder from a silicate cement and acid etching with phosphoric acid, was used. However only one-third of the sealants were intact after 12 months because the material hydrolyzed in the presence of moisture. The next group of materials was based on polyurethane technology, which has the potential to contain and release fluoride. However, they were removed from the market due to unsatisfactory retention rates (Newbrun *et al.* 1974; Rock 1974; Murray and Williams 1975).

Materials for sealants

Ideal sealants

The desired clinical outcomes from the use of sealants are to prevent the establishment and stop the progression of carious lesions. However, to reliably prevent caries on any surface, the technique must provide good retention, a long-term seal and be non-technique sensitive so that it can be applied by both dentists and dental auxiliaries such as hygienists and therapists. The requirements of an

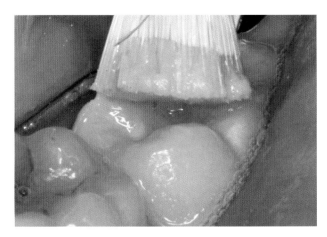

Figure 17-11 Surface of the tooth is cleaned using a slurry of pumice and water.

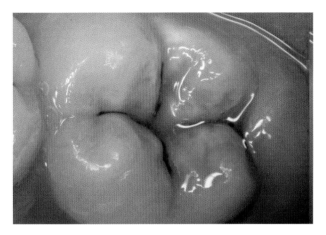

Figure 17-12 Cotton roll isolation is essential. The tooth is washed then a surface conditioner is applied for 10 seconds.

ideal material include biocompatibility, low viscosity, low solubility, esthetically acceptable, and reasonably visible to facilitate reassessment.

There are two main types of materials that can be used as sealants: unfilled or lightly filled composite resins and glass ionomers. Neither of these can be regarded as ideal so the selection of which material to use will be driven by the requirements of each case.

Over time both groups have evolved, and today there are subdivisions within these two, the compomers and resin modified glass ionomers (Mount *et al.* 2009). The common denominators are that both groups are tooth colored and can adhere to tooth surfaces but beyond that, the differences are profound, and it is important for clinicians to understand the advantages and disadvantages of each so they can choose the most suitable material for the situation and then handle it correctly.

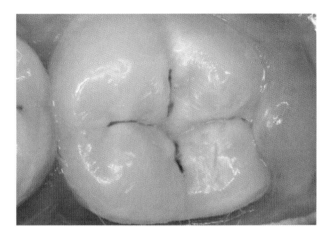

Figure 17-13 The conditioner is washed off with water then dried. Adequate field control is essential.

Glass ionomer sealants: placement protocol

The main advantage of the glass-ionomer cement is its ability to chemically adhere to the tooth surface with minimal preparation (Ngo *et al.* 1997). The placement protocol starts with cleaning the surface with an oil-free slurry of pumice and water, applied with a speed reducing handpiece at 400 rpm (Figure 17-11). The pumice is washed off using an air/water spray from a triple syringe for 10 seconds. Tooth isolation is essential. Even though glass ionomer is tolerant to some moisture, a dry field is essential to obtain maximum retention. The tooth surface is then treated with a surface conditioner, an aqueous solution containing between 10 and 20% polyacrylic acid for 10 seconds. Polyacrylic acid is a mild acid, and it forms the backbone for cross-linking in the final glass ionomer. This diluted version does not etch the enamel but rather prepares it by increasing surface energy to improve wetting of the glass-ionomer sealant and improve

adhesion (Figure 17-12). Even though glass ionomer is a water-based material and is relatively not technique sensitive, the working field has to be dry right through the procedure. Cotton roll isolation can be adequate in most cases (Figure 17-13). After placement, it is important to protect the immature glass ionomer with a thin coat of unfilled resin. It is important to maintain water balance within the material, and if not done properly, surface crazing will compromise both wear resistance and solubility (Ngo 2010). This can be illustrated by the slight crazing of the mesial part of the sealant in the time it took to record this series (Figure 17-14).

The main advantages of glass-ionomer cement are ion exchange adhesion to tooth structure, fluoride release, and technique tolerance. It is the only group of dental materials with true chemical adhesion (Ngo *et al.* 2006). The well-recognized anti-caries effect of glass ionomer can be attributed to both long-term fluoride release and

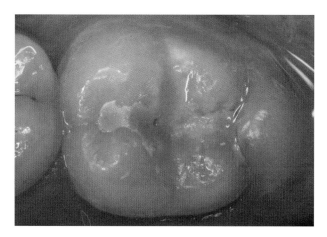

Figure 17-14 A high fluoride-releasing, glass-ionomer sealant that sets within 90 seconds is placed. Surface crazing can be seen on the mesial section.

recharge and the presence of strontium in the later generations of glass ionomers (Ngo 2010). Recently, fluoride release has been a more intentional part of the development of products. For example, Fuji IX Extra and Fuji Triage (VII) (GC Corporation, Tokyo, Japan) are two products that are designed to release substantially more fluoride than the earlier generations of glass-ionomer cements. Initial studies report that fluoride is released primarily during the first weeks after placing the restoration, although a sustained released has been measured for years (Swartz *et al.* 1984; Swartz *et al.* 1984; Forsten 1995; Forsten 1998).

Of the total amount of fluoride in the set cement, only a small fraction is available for release. Walls (1986) pointed out that unless the ions are important to the matrix structure, then their loss need not be harmful to the physical properties of the cement. The pattern and total amount released is not dependent on the total fluoride content of the cement, but it is partly controlled by the amount of sodium that is available to re-establish electron neutrality in the cement.

Even when fully set, glass-ionomer cements release apatite-forming ions into an aqueous environment. This tends to happen as an exchange process, so it can also be recharged. It has been shown that conventional glass-ionomer cements release sodium, fluoride, silica, and calcium or strontium (Wilson *et al.* 1985; Ngo 2010). Wilson studied this over a period of 20 months and found that these species were still being released at the end of the experimental period, albeit at a diminished rate. Although many studies have reported a sustained release of fluoride from set glass ionomer, its mechanism is still not completely understood. It is generally accepted that there may be two reactions involved. First a short-term reaction of high fluoride release corresponding to

initial elution due to the maturation process, during which fluoride ions are released from the surface as well as from within the bulk of material. The surface process peters out after a while leaving the bulk diffusion process to continue over a long period in an apparently inexhaustible fashion. The second reaction is a long-term low release of fluoride, which can be attributed to equilibrium diffusion processes.

Since the fluoride is not an integral part of the matrix of the cement, its release is not deleterious to the physical properties. It has been suggested that there is, in fact, a fluoride exchange available, with fluoride ions returning to the cement from external applications of fluoride if the fluoride gradient is in the right direction (Cranfield *et al.* 1982). This exchange also occurs with other species. For example, strontium from the matrix will be exchanged with calcium from the environment (Ngo 2010).

Resin sealants

The resin-based materials will adhere to etched enamel and dentine through micro-mechanical interlocking, and this requires a material of low viscosity with good flowability. Because resin sealants have low viscosity, they do not need an adhesive, however, restorative composite resins require a bonding agent due to the high viscosity of the materials. The current generation of resin sealants is based on the dimethacrylate monomers that were introduced to dentistry by Bowen (1970). They contain either a bis-GMA dimethacrylate or a urethane dimethacrylate. Apart from the monomers, resin fissure sealants can also be differentiated based on filler content (filled or unfilled), appearance (clear, tinted, opaque, or color changing), mode of setting initiation (chemical or visible light cure), and fluoride release. These variations do not seem to affect clinical performance, and the selection of which material to use can be based on the operator's or patient's preference.

Resin sealant: placement protocols

When a resin sealant is used, moisture control is of utmost importance. The tooth must be fully erupted with the distal operculum below the distal marginal ridge, as illustrated in Figure 17-15. In an ideal situation, a rubber dam should be used. However, for many young children an acceptable alternative is a combination of cotton roll isolation, high-speed suction, and a well-trained dental assistant using four-handed dentistry.

The area to be treated needs to be cleaned thoroughly with pumice and water (Figure 17-15). An etchant of 37% phosphoric acid is applied for 20 seconds. Ensure that no large air voids are trapped under the acid. After a few seconds, small bubbles can be seen forming inside

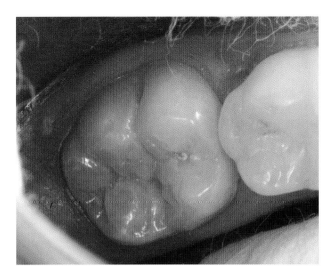

Figure 17-15 Tooth was cleaned with pumice and water then washed thoroughly and dried.

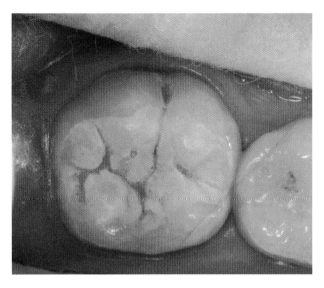

Figure 17-17 After washing, the surface must present a frosty appearance, including the buccal pit.

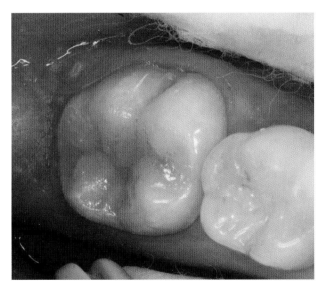

Figure 17-16 Acid etch is applied to the entire occlusal pits and fissures as well as the buccal pit.

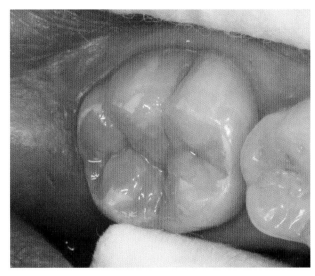

Figure 17-18 Due to the presence of some debris inside the fissure (Figure 17-17), a primer is applied to achieve deeper penetration of the sealant.

the liquid indicating that the acid is working (Figure 17-16). After washing and drying using a triple syringe, the surface should be examined thoroughly. An even, frosty appearance should now be obvious (Figure 17-17). If there are areas at or near the opening of the pits and fissures that do not have the frosty look, then etch again. A lack of etch may be due to the aprismatic enamel layer, which was described previously. Alternatively there may be organic debris still inside the fissures that can be physically removed (Simonsen 1980). Another alternative is to apply a primer to facilitate resin penetration (Figure 17-18) (Feigal *et al.* 2000). Finally Figure 17-19 shows a well-placed fissure sealant.

When to use glass-ionomer sealants?

This section offers suggestions where glass ionomer is the material of choice.

In 1974, McLean and Wilson (1974) introduced the first glass-ionomer fissure sealant and carried out a clinical trial, which reported a good retention rate of 84% at the 1-year recall and 78% at the 2-year mark. Despite this initial success, results of later clinical trials were not consistent. McKenna and Grundy (1987) reported an 82% retention rate after 1 year; however, Boksman *et al.* (1993) reported a total loss within 6 months. The routine use of glass-ionomer sealants only received guarded

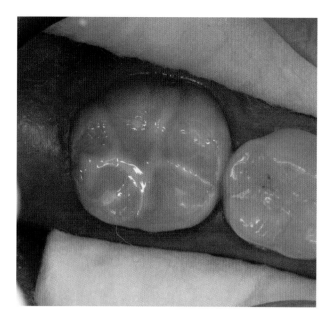

Figure 17-19 A well-placed pit and fissure sealant.

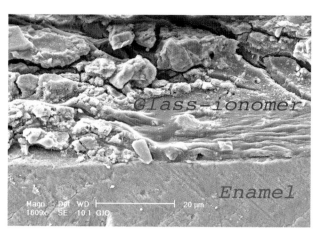

Figure 17-20 As glass-ionomer bonds to the tooth by chemical means, and tends to fail cohesively, there is always a layer of glass ionomer remaining on the tooth surface or in the fissure.

recommendation in a recent systematic review: "Glass ionomer cement may be used as an interim preventive agent when there are indications for placement of a resin-based sealant but concerns about moisture control may compromised such placement" (Beauchamp *et al.* 2008). This may be due to the poor retention rate that was reported in some studies (Mejare and Mjor 1990; Boksman *et al.* 1993). It is important to recognize that the earlier studies used a first generation glass-ionomer cement fissure sealant, Fuji III, which has long been superseded by later generations of glass ionomer, with much better physical and mechanical properties.

Most literature reviews recognize the role of a glass-ionomer sealant; however, based on the good retention rate of resin fissure sealants, most authors maintains that the material of first choice is a resin-based sealant (Simonsen 2002; Azarpazhooh and Main 2008; Beauchamp *et al.* 2008). This is surprising when there is evidence to suggest that there is a superior caries prevention effect despite the poor retention (Arrow and Riordan 1995; Simonsen 2002; Beiruti *et al.* 2006). Mejare and Mjor (1990) were the first to clinically evaluate the retention rate and caries prevention effect of a glass-ionomer sealant and two resin fissure sealants. Scoring was done both clinically and with replicas. The resin sealants were retained better than the glass ionomers, however, 5% of the resin-sealed surfaces developed lesions. For the glass-ionomer sealants, 84% were judged totally missing during the clinical examination, but the replicas revealed a retained layer of glass ionomer within the fissures and no caries lesions at all. The caries protective effect can be explained by the presence of remaining glass-

ionomer on the surface, which protects the tooth both physically and chemically, through fluoride release. This has been confirmed in later studies, with Arrow estimating that a glass-ionomer sealed tooth has 19% chance of becoming carious when compared with a resin-sealed tooth even when the glass-ionomer sealant was considered to be defective (Komatsu *et al.* 1994; Arrow and Riordan 1995; Forss and Halme 1998). This feature of glass ionomer has been known for a while by researchers who studied the interface between glass ionomer and enamel or dentin (Figure 17-20) (Ngo *et al.* 1997).

Based on the above studies, the following recommendations can be made:

1. The caries preventive effect of glass ionomer is due to the fact that there is always an ion exchange layer remaining on the surface after bulk loss.
2. Glass ionomer is more technique tolerant so should be considered when:
   - Four-handed dentistry is not available
   - Lack of patient's full co-operation
   - There is bleeding or gingival fluid seepage
   - Moisture control is compromised
3. Light curing is not available.
4. Repair may be required, at a later date, because there is chemical bonding between old and new glass ionomer.
5. Glass ionomer is best suited for protecting erupting teeth when it is inserted under the operculum.

Preventing caries in erupting teeth: surface protection with glass inomer cement, a "pre-fissure sealant" procedure

The first suggestion that an erupting tooth should be protected from occlusal caries was made by Hyatt (1923) when he suggested that the occlusal surface of an erupting tooth should be sealed with zinc phosphate cement as soon as possible. However, he also suggested that when the tooth is sufficiently erupted, a Class I amalgam should be placed to prevent the fissure from becoming carious. Fortunately, this concept did not gain popularity even though the eradication of enamel fissures was once again discussed by Bodecker (1929).

Today, it is well accepted that a preventive regimen, commencing when the first permanent teeth begin to erupt, is essential for overall caries prevention. The emerging, newly formed, immature enamel surface is vulnerable to caries attack and as the process of eruption is relatively lengthy, a few preventive methods can be instituted during this period to reduce the caries risk. First, tooth brushing with fluoridated toothpaste performed twice daily, using a soft brush to scrub the occlusal surfaces of the emerging teeth can remove the biofilm. Daily rinsing with 0.2% fluoride solution will further decrease the caries risk (Carvalho *et al*. 1991). In addition, the child's diet should be monitored to reduce frequency of sugar consumption. However, the most important risk factor to consider is the fact that the enamel under the operculum cannot be cleaned by the child or parents due to lack of access.

Obtaining a dry field on a partially erupted tooth is not possible so the only material that can be used for this purpose is a fast-setting, high-fluoride-releasing, conventional glass ionomer. Although the retention rate of glass ionomer cement (GIC) sealants may be less compared to resin sealants, GICs are less sensitive to moisture and the sealants can provide additional fluoride, which can be replenished from the fluoride rinses (Salar *et al*. 2007). When the teeth are fully erupted, the need to place a long term sealant can be reassessed.

The procedure to apply glass ionomer under the operculum is also called a "pre-fissure sealant," and is designed to provide protection during the entire eruption period of a permanent molar. The alternative is intensive professional intervention with regular recalls and repeated applications of fluoride varnish.

The tooth to be treated was previously illustrated in Figure 17-9. The material used in this case was a fast-setting (90 seconds), high-flow, high-fluoride-releasing glass ionomer. It is pink in color so the treated surface can be easily identified and monitored, and the color is a marker for the temporary "pre-fissure sealant" treatment. When the tooth becomes fully exposed, a decision on further treatment can be made.

Placement protocol

The area should be isolated using cotton rolls and high volume suction. Debris can be gently removed from under the operculum and the tooth surface treated with conditioner using a small micro-brush (Figure 17-21). The glass

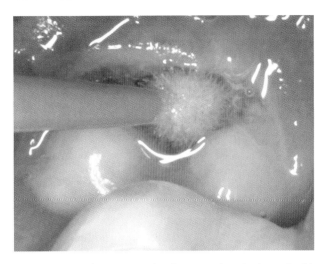

Figure 17-21 The space under the operculum is cleaned with conditioner and a micro-brush.

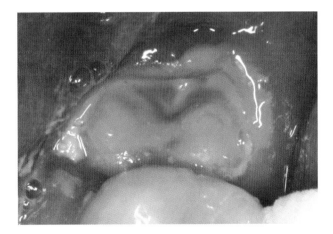

Figure 17-22 Fuji 7 is applied to the space under the operculum and on to the occlusal surface of this erupting molar.

ionomer is then used to cover the entire exposed surface of the erupting tooth as well as the space under the operculum. It will now remain until the tooth becomes fully exposed. The excess glass ionomer as seen in Figure 17-22 will be removed with tooth brushing after the session.

Sealing over caries lesions

Clinicians are often concerned regarding the inadvertent sealing of surfaces that are already carious because of the possibility that sealed lesions will remain active. However, studies have shown that carious lesions that are effectively sealed do not progress for as long as 10 years (Mertz-Farihurst *et al*. 1998; Ricketts *et al*. 2006). Sealed lesions generally become arrested because the microorganisms do not remain vital within the lesion and what bacteria remain are not capable of maintaining progression of the lesion (Going *et al*. 1978). In addition, the acid-etching process alone can reduce the bacterial load by 100% (Jensen and Handelman 1980). All of the evidence suggests that the sealing of caries is not likely to result in progression of the lesion for as long as the seal is intact (Handelman *et al.* 1985).

Nevertheless, because a small percentage of sealants do not have full marginal integrity, it may be prudent at the initial examination to check radiographs for the presence of dentinal caries beneath the enamel surface. Furthermore, as the sensitivity and specificity of visual-tactile examinations range from 80–90%, the possibility of not detecting occlusal caries using probe and visual examination may be clinically significant. If dentinal caries is detected at initial examination, the lesion should be managed according to guidelines for minimal intervention dentistry (Mount and Ngo 2000; Tyas *et al.* 2000), and when appropriate, a preventive resin restoration should be the treatment of choice (Simonsen 1980).

Sealants for proximal enamel surfaces

Adhesive resins can be applied for sealing early carious enamel lesions on proximal surfaces in order to arrest their progression. Clinical trials in adults have reported caries progression of only 22% in treated proximal surfaces compared to 47 and 68% of control teeth after 18 months and 3–4 years, respectively (Martignon *et al.* 2009). Although no studies are available, the proximal sealant technique is likely to be suitable for the primary dentition as the progression of enamel caries into dentine occurs relatively quickly, and the timely placement of sealants can halt progression of the lesions. However, this technique may be hampered by the requirement for separation of the teeth prior to placement of the sealants and the need for repeated radiographs at initial and periodic examinations to check for progression of the lesions.

Sealants for infiltration into proximal early enamel lesions

The concept of sealing the proximal enamel lesion can be considered to be an extension of fissure sealing. If it is possible to etch occlusal enamel then it is possible to etch and seal proximal enamel and increase its stability in cariogenic environments. The technique involves separating the approximal tooth surfaces by wedging, acid etching of surface with 15% hydrochloric acid for 120 seconds to erode the surface, followed by infiltrating the surface with a resin. Early clinical data on the primary dentition have demonstrated a rate of progression of caries of approximately 31% and 11% after 12 and 18 months, compared to a rate of 61% and 38% using topical fluoride and oral hygiene instruction, respectively (Ekstrand *et al.* 2010). This technique was proposed as a treatment for non-cavitated incipient lesions on proximal surfaces, and the most challenging part is to how to gain access to these areas.

Smooth surface sealant: A new concept for consideration

In the permanent dentition, while there is evidence that prevalence rates of caries have stabilized, longitudinal data have indicated that the proximal surface caries constitute approximately 30% of caries in children at age 13 years (Mejare *et al.* 2004). This percentage increases steadily to more than 40 and 50% at 19 and 27 years of age, respectively.

Therefore, a strong case can be made for the prevention of caries on the proximal surfaces of the teeth, and the authors propose a method for preventing smooth/proximal caries in children based on the concept of sealing susceptible surfaces. The large involvement of the exposed smooth surfaces in the primary dentition and the proximal surfaces in caries of the permanent dentition in children from 12 to 18 years suggests that a significant proportion of caries in children can be eliminated by preventing caries on these surfaces.

The high effectiveness of sealants in preventing caries in pits and fissures is well established by randomized clinical trials and cost-benefit analyses. However, such preventive measures have not been tested in the prevention of smooth surfaces caries. Of all the smooth surfaces, the proximal surfaces are at highest risk for caries due to the presence of contact areas that act as areas of stagnation that are difficult to reach by toothbrush and accessible only by flossing. In high-risk children, caries on the proximal surfaces can be visible approximately 12–18 months after the establishment of the contacts in the posterior teeth.

Traditional approaches for preventing proximal lesions such as flossing and rinsing with fluoride usually have limited success because they rely heavily on patient compliance (Alm *et al.* 2007). More recently, treatment of proximal caries has been focused on arresting initial caries by sealing these lesions with low viscosity resins (Ekstrand *et al.* 2010). Although early success has been reported, this technique requires the operator to gain access to the proximal lesions using physical separation of the teeth. This technique usually involves two appointments, so it is not practical for young children.

An alternative method would be to seal the teeth while it is possible to gain access to the proximal smooth surfaces before the contacts with adjacent teeth are established. There are a few stages in the development of the primary and permanent dentitions that provide windows of opportunity to gain such access to specific proximal surfaces of the posterior teeth.

Placement protocol

An opportunity to seal the proximal surfaces of the first molars would be toward the end of the mixed dentition

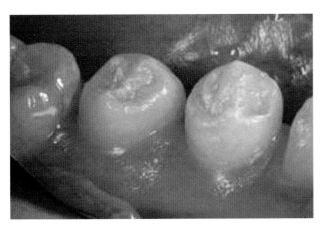

Figure 17-23 There is already a white spot lesion on the mesial surface of the first molar (*green arrow*) there is also easy access to the other proximal surfaces.

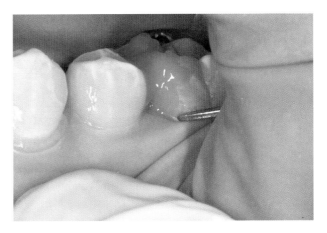

Figure 17-25 All proximal surfaces are acid etched.

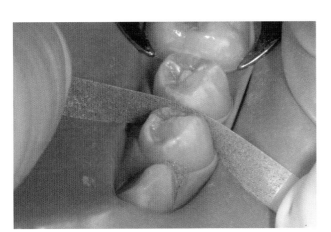

Figure 17-24 The proximal surfaces were cleaned with an abrasive strip.

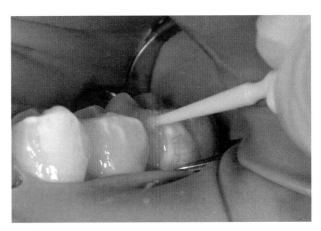

Figure 17-26 A hard-wearing, nano-filled resin was applied then light cured.

stage. As depicted in the case above, the premolars are fully erupted but there is relatively easy access to all proximal surfaces. There is a white spot lesion that was probably formed during the time when the primary molar was present (Figure 17-23). Rubber dam isolation is applied and the exposed surfaces are cleaned using an abrasive strip (Figure 17-24). All proximal surfaces are prepared with the application of 37% phosphoric acid for 20 seconds, then washed and dried with a triple syringe (Figure 17-25). A hard-wearing nano-filled resin is applied as a sealant, then light cured (Figure 17-26). It is important to ensure that there is no overhang of the material after placement.

Conclusions

As occlusal caries constitutes a significant proportion of caries in children and adolescents, preventing caries on the occlusal surfaces will substantially reduce the overall caries rates. Sealants are now well established as a

method of caries prevention on pits and fissures of the molar teeth, and are particularly suitable on occlusal surfaces that have steep cuspal inclines and deep and complex fissures that are highly predisposed to caries. In fully erupted teeth, the acid etch technique using resins is associated with high rates of retention and caries prevention. In partially erupted teeth, glass-ionomer cements are the materials of choice because they form chemical bonds to enamel and dentine and are more moisture tolerant and release fluoride, which may provide additional caries prevention. Most pit and fissure sealants inserted using the acid etch technique can be expected to have a retention rate of over 90% in the first 5 years; however, there is no evidence to suggest that there is a significant difference in the caries preventive effect between the two material groups. Further study is recommended.

Future improvements in adhesive materials may make possible the placement of sealants under non-ideal conditions and the production of sealant materials with enhanced retention and caries prevention through the combination release of fluoride- and apatite-forming ions.

In this chapter, the authors further extended the traditional concepts of sealants to propose a method of sealing smooth surfaces (for example, the proximal surfaces of molars during windows of opportunity that present when the teeth are partially erupted and before the establishment of contacts with adjacent teeth). Together with the established methods of caries prevention such as topical fluoride, these exciting innovations in sealant applications will contribute further to decreasing caries in children. Sealants should be reviewed regularly and be part of a comprehensive prevention strategy, which includes both population and individual risk assessment.

References

Ahovuo-Saloranta, A., Hiiri, A., Nordblad, A., et al. (2008) Pit and fissure sealants for preventing dental decay in the permanent teeth of children and adolescents. *Cochrane Database Systematic Reviews*, 2008(4), CD001830.

Alm, A., L.K. Wendt, L.K., Koch, G., et al. (2007) Prevalence of approximal caries in posterior teeth in 15-year-old Swedish teenagers in relation to their caries experience at 3 years of age. *Caries Research*, 41, 392–398.

Arrow, P. and Riordan, P.J. (1995) Retention and caries preventive effects of a GIC and a resin-based fissure sealant. *Community Dentistry and Oral Epidemiology*, 23, 282–285.

Ast, D.B., Bushel, A., Chase, H.C., et al. (1950) Clinical studies of caries prophylaxis with zinc chloride and potassium ferrocyanide. *Journal of the American Dental Association*, 41, 437–442.

Azarpazhooh, A. and Main, P.A. (2008) Pit and fissure sealants in the prevention of dental caries in children and adolescents: a systematic review. *Canadian Dental Association Journal*, 74, 171–177.

Beauchamp, J., Caufield, P.W., Crall, J.J., et al. (2008) Evidence-based clinical recommendations for the use of pit-and-fissure sealants: a report of the American Dental Association Council on Scientific Affairs. *Journal of the American Dental Association*, 139, 257–268.

Beiruti, N., Frencken, J.E., van't Hof, M.A., et al. (2006) Caries-preventive effect of resin-based and glass ionomer sealants over time: a systematic review. *Community Dentistry and Oral Epidemiology*, 34, 403–409.

Beltran-Aguilar, E.D., Barker, L.K., Canto, M.T. et al. (2005) Surveillance for dental caries, dental sealants, tooth retention, edentulism, and enamel fluorosis—United States, 1988–1994 and 1999–2002. *Morbidity and mortality Weekly Report; Surveillance Summary*, 54, 1–43.

Bodecker, C.F. (1929) The eradication of enamel fissures. *Dentistry Items International*, 51, 859.

Boksman, L., McConnell, R.J. Carson, B., et al. (1993) A 2-year clinical evaluation of two pit and fissure sealants placed with and without the use of a bonding agent. *Quintessence International*, 24, 131–133.

Borem, L.M. and Feigal, R.J. (1994) Reducing microleakage of sealants under salivary contamination: digital-image analysis evaluation. *Quintessence International*, 25, 283–289.

Bowen, R.L. (1963) Properties of a silica-reinforced polymer for dental restorations. *Journal of the American Dental Association*, 66, 57–64.

Bowen, R.L. (1970) Crystalline dimethacrylate monomers. *Journal of Dental Research*, 49, 810–815.

Brown, L.J. and Selwitz R.H. (1995) The impact of recent changes in the epidemiology of dental caries on guidelines for the use of dental sealants. *Journal of Public Health Dentistry*, 55 (5 Spec No), 274–291.

Burt, B.A. (1998) Prevention policies in the light of the changed distribution of dental caries. *Acta Odontologica Scandinavica*, 56, 179–186.

Carvalho, J.C., Ekstrand, K.R. Thylstrup, A., et al. (1989) Dental plaque and caries on occlusal surfaces of first permanent molars in relation to stage of eruption. *Journal of Dental Research*, 68, 773–779.

Carvalho, J.C., Ekstrand, K.R. Thylstrup, A., et al. (1991) Results after one year of non-operative occlusal caries treatment of erupting permanent first molars. *Community Dentistry and Oral Epidemiology*, 119, 23–28.

Carvalho, J.C., Thylstrup, A., Ekstrand, K.R., et al. (1992) Results after 3 years of non-operative occlusal caries treatment of erupting permanent first molars. *Community Dentistry and Oral Epidemiology*, 20, 187–192.

Choi, J.W., Drummond, J.L. Dooley, R. et al. (1997) The efficacy of primer on sealant shear bond strength. *Pediatric Dentistry*, 19, 286–288.

Cranfield, M., Kuhn, A.T., Winter, G.B. (1982) Factors relating to the rate of fluoride-ion release from glass-ionomer cement. *Journal of Dentistry*, 10, 333–341.

Cueto, E.I. and Buonocore, M.G. (1967) Sealing of pits and fissures with an adhesive resin: its use in caries prevention. *Journal of the American Dental Association*, 75, 121–128.

Eccles, M.F. (1989) The problem of occlusal caries and its current management. *New Zealand Dental Journal*, 85, 50–55.

Ekstrand, K.R., Bakhshandeh, A., Matignon, S. (2010) Treatment of proximal superficial caries lesions on primary molar teeth with resin infiltration and fluoride varnish versus fluoride varnish only: efficacy after 1 year. *Caries Research*, 44, 41–46.

Ekstrand, K.R., Nielsen, L.A., Carvalho, J.C., et al. (1993) Dental plaque and caries on permanent first molar occlusal surfaces in relation to sagittal occlusion. *Scandinavian Journal of Dental Research*, 101, 9–15.

Feigal, R.J., Musherure, P., Gillespie, B., et al. (2000) Improved sealant retention with bonding agents: a clinical study of two-bottle and single-bottle systems. *Journal of Dental Research*, 79, 1850–1856.

Forss, H. and Halme, E. (1998) Retention of a glass ionomer cement and a resin-based fissure sealant and effect on carious outcome after 7 years. *Community Dentistry and Oral Epidemiology*, 26, 21–25.

Forsten, L. (1995) Resin-modified glass ionomer cements: fluoride release and uptake. *Acta Odontolologica Scandinavica*, 53, 222–225.

Forsten, L. (1998) Fluoride release and uptake by glass-ionomers and related materials and its clinical effect. *Biomaterials*, 19, 503–508.

Going, R.E., Loesche, W.J., Grainger, D.A., et al. (1978) The viability of microorganisms in carious lesions five years after covering with a fissure sealant. *Journal of the American Dental Association*, 97(3), 455–462.

Handelman, S.L., Leverett, D.H., Iker, P.H. (1985) Longitudinal radiographic evaluation of the progress of caries under sealants. *Journal of Pedodontics*, 9, 119–126.

Handelman, S.L. and Shey, Z. (1996) Michael Buonocore and the Eastman Dental Center: a historic perspective on sealants. *Journal of Dental Research*, 75, 529–534.

Hebling, J. and Feigal, R.J. (2000) Use of one-bottle adhesive as an intermediate bonding layer to reduce sealant microleakage on saliva-contaminated enamel. *American Journal of Dentistry*, 13, 187–191.

Hitt, J.C. and Feigal, R.J. (1992) Use of a bonding agent to reduce sealant sensitivity to moisture contamination: an in vitro study. *Pediatric Dentistry*, 14, 41–46.

Holst, A., Braune, K., Sullivan, A. (1998) A five-year evaluation of fissure sealants applied by dental assistants. *Swedish Dental Journal*, 22, 195–201.

Hyatt, T. (1923) Prophylactic odontomy. *Dental Cosmos*, 65: 234–241.

Jensen, O.E. and Handelman S.L. (1980) Effect of an autopolymerising sealant on viability of microflora in occlusal dental caries. *Scandinavian Journal of Dental Research*, 88, 382–388.

Klein, H. and Knutsan, J.W. (1942) Studies on dental caries. XIII Effect of ammonical silver nitrateon caries in first permanent molars. *Journal of the American Dental Association*, 29, 1420–1426.

Komatsu, H., Shimokobe, H., Kawakami, S., *et al.* (1994) Caries-preventive effect of glass ionomer sealant reapplication: study presents three-year results. *Journal of the American Dental Association*, 125, 543–549.

Locker, D., Jokovic, A., Kay, E.J. (2003) Prevention. Part 8: The use of pit and fissure sealants in preventing caries in the permanent dentition of children. *British Dental Journal*, 195, 375–378.

Marsh, P.D. (1994) Microbial ecology of dental plaque and its significance in health and disease. *Advances in Dental Research*, 8, 263–271.

Martignon, S., Chavarria, N., Ekstrand, K.R. (2009) Caries status and proximal lesion behaviour during a 6 year period in young adult Danes: an epidemiological investigation. *Clinical Oral Investigation*, 14, 383–390.

McKenna, E.F. and Grundy, G.E. (1987) Glass ionomer cement fissure sealants applied by operative dental auxiliaries—retention rate after one year. *Australia Dental Journal*, 32, 200–203.

McLean, J.W. and Wilson, A.D. (1974) Fissure sealing and filling with an adhesive glass-ionomer cement. *British Dental Journal*, 136, 269–276.

Mejare, I. and Mjor, I.A. (1990) Glass ionomer and resin-based fissure sealants: a clinical study. *Scandinavian Journal of Dental Research*, 98, 345–350.

Mejàre, I., Stenlund, H., Zelezny-Holmlund, C. (2004) Caries incidence and lesion progression from adolescence to young adulthood: a prospective 15-year cohort study in Sweden. *Caries Research*, 38, 130–141.

Mertz-Farihurst, E.J., Curtis, J.W., Ergle, J.W., *et al.* (1998) Ultraconservative and cariostatic sealed restorations: results at year 10. *Journal of the American Dental Association*, 129, 55–66.

Meyer-Lueckel, H. and Paris, S. (2008) Progression of artificial enamel caries lesions after infiltration with experimental light curing resins. *Caries Research*, 42, 117–124.

Mount, G.J. and Ngo, H. (2000). Minimal intervention: early lesions. *Quintessence International*, 31, 535–546.

Mount, G.J., Tyas, M.J., Ferracane, J.L., *et al.* (2009) A revised classification for direct tooth-colored restorative materials. *Quintessence International*, 40, 691–697.

Murray, J.J. and Williams, B. (1975) Fissure sealants and dental caries: a review. *Journal of Dentistry*, 3, 145–152.

Newbrun, E., Plasschaert, A.J. König, K.G., *et al.* (1974) Progress of caries in fissures of rat molars treated with occlusal sealants. *Journal of the American Dental Association*, 89, 121–126.

Ngo, H. (2010) Glass-ionomer cements as restorative and preventive materials. *Dental Clinics of North America*, 54, 551–563.

Ngo, H. and Gaffney, S. (2005) Risk assessment in the diagnosis and management of caries. In: *Preservation and Restoration of Tooth Structure* (Eds. G.J. Mount and W.R. Hume), pp. 61–82, Knowledge Book and Software, Brighton, UK.

Ngo, H., Mount, G.J., Peters, M.C. (1997) A study of glass-ionomer cement and its interface with enamel and dentin using a low-temperature, high-resolution scanning electron microscopic technique. *Quintessence International*, 28, 63–69.

Ngo, H.C., Mount, G., McIntyre, J., *et al.* (2006) Chemical exchange between glass-ionomer restorations and residual carious dentine in permanent molars: an in vivo study. *Journal of Dentistry*, 34, 608–613.

Oong, E. M., Griffin, S. O., Kohn, W.G. (2008) The effect of dental sealants on bacteria levels in caries lesions: a review of the evidence. *Journal of the American Dental Association*, 139, 271–278; quiz 357–278.

Ricketts, D.N., Kidd, E.A. Innes, N., *et al.* (2006) Complete or ultra-conservative removal of decayed tissue in unfilled teeth. *Cochrane Database Systematic Reviews*, 3: CD003808.

Rock, W.P. (1974) Fissure sealants. Further results of clinical trials. *British Dental Journal*, 136, 317–321.

Salar, D.V., Garcia-Godoy, F., Flaitz, C.M., *et al.* (2007) Potential inhibition of demineralization in vitro by fluoride-releasing sealants. *Journal of the American Dental Association*, 138, 502–506.

Simonsen, R. (1991) Retention and effectiveness of dental sealants after 15 years. *Journal of the American Dental Association*, 122, 34–42.

Simonsen, R.J. (1980) Preventive resin restorations: three-year results. *Journal of the American Dental Association*, 100(4), 535–539.

Simonsen, R.J. (2002) Pit and fissure sealant: review of the literature. *Pediatric Dentistry*, 24, 393–414.

Smith, D.C. (1967) Protection of silicate restorations from contaminaton by moisture. *British Dental Journal*, 122, 382–386.

Stiles, H.M., Ward, G.T., Woolridge, E.D., *et al.* (1976) Adhesive sealant clinical trial: comparative results of application by a dentist or dental auxiliaries. *Journal of Preventive Dentistry*, 3, 8–11.

Swartz, M.L., Phillips, R.W., Clark, H.E. (1984) Long-term F release from glass ionomer cements. *Journal of Dental Research*, 63, 158–160.

Symons, A.L., Chu, C.Y., Meyers, I.A. (1996) The effect of fissure morphology and pretreatment of the enamel surface on penetration and adhesion of fissure sealants. *Journal of Oral Rehabilitation*, 23, 791–798.

Thomson, J.L., Main, C., Gillespie, F.C., *et al.* (1981) The effect of salivary contamination on fissure sealant—enamel bond strength. *Journal of Oral Rehabilitation*, 8, 11–18.

Thylstrup, A. and Qvist V. (1987) Principal enamel and dentine reactions during caries progression. In: *Dentine and dentine reactions in the oral cavity*. (Eds. A. Thylstrup, S. A. Leach, V. Qvist), pp. 3–16, IRL Press, Oxford, UK.

Tyas, M.J., Anusavice, K.J., Frencken, J.E., *et al.* (2000) Minimal intervention dentistry—a review. FDI Commission Project 1–97. *International Dental Journal*, 50, 1–12.

Walls, A.W. (1986) Glass polyalkenoate (glass-ionomer) cements: a review. *Journal of Dentistry*, 14, 231–246.

Wilson, A.D., Groffman, D.M., Kuhn, A.T. (1985) The release of fluoride and other chemical species from a glass-ionomer cement. *Biomaterials*, 6, 431–433.

Zero, D. T., Fontana, M., Martínez-Mier, E.A. *et al.* (2009) The biology, prevention, diagnosis and treatment of dental caries: scientific advances in the United States. *Journal of the American Dental Association*, 140 (Suppl 1), 25S–34S.

18

Strategies for remineralization

Laurence J. Walsh

Introduction

Fluoride has been the gold standard for remineralization in clinical practice; however, over the past 2 decades new strategies for enhancing the uptake of fluoride into dental hard tissues and for incorporating other ionic components needed for forming apatite minerals have been developed. This chapter provides a summary of such methods and how they have been deployed into clinical practice.

Light-activation of fluoride uptake

All dental clinicians are familiar with the use of topical fluorides for caries prevention in adults, however, the concept of enhancing fluoride uptake into tooth structure by using intense light immediately after topical fluoride application is less well known, despite this suggestion having been in the dental literature since the late 1980s (Tagomori and Morioka 1989). More than 30 studies over the past 35 years have shown that laser energy, either used alone or in combination with topical fluoride therapies, can increase the resistance of tooth structure to mineral loss from the organic acids involved in dental caries. It is now realized that the concept of light-activated uptake of fluoride into enamel is not specific to lasers but applies equally well to other intense near-monochromatic light sources, such as light emitting diodes (LED). It is now realized that the combination of fluoride topical treatment immediately followed by intense light exposure enhances fluoride uptake into enamel, causes the formation of fluorapatite even under neutral pH conditions, and lowers the critical pH at which enamel and dentin dissolution occurs.

Caries prevention with light-activated fluoride

Light-activated fluoride (LAF) can reduce susceptibility of both enamel and root surfaces to cariogenic challenges posed by lactic, pyruvic, and other organic acids, as well as to erosive challenges, such as those posed by gastric contents and acidic beverages (Hicks *et al.* 1993; Hossain *et al.* 2002). Using LAF therapy, clinicians can help to reduce the likelihood of caries and erosion. Even if caries does develop and progress, the depth of the lesion at a treated enamel or root surface site will be reduced by as much as one-half compared with an untreated site. In other words, LAF can be applied to prevent caries from developing, as well as to reduce the progression rate of existing lesions on the enamel and root surfaces of teeth.

Laboratory studies using caries models that employed the visible blue argon ion laser (230 milliWatts for 10 seconds) for LAF have shown a reduction in lesion depth by 15% and an even greater reduction of 33–46% in the speed of lesion progression (Westerman *et al.* 2002). LAF using 2% neutral sodium fluoride with blue light gave a reduction in lesion progression of 29%; reductions of between 31 and 50% in caries initiation and progression have been reported in other studies using similar exposure parameters (Hicks *et al.* 1993; Westerman *et al.* 1994; Flaitz *et al.* 1995; Blankenau *et al.* 1999). Reported lesion depth reductions using blue light combined with 1.23% acidulated phosphate fluoride (APF) range from 25–55% (Hicks *et al.* 1995; Anderson *et al.* 2000).

Clinical studies of LAF for preventing enamel and root surface caries in high-risk patients have confirmed that the positive effects seen in laboratory models translate directly to the clinical setting. These clinical

Comprehensive Preventive Dentistry, First Edition. Edited by Hardy Limeback.
© 2012 John Wiley & Sons, Ltd. Published 2012 by John Wiley & Sons, Ltd.

studies have also shown protective effects of LAF on root surface dentin in xerostomic patients, as well as evidence of caries arrest and reversal for incipient lesions on cervical surfaces (Walsh 1994; Blankenau *et al.* 1999; Vlacic, Meyers, and Walsh 2007).

Action spectrum of light-activated fluoride: which light to use?

Recent studies have examined systematically the action spectrum of LAF to determine the optimal wavelengths of light. Early work on LAF had employed the visible blue argon ion laser (488 nm), which is similar in wavelength to an LED or halogen curing light (470–500 nm). It soon became apparent that the synergistic effect of laser irradiation and topical fluoride on the tooth surface was not confined to the argon laser, with the benefits of LAF with the Nd:YAG and carbon dioxide lasers in terms of increased caries resistance of enamel being reported by a number of studies (Tagomori and Morioka 1989; Zhang, Kimura, and Matsumoto 1996; Featherstone *et al.* 1998). Laboratory studies have shown that enhanced protection against both cariogenic and erosive challenges can be gained using LAF with seven commonly available laser wavelengths, as well as by LEDs with comparable emission characteristics (Vlacic *et al.* 2007; Vlacic, Meyers, and Walsh 2007). These treatments were found to prevent softening of tooth structure following either short- or long-term exposure to acids, as determined used microhardness testing. These finding suggested that partial conversion of the enamel surface to fluorapatite was achieved using LAF, causing a corresponding reduction in the critical pH, which gives enhanced protection from cariogenic challenges and reduced softening from stronger corrosive acids such as those found in gastric reflux diseases.

Mechanisms of action of LAF

The mechanisms by which the LAF protective effect is achieved has been the subject of much discussion in the literature. Several physico-chemical changes have been shown to occur during LAF treatment (Table 18-1).

Table 18-1 Multiple mechanisms for light-activated fluoride therapy

Enhanced deposition of calcium fluoride
Swelling and denaturation of proteins on the tooth surface
Formation of micro spaces in tooth structure
Greater affinity for calcium, phosphate, and fluoride ions
Trapping of minerals in the subsurface
Formation of tri-calcium phosphate
Sealing of surface pores
Conversion of hydroxyapatite to fluorapatite

Scanning electron microscopic examination of enamel treated with blue light shows subtle modifications including sporadic globular deposits and reduced surface micro-porosities. The lased surface has a greater affinity for calcium, phosphate, and fluoride ions, and the enhanced accumulation of these optimizes its resistance to a cariogenic attack.

The original suggestion that more fluoride may be incorporated chemically into enamel mineral when topical fluoride exposure was followed by intense light was proposed in 1989. This concept, which has also been termed "photonic conversion" has evolved over the following 20 years. Greater retention of fluoride in the enamel surface after *in vivo* LAF treatment has been demonstrated formally with use of visible blue light from the argon laser, compared with both untreated enamel and topical fluoride treatment alone (Nammour *et al.* 2003). Moreover, recent laboratory studies (Vlacic *et al.* 2007a; Vlacic, Meyers, and Walsh 2007c) have shown that both LAF and laser alone have beneficial effects on enamel microhardness, unlike fluoride therapy alone, with LAF giving the greatest positive effect.

In addition to physical effects on the tooth surface, the intriguing possibility also exists that LAF may induce chemical changes in tooth structure, such as partial conversion of various forms of carbonated apatite or hydroxyapatite to fluorapatite, thereby conferring the increased resistance to acid dissolution that has been documented in both caries and erosion models. A recent study (Vlacic *et al.* 2008) explored whether photonic conversion occurred, using the surface analytical technique of X-ray photoelectron spectroscopy (XPS), in which a monochromatic source of X-rays is focused on the surface of the sample, under high vacuum conditions, thereby liberating electrons. By measuring the kinetic energy of the emitted electrons, their binding energy can be determined and from this, the chemical structure of the material can be deduced. XPS provides both quantitative and qualitative data regarding atomic composition and chemical structure.

The findings from XPS analysis of topical fluoride and LAF therapies can be summarized as follows. Acidulated fluoride causes a decrease in the phosphorous concentration and a high concentration of fluorine at the surface through deposition of calcium fluoride (fluorine binding energy 684.8 eV). Treatment with neutral sodium fluoride gel only gives fluorine with a peak binding energy of 684.5 eV, which is due to physical trapping of sodium fluoride. When neutral sodium fluoride gel is followed immediately by light, fluorapatite is formed in the outer layers, as shown by an altered fluorine to calcium atomic ratio, a high oxygen to fluorine atomic ratio, and

Table 18-2 Changes in atomic ratios with LAF therapy on dentin

Material	F:Ca ratio	Ca:P ratio
Fluorapatite	0.25	1.67
Calcium fluoride	2.0	–
Unlased dentin	0	1.69
NaF topical fluoride	0.28	1.72
LAF	0.27	1.49

a fluorine binding energy of 684.6 eV, which corresponds to fluorapatite (Table 18-2).

The formal documentation of the transformation of hydroxyapatite to fluorapatite following LAF explains the reduced solubility under acidic challenges and increased resistance to acid dissolution. The XPS study also illustrates the importance of the combination effect, since topical application of sodium fluoride gel to dentin, under identical conditions but in the absence of laser irradiation, did not result in transformation.

Root surface treatment

Treatment of root surfaces is a particular area where the combination of light with fluoride can be of benefit, with reductions in lesion depth of up to 54% for root surfaces in teeth that had been treated with APF gel (1.23% fluoride) and visible blue light (200 milliWatts for 10 seconds) in combination (Hicks *et al.* 1997). The combination of blue light and fluoride resulted in a synergistic effect, with a greater reduction in lesion depth than either laser alone or fluoride alone. This may be due in part to the trapping of the more soluble mineral phases, effectively limiting the formation of a carious lesion. Root surfaces that have been exposed to APF gel alone have a homogeneous surface coating, with sporadic granular deposits of calcium fluoride (<1 micron in diameter). Irradiation of the root surface with blue light and fluoride increases both granular and globular deposits of calcium fluoride (1–2 microns in dimension) and micro-porosities (<1 micron in diameter) (Westerman *et al.* 1999). The latter may further enhance uptake of fluoride.

LAF and sensitivity

The concept of surface alterations by LAF, such as blockage of dentinal tubules, has now been demonstrated formally *in vitro* by environmental SEM studies of LAF therapy applied at the dentin-enamel junction using a variety of fluoride vehicles combined with KTP or carbon dioxide lasers (Goharkay *et al.* 2007). Of note, fluoride treatments with stannous fluoride gel, amino fluoride solution, or fluoride varnish did not cause closure of dentin tubules, while LAF treatment caused partial or total occlusion, providing an explanation for the desensitizing effect of LAF when used clinically.

Clinical protocols

The basis of the clinical protocol for LAF is the conventional in-office topical fluoride therapy, beginning with appropriate isolation of the teeth and removal of any gross plaque deposits by professional prophylaxis. Either neutral or acidulated sodium fluoride gel may be used, and this is applied onto the teeth with a cotton bud or microbrush. Neutral sodium fluoride is preferred because there is no risk of sensitivity, erosion, or damage to tooth-colored restorations. The color and viscosity of the gel does not affect the activation process. Fluoride ionic concentrations of 9,000–12,300 ppm have been shown to be effective.

The gel is irradiated while in place on the tooth surface in a non-contact manner with a spot size of 5 to 8 mm. The light source can be operated in continuous or pulsed mode, however, it is necessary to achieve an energy density of 15 Joules per square cm, which is the optimal value as shown in laboratory and clinical studies. With a halogen curing light with a nominal optical power of 500 mW, this translates into an exposure time of 30 seconds. With LED curing lights of greater optical power, an exposure time of 20 seconds will suffice, if continuous emission mode is used. Exposure parameters for a wide range of lasers have been published (Vlacic *et al.* 2007a; Vlacic *et al.* 2007b); however, most dental practitioners will find it easier to use their curing light for activation of fluoride. The gel is not touched by the light source, and there is no visible change in either the gel or the tooth during the treatment. The patient then expectorates the fluoride gel or it is removed by gentle irrigation with a triple syringe combined with high velocity evacuation.

LAF therapy can be repeated without adverse effects on the tooth structure or the dental pulp, since there are minimal changes at the level of the dental pulp when the energy density is maintained at the correct rate for both visible and near infrared lasers and intense light sources including LED curing lights (Weerakoon *et al.* 2002).

In conclusion, LAF can be delivered using the existing clinical armamentarium of a curing light, or using other intense light sources such as a KTP or argon laser, to provide an additional benefit beyond conventional fluoride therapy by irradiating fluoride gel while it is still present on the tooth surface.

Factors that influence remineralization

Remineralization is the natural repair process for non-cavitated lesions, and relies on calcium and phosphate

Table 18-3 Some key proteins that stabilize calcium and phosphate

Saliva
  Statherin
  Acidic proline-rich proteins
  Histatins

Milk
  Alpha caseins
  Beta caseins

Hard tissues
  Ameloblastin
  Enamelin
  Osteopontin
  Bone sialoprotein
  Dentin sialoprotein

ions assisted by fluoride to rebuild a new surface on existing crystal remnants in subsurface lesions remaining after demineralization. These remineralized crystals are less acid soluble than the original mineral.

Calcium availability is the singular limiting factor in enamel remineralization, and this is underpinned by the low solubility of calcium phosphates, particularly in the presence of fluoride ions and calcium fluoride compounds. The majority of calcium compounds are very insoluble, and the calcium phosphates are particularly so. Many laboratory remineralizing solutions contain only 1 to 3 mM calcium ions, together with phosphate ions (in various ratios from 1:1 to 1.66:1). Fluoride ions may also be included at levels of up to 1 ppm. A key point is that higher ionic concentrations cannot be used because of the inherent instability of these solutions. Moreover, all such solutions fail to localize the ions at the tooth surface in sufficient concentrations to promote enamel subsurface remineralization *in vivo* (Cochrane *et al.* 2010).

Consequently, an important component of saliva that influences remineralization is the phosphoproteins that regulate calcium saturation of the saliva. As well, the early pellicle glycoproteins, acidic proline-rich proteins and statherin, promote remineralization of the enamel by attracting calcium ions (Table 18-3).

Differences in calcium concentration have important implications for the critical pH and for the possibility of remineralization, since the latter will not occur when the degree of saturation of saliva with respect to tooth mineral is low (Aiuchi *et al.* 2008). In other words, remineralization may be enhanced by providing low levels of bio-available calcium and phosphate ions, in conjunction with minimal amounts of fluoride. Sub-ppm levels of fluoride (<1 ppm) act as a catalyst and influence reaction rates with dissolution and transformation of the

various calcium phosphate mineral phases that are within tooth structure and resident within plaque adjacent to tooth surfaces (Hicks *et al.* 2004).

Saliva, enamel, bone, cementum, dentin, and milk contain closely related phosphoproteins that bind and stabilize calcium and phosphate, orchestrating the behavior of these ions in a pH dependent fashion. In fact, statherins in saliva, casein phosphoproteins in commercial Recaldent™ products, and phosphoproteins in tooth structure share remarkable similarity. When hard tissues are demineralized, the phosphoproteins that remain influence the ability of this tissue to remineralize (Clarkson *et al.* 1998).

Beta Tricalcium Phosphate (TCP)

Tricalcium phosphate has the chemical formula $Ca_3(PO_4)_2$, and TCP exists in two forms, alpha and beta. Alpha TCP is formed when human enamel is heated to high temperatures, and is relatively insoluble in water. Crystalline beta TCP can be formed by combining calcium carbonate and calcium hydrogen phosphate, and heating the mixture to over 1,000°C for 1 day, to give a flaky, stiff powder. The average size of the TCP particles can then be adjusted by milling them. Typically, particles range from 0.01 to 5 microns in size. Beta TCP is even less soluble than alpha TCP, and thus in an unmodified form is unlikely to provide bio-available calcium.

Nevertheless, TCP has been studied as one possible means for enhancing levels of calcium in plaque and saliva. Some small effects on free calcium and phosphate levels in plaque fluid and in saliva have been found when an experimental gum with 2.5% alpha TCP by weight was chewed, when compared to a control gum without added TCP (Vogel *et al.* 1998). A significant problem with such uses of TCP is the formation of calcium-phosphate complexes, or if fluorides are present, formation of calcium fluoride, which would inhibit remineralization by lowering the levels of bioavailable calcium and fluoride. For this reason, TCP levels in remineralizing products have to be kept very low, in the order of less than 1%. The amount of material released from TCP under normal salivary pH conditions is very low, and sustained contact with highly acidic saliva would be required to cause sufficient dissolution of TCP particles to liberate ions for remineralization. Moreover, to achieve dissolution of the calcium phosphate phase into saliva, the saliva must be under-saturated with respect to that crystalline phase, which would normally not be the case (Cochrane *et al.* 2010).

TCP can be combined with a ceramic such as titanium dioxide, or other metal oxides, in order to limit the interaction between calcium and phosphate, and make the material more stable in solution or suspension. An alloy of TCP and a metal oxide can be created by mechanical alloying, during which fracturing and the cold welding of particles occurs. There is some laboratory evidence using demineralized bovine enamel pH cycling models that shows increased surface microhardness after treatment with TCP-titania alloys (Ingram *et al.* 2005).

A further development of this concept is to coat particles of TCP or TCP alloys with sodium lauryl sulphate (SLS) or other surfactants, with carboxylic acids (such as fumaric acid), polymers, or copolymers. Such organic coatings can be applied by pulverizing the TCP or TCP alloy together with the coating material in a planetary ball mill for several days (Karlinsey and Mackey 2009). The intention is that the organic coating on the TCP prevents undesirable interactions with fluoride. The organic component subsequently dissolves away when placed in saliva, to leave the particles active. TCP particles coated with SLS are the basis for the fluoride dentifrices in the 3M-Espe ClinPro Tooth Cream™ product range. An organically modified TCP technology should operate best at neutral or slightly alkaline pH. As with TCP alloys, there is some laboratory evidence using bovine enamel models that shows increased surface microhardness, and fluoride incorporation into the outer layers of the enamel (Lussi *et al.* 2008). It is not yet known what effects are achieved in the enamel subsurface, the region of greatest interest in terms of remineralization therapies. The limited available data at present indicate only limited release of calcium is achieved during clinical use (Reynolds *et al.* 2010). It is not yet known what the potential is for TCP alloys or organically modified TCP in terms of remineralization.

Bioactive glass containing calcium sodium phosphosilicate (NovaMin™)

NovaMin™ is a bioactive glass that in aqueous solutions, comprises 45% SiO_2, 24.5% Na_2O, 24.5% CaO, and 6% P_2O_5. Of these components, ionic forms of calcium and phosphorus may potentially contribute to remineralization. NovaMin™ has been incorporated into a number of products, including dentifrices and gels. It is unclear at present what proportion of the released calcium and phosphate ions are bio-available, and how they interact with fluoride and with salivary components. The material has attracted some interest both as a desensitizing agent (by occluding dentin tubules) and as a potential remineralizing agent for enamel white spot lesions, although there is as yet no published evidence to support such a clinical application.

Unstabilized calcium and phosphate salts with sodium fluoride (Enamelon™)

In this technology, the calcium salts are separated from the phosphate salts and sodium fluoride by a plastic divider in the center of the dentifrice tube. There is a modest evidence base for Enamelon™, with five laboratory studies, three rat caries trials, and four clinical trials. There is evidence of a caries inhibitory action of Enamelon™ dentifrice in a rat dental caries model (Thompson *et al.* 1999). Similarly, clinical studies have indicated that the incidence of root surface caries in radiotherapy patients using Enamelon™ dentifrice over 12 months was less than in those using a conventional fluoride dentifrice, and the reduction seen was comparable to that gained by daily use of stannous fluoride gel in trays (Papas *et al.* 1999; Papas *et al.* 2008). An important technical issue with Enamelon™ is that the calcium and phosphate ions are not stabilized, allowing the two to combine into insoluble precipitates before they come into contact with saliva or enamel.

Amorphous calcium phosphate

The macromolecule amorphous calcium phosphate (ACP) was developed by the American Dental Association Health Foundation at their Paffenbarger facility in Maryland. When applied topically, ACP may flow onto the tooth surface and penetrate into microscopic surface defects, altering the smoothness and luster of the enamel surface, and giving some cosmetic improvements in dimpled, abraded, or etched tooth enamel (Charig *et al.* 2004; Litkowski *et al.* 2004). A surface impregnated with ACP in this manner would, paradoxically, reduce surface porosity and thus reduce the likelihood of achieving deep penetration of mineral into subsurface defects and white spot lesions.

ACP hydrolyzes under physiological temperatures at a pH of 7.4 to form octacalcium phosphate and an intermediate, and then apatite. Through this mechanism, a thin surface coating of hydroxyapatite over the original tooth surface may be achieved as a purely surface phenomenon. This surface action explains why ACP has desensitizing actions (Tung and Eichmiller 1999; Tung and Eichmiller 2004).

The stability of ACP in dental products is an issue, with single-phase ACP systems formulated without water, to keep the ACP reacting to form apatite. This problem arises because ACP is the least stable calcium phosphate compound, whereas apatites are the most stable. An alternative approach that has been tried is to separate the calcium and phosphate components and mix these during dispensing immediately prior to use. The challenge here is controlling the process using pH, for example through the bicarbonate and phosphate buffer systems or via dissolved carbon dioxide gas. If the pH is raised above 4.5, stability of calcium and phosphate ions reduces dramatically, and ACP will precipitate. This could be undertaken by mixing acidic calcium solutions with basic phosphate and carbonate solutions using a dual dispensing system.

Dicalcium phosphate dehydrate

Dicalcium phosphate dehydrate (DCPD) has been used in some fluoride dentifrices to attempt to enhance the remineralizing effects of the fluoride component. Examination of plaque fluid indicates that inclusion of DCPD increases the levels of free calcium ions in plaque fluid, which is normally undersaturated with respect to DCPD, thus allowing DCPD to dissolve in the mouth. There is evidence of an elevated calcium level in plaque fluid 12 hours after brushing with such a dentifrice, when compared to conventional silica dentifrices, and of some incorporation of this calcium into the outer enamel (Sullivan *et al.* 1997).

Other calcium compounds

Because an inverse relationship exists between plaque calcium concentrations and dental caries risk, a range of other calcium compounds have been added to oral care products in an attempt to promote remineralization. In fact, elevated plaque calcium levels have the potential to elevate plaque fluoride levels, a second parameter also linked to reduced dental caries experience (Lynch and ten Cate 2005).

Calcium peroxide has been added to bleaching gels, while dicalcium phosphate, calcium carbonate, calcium chloride, calcium gluconate, calcium glycerophosphate, and calcium lactate have been added to dentifrices, gels, and chewing gums. Of these, calcium lactate and calcium gluconate are the most soluble in water, with solubilities of 9.3 and 3.0 g/100 mL, respectively. The key problems encountered have been the limited bioavailability of calcium, interactions with fluoride compounds in the products, and the poor solubility and palatability of these calcium compounds, since inorganic calcium salts typically taste chalky or astringent.

Similar comments apply to the incorporation of calcium compounds into drinks to reduce their erosive potential. Some calcium salts have been added to erosive drinks to increase calcium levels and reduce surface softening caused by these beverages, but other than adding CPP-ACP, it is not readily possible to gain dramatic increases in calcium levels in the most erosive foods and beverages, because of the inherent instability of calcium compounds.

Recaldent™ (CPP-ACP Nanocomplexes)

Other than fluoride, Casein Phosphopeptide-Amorphous Calcium Phosphate (CPP-ACP) is the most extensively researched remineralization technology, and is used widely in chewing gums such as Recaldent® gum and Trident Xtra Care®, and in topical tooth creams such as MI Paste™ and GC Tooth Mousse™. The clinical use of this technology is supported by a large body of literature including a number of systematic reviews, the highest form of evidence in the pyramid of evidence-based practice. A 2009 meta-analysis (Yengopal and Mickenautsch 2009) identified more than 120 journal articles on CPP-ACP technology, which included animal model studies, *in situ* clinical studies, and randomized clinical trials.

This unique naturally derived protein-based remineralizing technology comprises specific phosphopeptides derived from milk caseins, which are complexed with amorphous calcium phosphate to form stable complexes. These nanoparticles are some 2 nm in diameter and have a large surface area for mineral exchange. The configuration of the ACP in the CPP-ACP complex differs completely from that found in macromolecular aggregates of ACP, as has been included in some current prophylaxis pastes and bleaching gels.

CPP-ACP technology was developed by Eric Reynolds and co-workers at the University of Melbourne, Australia, and first became available in forms without fluoride. More recently, a formulation with incorporated fluoride to a level of 900 ppm (MI Paste Plus™, GC Tooth Mousse Plus™) has become available. The author was involved in developing a number of the clinical protocols for using 10% CPP-ACP tooth creams in clinical dental practice (Walsh 2007a). Today, a range of clinical applications for such topical creams is in used globally (Table 18-4).

Table 18-4 Applications of topical CPP-ACP cream

Prevention
- Caries prevention in high caries risk patients
- Caries prevention during fixed orthodontic treatment

Treatment of enamel
- Reversal of carious white spot lesions
- Reversal of orthodontic decalcification
- Reversal of mild and moderate fluorosis
- Reversal of mild white developmental opacities
- Reversal of enamel opacity from excessive bleaching

Treatment of dentin and root surfaces
- Desensitization of cervical dentin
- Prevention of root surface caries in high risk patients

Mechanisms of action

The genesis of this technology relates to the problem of stabilizing calcium ions so that bioavailable calcium can be delivered when needed. This is a major biological challenge that impacts all dental hard tissues as well as other hard tissues in the body. Understanding this natural process of calcium stabilization, transport, and delivery by phosphoproteins led to the identification of particular peptide sequences from bovine milk casein, which have caries preventive actions and form the framework of nanocomplexes with unique remineralizing properties.

Within milk, the casein phosphopeptides stabilize calcium and phosphate ions through the formation of complexes. The calcium phosphate in these complexes is biologically available for intestinal absorption, and the same concept has now been applied to create materials with bio-available calcium and phosphate in the appropriate form and molecular ratio for remineralization of subsurface lesions in enamel. Clusters of phosphorylated seryl residues are responsible for the interaction that occurs in bovine milk between the caseins and calcium phosphate, and this in turn results in the formation of casein micelles (Cross *et al.* 2005).

CPP-ACP is in essence a protein nanotechnology containing and releasing calcium, phosphate, and fluoride ions, which puts this into a different class from other remineralizing agents that are fundamentally mineral technologies. The ACP forms around the phosphopeptides, and thus is structurally quite different to the ACP macromaterial described above. The precise ratio is 144 calcium ions plus 96 phosphate ions and 6 peptides of CPP. The nanocomplexes form over a pH range from 5.0 to 9.0. Compared to plain, alloyed, or organically modified TCP materials, the particles of CPP-ACP are much smaller and of different composition. Most importantly, the remineralizing actions work effectively at acidic pH levels (down to pH 4.0) as well as in the neutral and alkaline ranges.

The casein phosphopeptides (CPP) are produced from a tryptic digest of the milk protein casein, then aggregated with calcium phosphate and purified by ultrafiltration. Under alkaline conditions the calcium phosphate is present as an alkaline amorphous phase complexed by the CPP.

The CPP bind to forming clusters of ACP in metastable solution, preventing their growth to the critical size required for nucleation and precipitation (Cross *et al.* 2007).

Under neutral and alkaline conditions, the casein phosphopeptides stabilize calcium and phosphate ions, forming metastable solutions that are supersaturated with respect to the basic calcium phosphate phases. The amount of calcium and phosphate bound by CPP increases as the pH rises, reaching the point where the CPP have bound their equivalent weights of calcium and phosphate.

Remineralizing actions

There is extensive clinical as well as laboratory evidence for the effects of CPP-ACP as a remineralizing agent, as well as a truly anti-cariogenic agent, with the latter being demonstrated in both animal and *in situ* human caries models. The material is pH responsive, with increasing pH raising the level of bound ACP and stabilizing free calcium and phosphate so that spontaneous precipitation of calcium phosphate does not occur. This is also inherently an anti-calculus action (Reynolds 1998).

CPP-ACP provides a highly effective means for elevating calcium levels in dental plaque fluid, something that is desirable for enhancing remineralization but is difficult to achieve by using calcium in other forms (Magalhães *et al.* 2007). In fact, in a mouth-rinse study that compared CPP-ACP and solutions of calcium phosphate, only the CPP-ACP-containing mouth rinse significantly increased plaque calcium and inorganic phosphate levels (Reynolds *et al.* 2003).

Of note, the extent of remineralization seen with Recaldent™ does not significantly correlate with levels of CPP-bound ACP or the degrees of saturation for hydroxyapatite, octacalcium phosphate, or ACP. Rather, there is a strong correlation between remineralization and the concentration of the neutral ion pair $CaHPO_4$. By stabilizing calcium phosphate in solution, the CPP maintain high-concentration gradients of calcium and phosphate ions and ion pairs into subsurface lesions, an effect that explains the high rates of enamel subsurface remineralization that can be achieved when these products are used in solutions, gums, lozenges, and creams (Reynolds 1997).

Anti-cariogenic actions

The delivery of simultaneous calcium, fluoride, and phosphate using Recaldent™ products that include fluoride provides an effective means of controlling the process of fluoride levels in dental plaque. These levels influence the behavior of bacteria as well as contribute to remineralization. The efficacy of these nanocomplexes as anti-cariogenic agents was first demonstrated in numerous animal and *in situ* human caries models, and then in clinical trials (Reynolds 1997; Reynolds 2008; Reynolds 2009). As well as being an effective anti-cariogenic agent for enamel caries (Llena, Forner, and Baca 2009), CPP-ACP has also been shown to prevent root surface caries in xerostomic patients (Vlacic 2007;

Vlacic, Meyers, and Walsh, 2007), and to be more effective than saliva for remineralization after either caries- and erosion-like assaults to the enamel (Cai *et al.* 2003). This point has important practical implications for stabilizing the oral environment in patients with dental caries or with dental erosion and underlying salivary dysfunction, in whom daily use of a topical CPP-ACP cream can have major benefits (Meyers 2008; Piekarz *et al.* 2008; Ranjitkar *et al.* 2009).

The anti-caries action of Recaldent™ involves actions other than suppressing demineralization and enhancing remineralization. There is increasing evidence that Recaldent™ may influence the properties and behavior of dental plaque through (1) binding to adhesion molecules on mutans streptococci and thus impairing their incorporation into dental plaque, (2) elevating plaque calcium ion levels to inhibit plaque fermentation, and (3) providing protein and phosphate buffering of plaque fluid pH, to suppresses overgrowth of aciduric species under conditions where fermentable carbohydrate is in excess (Reynolds and Walsh 2005). Intra-oral application of a topical cream containing CPP-ACP immediately before a sucrose challenge has been shown to reduce plaque acid production (Caruana *et al.* 2009).

Delivery systems

CPP-ACP incorporated into chewing gum, lozenges, and mouth rinses has been shown to remineralize enamel subsurface lesions in numerous human *in situ* studies (Manton *et al.* 2008). CPP-ACP has also been used in dentifrices (Rao *et al.* 2009).

The addition of CPP-ACP to existing foods has been shown to enhance their dental health benefits. Enhanced remineralization of enamel subsurface lesions has been shown when CPP-ACP is added to bovine milk at levels of 2.0 or 5.0 g/liter. At an intake level of 200 mL of milk once daily for each week day over 3 consecutive weeks, gains in mineral content of 70 and 148%, respectively, occurred relative to the normal milk control (Walker *et al.* 2006).

CPP-ACP added to acidic beverages has been shown to abrogate their erosive effects. A key factor in such an approach is to estimate the lowest concentration of CPP-ACP, which can be added to erosive drinks to eliminate the risk of erosion to enamel. Past research work on this topic has explored this issue using Powerade™, to which was added varying amounts of CPP-ACP from 0.063% up to 0.25%. Analysis of the surface characteristics of enamel slabs in the laboratory setting using stereomicroscopy, scanning electron microscopy, and surface profilometry demonstrated that adding CPP-ACP at 0.25% raised the pH from 2.70 to 3.90, and lowered the titratable acidity from 1.83 to 1.36. Enamel loss from etching reduced from 3.87 μm to 0.19 μm, which was identical to enamel samples kept in distilled water (0.25 μm). A reduction in the erosive step defect occurred at concentrations down to 0.09%. Thus, the erosive potential of Powerade™ was attenuated or eliminated completely by the addition of low concentrations of CPP-ACP (Ramilingham *et al.* 2005).

CPP-ACFP nanocomplexes

Casein phosphopeptides containing the cluster sequence-Ser(P)-Ser(P)-Ser(P)-Glu-Glu- bind fluoride as well as calcium and phosphate, and thus can also stabilize calcium fluoride phosphate as soluble complexes. These complexes are designated CPP-ACFP. Studies of such nanocomplexes based on the casein alpha-S1 peptide fragment 59–79 have revealed a particle size of some 2 nm and stoichiometry of one peptide to 15 calcium, 9 phosphate, and 3 fluoride ions (Cross *et al.* 2004). By stabilizing ACFP, additive effects on remineralization are achieved compared with the fluoride or CPP-ACP alone.

Clinical studies of mouth rinses and dentifrices containing CPP-ACP and fluoride have provided interesting insights into the synergy between these. For example, addition of CPP-ACP to a fluoride mouth rinse increases the incorporation of fluoride into dental plaque biofilm. A dentifrice containing CPP-ACP with fluoride provides remineralization, which is superior to both CPP-ACP alone and to conventional and high fluoride dentifrices (Reynolds *et al.* 2008). This synergy between CPP-ACP and fluoride had been identified in laboratory studies using Recaldent™ creams, which showed that preparations without fluoride remineralized initial enamel lesions better when applied as a topical coating after the use of a fluoride dentifrice (Kumar *et al.* 2008). In the absence of such "environmental" fluoride, the predominant mineral that will be formed in enamel subsurface lesions during remineralization with CPP-ACP will be hydroxyapatite.

It is now known that CPP can stabilize high concentrations of calcium, phosphate, and fluoride ions at all pH values from 4.5 up to 7.0, and the ability to remineralize enamel subsurface lesions was observed at all pH values in this range, with a maximal effect at pH 5.5 (Cochrane *et al.* 2008). In fact, at pH values below 5.5, CPP-ACFP produces greater remineralization than CPP-ACP, and the major product formed when remineralization is undertaken with CPP-ACFP is fluorapatite, which is highly resistant to acid dissolution. In either event it appears that mineral formation is optimized, since acid challenge of lesions after remineralization with CPP-ACP or CPP-ACFP gives demineralization underneath the remineralized zone, indicating that the remineralized mineral was more resistant to subsequent acid challenge (Iijima *et al.* 2004).

Treatment of white spot lesions

Because CPP-ACP nanocomplexes act as biological calcium phosphate delivery vehicles, they are able to boost levels of bio-available calcium and phosphate in saliva and plaque fluid without causing indiscriminate precipitation of calcium salts. This makes this material particularly effective in the remineralization of early enamel carious lesions (Figure 18-1) and in the treatment of other types of enamel opacities (shown also in subsequent figures) (Walsh 2007; Morgan *et al.* 2008).

Current treatment protocols using Recaldent™ tooth creams are based on the neutral ion species gaining access to the subsurface lesion through a porous enamel surface. This is the reason why arrested white spot lesions should have a surface etching treatment before remineralization with Recaldent™ topical creams. Such a treatment, either alone or combined with gentle pumicing, will remove approximately 30 microns of surface enamel but will not cause further mineral loss from the subsurface zone of the white spot lesion (Peariasamy *et al.* 2001).

Unlike fluoride treatments with conventional dentifrices (1,000 ppm) that deposit surface mineral but do not eliminate a white spot lesion (Al-Khateeb *et al.* 2000), Recaldent™ has been shown to cause regression of lesions, with a large-scale 2-year clinical trial with 2,720 adolescent subjects demonstrating regression of proximal carious lesions on sequential standardized digital bitewing radiographs. Those chewing the CPP-ACP gum were also less likely to show caries progression of approximal caries relative to a control sugar-free gum (Morgan *et al.* 2008).

Early case reports of using 10% CPP-ACP cream to achieve visible reversal of enamel white spot lesions (WSL) in young adult patients in Australia (Walsh 2003; Walsh 2007a) and later in Japan (Reynolds and Walsh 2005; Walsh 2007b), Europe (Ardu *et al.* 2007), and North America (Milnar 2007) have been followed by randomized controlled clinical trials in patients with naturally occurring WSL (Andersson *et al.* 2007; Bailey *et al.* 2009; Zhou *et al.* 2009). By the end of 2010, nine such clinical trials had been conducted across a range of locations: Melbourne, Brisbane, Tokyo, Halmstad, Changchun, and Istanbul. Each of these had shown regression of WSL by topical CPP-ACP cream, bringing this application to prominence in clinical practice. In all of these studies, remineralization of WSL by CPP-ACP was accompanied by improved translucency and reduced opacity of the white spot lesions, which occurred gradually as reversal occurs and mineral content increases.

It is now realized that optimal treatment results for WSL are obtained when pre-treatment is undertaken to maximize the penetration of ions into the deeper parts of

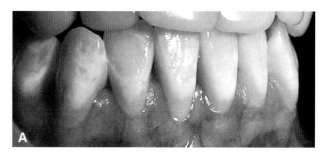
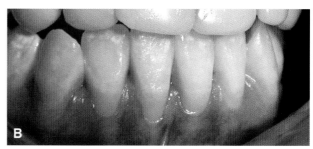
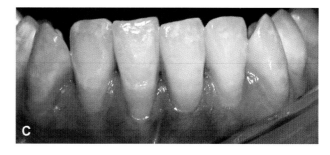
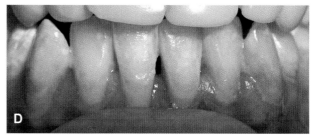

Figure 18-1 Visible reversal of carious white spot lesions (WSL) using topical CPP-ACP crème (GC MI Paste ™ / Tooth Mousse ™). A, Baseline situation in an irradiated xerostomic cancer patient who developed extensive areas of decalcification during a period of prolonged hospitalization. After discharge the patient had been placed on an intensive preventive program which included a high dose fluoride dentifrice, which had arrested the lesions. B, Two 30 second acid etching treatments were undertaken to increase surface porosity of the lesions, and CPP-ACP crème applied onto the teeth with a finger each night before retiring, for 7 months, and then discontinued. Visible reversal of WSL can be seen at the 7 month review appointment. C, A clinical review after a further six months shows the short-term stability of the result. D, The 2 year post-treatment situation. The treated enamel retained a normal appearance during a further 4 years of follow-up.

the enamel lesion. For inactive WSL (which typically have a shiny surface), pre-treatment is recommended, which can be in the form of a 15-second etch with 37% orthophosphoric acid, etching combined with gentle micro-abrasion (using fine flour of pumice), or the application of carbamide or hydrogen peroxide in an in-office bleaching procedure (Figure 18-1). Active WSLs, which have a frosty surface, do not require pre-treatment; however, it is important that patients remove gross deposits of plaque from the area before applying the cream.

Although bleaching appears to be an effective method of deproteinating the surface of WSL to increase porosity inter-prismatically, and is a viable alternative to acid etching, there is considerable scope to develop other methods to enhance penetration and increase the surface porosity (Cochrane *et al.* 2010).

Cases of reversal of moderate fluorosis using topical CPP-ACP cream have also been presented (Figure 18-2 and Figure 18-3) (Walsh 2003; Reynolds and Walsh 2005; Walsh 2007a; Ng and Manton 2007), as well as reversal of

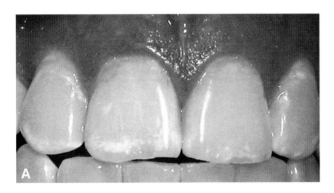

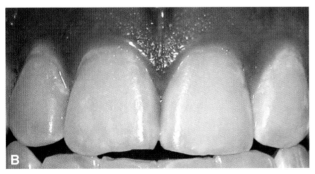

Figure 18-2 CPP-ACP topical treatment of mild fluorosis. A, Baseline clinical situation, showing a typical "snow-capping" pattern of opacity on the incisal third of the labial enamel of the teeth. The labial enamel surfaces of all anterior teeth were then treated using a 3 minute etch with orthophosphoric acid under constant agitation, followed by gentle application of fine flour of pumice using a rubber prophylaxis cup at 1400 rpm for 20 seconds per tooth. The patient applied CPP-ACP crème to the teeth each night for 4 weeks. B, Clinical situation after 4 weeks, with no opacities evident.

developmental white spots caused by altered enamel mineralization (Figure 18-4 and Figure 18-5), and post-eruptive opacities due to excessive bleaching (Walsh 2007a; Walsh 2007b; Walsh 2008a). Such treatments can be undertaken in a series of stages, with prolonged etching (3 minutes with 37% orthophosphoric acid) followed by pumice microabrasion of the enamel repeated at 4- to 6-week intervals several times until the desired effect is achieved. The patient applies CPP-ACP cream daily during the treatment. Fortunately, CPP-ACP treatment does not affect bleaching or interfere with bonding of resin composites to tooth structure (Adebayo, Burrow, and Tyas 2008; Adebayo *et al.* 2009), allowing topical treatments of enamel lesions to be incorporated into a range of esthetic dental treatments.

Clinical applications and protocols

In most preventive protocols, topical cream containing CPP-ACP is applied daily in a pea-size amount using a clean finger to the labial surfaces of the teeth immediately before bed (Figure 18-4). By dissolving slowly, the material contributes bioavailable calcium and phosphates to the saliva, and is able to promote remineralization at a time when salivary defenses are at their lowest point.

A home bleaching tray can also be used to apply the cream, as an alternative to using the finger application technique. The tray containing the cream should be held in place for 5 minutes, then removed, and the tongue used to spread the cream across the tooth surfaces. The mixture of saliva and topical cream should be retained in the mouth for a further 3 minutes before expectoration. The rationale for this is to allow sufficient contact between the saliva and the material, which facilitates release of ions.

The release of ions from topical CPP-ACP creams at neutral pH is rapid, with calcium ion release into water occurring in a saturating exponential manner, with approximately 95% release after 15 minutes. Because of this rapid release, when the cream is applied to tooth surfaces there will be a rapid increase in calcium ion concentration in the plaque fluid and saliva. Their supersaturation for calcium with respect to tooth enamel drives remineralization and prevents mineral loss. The level of water-soluble calcium released from MI Paste™ or MI Paste Plus™ topical creams (321.8 ± 2.6 μmol/g) is some 14 times or greater than that from NovaMin®, Clinpro™ Tooth Crème, Clinpro™ 5000, and Remin Pro, as shown in tests by several research groups conducted during 2009 and 2010 using both neutral and acidic solutions to trigger ion release.

Topical CPP-ACP creams without fluoride can be used in patients of all ages because the material is

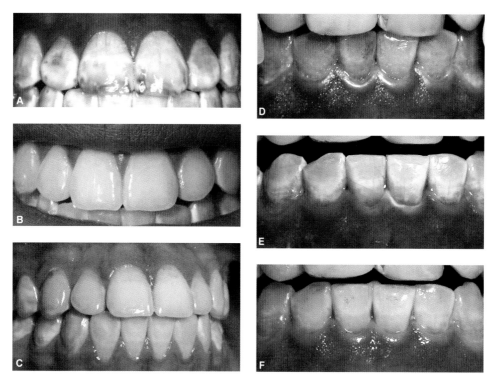

Figure 18-3 Topical CPP-ACP treatment of moderate fluorosis. A, Initial presentation of moderate fluorosis, with intense opacity of the enamel and some surface pitting. The patient underwent three etching/microabrasion treatments of the maxillary and mandibular anterior teeth, and applied CPP-ACP crème each night to the labial surfaces of all teeth. B and C, Clinical situation after 18 months. This result has been stable over the following 8 years. Note the less dramatic treatment outcome on the bicuspids, which did not undergo surface preparation. D, Baseline situation in a patient with moderate fluorosis and intense intrinsic discolouration from tetracycline. Because of the tetracycline staining, the fluorosis is not easy to identify. E, The fluorosis is readily evident once the tetracycline compounds have been eliminated by in-office power bleaching using a photodynamic laser method (KTP laser with Smartbleach ™ gel). The bleaching treatment creates sufficient surface porosity that no further surface treatment of the teeth. A small area of gingival irritation is present on the mandibular left central incisor which is caused by the gel used with the laser treatment. The patient applied CPP-ACP crème each night for 4 weeks after the in-office bleaching treatment. F, The opacities are fully reversed after 4 weeks. Figures 18-3 a and b from Reynolds & Walsh (2005) are used with permission from Knowledge Books and Software.

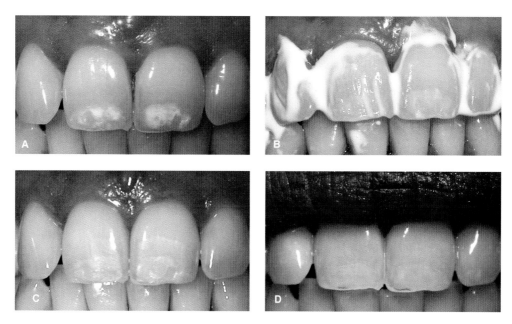

Figure 18-4 Topical CPP-ACP treatment of diffuse enamel opacities on both maxillary central incisors caused by a localized disturbance to enamel formation. A, Initial clinical situation. B, The areas were etched for 30 seconds and subjected to mild abrasion using pumice. The patient then applied CPP-ACP crème each night to the teeth. An initial treatment was undertaken in the dental office. C, The situation has improved considerably at the 4 week review. A further etching/microabrasion step was performed at this stage, and the patient continued the CPP-ACP treatment for a further 2 weeks. D, Final result after 6 weeks of daily treatment.

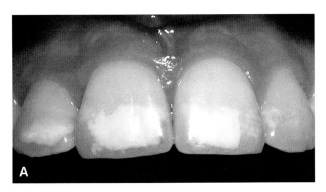

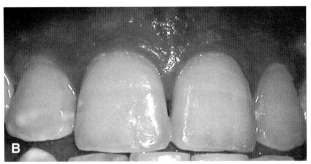

Figure 18-5 Topical CPP-ACP treatment of well demarcated enamel opacities caused by a systemic factor which influenced enamel formation. A, Initial clinical situation showing intense opacities on all maxillary incisors. The areas were etched for 30 seconds and subjected to mild abrasion using pumice. The patient then applied CPP-ACP crème each night to the teeth for a total of 12 months. The surface preparation treatment was repeated at six months. B, Final result at the 12 month review. Some faint opacities remain on the right lateral incisor. The enamel of the remaining teeth appears completely normal.

classified as safe to ingest. Topical CPP-ACP creams containing fluoride are used where indicated in children aged 7 years and above.

Etching and gentle enamel microabrasion followed by topical CPP-ACP cream has been shown to exert subtle effects on the optics of human enamel. This tooth-lightening concept is based on enhanced reflection of short wavelength (blue) reflection and scatter of enamel, and reduced enamel transmission of yellow light and absorption of red light (Walsh 2008b). This procedure can precede in-office or at-home whitening treatments, to establish optimal enamel properties and aesthetics, or can follow other cosmetic treatments.

Desensitizing cervical dentin

Emerging literature regarding the use of topical CPP-ACP products for treating cervical dentinal hypersensitivity exists, with five randomized controlled trials now having been undertaken. Together, these demonstrated that daily application of topical cream containing CPP-ACP reduced sensitivity to air, osmotic, thermal, and

tactile stimuli, with an effectiveness equal to that of potassium nitrate dentifrice (Walsh 2010).

CPP-ACP in chewing gums

The inclusion of CPP-ACP in chewing gums (such as Recaldent® and Trident Xtra Care®) is an effective caries preventive measure. Early studies of this approach used *in situ* studies (Cai *et al.* 2003) and then progressed to randomized, double blind cross-over designs to compare gums containing CPP-ACP with several commercial sugar-free gums. Subjects in these studies chewed the various gums for a 20-minute period four times per day for 14 days. By using paired enamel half slabs, precise determinations of mineral levels could be made. These studies showed that CPP-ACP gum produced 75–107% more remineralization than sugar-free gums. It is well known that xylitol-based gums reduce the caries increment but have little or no effect on approximal caries. In contrast, gums containing CPP-ACP are highly effective at remineralizing WSL, and were shown to arrest and reverse approximal lesions in a large-scale clinical trial involving more than 2,900 subjects (Morgan *et al.* 2008).

Recaldent® gum is ideally suited to both child and adult patients where a lifestyle activity is linked to sub-clinical dehydration, and the patient suffers the problems from depressed salivary pH and flow under resting conditions (Walsh 2007c). Because gum can be incorporated into a range of outdoor and exerting activities, the introduction of Recaldent® gum should be considered for patients who undertake strenuous activity, for example, outdoor exercise, outdoor work, or gym training sessions (Walsh 2007d). The timing is important since the stimulation of salivary flow achieved by the gum will occur at a time when otherwise resting flow and pH would be depressed. Recaldent® gum provides an excellent preventive effect, and is easily incorporated into a busy modern lifestyle.

Disclosure

In addition to serving as product consultant for Colgate and Johnsons and Johnson, Dr. Walsh has served as a paid consultant for GC Australasia to develop educational materials relating to CPP-ACP and as a paid guest lecturer for GC America in US dental schools on topics related to diagnostics, minimally invasive dentistry, and preventive dentistry. He developed the MI Paste protocols in his private practice, which GC America uses with permission but without additional remuneration. Dr. Walsh receives royalties for other GC America diagnostic products that he invented. A research group in 2010 at Dr. Walsh's dental school received competitive research funds to assist the Co-operative Research

Centre for Oral Health in Melbourne, where MI Paste and its predecessor Tooth Mousse was developed, to conduct additional studies on CPP-ACP technology.

References

Adebayo, O.A., Burrow, M.F., Tyas M.J. (2008) Dentine bonding after CPP-ACP paste treatment with and without conditioning. *Journal of Dentistry*, 36, 1013–1024.

Adebayo, O.A., Burrow, M.F., Tyas M.J. (2009) An SEM evaluation of conditioned and bonded enamel following carbamide peroxide bleaching and casein phosphopeptide-amorphous calcium phosphate (CPP-ACP) treatment. *Journal of Dentistry*, 37, 297–306.

Aiuchi, H., Kitasako, Y., Fukuda, Y., *et al.* (2008) Relationship between quantitative assessments of salivary buffering capacity and ion activity product for hydroxyapatite in relation to cariogenic potential. *Australian Dental Journal*, 53, 167–171.

Al-Khateeb, S., Exterkate, R., Angmar-Månsson, B., *et al.* (2000) Effect of acid-etching on remineralization of enamel white spot lesions. *Acta Odontologica Scandinavica*, 58, 31–36.

Anderson, J.R., Ellis, R.W., Blankenau, R.J., *et al.* (2000) Caries resistance in enamel by laser irradiation and topical fluoride treatment. *Journal of Clinical Laser Medicine and Surgery*, 18, 33–36.

Andersson, A., Skold-Larsson, K., Hallgren, A., *et al.* (2007) Effect of a dental cream containing amorphous cream phosphate complexes on white spot lesion regression assessed by laser fluorescence. *Oral Health and Preventive Dentistry*, 7, 229–233.

Ardu, S. Castioni, N.V., Benbachir, N., *et al.* (2007) Minimally invasive treatment of white spot enamel lesions. *Quintessence International* 38, 633–636.

Bailey, D.L., Adams, G.G., Tsao, C.E. *et al.* (2009) Regression of post-orthodontic lesions by a remineralizing cream. *Journal of Dental Research*, 88, 1148–1153.

Blankenau, R.J., Powell, G.L., Ellis, R.W., *et al.* (1999) *In vivo* caries-like lesion prevention with argon laser: pilot study. *Journal of Clinical Laser Medicine and Surgery*, 17, 241–243.

Cai, F., Shen, P., Morgan, M.V. *et al.* (2003) Remineralization of enamel subsurface lesions *in situ* by sugar-free lozenges containing casein phosphopeptide-amorphous calcium phosphate. *Australian Dental Journal*, 48, 240–243.

Caruana, P.C., Mulaify, S.A., Moazzez, R., *et al.* (2009) The effect of casein and calcium containing paste on plaque pH following a subsequent carbohydrate challenge. *Journal of Dentistry*, 37, 522–526.

Charig, A., Winston, A., Flickinger, M. (2004) Enamel mineralization by calcium-containing-bicarbonate toothpastes: assessment by various techniques. *Compendium of Continuing Education in Dentistry*, 25 (Suppl 1), 14–24.

Clarkson, B.H., Chang, S.R., Holland, G.R. (1998) Phosphoprotein analysis of sequential extracts of human dentin and the determination of the subsequent remineralization potential of these dentin matrices. *Caries Research*, 32, 357–364.

Cochrane, N.J., Cai, F., Huq, N.L. *et al.* (2010) New approaches to enhanced remineralization of tooth enamel. *Journal of Dental Research*, 89, 1187–1197.

Cochrane, N.J., Saranathan, S., Cai, F., *et al.* (2008) Enamel subsurface lesion remineralisation with casein phosphopeptide stabilised solutions of calcium, phosphate and fluoride. *Caries Research*, 42, 88–97.

Cross, K.J., Huq, N.L., Palamara, J.E., *et al.* (2005) Physicochemical characterization of casein phosphopeptide-amorphous calcium phosphate nanocomplexes. *Journal of Biological Chemistry*, 280, 15362–15369.

Cross, K.J., Huq, N.L., Reynolds, E.C. (2007) Casein phosphopeptides in oral health—chemistry and clinical applications. *Current Pharmaceutical Design*, 13, 793–800.

Cross, K.J., Huq, N.L., Stanton, D.P., *et al.* (2004) NMR studies of a novel calcium, phosphate and fluoride delivery vehicle-alpha(S1)-casein(59–79) by stabilized amorphous calcium fluoride phosphate nanocomplexes. *Biomaterials*, 25, 5061–5069.

Featherstone, J.D., Barrett-Vespone, N.A., Fried, D., *et al.* (1998) CO_2 laser inhibitor of artificial caries-like lesion progression in dental enamel. *Journal of Dental Research*, 77, 1397–1403.

Flaitz, C.M., Hicks, M.J., Westerman, G.H., *et al.* (1995) Argon laser irradiation and acidulated phosphate fluoride treatment in caries-like lesion formation in enamel: an *in vitro* study. *Pediatric Dentistry*, 17, 31–35.

Goharkay, K., Wernisch, J., Schoop, U., *et al.* (2007) Laser treatment of hypersensitive dentine: comparative ESEM investigations. *Journal of Oral Laser Applications*, 7, 211–223.

Hicks, M.J., Flaitz, C.M., Westerman, G.H., *et al.* (1993) Caries-like lesion initiation and progression in sound enamel following argon laser irradiation: an *in vitro* study. *Journal of Dentistry for Children*, 60, 201–206.

Hicks, M.J., Flaitz, C.M., Westerman, G.H., *et al.* (1995) Enamel caries initiation and progression following low fluence (energy) argon laser and fluoride treatment. *Journal of Clinical Pediatric Dentistry*, 20, 9–13.

Hicks, M.J., Flaitz, C.M., Westerman, G.H., *et al.* (1997) Root caries *in vitro* after low fluence argon laser and fluoride treatment. *Compendium of Continuing Education in Dentistry*, 18, 543–548.

Hicks, J., Garcia-Godoy, F., Flaitz, C. (2004) Biological factors in dental caries: role of remineralization and fluoride in the dynamic process of demineralization and remineralization (part 3). *Journal of Clinical Pediatric Dentistry*, 28, 203–214.

Hossain, M.M., Hossain, M., Kimura, Y., *et al.* (2002) Acquired acid resistance of enamel and dentin by CO_2 laser irradiation with sodium fluoride solution. *Journal of Clinical Laser Medicine and Surgery*, 20, 77–82.

Iijima, Y., Cai, F., Shen, P., *et al.* (2004) Acid resistance of enamel subsurface lesions remineralized by a sugar-free chewing gum containing casein phosphopeptide-amorphous calcium phosphate. *Caries Research*, 38, 551–556.

Ingram, G.S., Agalamanyi, E.A., Higham, S.M. (2005) Caries and fluoride processes. *Journal of Dentistry*, 33, 187–191.

Karlinsey, R.L. and Mackey, A.C. (2009) Solid-state preparation and dental application of an organically modified calcium phosphate. *Journal of Material Science*, 44, 346–349.

Kumar, V.L., Itthagarun, A., King, N.M. (2008) The effect of casein phosphopeptide-amorphous calcium phosphate on remineralization of artificial caries-like lesions: an *in vitro* study. *Australian Dental Journal*, 53, 34–40.

Litkowski, L.J., Quinlan, K.B., Ross, D.R., *et al.* (2004) Intraoral evaluation of mineralization of cosmetic defects by a toothpaste containing calcium, fluoride, and sodium bicarbonate. *Compendium of Continuing Education in Dentistry*, 25 (Suppl 1), 25–31.

Llena, C., Forner, L., Baca, P. (2009) Anticariogenicity of casein phosphopeptide-amorphous calcium phosphate: a review of the literature. *Journal of Contemporary Dental Practice*, 10, 1–9.

Lussi, A., Megert, B., Eggenberger, D., *et al.* (2008) Impact of different toothpastes on the prevention of erosion. *Caries Research*, 42, 62–67.

Lynch, R.J. and ten Cate, J.M. (2005) The anti-caries efficacy of calcium carbonate-based fluoride toothpastes. *International Dental Journal*, 55 (Suppl 1), 175–178.

Magalhães, A.C., Furlani, T.A., Italiani. F.M., *et al.* (2007) Effect of calcium pre-rinse and fluoride dentifrice on remineralisation of artificially demineralised enamel and on the composition of the dental biofilm formed in situ. *Archives of Oral Biology*, 52, 1155–1160.

Manton, D.J., Walker, G.D., Cai, F., *et al.* (2008) Remineralization of enamel subsurface lesions in situ by the use of three commercially available sugar-free gums. *International Journal of Paediatric Dentistry*, 18, 284–290.

Meyers, I.A. (2008) Diagnosis and management of the worn dentition: risk management and prerestorative strategies for the oral and dental environment. *Annals of the Royal Australasian College of Dental Surgeons*, 19, 27–30.

Milnar, F.J. (2007) Considering biomodification and remineralization techniques as adjuncts to vital tooth-bleaching regimens. *Compendium of Continuing Education in Dentistry*, 28, 234–240.

Morgan, M.V., Adams, G.G., Bailey, D.L., *et al.* (2008) The anticariogenic effect of sugar-free gum containing CPP-ACP nanocomplexes on approximal caries determined using digital bitewing radiography. *Caries Research*, 42, 171–184.

Nammour, S., Demortier, G., Florio, P., *et al.* (2003) Increase of enamel fluoride retention by low fluence argon laser *in vivo*. *Lasers in Surgery and Medicine*, 33, 260–263.

Ng, F. and Manton D.J. (2007) Aesthetic management of severely fluorosed incisors in an adolescent female. *Australian Dental Journal*, 52, 243–248.

Papas, A., Russell, D., Singh, M., *et al.* (1999) Double blind clinical trial of a remineralizing dentifrice in the prevention of caries in a radiation therapy population. *Gerodontology*, 16, 2–10.

Papas, A., Russell, D., Singh, M., *et al.* (2008) Caries clinical trial of a remineralizing toothpaste in radiation patients. *Gerodontology*, 25, 76–88.

Peariasamy, K., Anderson, P., Brook, A.H. (2001) A quantitative study of the effect of pumicing and etching on the remineralisation of enamel opacities. *International Journal of Paediatric Dentistry*, 11, 193–200.

Piekarz, C., Ranjitkar, S., Hunt, D. *et al.* (2008) An *in vitro* assessment of the role of Tooth Mousse in preventing wine erosion. *Australian Dental Journal*, 53, 22–25.

Ramilingham, L., Messer, L.B., Reynolds, E.C. (2005) Adding casein phosphopeptide-amorphous calcium phosphate to sports drinks to eliminate *in vitro* erosion. *Pediatric Dentistry*, 27, 61–67.

Ranjitkar, S., Kaidonis, J.A., Richards, L.C., *et al.* (2009) The effect of CPP-ACP on enamel wear under severe erosive conditions. *Archives of Oral Biology*, 54, 527–532.

Rao, S.K., Bhat, G.S, Aradhya, S., *et al.* (2009) Study of the efficacy of toothpaste containing casein phosphopeptide in the prevention of dental caries: a randomized controlled trial in 12- to 15-year-old high caries risk children in Bangalore, India. *Caries Research*, 43, 430–435.

Reynolds, E.C. (1997) Remineralization of enamel subsurface lesions by casein phosphopeptide-stabilized calcium phosphate solutions. *Journal of Dental Research*, 76, 1587–1595.

Reynolds, E.C. (1998) Anticariogenic complexes of amorphous calcium phosphate stabilized by casein phosphopeptides: a review. *Special Care in Dentistry*, 18, 8–16.

Reynolds, E.C. (2008) Calcium phosphate-based remineralization systems: scientific evidence? *Australian Dental Journal*, 53, 268–273.

Reynolds, E.C. (2009) Casein phosphopeptide-amorphous calcium phosphate: the scientific evidence. *Advances in Dental Research*, 21, 25–29.

Reynolds, E.C., Cai, F., Cochrane, N.J., *et al.* (2008) Fluoride and casein phosphopeptide-amorphous calcium phosphate. *Journal of Dental Research*, 87, 344–348.

Reynolds, E.C., Cai, F., Shen, P., *et al.* (2003) Retention in plaque and remineralization of enamel lesions by various forms of calcium in a

mouthrinse or sugar-free chewing gum. *Journal of Dental Research*, 82, 206–211.

Reynolds, E.C., Cai, F., Shen, P. *et al.* (2010) Comparison of Tooth Mousse (MI Paste) with Clinpro in situ. *Journal of Dental Research*, 89 (Sp Iss B), 3645. (www.dentalresearch.org)

Reynolds, E.C. and Walsh, L.J. (2005) Additional aids to the remineralization of tooth structure. In: Preservation and Restoration of Tooth Structure. (Eds. G.J. Mount and W.R. Hume, 2nd edn. pp. 111–118. Knowledge Books and Software. Brighton Queensland AU).

Sullivan, R.J., Charig, A., Blake-Haskins, J., *et al.* (1997) *In vivo* detection of calcium from dicalcium phosphate dihydrate dentifrices in demineralized human enamel and plaque. *Advances in Dental Research*, 11, 380–387.

Tagomori, S. and Morioka, T. (1989) Combined effects of laser and fluoride on acid resistance of human dental enamel. *Caries Research*, 23, 225–231.

Thompson, A., Grant, L.P., Tanzer, J.M. (1999) Model for assessment of carious lesion remineralization, and remineralization by a novel toothpaste. *Journal of Clinical Dentistry*, 10 (Spec Iss 1), 34–39.

Tung, M.S. and Eichmiller, F.C. (1999) Dental applications of amorphous calcium phosphates. *Journal of Clinical Dentistry*, 10 (Sp Iss 1), 1–6.

Tung, M.S. and Eichmiller, F.C. (2004) Amorphous calcium phosphates for tooth remineralization. *Compendium of Continuing Education in Dentistry*, 25 (Suppl 1), 9–13.

Vlacic, J. (2007) *In vivo* and *in vitro* investigations of laser and non-laser therapies in treatment of root surface erosion and root surface caries. PhD thesis, The University of Queensland, Brisbane, AU.

Vlacic, J., Meyers, I.A., Kim, J., *et al.* (2007a) Laser-activated fluoride treatment of enamel against an artificial caries challenge: comparison of five wavelengths. *Australian Dental Journal*, 52, 101–105.

Vlacic, J., Meyers, I.A., Walsh, L.J. (2007b) Laser-activated fluoride treatment of enamel as prevention against erosion. *Australian Dental Journal*, 52, 175–180.

Vlacic, J., Meyers, I.A., Walsh, L.J. (2007c) Combined CPP-ACP and photoactivated disinfection (PAD) therapy in arresting root surface caries: a case report. *British Dental Journal*, 203, 457–459.

Vlacic, J., Meyers, I.A., Walsh, L.J. (2008) Photonic conversion of hydroxyapapite to fluorapatite: a possible mechanism for laser-activated fluoride therapy. *Journal of Oral Laser Applications*, 8, 95–102.

Vogel, G.L., Zhang, Z., Carey, C.M., *et al.* (1998) Composition of plaque and saliva following a sucrose challenge and use of an alpha-tricalcium-phosphate-containing chewing gum. *Journal of Dental Research*, 77, 518–524.

Walker, G., Cai, F., Shen, P., *et al.* (2006) Increased remineralization of tooth enamel by milk containing added casein phosphopeptide-amorphous calcium phosphate. *Journal of Dairy Research*, 73, 74–78.

Walsh, L.J. (1994) Clinical evaluation of dental hard tissue applications of carbon dioxide lasers. *Journal of Clinical Laser Medicine and Surgery*, 12, 11–15.

Walsh, L.J. (2003). Tooth Mousse Portfolio. GC Asia Dental Pte Ltd. Singapore.

Walsh, L.J. (2007a) Tooth Mouse: anthology of applications. GC Asia Pte Ltd. Singapore.

Walsh, L.J. (2007b) White spots. GC Asia Dental Pte Ltd. Singapore.

Walsh, L.J. (2007c) Clinical aspects of salivary biology for the dental clinician. *International Dentistry*, 2, 16–30.

Walsh, L.J. (2007d) Clinical applications of Recaldent products: which ones to use where. *Australasian Dental Practice*, 18, 144–146.

Walsh, L.J. (2008a) Application of the System for Total Environmental Management (STEM) to dysmineralization, dental erosion and tooth wear. *Australasian Dental Practice*, 19, 52–58.

Walsh, L.J. (2008b) Tooth lightening: a new concept for maximizing surface aesthetics. *Australasian Dental Practice*, 19, 48–50.

Walsh, L.J. (2010) The effects of GC Tooth Mousse on cervical dentinal sensitivity: a controlled clinical trial. *International Dentistry*, 5, 16–23.

Weerakoon, A.T., Meyers, I.A., Symons, A.L., *et al.* (2002) Pulpal heat changes with newly developed resin photopolymerization systems. *Australian Endodontic Journal*, 28, 108–111.

Westerman, G.H., Flaitz, C.M., Powell, G.L., *et al.* (2002) Enamel caries initiation and progression after argon laser irradiation: *in vitro* argon laser systems comparison. *Journal of Clinical Laser Medicine and Surgery*, 20, 257–262.

Westerman, G.H., Hicks, M.J., Flaitz, C.M., *et al.* (1994) Argon laser irradiation in root surface caries: *in vitro* study examines laser's effects. *Journal of the American Dental Association*, 125, 401–407.

Westerman, G.H., Hicks, M.J., Flaitz, C.M., *et al.* (1999) Combined effects of acidulated phosphate fluoride and argon laser on sound root surface morphology: an *in vitro* scanning electron microscopy study. *Journal of Clinical Laser Medicine and Surgery,* 17, 63–68.

Yengopal, V. and Mickenautsch, S. (2009) Caries preventive effect of casein phosphopeptide-amorphous calcium phosphate (CPP-ACP): a meta-analysis. *Acta Odontologica Scandinavica*, 21, 1–12.

Zhang, C., Kimura, Y., Matsumoto, K. (1996) The effects of pulsed Nd:YAG laser irradiation with fluoride on root surface. *Journal of Clinical Laser Medicine and Surgery*, 14, 399–403.

Zhou, C.H., Sun, X.H., Zhu, X.C. (2009) Quantification of remineralized effect of casein phosphopeptiode-amorphous calcium phosphate on post-orthodontic white spot lesion. *Shanghai Kou Qiang Yi Xue*, 18, 449–454.

19

Oral health promotion in infants and preschool age children

Gajanan Vishwanath (Kiran) Kulkarni

Introduction

The majority of oral and dental problems encountered in children are completely preventable. Problems that are not preventable usually have a genetic or systemic component. Fortunately, these problems occur infrequently. The focus of this chapter is on oral health promotion in young children. Development of good oral health in children starts with a healthy pregnancy and continues right from birth through infancy, toddlerhood, and all of the preschool years. Preliminary evidence from ongoing research suggests that an individual's pattern of adult health/disease might be set in early childhood from unique combinations of genetic predisposition and environmental exposures during early development. This underscores the importance of maintaining good oral health from birth.

The most common oral problems encountered in young children

The most common oral problems encountered by young children can be broadly categorized into four areas. In decreasing order of frequency of occurrence, they are as follows:

Dental caries and associated infections (Figure 19-1)
Malocclusions arising from oral habits (Figure 19-2)
Injuries to the mouth and teeth (Figure 19-3)
Oral and dental pathology of developmental origin (Figure 19-4)

The problems listed above are in descending order of frequency. The vast majority of dental visits where

definitive dental treatment is needed arise from primary teeth being affected by dental caries or the sequelae of advanced dental caries. Sequelae include pulpitis from deep caries and periapical infections that may lead to more extensive infections manifesting as facial cellulitis. From the above four categories, it is important to appreciate that except for problems of developmental origin, most problems are preventable.

Prevention of oral problems

Strategies for parents

Ensuring good oral health in children starts with a healthy pregnancy. Good parental health, especially maternal health during pregnancy, is essential for normal development of the oral cavity including the primary and permanent teeth. For example, smoking by the mother during pregnancy is a well-known risk factor for the development of oral clefts (Chung et al. 2000), which in turn is a risk factor for dental caries (Tanaka et al. 2010). The relationship between smoking and dental caries in children was until recently shown to be an association (See also Chapter 1.) Children whose mothers smoked during pregnancy or those exposed to environmental tobacco smoke after birth have been shown to experience higher levels of dental caries (Aligne et al. 2003; Tanaka et al. 2010). More recent research suggests that components of tobacco smoke can alter organisms in the dental biofilm and thereby possibly render them more cariogenic (Zonuz et al. 2008). It is therefore incumbent upon parents to ensure that their unborn and born children are not exposed to tobacco products so as not to increase the risk of oral defects and dental caries.

Comprehensive Preventive Dentistry, First Edition. Edited by Hardy Limeback.
© 2012 John Wiley & Sons, Ltd. Published 2012 by John Wiley & Sons, Ltd.

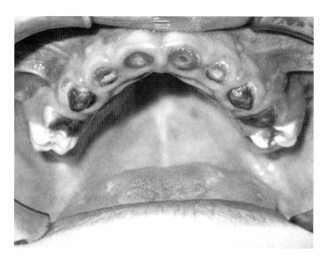

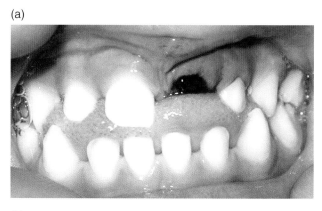

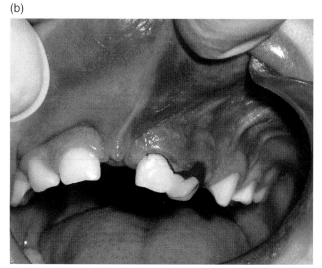

Figure 19-1 Severe early childhood caries showing several carious teeth associated with periapical infections.

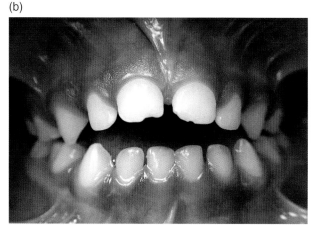

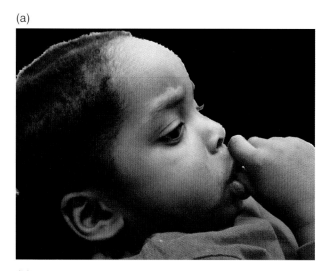

Figure 19-2 (a) Child engaging in the non-nutritive habit of thumb sucking. (b) Dental occlusion of the child in Figure 19-2a showing typical anterior open bite extending posteriorly to the first primary molars. Note that the open bite is more pronounced on the right, which is consistent with the right hand thumb engaged in the habit.

Figure 19-3 Injuries to the mouth and teeth. (a) Oral injury showing the maxillary left primary incisor intruded into the gums. Note that this injury can easily be mistaken for an avulsion injury where a tooth is knocked out of the socket. (b) Subluxation of primary teeth associated with alveolar fracture showing widespread soft tissue hematoma and gingival bleeding. In such cases of severe injury in young children, one must always rule out possible child abuse.

Strategies for all caregivers

Dental caries remains the most common oral problem in preschool age children. Dental caries is a bacterial disease. At birth the oral cavity is essentially sterile. Over time the oral cavity is colonized by bacteria that are acquired from the environment and from other human hosts. Bacteria that cause dental caries are usually passed from parent to child, usually the parent who is most in contact with the child during infancy and toddlerhood. The probability and timing of transfer of the bacteria from the parent's mouth to the mouth of the child are influenced by the levels of those bacteria in the parent's mouth. Higher levels of bacteria are found in individuals with multiple cavities and/or fillings or a generally poor state of oral hygiene. Bacteria in

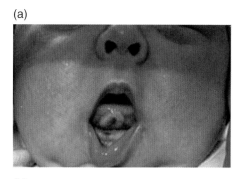

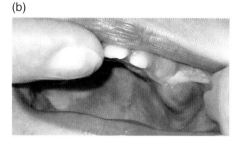

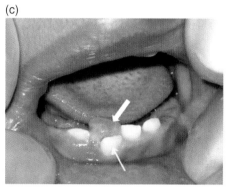

Figure 19-4 (a) Ulcer on the ventral surface of the tongue from the tongue rubbing on a prematurely erupted mandibular incisor in a neonate. (b) Bluish swelling overlying an erupting maxillary primary molar in a toddler. Termed eruption hematomas, these are benign, asymptomatic, and self-limiting entities that frequently alarm parents. (c) Large soft tissue mass (*white arrow*) in a 9-month old infant causing displacement of the mandibular left central incisor (*yellow arrow*). Such entities although rare, must receive prompt dental attention to restore normal oral and dental development.

saliva are transferred by directly kissing the baby on the mouth or sharing food or utensils. Therefore, parents can take the following steps to reduce the transfer of organisms:

- Maintain good oral hygiene themselves.
- Treat all active disease including cavities.
- Do not kiss the baby directly on the mouth.
- Do not share food or utensils with the baby.
- Reduce levels of bacteria in their own mouths by using mouthwashes or by chewing xylitol-containing gum.

Strategies for dental professionals

Dental professionals have several options at their disposal to prevent caries and treat incipient caries without resorting to conventional restorative treatments. Most in-office treatments involve the application of topical fluoride. These topical fluorides are available in varying strengths based on the fluoride concentrations, the vehicles containing the fluorides, and the modes of application. As a rule, these in-office topical fluoride products provide a high local concentration of ionic fluoride at the time of application, which is then sustained for several hours. For children with established caries or those determined to be at high risk for caries, the most effective form of topical fluoride has been shown to be fluoride varnish. Fluoride varnish typically contains 5% sodium fluoride in a synthetic varnish, which provides substantivity to the actions of fluoride.

Newer in-office products that are not fluoride based are currently being studied. One such product is a 2% chlorhexidine-containing varnish. At high concentration, chlorhexidine is bactericidal. When applied to teeth, the chlorhexidine varnish suppresses all oral bacteria including cariogenic bacteria. In a limited number of clinical trials and over a limited time period, this has been shown to be an effective strategy for preventing early childhood caries. The question of whether it is better to build resistance in the tooth via fluoride or reduce the caries challenge by suppressing cariogenic bacteria or have some combination of both approaches has yet to be definitively answered.

Public health measures

Most departments of public health have free screening programs for preschool-age children. In some jurisdictions, such screening programs are mandated by state governments. However, these programs do not usually address the needs of infants or their parents. Public health measures that can benefit young children include diet and nutrition counseling for prenatal and postnatal women and assistance with breastfeeding. There is still a lack of awareness among parents regarding feeding practices in infants and young children. Dental public health can play a significant role in raising the awareness among young parents about healthy snacks and especially the risks of drinks sweetened with sucrose in the very young. Campaigns for promoting the consumption of water or milk as alternatives to sweetened beverages can go a long way in reducing early childhood caries.

Public health can also contribute in the area of developing public policy regarding oral health and hygiene for preschool age children who are in full-day childcare. With the trend in public education toward early childhood learning, more and more young children are spending increasing amounts of time in classrooms and childcare centers. There is a lack of policies, guidelines, and support for implementation of oral hygiene routines for children of different ages in supervised care settings (Gartsbein *et al.* 2008; Gartsbein *et al.* 2009). A ten-point policy for such settings has been suggested by the author and is outlined in the following section.

An effective model for oral health promotion in infants and young children using the 'baby oral health: pregnancy through childhood' video

In-office and community-based models for oral health promotion

A unique model for oral health promotion from birth to preschool age has been developed and described in the literature (Alsada *et al.* 2005). The model is based on a video (Figure 19-5) developed by the author. It can be previewed at the following Website: http://www.utoronto.ca/dentistry/newsresources/kids/index.html.

The 'Baby Oral Health' video (Figure 19-5) contains the following chapters:

1. The AV Aid Contents
2. Healthy Pregnancy
3. Teeth Development
4. Nutrition
5. Oral Hygiene
6. Fluoride
7. Bacterial Transmission and Acquisition
8. Night Feeding Habits
9. Early Childhood Caries
10. Oral Habits
11. Prevention of Injuries
12. First Dental Visit
13. Regular Dental Visits

The video is short but covers all topics relevant to the oral health of infants and children. It also makes use of simple language to maintain audience attention and interest and to be as broad reaching as possible. The AV aid emphasizes the importance of a healthy pregnancy to the oral and dental health of the infant by informing the target audience about the timing of the development of primary teeth, the importance of a healthy diet, and the negative effects of nonprescription drugs, smoking, and alcoholic drinks. The literature has demonstrated a relation between smoking during pregnancy and low birth weight and between smoking in the household and increased risk of caries in children of those households. Congenital malformations that have been linked to the use of certain drugs and alcoholic drinks during

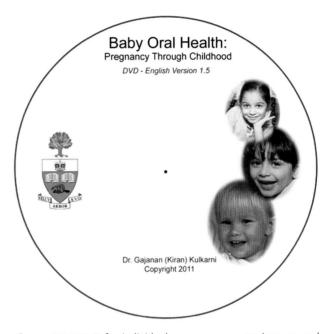

Figure 19-5 DVD for individual or group presentations on oral health promotion in infants and young children. Audiovisual aids such as this provide the simplest and most effective means of communicating dental concepts to lay parents.

pregnancy are also highlighted. The growth and development of baby teeth are illustrated with emphasis on the pattern of eruption, normal number of baby teeth, presence of primary spacing, and proximity to the underlying developing permanent teeth. Most laypersons do not appreciate the fact that permanent tooth development commences at or slightly before birth. Advice is provided for the management of teething, which is of significant concern to many parents.

The importance of a healthy diet and nutrition in keeping with the Canadian Health and Food Group Recommendations is stressed. The role of cariogenic food types in caries development is also illustrated. Proper oral hygiene practices are presented, starting with cleaning of edentulous alveolar ridges in infants with gauze to familiarize them with mouth-cleaning routines and to reduce the level of oral microorganisms. The position and techniques for infant oral hygiene are demonstrated. Also, facts regarding dental plaque are explained and visually reinforced with images of plaque on primary teeth after the application of a disclosing dye. The importance and appropriate use of fluoride are presented. Advice is provided regarding the appropriate timing of fluoride introduction in young children to maximize the preventive aspects while reducing the chances of fluoride toxicity. The audience is informed about the availability of fluoride in drinking water and advised to seek professional consultation when the local water supply is not fluoridated.

The transmission and acquisition of oral bacteria and the concept of this as an infectious disease is introduced. The audience is shown how practices such as kissing and sharing of eating utensils can promote caregiver-to-child transmission of oral bacteria. Parents and caregivers are also advised about the importance of maintaining their own good level of oral hygiene to minimize or delay the chance of their children being infected. Night bottle feeding and prolonged ad-lib breastfeeding, especially at night, with lack of appropriate oral hygiene, are identified as major causes of early childhood caries. Weaning to a sipping or regular cup is advised by 12 months of age. The audience is warned that ad-lib drinking from a sipping cup can also place the child at risk for dental caries. The causes of early childhood caries (ECC), complications, and the complexity and cost of treatment are graphically shown to increase the impact and retention of the information.

A short segment of the video deals with oral habits and their role in normal development, including the timing and need for intervention to prevent the development of permanent dental and skeletal effects. Specific measures for the prevention of orofacial trauma are presented as an integral part of overall prevention. Emphasis is placed on home safety, use of appropriate car seats, and protection during sports and outdoor play. Consequences of injuries to the oral region and primary teeth are shown.

As an essential part of oral health prevention, the importance of having a "dental home" for young children is explained. The American Academy of Pediatric Dentistry defines the dental home as the ongoing relationship between the dentist and the patient, inclusive of all aspects of oral health care delivered in a comprehensive, continuously accessible, coordinated, and family-centered way (Poranganel *et al.* 2006). Establishing the dental home starts with the baby's first dental visit. The rationale for and nature of the early first dental visit is explained and illustrated as it pertains to improving general health. The knee-to-knee examination position is shown as one approach that can be used when dealing with difficult young children. Although this AV aid was designed for self-directed, interactive education with distinct "chapters," we found that it is most effective when administered by a health professional in a directed learning setting. The educator can pause the video between segments to review material and address questions that might be raised. Audience participation can also be enhanced by inviting parents to relate their own experiences and expectations for their children.

The uniqueness of this approach to oral health promotion in very children lies in the fact that it provides

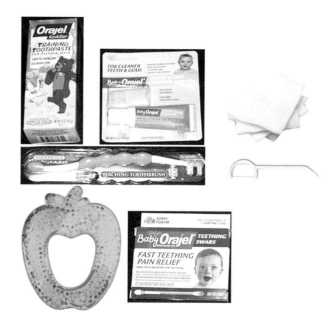

Figure 19-6 Oral health aids for infants and toddlers. Shown are 'Safe-to-Swallow' toothpaste, a combination of infant toothpaste and toothbrush worn on the parents' finger, disposable gauze pieces, dental flosser, teething ring, medication for easing the pain of teething.

comprehensive anticipatory guidance regarding oral health through a directed learning experience using an evidence-based audio-visual aid. The video provides standardized teaching for lay audiences and contains practical messages for parents to implement at home. This medium of 'edutainment' does not require active participation from the audience. As the information is visually vivid, it is widely accepted among diverse cultural and linguistic backgrounds for individual or group education sessions. The target audiences are parents, caregivers, and all professionals who interact with preschool-age children. This model can be easily learned and used by any health professional who deals with young children; it does not require specialized knowledge of dentistry. The novel features of the model are that it uses anticipatory guidance to focus the attention of young parents and direct caregivers on positive behaviors. It also promotes a broad approach to achieving overall oral health by preventing negative behaviors in a timely fashion.

The most effective mode of presentation to an audience follows the steps listed below:

1. Video introduced
2. Two to three segments shown then paused
3. Salient points reviewed and reemphasized
4. Audience asked to relate their experiences or to ask questions
5. Techniques and products (Figure 19-6) demonstrated

Answering questions about oral health of infants and toddlers, most frequently asked by parents

First-time parents frequently have questions or concerns regarding their children's oral health. Those questions/concerns generally follow the chapters in the 'Baby Oral Health video. Responses to those questions or concerns are provided below and are grouped under the headings that correspond to the segments that appear in the accompanying video. The answers are deliberately in non-technical language so that presenters with diverse professional backgrounds can use them verbatim and reach as wide an audience as possible. Some answers will change with improvement in our scientific understanding of issues, which in turn will influence public policies. Although some of the answers will change with time, health promoters should modify their responses bearing in mind that the answers meet the following criteria:

1. Be accurate, in accordance with current policies and guidelines
2. Must be comprehensive but not too lengthy
3. Not be academic, but in terms that lay parents can understand
4. Be practical, so that parents can put advice into practice
5. Be engaging

Growth and development of baby teeth

Can the mother's health during pregnancy affect the baby's mouth and teeth? How?

The baby's mouth and teeth start developing during early pregnancy. Certain problems during pregnancy can adversely affect the baby's mouth and teeth. A healthy pregnancy can be assured by having a well-balanced diet supplemented with prenatal vitamins as advised by the doctor. Smoking or drinking alcohol during pregnancy and taking some medications have been shown to predispose babies to certain oral and dental problems. One common example of such a birth defect is cleft lip and palate. It is advisable to ask your doctor before taking any medications. It is important for the mother to keep a healthy mouth, brush and floss every day, see the dentist regularly, and avoid sugary and sticky foods that may cause caries. The mother should also ensure that she does not have any cavities or gum problems that need urgent care or that are likely to get worse and require treatment during pregnancy. Certain oral conditions experienced by the mother during pregnancy have been shown to be associated with problems in the baby's health including the mouth and teeth.

When does the first baby tooth appear in the child's mouth?

The baby's first teeth usually appear around 6–7 months, but it can be much earlier or later (4–12 months). Typically, the bottom two front teeth appear first. Less frequently, the top two teeth appear first.

Can babies be born with teeth?

Rarely, babies are born with teeth. When they do appear, these teeth are called neo-natal or natal teeth. These teeth can occasionally cause problems with nursing and have to be removed.

How many baby teeth does a child get?

Normally the total number of baby or primary teeth is 20. However, a small percentage, about 1–2% of children are born with missing teeth or with additional teeth. Missing baby teeth frequently are associated with missing permanent teeth. Additional baby teeth are not necessarily associated with additional permanent teeth. Both missing teeth and additional teeth can lead to problems with the development of proper occlusion in the permanent teeth and should be monitored by dental professionals and treated at the appropriate times to minimize the impact on the permanent bite.

When should a parent be concerned about the late growth of baby teeth?

It is not uncommon for some babies to get their teeth later. They can be delayed by as much as a year. One should consult a dentist if the teeth are delayed by more than a year or if you are otherwise concerned. If the teeth haven't started growing or cannot be felt under the gums, the dentist might consider taking an X-ray to confirm that the teeth are present. There are a few rare but serious conditions that are associated with either late or non-development of baby teeth. One such condition is called ectodermal dysplasia where children grow few if any teeth, and those that grow are abnormal.

Why do babies drool?

Drooling is normal. It usually starts around 2–3 months. Babies use their mouth and tongue to experience the environment early in life before their senses of smell, sight, and touch develop to the point that they do not need to use their mouth. Therefore, the tongue is forward in the mouth. Saliva production is stimulated during teething, which coincides with their drooling. Also their swallowing has not matured, so the saliva tends to pool in the mouth and dribble out. Drooling gradually stops as the front teeth grow, the tongue goes further back in the mouth, and the infant learns to swallow. Drooling beyond a certain age could be a sign of delayed development and should be checked by a physician.

My child is three and a half years old and has an underbite. Do we need to worry?

You should have your child's bite checked by a specialist who is experienced in such problems because these are not common or routinely treated by all dentists. Some underbites are best treated early, even during the child's baby teeth stages if the child can cooperate with the treatment. Many of these treatments work best in young children when their jaws are developing. Moreover correcting the bite back to normal will give them the best possibility of developing a normal bite as they transition into their permanent teeth.

Diet and Nutrition

What are foods or snacks that can affect a child's baby and adult teeth?

In general, foods that have natural sugar or cooked starch can affect teeth, especially if eaten frequently and in between meals. Examples of healthy snacks include fruits and vegetables, unsweetened milk, yogurt, cheese, and other dairy products. In older children, nuts and seeds can be excellent snacks. Some examples of snack foods that are not tooth friendly include sticky candies and cookies, bread with sweet jams and jellies, and potato chips. The child's eating of these snack foods should be monitored by the parents, restricted in frequency, amounts, and timing, and most importantly followed by appropriate oral hygiene.

What are good drinks for children?

Water is the best drink after and between meals. Unsweetened milk is also a good for young children's general and dental health. However, children should not be put to bed with milk or formula. Drinks such as juices and soda pop drinks such as colas have added sugars and can cause cavities in teeth. It is better for children to eat fresh fruit than drink fruit juice.

What types of food cause tooth decay?

Foods that contain one or more types of sugar or starches can cause tooth decay. Among these are foods that are sticky on teeth and that are more likely to cause cavities as opposed to those that are easily removed from teeth. The most important thing to remember is how long foods stay in the mouth and how frequently they are eaten.

Nighttime feeding habits

What should I do if the baby cries to feed at night?

If the baby is hungry and it has been a while since the last feeding, then you may feed the baby. After feeding

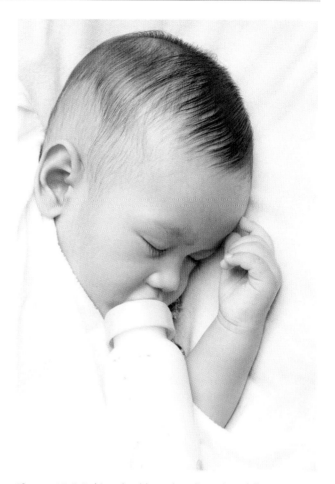

Figure 19-7 Babies should not be allowed to fall asleep with a bottle of milk, juice, or other sweet drinks. © 2011 *Twinpossible. com.* Used with permission.

the baby, clean the baby's mouth by gently wiping inside of the mouth and gums with moist, soft gauze. Often children use the bottle for comfort and to fall asleep. If the baby is crying at night and recently was fed, then you may give a bottle with only water in it. Giving milk or juice for nighttime feeding increases the risk of getting cavities especially if you do not follow the feeding by cleaning the teeth before the baby falls asleep (Figure 19-7).

When should weaning from a baby bottle to a training cup occur?

Weaning from a baby bottle to a training cup should occur by 1 year of age, transitioning to a regular cup depending on the child's skill thereafter. This is intended to avoid teeth from bathing in sweet drinks for prolonged periods, which occurs with a baby bottle because the child can take in only small volumes at a time.

Oral hygiene in infants and young children

When should cleaning my baby's mouth start?

Cleaning your baby's teeth should start as soon as possible, from birth. Babies will accept this when they have started gaining weight, typically after the first month.

What should I use to clean my baby's mouth?

You should use a clean wet baby washcloth or a piece of gauze. Unlike washcloths that need to be washed and dried regularly, pieces of gauze can be disposed of after a single use. Gauze pieces sweetened with xylitol, which is a sugar substitute, can also be purchased. These have been shown to be effective in preventing cavities in baby teeth, and the children accept the cleaning more readily because of the sweet taste.

When should I start brushing my baby's teeth?

Brushing should start soon after the eruption of the first baby teeth. A soft-bristled toothbrush designed specifically for infants should be used.

How often should I brush my baby's teeth?

Ideally, brush your baby's teeth after each feeding. The mouth and teeth should also be cleaned after breastfeeding.

Should she/he brush in the day-care center?

Children should brush in day-care centers especially if they are there for the entire day. If the daycare has a toothbrushing program, parents should consent to their children participating in the program. Ideally, the habit of toothbrushing should become a routine that is best established early in life. Young children in daycare settings are given 'nap or quiet times,' which typically follow a midday meal. To avoid children sleeping with food on their teeth, which promotes tooth decay, their teeth should be cleaned before they fall asleep.

Why doesn't my child's day-care center have a tooth-brushing routine?

They might not have enough resources. For a successful tooth-brushing program, the daycare must have age-appropriate sinks with running water, teachers who will aid or supervise the children, and a proper place for the children to store their brushes. If your child's daycare does not have a policy, parents can suggest having one. Typically this is dependent on the person in charge.

If we were to suggest that our baby's day care have a tooth-brushing policy, what should it include?

The basic tenets of the policy should be that all children are allowed and encouraged to brush their teeth on a voluntary basis, and that this should be practiced in a hygienic manner.

The author suggests the following 10-point policy:

1. Dental professionals should identify children at high risk for caries and recommend tooth brushing during school hours.
2. All children should be allowed to brush while in daycare, especially those identified as being at high risk by dental professionals.
3. All children should be encouraged to brush.
4. An adult should supervise the tooth-brushing activities, especially if toothpaste is used.
5. Following toothbrushing, children should be encouraged to rinse with water using individual disposable cups.
6. Tooth brushing should be practiced after meals and/or snacks, especially before children's naptime.
7. All daycares should have appropriate sinks suitable for tooth brushing.
8. Sinks should be sanitized before and after brushing activities.
9. Toothbrushes should be individually stored with the child's belongings
   or
10. For toothbrushes stored within the daycare center, each toothbrush should be labeled with child's name, washed, dried, and stored in a sanitary unit so as not to contact another toothbrush in order to prevent cross-infection.

How long should I brush my child's teeth?

Teeth should ideally be brushed long enough to remove plaque from all tooth surfaces, which in young children with all 20 baby teeth can take about 2 minutes (Figure 19-8).

How should I brush my children's teeth?

For infants and toddlers, you can brush their teeth while they lie on a sofa or bed with their head in your lap or in the crook of your elbow. This position of the child allows the parent to see all of their teeth especially their top teeth better than when they are standing up. Older children's teeth can be brushed while standing. Place the toothbrush where the teeth and the gum meet and do circular movements or sweep down toward the chewing

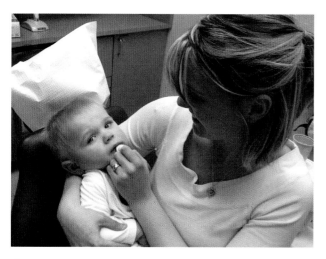

Figure 19-8 Parent cleaning the infant's mouth and teeth with a piece of gauze.

surface of the teeth. Make sure to pass through all the outer surfaces, then the inner surfaces (where the tongue is), and the chewing surfaces. It is best to follow all the teeth in an orderly sequence to avoid skipping any teeth or surfaces.

What brush should I use?

Use a soft toothbrush that is the appropriate size for the age of your child. The brush head of a child-size toothbrush is smaller than that of an adult toothbrush. A smaller head is important for reaching the child's back teeth without discomfort. Any toothbrush that meets these criteria will do the job. A more expensive toothbrush or an electric toothbrush does not necessarily mean that it is better. Proper use for a sufficiently long time is more important than the type of brush.

By what age can she/he brush her/his own teeth?

Children can start to use a toothbrush when they are able to demonstrate good hand/eye coordination. Cues for this include being able to draw pictures, write legibly, or eat with a fork and knife. As your child ages, encourage him to brush on his own, but supervise and assist him at least once per day to ensure that all tooth surfaces are being thoroughly brushed. There is no set age for being able to brush on your own. It is determined by the child's ability to complete the task properly without any assistance. Most children are up for the task between 5 to 8 years of age.

Do I need to floss my child's teeth? How?

Flossing is important when two teeth are in tight contact and the bristles of a toothbrush cannot clean in between. Usually the spaces between baby teeth are large enough

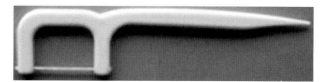

Figure 19-9 Dental flosser.

to be properly cleaned with a toothbrush. If there are tight contacts between your child's teeth (more common as she ages), you should floss them. Most children lack the coordination to floss their own teeth, so it is a task you will need to complete. To floss your child's teeth, first wash your hands. Then take about 15 centimeters (or 6 inches) of dental floss and wrap it around your middle fingers until there is only a short length of floss between them, about 2 centimeters (1 inch). This way, your thumbs and index fingers are free to hold and manipulate the floss. Handle the short length with your thumbs and index fingers and floss between two teeth at a time. You must stick your hands inside your child's mouth to do this properly. The flossing motion is up and down, not seesaw, along the sides of the teeth. A much easier option is to use a 'flosser,' which is a piece of floss on a small handle (Figure 19-9).

When should I floss his/her teeth?

Ideally, you will floss your child's teeth at least once per day, preferably before bedtime, until she is able to complete the task properly without any assistance.

The kids don't want to brush when they are sick and feverish. What should we do?

Maintaining good oral hygiene during bouts of illness is very important even if the child eats very little. When you are sick, your immune system can be overworked and weakened. Often illnesses in early childhood are caused by bacteria from the mouth. It is important to disinfect the brush between brushings during illness. Disinfection or changing to a new toothbrush has been shown to reduce the time required by the child to recover from the illness as bacteria are not re-introduced from the toothbrush back into the mouth.

My baby gets frequent ear infections. Is there a relationship between his mouth and ears?

Yes, there is a relationship between the ears and mouth. Although not visible, there is a tube that connects the inner ear to the nasal cavity, which connects to your mouth at the back of your throat. Bacteria in your mouth can track up the nose, through this tube, and into the middle ear where they can cause infection. It has been shown that children who have poor oral hygiene and lots of cavities and poor gums have a higher chance of getting ear infections.

Is there something we can do to reduce the length of time it takes before she gets well?

To reduce the length of time to recovery, keeping your child's mouth clean during the course of the illness is important. Infections can cause an increase in body temperature and dryness of the mouth. This results in very adherent plaque. Toothbrushing is critical even if children do not eat as usual during their illnesses. If the child is taking antibiotics for ear infections or other infections, the antibiotics are sweetened with sugar syrup. It is very important to brush your child's teeth after taking each dose of these sweetened medications, especially before bed. Lastly, disinfecting the toothbrush between brushings and allowing it to dry between brushings prevents reintroducing bacteria that grow on wet toothbrushes back into the mouth.

Which is the most important cleaning time?

The most important time to brush is right before the child sleeps. This could be the long nighttime sleep or the shorter daytime nap. During sleep the mouth is dry because salivation temporarily slows down. Saliva is important because it contains buffers that counteract the acid produced by bacteria living in our mouths. If a child goes to bed without brushing her teeth, the lingering food and plaque have greater potential to cause damage. While we sleep, our teeth are at greater risk for bacterial attack.

What is the best/easiest way to brush a baby's teeth?

It is easiest to clean an infant or young child's mouth and teeth when they are reclining either in the crook of your arm or with their head resting in your lap (Figure 19-10). This cleaning can be done in any room in the house. In the beginning you may find that the bathroom is not always ideal or necessary. Brushing in infancy or early childhood can be carried out either without toothpaste or with toothpaste that is safe to swallow and therefore there is no need for the child to spit. For older toddlers and preschoolers, approach your child from behind, like you are brushing your own teeth. Use a soft bristled, child-sized toothbrush and brush all food debris and/or plaque toward the biting surface. Ensure that each tooth and all surfaces are given equal attention. Ensure that the tooth touches the gums and teeth are thoroughly cleaned at the gumline.

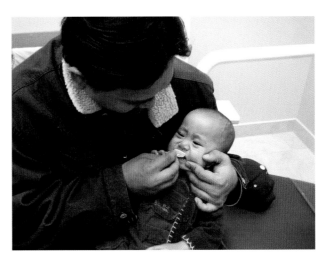

Figure 19-10 Positioning infants for oral hygiene.

Sometimes my kid's mouth has a bad smell. This is especially bad when he wakes up. What should I do?

Bad breath is mainly caused by oral bacteria, especially bacteria that causes gum disease. Bacteria are present on visible parts of teeth, below the gumline, and between teeth. Bacteria living on the tongue can also cause bad breath. To prevent bad breath in children, make sure to brush and floss regularly as described above. Also brush the top of the tongue. The back of the tongue is home to the most odor-producing bacteria. If the smell does not improve, make an appointment for your child to see his dentist who will rule out the presence of any cavities and gum disease. On rare occasions, bad breath can originate from the digestive or respiratory passages, which need to be examined by a physician.

I will have to make toothbrushing or flossing seem like fun at first. Any suggestions?

Children love routines and repetition. If oral hygiene is made a part of their routine right from the beginning, this will become relatively easy. This routine will evolve as the child gets older, but the regularity of the routine should be maintained. Older kids will enjoy if you incorporate games, stories, or songs. Praise and positive enforcement are sufficient rewards for young children. If you are not using toothpaste and the child does not have to spit, you could brush the child's teeth while she/he is watching television, wherever that might be. It is important to stress that thorough cleaning is more important than using a toothpaste.

Toothpastes and fluoride

What is fluoride?

Fluoride is a chemical element found in nature and is common in water, foods, and soil. Fluoride has two basic functions when it comes to protecting our teeth. Some fluoride-containing compounds when applied to teeth build resistance in teeth to prevent tooth decay by making the teeth less susceptible to acid attack. Also it promotes remineralization (rebuilding of tooth enamel from the calcium and the phosphate in the saliva).

When should you start using toothpaste with fluoride for cleaning my child's teeth?

You may begin to use toothpaste with fluoride when your child is capable of spitting and you are reasonably assured that he does not swallow toothpaste. Typically this can occur around 2 to 3 years of age; each child is different. Your dentist may advise a different age to start using fluoridated toothpaste based on your child's specific needs and risks for getting cavities.

Should we use kids' toothpaste or regular adult toothpaste?

Adult toothpastes typically contain a number of ingredients that are unnecessary for younger children. There is a difference in the amount of fluoride in children's and adult toothpaste. Adult toothpaste has approximately twice the amount of fluoride as children's toothpaste. Children's toothpaste has been shown to provide less protection from cavities than children's toothpaste in high-risk children. Also children's toothpastes are formulated for children's taste. Therefore they are more likely to swallow children's toothpaste than adult toothpaste. The only important and necessary ingredient in toothpaste is fluoride. The choice of toothpaste should be made in consultation with your dentist. Avoid using toothpastes with strong flavoring agents. Mint may be too spicy for your little one, which could cause him to reject toothbrushing. Whitening toothpastes are not indicated for children because they may contain abrasive agents that could wear or damage children's teeth.

How much toothpaste should one use for brushing a child's teeth?

Use a smear of toothpaste to brush the teeth of a child less than 2 years of age. For the 2- to 5-year-old child, dispense a pea-size amount of toothpaste (Figure 19-11). Even as an adult, a pea-sized amount of toothpaste is all you need.

What happens if they swallow toothpaste?

Discourage swallowing of toothpaste. If preschool-age children use toothpaste, an adult should supervise

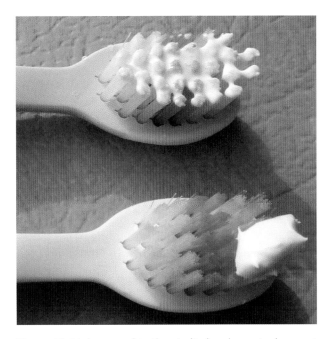

Figure 19-11 A smear of toothpaste (*top*) and pea-sized amount (*bottom*).

brushing to ensure that the children are not swallowing the toothpaste. It is important to avoid swallowing of toothpaste to avoid ingesting fluoride, which can cause defects in the permanent teeth that are developing during this period. If a child eats a significant amount of toothpaste, he could have nausea and stomach pain. Note both the time he swallowed the toothpaste and the amount he swallowed. Have him drink a glass of milk. If symptoms worsen, such as dizziness or throwing up violently, call your poison control center.

What about fluoride in drinking water?

Fluoride in drinking water was an effective and inexpensive method of preventing cavities for the general population when cavities were very common. However, it is now known that it is not essential to swallow fluoride to get the benefit of preventing cavities. Depending on where you live, you may or may not have fluoride in the drinking water.

Will boiling the water remove fluoride from it?

No. Boiling the water does not remove the fluoride from the water.

Can you use it for making formula?

Where fluoride is added to drinking water, it should not be used to make infant formula or other food for children younger than 2 years of age. This is intended to avoid children from getting permanent teeth that have spots or defects on permanent teeth that are growing during that period.

Tooth decay in baby teeth
What causes early baby tooth decay?

Early baby tooth decay, also called early childhood caries (ECC), is caused by acids produced by oral bacteria that use sugars from foods. The acids dissolve calcium from teeth, which results in cavities. Foods and drinks that contain natural sugars or cooked starches that stay on the teeth for prolonged periods of time cause ECC and are especially bad for the teeth.

Can breastfeeding cause or contribute to tooth decay?

This is a controversial topic. Breastfeeding is best for the baby and mother for the numerous health benefits. However, when breastfeeding is provided on demand to the baby and combined with formula or other semi-solid foods, it can cause tooth decay. This is especially true if the baby is allowed to fall asleep while nursing. If milk is allowed to stagnate on teeth, then the repeated and prolonged exposure leads to tooth decay.

The controversy arises from the many articles that report that breast milk does not cause cavities. This might be true in laboratory experiments, but it is not true in real-life situations. Moreover, it is impossible to conduct valid clinical trials where a group of women are deliberately prohibited from breastfeeding for the sake of an experiment. Putting aside this academic debate, the best practice is to breastfeed the baby providing it with all of the benefits of breastfeeding, but following it up with cleaning of the mouth before the baby falls asleep, which avoids the problems of tooth decay.

Does second-hand smoke in the household increase the risk for a child getting cavities?

Yes. It appears that children who are exposed to second-hand smoke have more mature plaque similar to adults. This may lead to higher counts of oral bacteria that cause cavities and gum disease. It can also increase your child's chances of staining of the teeth, bad breath, asthma, emphysema, and possibly cancer.

What is third-hand smoke? Would it be as bad as second-hand smoke?

Third-hand smoke is tobacco smoke contamination that remains after the cigarette has been extinguished. Toxins from smoke linger in carpets, sofas, clothes, and other materials hours or even days after a cigarette is put out. This is a health hazard for infants and children. As discussed above, infants tend to explore through their mouth. Third-hand smoke can be introduced into the mouth by children putting their fingers or toys in the mouth that are contaminated with those toxins.

Baby's first dental visit
When should I take my child to the dentist for his/her first dental visit?

The first dental visit should occur shortly after the first tooth erupts and no later than the child's first birthday.

Why so early? My baby barely has any teeth. What is the purpose of this visit?

The baby's first dental visit is as important as the well-baby visit with baby's medical doctor. There are three goals of the first dental visit: (1) to record the child's birth history and her current state of health; (2) to check the child's mouth and teeth; and (3) to get information and guidance to correct existing problems prevent any impending problems based on the child's individual risk. This will also set up an appropriate frequency of future visits. An additional benefit of this early visit is that the child gets used to the dentist and the dental office setting when no treatment is necessary so that she/he is more likely to have a pleasant experience and not have any fears that many children have associated with visiting the dentist.

My baby cries whenever a stranger looks at her. A 'stranger' who wants her to open her mouth will be terrifying for her. What do you suggest?

It is natural for a baby to cry or shy away from strangers. It is okay for a baby to cry if a practitioner examines the baby's mouth. Crying does not indicate that the baby is in pain or will be traumatized in the long run. If the parent comforts the child immediately after the examination, the baby will be back to herself in no time. With time and age, the baby will understand and cooperate without crying. We suggest using a knee-to-knee position (Figure 19-12). This optimal position allows you (the parent) to hold your baby, while the dentist looks inside the mouth. The parent gently holds the baby's

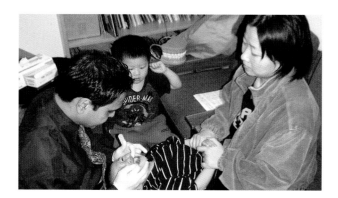

Figure 19-12 Baby's first dental visit. Knee-to-knee examination of an infant.

hands as the dentist looks inside the mouth. It is normal for the baby to cry during the examination.

Why do babies put everything they can hold in their mouth?

From birth through infancy and early toddlerhood, children explore their environment through their mouth. The mouth with its senses of touch, taste, and smell are more sensitive than those of sight or sound at those early stages of development.

My 3-year old loves his soother and keeps it in his mouth much of the day. What are some tips to make it easier for him to give it up? People are starting to comment, and I'm worried that kids might make fun of him.

Children have a psychological need to suck. Soothers provide a sense of comfort for young children. Most children will spontaneously stop the habit after 3 years of age possibly due to peer pressure. If by age 4 or 5 he has not stopped, then we suggest behavior modification therapy and counseling. If by age 5 or 6 he has not stopped, then we suggest appliance therapy with counseling.

Will I have to leave my child alone with the dentist if I take her for an appointment?

Absolutely not. You're always welcome in the operatory while your child is being treated. Most practitioners who are trained and comfortable treating young children prefer that. This is obviously beneficial for child but also for the parent and the practitioner. If you are nervous or have fears of your own, your child will sense that easily. In those circumstances, it will be your choice to stay outside. Nowadays no parent should be required to leave their child alone for their appointment. This is the current norm.

My child has a lot of fears right now. How can I prepare her for a visit to the dentist?

It is normal for a child to have fears; however, there are ways to prepare your child for a visit to the dentist. First, do not use words like hurt, pain, needle, drill, and other similar words. These words only increase the fear for your child. Second, try not to pass on your own fears or anxiety to your child because they may pick up on your emotions and become fearful. Your calm, reassuring, and comforting demeanor will help allay much of the child's anxiety. Third, inform your child that she is going to see a dentist who will 'count her teeth.'

Bacteria in the child's mouth

How are bacteria that cause cavities transmitted to children?

The main way bacteria get transmitted to children is from the mother or another caregiver, such as a grandmother or nanny. It is transmitted through saliva from kissing on the mouth, sharing foods or utensils such as spoons, or fingers from mother's mouth to child's mouth. The other way is from siblings or other children through sharing of foods, utensils, pacifiers, or sucking on shared toys.

What happens if parents have cavities or bad teeth?

If parents have cavities, then there is active disease in the mouth. That means that the parents have high levels of bacteria in their mouths that can be passed on to their children. It is important for the parents to see the dentist to have cavities and other dental problems fixed as early as possible.

What if the children are cared for by nannies or grandparents, or are in day-care centers?

Bacteria can be passed on from any caregiver, not just the parents. It is important for all caregivers to maintain optimal oral health and hygiene to minimize or delay bacterial transmission to the child.

Can we do something to prevent children from getting bacteria in their mouth?

One can prevent or delay children getting bacteria in their mouths by avoiding kissing children directly on their mouths and by not sharing foods or utensils with children. Ensure that parents and any other caregiver maintain optimal oral hygiene. Parents and caregivers can take specific steps to reduce bacteria in their own mouths. Proven strategies include certain antibacterial mouth rinses or chewing Xylitol-containing chewing gum.

Habits

Do oral habits such as thumb sucking and pacifier use affect the baby's teeth and jaws?

Thumb sucking and pacifier use may affect the position of your baby's teeth. The extent of the effect depends on the frequency, duration, and intensity of the habit. In general, if the child uses the pacifier many hours per day for a long period of time (usually beyond 3 years of age), the effect on the position of the teeth will be more pronounced. Thumb sucking and pacifier use will usually cause the upper front teeth to move forward, and the upper and lower front teeth may not overlap each other, leaving an opening in the front teeth. On the other hand, the sucking action of the cheeks pushes the back teeth in and can cause a crossbite on one or both sides. Initially the habits affect the teeth and later will affect the jaws.

How can I get my child to stop the habit?

Most children give up habits naturally. However, if the child persists with the habit that is affecting his bite, attempts to stop the habits should be made. It is best to postpone these attempts until such time as the child is mentally ready to quit the habit. Nagging a younger child before that stage might result in the child learning to ignore verbal instructions from parents. A couple of proven strategies to get children to stop include the use of a reward system and having the child sleep in pajamas with mitts attached to the ends of the sleeves. Using bitter or spicy liquids on the nails have limited success.

We have tried many of the remedies you have mentioned but none work. Can you do something?

Beyond a certain age and especially if the bite or jaws are being affected, the dentist can provide fixed or removable appliances that act as reminders to the child to stop the habit and deprive the pleasure and comfort to the child who eventually loses interest in the habit. The child needs to know and understand that this is not a punishment but only a reminder.

At what age should the child stop the habit?

Stopping the habit should be initiated after the child has a complete set of 20 baby teeth, typically by 3 years of age. If the habit has stopped before the age of 4 years, some bite problems can self correct. Trying to stop a pacifier habit in a very young child can inadvertently cause the child to start sucking his thumb or fingers, which is harder to break. Hence, heed the caution to make sure that the child is mentally ready to give up the habit for good.

My child sucks his thumb and pulls out his hair with the other. Are they related? What should we do?

Yes, they are probably related. The child has learned to associate the two actions with his feeling of comfort and self satisfaction. Often, stopping one might lead to stopping the other. Home remedies or dental remedies should be initiated as described above.

My child has the habit of biting his nails. Will it damage his teeth? How can I stop him doing that?

Nail biting is not known to damage the teeth. Usually you can't stop a habit unless your child wants to as well. You can use some of the strategies discussed above to stop them sucking their thumbs or fingers.

My child has the habit of sucking her lower lip. How can I get her to stop?

Where the habit is affecting the bite, jaws, or the lip itself, the dentist can place an appliance that can aid in the cessation of the habit.

My toddler has a tantrum when someone wants him to do something he doesn't want to do. I can't see how I could bring him to a dentist without that happening?

It most likely will happen, but sometimes we have to do things that are good for us and that we don't like for our own good. Is your child in pain? If not, this would be the best time to see him because it would be a non-invasive procedure and he can leave with a positive experience. Children should be expected to act their age and your child's dentist should be competent to help you and your child avoid or cope with it if it does happen.

Injuries to the mouth and teeth

What are the different oral or dental injuries an infant or child can suffer?

Injuries to the head and primary teeth usually result from falls and collisions as the child becomes more independently mobile. Falls on the face will injure the mouth and teeth. Injuries to the mouth can cause bruising, cuts, and bleeding. Injuries to teeth can cause them to be loose, painful, chipped, or knocked out of the socket. The bite may also get changed. Another serious injury to the mouth can result from a young child chewing on a live electric wire, which results in electric burns. Young children can also injure their mouth or gums with improper use of a toothbrush.

How can I make the home environment safe to prevent injuries?

To make the home safer you need to eliminate from his reach anything that may pose a danger to him, by raising it above his reach, locking it, or eliminating it altogether. Medicines, cleaning supplies, and small articles should all be out of his reach. Heavy objects such as bookcases should be secured to the wall, electric cords should not be in his reach, and it is recommended to use plug covers and stair gates. To prevent scalds always keep coffee and

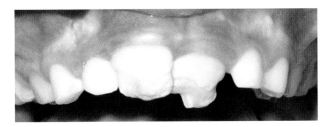

Figure 19-13 The permanent central incisors are hypoplastic and discolored due to severe trauma to the primary teeth in infancy.

tea cups out of his reach as well as pots with hot water. Walking around the house in socks can be very slippery and dangerous for a child who is learning to walk. Baby walkers should be avoided. Equipment for the baby's use, such as playpens or car seats, should be checked to ensure that they have not been recalled for safety reasons.

What happens if a baby injures her teeth?

Injuries to baby teeth can damage developing permanent teeth (Figure 19-13).

The roots of the baby teeth are close to the developing permanent teeth; therefore, an injury to the baby teeth can potentially affect the permanent teeth. You should contact a dentist immediately to have a consultation and treatment if necessary. Depending on the extent of the injury and even if it seems that the injury itself did not cause any harm, the dentist may decide to schedule recall exams to observe for outcomes. Some injuries might necessitate removal of baby teeth.

Should we put back knocked out baby teeth?

Knocked out baby teeth should not be put back either by caregivers or dentists. If you put the baby tooth back, it might harm the permanent tooth and affect its development. Knocked out permanent teeth, in contrast, should be put back immediately by anyone who is present at the time of the injury.

What first aid should we provide?

Remain calm and calm the child because the child will react to the injury, the pain, and the blood. Clean the child's face with a clean damp cloth or gauze and try to stop the bleeding.

What should we do if there is bleeding from the mouth?

To stop the bleeding, let him bite gently on the cloth or hold it for him in place. In infants, a pacifier can help to soothe the child and also aid in controlling the bleeding. You can provide age-appropriate pain relief. See the dentist as soon as possible.

Sometime ago, our child fell at the day-care center. Now his two front teeth are turning black. What should we do?

Teeth can turn color shortly after being hurt or much later. This occurs due to bleeding inside the tooth. You should contact a dentist for children to have the teeth checked. The dentist will check the teeth and will probably take an X-ray of the teeth to see the root and the surrounding bone. Depending on the findings, the dentist will decide on a recall schedule for observation or treatment. The options include no treatment but periodic observation, baby root canal treatment, or removal of the tooth if there is risk of damage to the permanent successor.

My son had beautiful teeth till he got hit by a swing and his teeth got pushed in. What should i do?

Contact a dentist as soon as possible to have the teeth checked and an X-ray taken. Teeth that are pushed in have a high risk of complications to the nerve and root and should be closely monitored. If these are baby teeth that were pushed in, there is also a risk of damage to the permanent teeth that are developing in the bone close to the roots of the baby teeth.

Regular dental care
How often should my child visit a dentist?

For a majority of children, twice a year check ups are suggested. However, every child is different, and some might need to see the dentist more often and some less. If your child is of increased risk of tooth decay, has unusual growth patterns, or has poor oral hygiene, he would benefit from more frequent appointments. Your child's need to see the dentist may change with time, and your pediatric or general dentist would re-evaluate this at each check up.

Do baby teeth need to be fixed? Can't we just pull them out? That's what we would do back home.

Yes, they need to be fixed. Cavities in baby teeth should be fixed for a number of reasons. Children need their baby teeth for eating, speech, and the proper development of permanent teeth. Extraction of teeth should be a last resort. Early loss of baby teeth can not only affect function but will also affect the appearance and esthetics and could lead to psychological problems in a young child who looks different from his/her peers. In our societal norms, it is not acceptable to leave problems in young children untreated especially if it affects their normal growth and development. In extreme circumstances, neglecting treatment of oral or dental conditions can have legal consequences to the caregivers.

How can I have them fixed if I can't pay for treatment?

Free dental treatment is provided through schemes provided by most western governments for anyone with limited means to pay for treatment of their children. Financial hardship should not be a reason to not seek timely treatment.

What can happen if the child's cavities are not taken care of reasonably promptly?

In the short term, children can experience pain, infections, swelling of the face, and the child getting generally ill, which will often require emergency treatment, sometimes in a hospital. Untreated cavities can result in the child eating poorly, being cranky, and missing school. In severe cases the child can fail to thrive. Extensive treatment is expensive and can require the use of sedation or general anesthesia. In the long term, children who experience severe disease very early in life also are known to be at a higher risk of disease in their permanent teeth and possibly have other medical problems. Untreated dental disease generally leads to a poor quality of life.

How do I know the teeth are infected?

You might see your child have pain that wakes them up in the night, pain that is spontaneous and isn't alleviated by analgesics, and facial swellings. A simple way to check for infections is to lift the lips and check for bumps or boils on the gum. Sometimes these are not visible and can only be seen when a dentist radiographs the teeth with an X-ray.

Oh yes, I have seen the bump over her tooth—it comes and goes but doesn't seem to bother her, except the first time. Is that something to be concerned about?

As it could affect the development of the permanent tooth, it should be treated promptly. Occasionally it can flare up, cause the face to swell painfully, and make your child sick and possibly require hospitalization.

What do we do if my child is complaining of pain in the mouth?

Try to find out the source of the pain. Common sources of pain in the mouth of children are pain during teething, cavities in teeth, or ulcers in the mouth. Try to avoid the food that irritates your child. If pain is from cavities then you should avoid sweet, cold, and sour foods. If the pain is caused by an ulcer, avoid spicy, hot, and acidic foods. Do not avoid brushing because most conditions tend to worsen with poor oral hygiene. Avoid sharp-tasting toothpastes. Pain medications that provide temporary relief should be swallowed and not applied to the teeth or ulcers. Have them examined by a dentist as soon as possible for definitive treatment of the problem.

How can we ease the discomfort of teething?

Children experience discomfort during teething from swollen gums. To ease the discomfort, it is important to keep the mouth clean. Massaging the gums during cleaning will ease discomfort somewhat. Application of cold to the gums will help. This can be achieved by letting the child bite on a piece of cold fruit such as a banana or on a cooled teething ring. Over the counter teething medications should be used sparingly and under dental or medical supervision.

Emergencies

When should my child be taken to a doctor/hospital?

The child should be taken to a hospital if he/she is not able to eat or drink because of pain, swelling, or injury. If there is a suspicion of a head injury, that must be examined before any oral or dental injury. If the child has facial swelling that is nearing or involving the eye, the child has difficulty swallowing or breathing, or generally appears listless and unwell, the child should be seen promptly by the child's physician. Children should be seen on an emergency basis if any of the following are noted: children who have experienced severe oral or dental injury/trauma that has caused significant bleeding; if the child is unable to close his mouth or bite together as before; if a tooth is broken and the broken piece cannot be found; if there is bleeding from the nerve of the tooth; and if teeth have moved out of their normal position or seem to have been knocked out. In cases where the child has suffered an injury that does not have a clear, obvious, or logical explanation, and the child is under the care of someone other than the primary caregiver, or when in doubt, seek professional guidance. If the injuries are clearly oral or dental and do not involve the head or any other part of the body, it is preferable to take the child to his/her primary dentist or pediatric dentist rather than an emergency department in a hospital. Many hospitals and emergency departments do not have dentists on staff who can provide the specialized treatment that is needed, and this can result in unnecessary delays in treatments of the dental injury.

References

Aligne, C.A., Moss, M.E., Auinger, P., *et al.* (2003) Association of pediatric dental caries with passive smoking. *Journal of the American Medical Association*, 289, 1258–1264.

Alsada, L., Sigal, M., Limeback, H., *et al.* (2005) Development and testing of an audio-visual aid for improvement of infant oral health through primary care giver education. *Canadian Dental Association Journal*, 71, 241, 241a–241h.

Chung, K.C., Kowalski, C.P., Kim, H.M., *et al.* (2000) Maternal cigarette smoking during pregnancy and the risk of having a child with cleft lip/palate. *Plastic and Reconstructive Surgery*, 105, 485–491.

Gartsbein, E. and Kulkarni, G. (2008) The need for an oral care policy in daycares: reasoning and direction. *Oral Health*, March: 30–34.

Gartsbein, E., Lawrence, H.P., Leake, J.L., *et al.* (2009) Lack of oral care policies in Toronto daycares. *Journal of Public Health Dentistry*, 69, 190–196.

Keene, K. and Johnson, R.B. (1999) The effect of nicotine on growth of Streptococcus mutans. *Mississippi Dental Association Journal*, 55, 38–39.

Kulkarni, G. (2010) Oral health promotion programs from infancy to childhood. *Canadian Dental Association Journal*, 75, 684–685.

Poranganel, L., Titley, K., Kulkarni, G. (2006) Establishing a Dental Home: A Program for Promoting Comprehensive Oral Health Starting from Pregnancy through Childhood. *Oral Health*, 96, 10–14.

Tanaka, K., Miyake, Y., and Sasaki, S. (2010) The Effect of Maternal Smoking During Pregnancy and Postnatal Household Smoking on Dental Caries in Young Children. *Obstetrics and Gynocology Survey*, 65, 15–17.

Zonuz, A.T., Rahmati, A., Mortazavi, H., *et al.* (2008) Effect of cigarette smoke exposure on the growth of Streptococcus mutans and Streptococcus sanguis: an in vitro study. *Nicotine and Tobacco Research*, 10, 63–67.

20

High-risk patients: the frail older adult living in long-term care homes

Mary-Lou van der Horst and Donna Bowes

Introduction: the need for better oral health care in long-term care

A significant proportion of the Canadian population is aging, and as a result, the profile of those who are being admitted to and reside in long-term care is also changing. For those adults who are over 65 years, 70% will require some long-term care services in their lifetime, and by age 80, one-third will require long-term care and more than one-half by age 90. Today, the average age of a long-term care resident is 83 years. Unfortunately, there has never been a strong emphasis on oral health in long-term care settings. No doubt, all long-term care residents would benefit from the expertise of oral health practitioners who specialize in, or have expertise in, geriatric dentistry or gerondontology. Studies, reviews, and reports consistently indicate the poor oral health among long-term care residents.

The majority of long-term care residents in the past were edentulous and received dental care infrequently, most often limited to emergency care with little or no focus to care aimed at retaining teeth through daily preventive oral hygiene regimes and use of restorative treatments. No longer is the focus of care on cure in long-term care but rather on maximizing the resident's quality of life by promoting and maintaining the resident's optimal physical, functional, cognitive, emotional, social, cultural, spiritual, and oral health. Venturing into long-term care can provide challenging opportunities for oral health care professionals who choose to work with this unique and demanding population. As residents' oral health problems worsen, dental treatments become increasingly difficult because many cannot tolerate lengthy procedures, and they or their families are unable to understand the need for or value of treatments. Every reasonable effort to prevent periodontal disease must be made to avoid the consequences of poor oral health in long-term care residents. Oral health is a care issue that transcends professional boundaries and long-term care provides a unique opportunity for collaboration and knowledge exchange in order to improve the oral health of residents.

What Is long-term care?

Long-term care is a complex, dynamic, changing, and collaborative care setting, and for many oral health practitioners it is an often overlooked, ignored, and misunderstood environment. The term "long-term care" is often used synonymously with the term "residential care facilities" in Canada. It refers to facilities with four or more beds that are funded, licensed, or approved by provincial/territorial departments of health and/or social services (Statistics Canada 2010a). Long-term care can encompass nursing homes, homes for the aged, lodges for senior citizens, residential homes, auxiliary hospitals, special care homes, rest homes, extra-mural (hospital-at-home) care, community health centres, and personal care homes (Figure 20-1).

In early 2008, there were 4,761 licensed residential care facilities across Canada. The industry generated revenues of $15.8 billion and expenses of $15.6 billion, with a resulting profit of $276.6 million or a mere 1.7% of total revenues. Of these 4,761 residential facilities, 2,183 provided dedicated care for 200,397 residents over the age of 65 years and generated $12.6 billion in revenues (Statistics Canada 2010a).

Comprehensive Preventive Dentistry, First Edition. Edited by Hardy Limeback.
© 2012 John Wiley & Sons, Ltd. Published 2012 by John Wiley & Sons, Ltd.

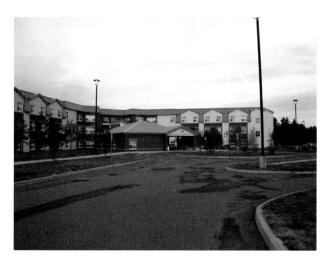

Figure 20-1 Typical long-term care group home. Courtesy of Lynda McKeown.

It is important to recognize that the key distinguishing feature of a long-term care home from other health care-funded settings is that it is *the home and primary residence of the resident*. Often referred to as "homes," long-term care facilities that serve the aged may be owned and/or operated by any of the following entities: provincial, territorial, or municipal governments; local, national, or international for-profit or non-profit, charitable, religious, cultural, ethnic, or community corporations or organizations. Long-term care homes are generally funded from a variety of sources, usually through the provincial or territorial government health insurance or social insurance plans, in combination with daily fees paid by residents, and/or additional funding from municipalities or operating/owner organizations.

The *Canada Health Act*, the federal legislation for publicly funded health care insurance, is designed to ensure that all eligible Canadian residents have reasonable access to insured health services on a prepaid basis, with no direct charges at the point of service. The Act requires that medically necessary hospital and physician services be fully covered. The provisions apply also to some parts of long-term residential care (nursing home intermediate care and adult residential care services), but the provinces and territories can determine what parts are publicly funded (Health Canada 2008; Fernandez and Spencer 2010). All provinces and territories pay a large portion of the costs of long-term care, but the private costs to long-term care residents differ considerably across jurisdictions with variations dependent on the household income level, marital status, and assets owned (Fernandez and Spencer 2010). For example, annually a low-income non-married long-term care resident in Prince Edward Island would have $20 discretionary spending money, while a low-income married couple

both in long-term care would have to pay an additional $456. A married couple in Quebec with sufficient assets would pay an additional $2,306 in costs whereas as a similar couple in Alberta would have $6,360 discretionary spending money; an average income couple with one spouse in care in Alberta would have $43,000 discretionary spending whereas a similar couple in Newfoundland would have $20,000 (Fernandez and Spencer 2010). The level of government funding and services provided per resident is set according to the severity of the residents' health issues and levels of need. Government funding for long-term care homes supports 24-hour nursing care, food, programming, and housekeeping/maintenance/laundry (Statistics Canada 2010a). Additional government funding is available to those who have insufficient money. When the resident's accommodation and care is fully funded by the government and once long-term care costs are reconciled, there may be a very small disposable monthly income remaining for the purchase of non-funded personal services such as dental care.

The provincial and territorial governments establish the licensing, standards for care and services provision, buildings, operations, and management. Many long-term care homes voluntarily participate in and achieve national accreditation standards in order to be recognized as "accredited" long-term care homes. Participating in accreditation demonstrates the long-term care home's commitment to quality health care to its staff, residents, families, and community. Approximately 75% of Ontario's long-term care homes are accredited with Accreditation Canada (Accreditation Canada 2010).

Who resides in long-term care homes?

A significant proportion of the Canadian population is aging, and as a result, the profile of those who are being admitted and who reside in long-term care is changing. There are 4.3 million Canadians over the age of 65 years, 73% are between the ages of 65 and 79 years, and 27% are 80 years and older. Immigrants account for approximately 28% of older adults and Aboriginal peoples about

1% (Public Health Agency of Canada 2010). Life expectancy has dramatically improved over the last century. Babies born today can expect to live to 100 years of age (Figure 20-2).

The growth of the older adult population over 65 years is expected to accelerate over the next 20 years and up to the early 2030s. By 2017 older adults will account for a larger proportion of the population than children under the age of 14 years, with the 90+-year-age group expected to triple in size (Ontario Ministry of Finance 2010). For those who live into their 80s and 90s, the cause of death is shifting from circulatory, respiratory, endocrine, and digestive diseases, and cancers to more nervous system, mental health behavioral issues (such as Alzheimer's disease, dementia), and injury (Public Health Agency of Canada 2010). Furthermore, the likelihood of frailty increases with age, and 20% of those 80 years and older are considered frail (Institute for Clinical Evaluative Science 2010). For those adults over 65 years, 70% will require some long-term care services in their lifetime and are estimated to need an average of 3 years of long-term care (Stevenson *et al.* 2010). Twenty percent are projected to need long-term care for up to 5 years, and 5% are projected to spend more than 5 years in a residential facility (O'Shaughnessy 2010) as shown in Table 20-1.

Approximately 7%, or about 1 in 30 Canadians aged 65 years or older, live in a long-term care home or home

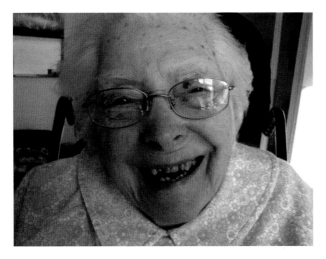

Figure 20-2 Photo of a centenarian who has retained most of her teeth. Courtesy of Lynda McKeown.

for the aged, increasing to 15% for those over 75 years (Public Health Agency of Canada 2006; CBC News 2007). About one-third of adults older than 80 years, and one-half of those over 90 years require long-term care (Rockwood *et al.* 1994). There were 242,977 people residing in Canada's 4,761 residential care facilities in early 2008, and occupancy rates across Canada average 95.9% (Statistics Canada 2010a). Yet, long-term care admission wait times are rising and in Ontario have doubled in the last 5 years. Worldwide, costs in long-term care have risen largely due to the increasing numbers of older persons who require total care (Institute for Clinical Evaluative Science 2010; Butler 2008). Many long-term care homes admit residents aged 18 years and older; however, the average age of a long-term care resident is 83 years (Ontario Ministry of Health and Long-term Care 2008). Older adults occupy the majority of the beds in long-term care homes with 76% of residents being over the age of 65 years. The rate of need for long-term care services is four times higher among adults age 85 and older, compared to adults age 65 to 84 (Avalere Health 2008). Females over the age of 80 years represent the greatest majority of residents at 43% (Table 20-1) (Statistics Canada 2010b). It is estimated that the marital status of Canadian long-term care residents is similar to that of the United States with 39% of male residents and 16% of female long-term care residents being married (Ness *et al.* 2004).

Residents' health conditions can be complex and unpredictable. Approximately 73% of residents have some form of cognitive impairment, and when dementia, depression, and delirium are accounted for, about 80% to 90% of resident have these mental health issues. Up to 60% of residents suffer from malnutrition and dehydration. Additional common conditions in long-term care include those associated with aging such as congestive heart failure, stroke, atherosclerosis, chronic obstructive lung disease, urinary incontinence, constipation, infections (for example, pneumonia, bladder), diabetes, arthritis, osteoarthritis, osteoporosis, cancer, prostate disease, Parkinson's disease, sensory/auditory/visual changes, skin changes (such as, bruising, pressure ulcers), mobility decline, falls, and injuries/fractures (Butler 2008; Ametanin *et al.* 2008).

Table 20-1 Percentage of aged residents in LTC homes in Canada (Stats Can 2010a)

All residents >65 years	Males >65 years	Females >65 years	All residents >80 years	Males >80 years	Females >80 years
76%	21%	55%	57%	14%	43%

> **Tip Box 20-2** Get to know the residents' profiles
>
> Understand the profile of long-term care residents and the adaptations that will need to be made in oral health care practices with these clients.
>
> A typical long-term care resident is female, in her 80s, frail, has multiple chronic conditions, takes multiple medications, has moderate Alzheimer's disease, is mobile but occasionally falls, and needs assistance with her personal care and daily activities. She may only need prompting to do her oral care but most likely has forgotten her oral care skills and may be resistive or refuse to have oral care done on the many care attempts by staff. As a result, her oral care is done infrequently.

> **Tip Box 20-3** What is the Resident Assessment Instrument – Minimum Data Set (RAI-MDS)?
>
> The RAI-MDS includes oral/dental status as a section of the assessment tool, but it underestimates the extent of oral health problems in long-term care residents.
>
> Since the late 1990s, researchers have expressed repeated concerns and alerted oral health care and health care professionals that RAI-MDS assessments identify few oral health problems. Researchers have found that the RAI-MDS consistently underestimated oral health problems for various reasons and unfortunately found a corresponding under-treatment of oral health conditions in long-term care residents. Oral health pain was poorly detected especially in those residents with dementia (Ettinger *et al.* 2000; Folse 2001; Cohen-Mansfield and Lipson 2002).

Older adults residing in long-term care homes receive more medications, including psychotropic medications, than their community-dwelling counterparts. There is massive use of prescription medications in long-term care with 23–28% of residents taking 12 or more prescription medications, which doubles the risk of adverse reactions compared to those taking five or less prescribed medications (Standing Committee on Public Accounts 2007). Many residents will have diminished capacity for decision making and therefore will have an individual designated by the resident (substitute decision-maker) who is lawfully authorized to make decisions on their behalf (such as a Power of Attorney). These decisions may include consent to treatment, approval of services, financial management, advanced care planning, and end-of-life care decisions.

How are care and services provided in long-term care homes?

Admission and assessments

Older adults generally enter long-term care due to cognitive decline, functional problems, physical decline, end-stage disease, or related issues. Long-term care homes provide health care services and accommodation for residents who are no longer able to live independently and require access to 24-hour nursing care and personal supervision within a safe and secure environment. About 43% of older adults over 65 years will have at least one long-term care home admission during their lifetime (Butler 2008; Ontario Ministry of Health and Long-term Care 2008). Pre-admission to long-term care homes is usually managed though a centralized government-funded organization to ensure fair and coordinated access based on eligibility criteria and urgency, usually determined using a common assessment tool such as the Resident Assessment Instrument-Minimum Data Set (RAI-MDS). The RAI-MDS for long-term care is an

accepted comprehensive, standardized, automated assessment instrument developed by interRAI, a not-for-profit research network operating in 30 countries. The information gathered enhances the management and quality of care and enables benchmarking across long-term care homes. The assessment evaluates the applicant's needs, preferences, and strengths. It records an extensive amount of information and includes health status, physical, cognitive, functional, and emotional status. The assessment generates real-time reports for staff to assist in individualized resident-focused holistic care planning and goal setting for new residents. Potential and actual care concerns are flagged for further investigation, an inter-professional approach is promoted, and better information analysis is provided to long-term care homes to enhance care decisions (CIHI 2005). Reassessments of the residents' health status are usually conducted quarterly plus any time their health status significantly changes (for example, critical illness, fractures).

There has never been a strong emphasis on oral health assessments in the long-term care setting. Long-term care regulations across Canada are usually vague, and although they often require a dental assessment upon admission, there is little direction given regarding the need for, and frequency of, follow-up; no indication of who should do the follow-up and whether decisions regarding dental care are to be deferred to the resident or family's personal choice or if the long-term care site is to be held accountable (MacEntee 2005). The oral/dental status and oral/nutritional status sections of the RAI-MDS address issues related to the resident's oral status that will trigger a Resident Assessment Protocol (RAP). RAPs are problem-oriented frameworks for additional assessment on problem identification items. The following seven items trigger a Dental Care RAP: debris in mouth prior to going to bed at night; having dentures/removable bridge; some or all of natural teeth are lost; broken, loose, or carious teeth present; inflamed/swollen or bleeding gums/oral abscesses/ulcers/rashes; no daily cleaning of teeth or dentures by resident or staff; and/or mouth pain (Ametanin *et al.* 2008).

There is an oral screening assessment tool for nondental care providers in long-term care homes that is more comprehensive than the RAI-MDS's seven triggers (Chalmers *et al.* 2005). The Oral Health Assessment Tool (OHAT) was developed for the *Best Practice Oral Health Model for Australian Residential Care and* designed to be a simple eight-category reliable and valid screening tool to assess the oral health of long-term care residents including those with dementia. Care providers found the OHAT to be user-friendly and prompted them to complete a more thorough oral exam as part of their overall health assessment processes. It is laid out in a table format and directs the assessor to the key components of oral health that need to be assessed (that is, lips, tongue, gums and tissues, saliva, natural teeth, dentures, oral cleanliness, and pain). In addition, the tool indicates normal and abnormal assessment findings, and when to refer the patient to an oral health professional. The OHAT was adapted with permission for Ontario's long-term care homes in 2007 (Figure 20-3).

Focus of care and services

The focus of care interventions and service provision in long-term care is to maximize the resident's quality of life by promoting and maintaining the resident's optimal physical, functional, cognitive, emotional, social, cultural, and spiritual health. The philosophical underpinning of a long-term care facility is that it is the home of the residents. Long-term care homes are not hospitals. In their long-term care home, residents are given the opportunity to live with dignity and respect no matter how frail they may be. To the best of their ability they are encouraged to continue the social roles and activities from which they have gained life satisfaction while receiving support to restore their self-care abilities. Most long-term care homes are linked to the health care system. Long-term care offers a broad range of support from minimal personal assistance with basic activities of daily living (ADL), to providing total care needs on a continuing basis. A wide variety of additional services including, but not limited to, medical, nursing, dietary, social, personal, supportive, and specialized care may also be offered. With the changing demographics, long-term care homes are admitting more older adults with multiple and complex care needs who require more specialized care and services than residents in the past (Ontario Ministry of Health and Long-term Care 2008; Chalmers *et al.* 2005; Sullivan-Marx and Gray-Micelli 2008).

Long-term care homes vary according to size and location. Although there are many small long-term care homes (such as those with fewer than 80 beds), the larger homes can be 200 to 400 beds in size. Specifics about the home such as room size, contents, and number of occupants, operations, management, staffing, records management, safety and risk management, quality improvement, medication administration, conditions to obtain a nursing home license, and other specifications vary according to the long-term care home's jurisdictional regulations. The main entrance generally has a reception and/or central welcome area. Space is designated for administrative and managerial offices, dining rooms/kitchen, nursing/care stations, medication storage, bathing areas, supplies and equipment storage, leisure/recreation, family lounge areas, and staff room/lockers. Newer long-term care homes may have additional space dedicated to hairdressing, spiritual services, library, and shared or rotational space for specialty services.

In Ontario, only 16% of long-term care homes have space available for use by oral health professionals, and less than 30% have all of the appropriate equipment for oral health care delivery (ODA 2008). Most long-term care homes are designed to have several contained resident home units/areas. These areas are often named a 'house,' 'home area,' or 'wing,' and will have a number of rooms clustered around a nursing/care station with a medication room, supplies area, bathing area, dining room, and lounges, and usually have regularly assigned staff to ensure consistency of care. There are 1-bed, 2-bed, and multiple bed rooms, usually with an attached wheelchair-accessible two-piece bathroom. Bedroom furniture is provided, and spouses may share a room. See Figure 20-4 for examples of residents performing their own oral hygiene.

There are designated secure areas so that those with dementia can wander freely and safely. Entry and exit security codes are necessary for those entering or leaving specific home units as well as for the main entry to the building. The security entry codes are usually posted at or near the entrances.

Each long-term care home has its unique organizational culture, beliefs, and values, and may focus on a specific niche market such as a particular cultural group. Residents are encouraged to decorate their rooms with personal belongings, small furniture items, and photographs. Long-term care homes usually have well-articulated mission and vision statements that guide their operations and care provision. They are multicultural environments for residents and staff. The cultural and linguistic challenges can sometimes be daunting for care providers.

ORAL HEALTH ASSESSMENT TOOL (OHAT) for LONG-TERM CARE

Resident:

Date:

Nursing Admission ○ Quarterly ○ 1 ○ 2 ○ 3

NOTE: A Star * and underline indicates referral to an oral health professional (i.e. dentist, dental hygienist, denturist) is required.

Category	0 = healthy	1 = changes	2 = unhealthy	Score	Action Required	Action Completed
Lips	Smooth, pink, moist	Dry, chapped, or red at corners	Swelling or lump, white/red/ulcerated patch; bleeding/ ulcerated at corners*		1=intervention 2 =refer	☐YES ☐ NO
Tongue	Normal, moist, pink	Patchy, fissured, red, coated	Patch that is red and/or white, ulcerated, swollen*		1=intervention 2 =refer	☐YES ☐ NO
Gums and Tissues	Pink, moist, Smooth, no bleeding	Dry, shiny, rough, red, swollen around 1 to 6 teeth, one ulcer or sore spot under denture*	Swollen, bleeding around 7 teeth or more, loose teeth, ulcers and/or white patches, generalized redness and/or tenderness*		1 or 2 = refer	☐YES ☐ NO
Saliva	Moist tissues, watery and free flowing saliva	Dry, sticky tissues, little saliva present, resident thinks they have dry mouth	Tissues parched and red, very little or no saliva present; saliva is thick, ropey, resident complains of dry mouth*		1=intervention 2 =refer	☐YES ☐ NO
Natural Teeth ☐ Y ☐ N	No decayed or broken teeth/ roots	1 to 3 decayed or broken teeth/roots*	4 or more decayed or broken teeth/ roots, or very worn down teeth, or less than 4 teeth with no denture*		1 or 2 = refer	☐YES ☐ NO
Denture(s) ☐ Y ☐ N	No broken areas/teeth, dentures worn regularly and name is on	1 broken area/tooth, or dentures only worn for 1 to 2 hours daily, or no name on denture(s)	More than 1 broken area/tooth, denture missing or not worn due to poor fit, or worn only with denture adhesive*		1 = ID denture 2 = refer	☐YES ☐ NO
Oral Cleanliness	Clean and no food particles or tartar on teeth or dentures	Food particles/ tartar/ debris in 1 or 2 areas of the mouth or on small area of dentures; occasional bad breath	Food particles, tartar, debris in most areas of the mouth or on most areas of denture(s), or severe halitosis (bad breath)*		1=intervention 2 =refer	☐YES ☐ NO
Dental Pain	No behavioral, verbal or physical signs of pain	Verbal and/or behavioral, signs of pain such as pulling of face, chewing lips, not eating, aggression*	Physical signs such as swelling of cheek or gum, broken teeth, ulcers, 'gum boil', as well as verbal and or behavioral signs*		1 or 2 = refer	☐YES ☐ NO
					Completed by:	

FOLLOW UP
☐ Oral Hygiene Care Plan - Date: _____   ☐ Oral Health Assessment to be repeated on - Date: _____

☐ Person and/or family/guardian refuses: a) ☐ Referral - Date: _____   b) ☐ Dental Treatment - Date: _____

2007 Halton Region's Health Department modified with permission Chalmers (2004)   Best Practice Coordinators in Long-Term Care Initiative

Available for download: www.halton.ca   Central South   Available for download: www.rgpc.ca

Figure 20-3 Oral Health Assessment Tool (OHAT) for Long-Term Care. Reprinted with permission from the Regional Geriatric Program Central.

(a)

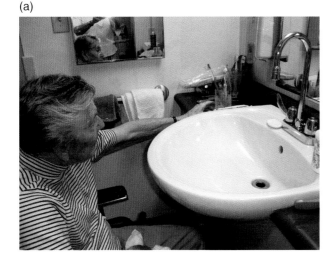

(b)

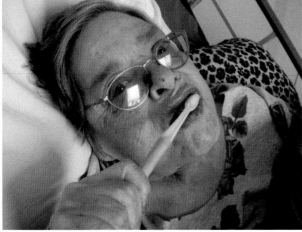

Figure 20-4 Residents conducting their own oral hygiene—one at a wheel-chair accessible sink (a) and the other in her bed (b). Courtesy of Lynda McKeown.

Staffing

All nursing care and supervision is provided by either registered nurses or registered practical nurses and personal care is provided by health care aide workers available on a 24-hour basis. Residents also have access to regular medical care, medical and treatment supplies and equipment, basic personal hygiene supplies, common use equipment such as wheelchairs, bedroom furniture, specialty programs, cleaning, laundry services, and three meals a day, plus snacks. Optional services are non-mandated services that are paid for by the resident and include hairdressing/barber, variety store, newspaper, dry cleaning, mending, ironing, non-prescription/not covered medications, and uninsured services such as specialized foot care, dental care, etc. External agencies may be contracted and involved in mandated care deliv-

> **Tip Box 20-4** What you can expect for a typical day. Is there time for mouth care?
>
> On a typical day, residents are awakened, toileted, dressed in a housecoat, and walked to or taken in a wheelchair to the dining room for breakfast at about 8:00 am. Nurses are busy administering medications. Residents eat, are coached, or are fed their breakfasts. The remainder of the morning is dedicated to completing morning hygiene care, nursing treatments and medications, mid-morning snacks, leisure/exercise, and excursion programs. Lunch is served from noon to 1:30 pm. The afternoon is spent providing nursing treatments and medications, completing hygiene care, attending leisure/social/exercise programs, other therapies, mid-afternoon snack, and afternoon napping. Outside agencies often arrive during the late morning or afternoons. Toileting happens usually before and after all meals. Supper is served around 5:00 to 6:00 pm. Often family visit in the afternoons, during dinner, and the evenings. Many residents begin requesting to go to bed at 8:00 pm. The evening is spent getting residents into their nightwear, toileting, serving snacks, and providing evening hygiene, medications, and treatments. Disruptions are minimized during the night.

ery as well as optional services provision. For example, a long-term care home may have a contract with a private dental company to provide annual oral health screening and emergency dental, care and serve as the preferred provider for residents who wish to have additional dental treatment (Chalmers *et al.* 2005; Sullivan-Marx and Gray-Micelli 2008).

In early 2008 residential care facilities providing care to the aged employed 179,582 full-time equivalents and generated $7.6 billion in wages and salaries. There is significant variability in the level, type, and cultural heritage of staff in long-term care homes. Approximately 75% of staff in long-term care homes are nonprofessional employees who are not licensed. These include personal support workers, health care aides, nursing aides, spiritual workers, therapy aides, dietary aides, housekeeping, maintenance, and leisure/activity staff. Yet, these staff members are responsible for providing the majority of the direct care and services including cleaning, maintenance, cooking, serving, and leisure activities of residents. The professional staff members who are governed by regulatory and professional standards, ethical codes of conduct, and organizational guidelines consisting of nurses, physicians, dieticians, occupational and physical therapists, speech language pathologists, social workers, and pharmacists make up the 25% balance of staffing. Long-term care homes must use a variety of approaches to schedule staff and maximize skill levels in order to provide care and services to complex and diverse

Table 20-2 Typical long-term care roles and responsibilities

Administrator	Operations, management team, external reporting, total budget
Director of Care/Nursing	Nursing management, manages and coordinates care provision throughout the long-term care home, nursing budget, often considered to be second in command below the administrator
Registered Nurses	Nursing care and treatments, coordinate personal care provision, coordinates care on the Resident Home Units, in-charge of the long-term care home when Director of Care/Nursing is off-site, onsite 24 hours a day, responsible for oral assessments (RAI-MDS)
Nurse Practitioners	Advanced nursing care provision, collaborate with physicians, can order some medications and treatments, may work in one home or many homes
Personal Support Workers	Provide personal care, may feed, on-site 24 hours a day, responsible for direct oral care
Medical Director	Medical care and treatments (±contracted position), may assess oral health on admission/ quarterly
Physicians	Medical care and treatments (usually general practitioners who continue to see residents who are still part of their medical practices, ± contracted position), may assess oral health on admission/quarterly
Dietitian	Nutritional, hydration status of residents (± contracted position)
Dietary Manager	Food operations, menu planning, mealtime provision, food budget
Dietary Aides	Food preparation, mealtime serving, ± feeding
Pharmacist	Medication dispensing system, medication consultation (± contracted position)
Occupational Therapists and Physical Therapists	Functional, physical, mobility, equipment and adaptation aid assessments, therapy programs (± contracted position)
Speech Language Pathologist	Swallowing and communication assessments (± contracted position)
Social Worker	Advocates, coordinate social assistance, family support (± contracted position)
Spiritual Worker	Spiritual program and counseling, family support (± contracted position)
Recreation/Leisure/Activity Manager	Coordinate, manage, and provide activity, leisure, recreational program, recreational budget
Recreation/Leisure/Activity Workers	Provide activity, leisure, recreational programming
Volunteers	Directed by Recreation Manager, assist with provision of leisure activities, may assist with feeding residents
Environmental Manager	Coordinates and manages the housekeeping, laundry, and maintenance services, environmental budget
Housekeeping, laundry and maintenance workers	Provide housekeeping, laundry and maintenance services
Family	May be involved with direct personal care such as feeding, oral hygiene care, may assist with additional residents
Other services	Contracted services, optional for purchase by resident, ± hair dressing, foot care, dental care

residents. This is especially challenging because the daytime hours from before breakfast to just after supper are when the bulk of the activities occur. Long-term care home medical directors, who are often general practitioners, schedule on-site visits and may provide services to more than one long-term care home (Statistics Canada 2010; Ontario Ministry of Health and Long-term Care 2008; Chalmers *et al.* 2005; Sullivan-Marx and Gray-Micelli 2008). Table 20-2 lists the more common roles and responsibilities in long-term care homes.

Plan of care—team collaboration

Collaborative teams composed of a combination of professionals, non-professionals, residents, and families are the most common model used in long-term care homes to oversee the provision of the broad range of care and services. Given the rapidly changing care needs, and diversity and complexity of long-term care residents, collaborative teamwork and effective communication skills are essential for achieving care goals and a better quality of life for residents. Teams must provide an environment of collegial support and assistance among members, as well as a willingness to learn from each other.

Each resident has a coordinated plan of care that is developed based on an interface between the various health professional assessments. Assessments are documented in clear, concise language and usually entered into an electronic chart. Reliable, validated assessment tools are preferred, with appropriate implementation strategies, evaluation, and ongoing monitoring, based on best practices and evidence-based care. Care goals are determined in collaboration with the resident and family. After the admission assessment, repeat comprehensive assessments occur quarterly and as necessary when there is a sudden change in health status. Staff members are challenged continuously to adapt optimal health care practices to meet each resident's preferences and unique needs.

In long-term care, it is important to always obtain consent before beginning each treatment. A treatment is defined as anything that is done for a therapeutic, preventative, palliative, diagnostic, cosmetic, or other health-related purpose and includes a course of treatment or plan of treatment. All care providers should review the laws or legislation related to consent for treatment and applicable legislation regarding substitute decision-makers. Long-term care homes have this information readily available. A resident's known wishes must always be respected in long-term care. Legal and ethical issues are common concerns that residents and families have regarding decisions for care and treatments, obtaining consent for the plan of care, including new or changed care, treatments, and therapies. Across Canada, there is a *Resident's Bill of Rights* that recognizes the balance of rights and responsibilities of providers, residents/families, and government. This Bill promotes residents' well-being, dignity, and safety, ability to appeal, and promotion of resident and family councils (Chalmers *et al.* 2005; Sullivan-Marx and Gray-Micelli 2008; Resident's Rights 2010). Contracted or private care providers should consider having a staff member from the long-term care home present with them when reviewing and discussing treatment plans, proposing treatment options, or providing care. Residents and family members generally trust and rely upon their care-giving staff to explain and discuss recommendations about treatments or care provision with them. Staff members are familiar with each resident, their preferences and individual unique behaviors, and understand how care can be best provided to gain cooperation or help them understand.

Best practices and quality care

A best practice is a technique or methodology that, through experience and research, has proven to reliably lead to a desired result. A commitment to using best practices in health care is a commitment to optimal use of knowledge and technology to ensure clinical outcome success. Best practices and/or evidence-based practice is about clinical decision making based on effective use of sound research to help with patient care, improve knowledge, competency, and skills in order to provide better patient care (DiCenso *et al.* 2005). Evidence-based practice integrates best research evidence with clinical expertise and patient values to facilitate clinical decision making. Identification and consideration of patient preferences and actions are central to evidence-based decision making (Sackett *et al.* 2000).

Over the past 10 years there has been an increasing focus on providing the long-term care sector and its individual health care clinicians with guidelines or algorithms that can structure and guide the diagnostic, treatment, and care interventions necessary for best practice. Clinicians must assume responsibility for implementing these guidelines and for providing the necessary components of practice derived from a combination of their education, experience, skills, and desire for quality care and optimal outcomes for long-term care residents. Examples of best practice or evidence-based guidelines used in long-term care include those from the American Medical Directors Association (AMDA), which is the professional association of medical directors, attending physicians, and others practicing in the long-term care continuum. The AMDA is dedicated to excellence in resident care and provides education, advocacy, information, and professional development to promote the delivery of quality long-term care medicine. Clinical practice guidelines for long-term care, protocols, tools and resources, journals, and other information are available on their Web site (American Medical Directors Association 2010). Other examples include nursing organizations dedicated to care of older adults that have created multiple best practices and evidence-based clinical guidelines. The Registered Nurses Association of Ontario has produced at least 44 best practice guidelines, many of which are inter-professional in focus, such as the Nursing Best Practice Guideline–Oral Health: Nursing Assessment and Intervention 2008 (Registered Nurses' Association of Ontario 2010). The University of Iowa has also produced several clinical practice guidelines such as the Oral Hygiene Care for Palliative Residents in Nursing Homes and Oral Hygiene Care for Nursing Home Residents with Dementia (University of Iowa 2010).

Implementing best practices and evidence-based guidelines to ensure quality of care and services is of vital importance (Leone 2010); however, complicating factors such as the high costs of long-term care and increasing numbers of frail older people combine to pose a significant dilemma for administration and staff alike in

Tip Box 20-5 A summary of the LTC environment

Uniqueness of long-term care	Challenges for oral health care professionals	Preparation
• Philosophy	• Operates as a home • It is not a hospital	• Limited health care resources available
• Design	• No or limited space for specialty services • Secured environment for residents	• Oral care treatments will need to be provided at the residents bedside • Bring portable equipment • Obtain the entry/exit codes
• Demographics	• More residents with complex care and services needs	• Learn the profile of the residents
• Organizational culture	• Mission and vision variations	• Respect the home's mission and vision
• Multicultural environment	• Cultural differences and linguistic barriers of residents and staff	• Understand your own cultural values, beliefs • Respect the resident's cultural beliefs and values • May require someone to interpret
• Staff	• Significant variability in the level and type of staff • Staff and families often express concerns of need for more staff	• Understand the staff composition and responsibilities • Connect with the Director of Care/Nursing • No or limited staff available to assist
• Team	• Inter-professional team model • Residents and families are part of the team	• Interaction with the team is critical • Resident and family make the final care decisions • Organize care to best meet the resident's needs and wishes
• Best practices and quality care	• Best practices, evidence-based care, valid reliable assessment tools are preferred by long-term care • Quality of care, measuring care outcomes	• Use valid reliable assessment tools • Use best practices, practices based in research evidence • Uphold practice standards • Measurement of care outcomes and care processes
• Consent and resident rights	• Consent is required before any treatment • Resident's known wishes must be respected	• Understand the laws or legislation related to consent for treatment and substitute decision-makers • Obtain consent before treatment • Be prepared to handle complaints

determining how best to undertake this endeavour. In the Canadian public health sector, the challenge is being addressed with an increasing focus on measurement of the quality of long-term care, whereas the focus in the private services area has been on competition and quality. A successful approach in the US has been the application of quality improvement of care. In particular it shows how the availability of public data has pushed the development of common indicators (Leone 2010). Starting with nursing homes, it has developed into a wider quality assurance exercise across all health care sectors and into other countries. The increasing use of RAI-MDS/interRAI in Canada has been a step to creating greater availability of resident-related data, homogenization of measurement, and narrowing of necessary and applicable quality indicators for long-term care. One of the original intended uses of MDS was not

just monitoring but also benchmarking of nursing home quality of care (Interrai 2010). The advantage of MDS-based quality indicators is that they are derived directly from the RAI assessment instrument and they are being used by government and long-term care homes to monitor their quality of care and for reporting. Nevertheless, the RAI system is only one approach, and the implementation of benchmarking will depend on national or provincial needs. Currently, there are no additional long-term care oral health quality indicators beyond RAI-MDS.

A quality improvement strategy under way across Ontario's long-term care sector is the *Residents First* initiative (Residents First 2010). This initiative is a first step to benchmarking on many indicators of quality (that is, outcome, process, balancing), provincially and in individual long-term care homes. *Residents First* is one of the most comprehensive and innovative quality improvement (QI) initiatives in Canada. It supports long-term care homes and their care teams in providing an environment for their residents that enhances their quality of life and helps them to manage complex change collaboratively, direct and create a culture of greater accountability, improve care and service care provision processes, standardize necessary processes, and achieve continuing improvements in residents' care and services. The initial five topics for quality improvement cover falls, continence, pressure ulcers, consistency of Personal Support Worker assignment, and emergency department utilization. As successes are achieved in the initial five topics, new topic areas will be introduced and hopefully provide an opportunity for other topics such as oral health to be considered.

What is the status of oral health in long-term care?

Studies, reviews, and reports consistently indicate the poor oral health status among long-term care residents and frail older adults (MacEntee *et al.* 1990; MacEntee 2005; Wyatt *et al.* 2006; Ettinger 2007; Scully and Ettinger 2007; Chalmers and Ettinger 2008; Canadian Dental Association 2009; Glassman 2010). See Figure 20-5.

Table 20-3 summarizes the extent of long-term care residents' poor oral health. The majority of long-term care residents in the past were edentulous and received dental care infrequently, often limited to emergency care with no emphasis on care aimed at retaining teeth through daily preventive oral care and use of restorative treatments (Peltola *et al.* 2004). As the oral health problems worsen in long-term care residents, dental treatments become increasingly difficult because many residents cannot tolerate lengthy procedures, and they, or their families, are unable to understand the reason for, or value of, treatment (Ontario Dental Association 2010). See Figure 20-6 for an example of a complete denture that has not been cleaned recently.

The overall rate of edentulism has been declining from 20.3% in 1972 to 13.9% in 2001 (Cunha-Cruz *et al.* 2007). Today, the trend is that Canadians are aging with a greater percentage of their natural teeth in place with 54.9–74.5% of adults between 60 and 79 years of age having some or all of their natural teeth (Statistics Canada 2010b). Long-term care can expect to see a shift to newly admitted residents having more intact teeth, dental restorations and implants, complex dental needs, and experience with receiving regular dental care and oral hygiene practices. Figure 20-7 shows a resident with porcelain crowns with retained roots where crowns of the teeth broke off.

(a)

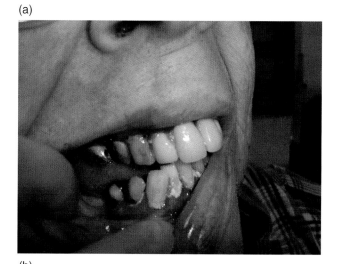

(b)

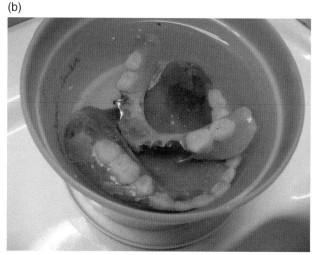

Figure 20-5 Typical hygiene in LTC. A mouth with existing teeth (a) and unclean dentures from a different patient soaking in a cup (b). Courtesy of Lynda McKeown.

Currently, the oral health status of long-term care remains poor along with many unmet dental needs, therefore, it is both inappropriate and inaccurate to continue to associate geriatric and long-term care residents' oral and dental care with denture care (Ettinger 2007). There will be an expectation from residents and families that their oral health will continue to be maintained.

Long-term care residents have complex co-morbid health conditions, take multiple medications, and continue to be at greater risk for many oral health issues (MacEntee *et al.* 1990; MacEntee 2005; Wyatt *et al.* 2006; CDA 2007; Ettinger 2007; Scully and Ettinger 2007; Chalmers and Ettinger 2008; CDA 2009; Glassman 2010). Periodontal disease is a common chronic oral inflammatory disease often found in long-term care residents. Periodontal disease directly increases the resident's risk of developing root caries and tooth loss with

Table 20-3 Prevalence of oral health issues of long-term care residents

Unmet dental needs	• 80% have unmet dental needs (Ettinger *et al.* 2000; Folse 2001) • 70% had not seen a dentist in 5 years (Frenkel *et al.* 2000) • 22% reported a current dental problem (Frenkel *et al.* 2000)
Mouth pain	• 56% have mouth pain (Ettinger *et al.* 2000; Folse 2001)
Carious, loose or broken teeth	• 32% have broken, loose, or carious teeth (Ettinger *et al.* 2000; Folse 2001) • 63% had root caries (Frenkel *et al.* 2000) • 37% were in need of restorations (Peltola *et al.* 2004) • 42% in need of extractions (Peltola *et al.* 2004)
Inflamed gums	• 37–46% have inflamed gums (Ettinger *et al.* 2000; Folse 2001) • 51% were in need of periodontal therapy (Peltola *et al.* 2004)
Teeth cleanliness	• 75% were unable to clean their teeth (Frenkel *et al.* 2000) • 2/3 of tooth surface was covered in plaque (Frenkel *et al.* 2000) • 82% had calculus present
Gingivitis	• Gingivitis noted was moderately severe (Frenkel *et al.* 2000)
Edentulism	• 42% were edentulous (Peltola *et al.* 2004)
Dentures	• 41% had removable dentures (Peltola *et al.* 2004) • 25% of dentures were in need of repair (Peltola *et al.* 2004)
Denture cleanliness	• 82% were unable to clean their dentures (Frenkel *et al.* 2000) • 64% had dentures cleaned by staff (Frenkel *et al.* 2000) • 19% had good denture hygiene (Peltola *et al.* 2004) • 95% wore unhygienic dentures (Frenkel *et al.* 2000)
Denture stomatitis	• 33% had denture stomatitis (Frenkel *et al.* 2000) • 25% had denture stomatitis (Peltola *et al.* 2004)

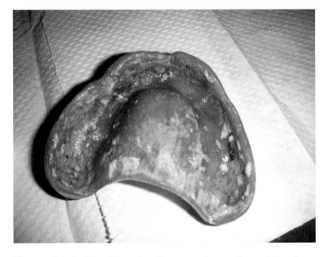

Figure 20-6 Complete that has not been cleaned in days. Courtesy of Lynda McKeown.

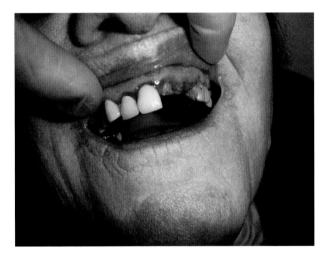

Figure 20-7 Resident with porcelain crowns retained roots where the crowns of the teeth broke off. Courtesy of Lynda McKeown.

resulting impaired chewing, eating, nutrition, and speech and reduced socialization and quality of life (MacEntee *et al.* 1990; MacEntee 2005; Wyatt *et al.* 2006; CDA 2007; Ettinger 2007; Boehm and Scannapieco 2007; Scully & Ettinger 2007; Chalmers and Ettinger 2008; CDA 2009; Glassman 2010). The pain associated with poor oral

health and ill-fitting dentures is often unrecognized thus affecting the residents' chewing ability and nutrition, causing unexplained weight loss. Research continues to directly link periodontal health to systemic health especially diabetes, cardiovascular disease (for example, stroke), lung disease (such as pneumonia), systemic infection, poor nutrition, pain, and other serious illnesses (MacEntee et al. 1990; MacEntee 2005; Wyatt et al. 2006; Coleman and Watson 2006; Ettinger 2007; CDA 2007; Scully and Ettinger 2007; Chalmers and Ettinger 2008; CDA 2009; Glassman 2010). More than 100 chronic diseases can affect the oral health of long-term care residents and in combination with multiple medications, increasing physical disability, reduced muscle strength, mobility loss, arthritis, cognitive impairment (such as dementia), tremors, stroke, Parkinson's disease, visual impairments, and difficulty swallowing make oral self-care extremely difficult, resulting in a rapid decline in the state of oral health (ODA 2010; Haumschild and Haumschild 2009). Table 20-4 provides a summary of 10 common systemic diseases (Peltola et al. 2004) and their influence on long-term care residents' oral health.

Bacterial pneumonia is one of the leading causes of death of long-term care residents. The link between periodontal disease, poor oral hygiene, and aspiration pneumonia is now well recognized through many studies (Limeback 1988; MacEntee et al. 1990; Frenkel et al. 2000; Terpenning 2005; MacEntee 2005; Wyatt et al. 2006; Ettinger 2007; Scully and Ettinger 2007; CDA 2007; Chalmers and Ettinger 2008; Bassim et al. 2008; CDA 2009; Haumschild and Haumschild 2009; Glassman 2010). The microorganisms that cause pneumonia are commonly found in significantly high concentrations in the dental plaque of older adults with periodontal disease. The dental plaque acts as a reservoir for the respiratory pathogens and can be aspirated into the lungs (Peltola et al. 2004). Aspiration pneumonia caused by bacteria-laden saliva from the dental plaque that accidentally enter the windpipe and travel to the lungs are the most threatening and dangerous consequence of poor oral hygiene for long-term care residents. An argument has been made by at least one prominent researcher that the cost of aspiration pneumonia as a nursing home complication to the health care system makes dental hygiene a potentially cost-saving and perhaps even a life-saving intervention (Terpenning 2005).

Research overwhelmingly indicates a shared association between periodontal disease and diabetes. Because long-term care residents with diabetes are particularly susceptible to contracting infections, they are at greater risk of developing periodontal disease. At the same time, oral infections can increase the severity of diabetes by increasing blood sugar levels, leading to such complications as premature degeneration of the eyes, kidneys, nerves, and blood vessels (Haumschild and Haumschild 2009).

A confirmed relationship between poor oral health and malnutrition in older adults also exists. Compromised oral health is one of the many barriers to achieving adequate food intake in older adults. Older adults with poor oral health do not benefit from being able to eat a much broader variety of nutritious foods due to their oral pain, discomfort, or tooth loss. In fact, the risk of malnutrition triples when the mouth is unhealthy (Haumschild and Haumschild 2009; Sheiham et al. 2002). The first signs of micronutrient deficiencies often are evident in the oral tissues (Moynihan 2007). Periodontal disease has been found to be causally related to a weight loss of 5% in older adults and as such may increase their risk of morbidity and mortality. Also, the number of teeth has been shown to be inversely related to weight loss. Older adults with more teeth experienced less periodontal disease and had at least two fewer teeth than those who were found to be weight stable (Weyant et al. 2004).

Many studies have confirmed that older adults with dementia have the worst oral health of all long-term care residents. They have more dental plaque, a higher debris index, poorer periodontal condition, higher coronal and root caries, more unrestorable teeth, and fewer filled and sound teeth (Chalmers et al. 2002; Chalmers et al. 2003). Possible risk factors identified for residents with dementia include salivary dysfunction, polypharmacy, multiple medical conditions, swallowing and dietary problems, functional dependence, oral hygiene care assistance, and poor use of dental care (Chalmers and Pearson 2005b). For residents with dementia, 60% have pain-causing dental conditions, which were found to be potentially life threatening because they often interfere with eating and lead to malnutrition (Cohen-Mansfield and Lipson 2002). In addition, older adults with cognitive impairment have more carious teeth, are more often edentulous, are not using or unable to use a denture, and have poorer denture hygiene than those who are healthy (Syrajala et al. 2007).

The risk for caries continues into old age, especially when medications disturb saliva and the frequency of sugar consumption increases. The percentage of teeth with decayed or filled root surfaces increases with each decade of adulthood, affecting more than half of remaining teeth by age 75 years (Winn et al. 1996). Tooth decay is more than three times greater for older adults than for those under 45 years and exceeds tooth decay rates of adolescents (CDA 2007; Chalmers and Ettinger 2008). Long-term care residents are at increased risk for caries because of the constant availability of sugary snacks such as muffins, cookies, and cakes, and as a result of their impaired ability to clear residual food from the mouth during meals, as well as issues with salivary flow and buffering capacity (MacEntee, et al. 1993). Frail older adults appear less aware of food debris, bacterial plaque, and gingivitis around their teeth, probably due to reduced proprioceptive awareness in or around the

Table 20-4 Common systemic diseases that influence oral health in long-term care

Diseases (Scully and Ettinger 2007)	Long-term care impact
Cognitive impairment Alzheimer disease Mental health	• Self-care prompting to total dependency for oral care hygiene • Increased resistance to oral care, responsive behaviors and resulting oral care neglect • Timing and repeat attempts of "short" oral procedure important, often requires two people • Confusion, communication problems, and loss of oral-self care skills • Pocketing food in mouth, difficulty swallowing, dry mouth • High risk for oral diseases • Restorative care difficult • Refusal to or forgets to wear denture, loses dentures
Diabetes	• Periodontal-diabetes systemic link greater than blood sugar control issues • Risk of infection, immunocompromised, • Wound susceptibility and reduced healing
Ischemic heart disease	• Reduced tolerance for oral procedures related to disease severity • Review ischemic heart disease status for severity, for example,. congestive heart failure, medication management, may tolerate procedures best when upright • Review anticoagulant therapy—bleeding gums • Dry mouth secondary to medications
Hypertension	• Reduced tolerance for oral procedures related to disease severity • Review medications—risk for hypotensive episodes • Dry mouth secondary to medications
Chronic obstructive pulmonary disease	• Reduced tolerance for oral procedures related to disease severity especially shortness of breath, best sitting upright • Mouth breather • Review medication therapy – corticosteroids, bronchodilators • Dry mouth secondary to medications
Stroke	• Extensiveness of paralysis on one side is variable • Physical, communication, mobility, chewing/swallowing, cognitive losses • Taking multiple medications, review anticoagulant therapy—bleeding gums • Dry mouth secondary to medications • May require two people for oral procedures • Pocketing food in mouth
Osteoporosis	• High risk for fractures • May need to adjust procedure position due to kyphosis • Risk for osteonecrosis of jaw in residents with compromised/severe oral and health status undergoing invasive dental procedures
Parkinson disease	• Involuntary movements • Increasing dependency for oral care hygiene • Review medication therapy • Dry mouth secondary to medications
Arthritis	• Reducing dexterity in hands for oral self-care, joint pain • Increasing dependency for oral care assistance • Reduced mobility • Taking multiple medications—may bleed easier
Head and neck cancer	• Reduced salivary flow after chemotherapy and radiation therapy • Mucositis, oral ulcers post therapy, need to manage discomfort, careful oral care • Need for oral care before cancer therapy

mouth. An increase in the onset of caries is evident among long-term care residents who have not had high levels of caries in the past, as well as those who have had extensive restorative care during their lifetime (Chalmers 2006).

Dental caries is also more common in older adults with xerostomia. With insufficient saliva to restore the oral pH and regulate bacterial populations, the mouth becomes quickly colonized with caries-related organisms (Gorovenko *et al.* 2009). Xerostomia is the sensation of having a dry mouth characterized by a reduction in, or complete loss of, salivary flow resulting in oral dryness and alterations in the composition of the saliva. This condition leads to problems with mastication, swallowing, speaking, taste acuity, and halitosis. There are a variety of causes such as irradiation treatment to the head and neck, uncontrolled diabetes, Sjögren's syndrome, and renal failure, however, the most common cause of salivary disorders is prescription and non-prescription medications (Chalmers 2006; Turner and Ship 2007; Gorovenko *et al.* 2009). Many systemic drugs prescribed for chronic conditions can cause adverse effects to the oral mucosa, the most common being hyposalivation. More than 80% of the most commonly prescribed medications can cause xerostomia. Long-term care residents tend to take more medications making them more susceptive to medication side effects and may experience xerostomia, bleeding disorders of the tissues, lichenoid reactions, tissue overgrowth, and/or hypersensitivity reactions. The most common of these adverse effects is dry mouth (hyposalivation, xerostomia), often leading to significant oropharyngeal disorders, pain, and impaired quality of life (for example, related to eating and speaking) (Ettinger 2007). Saliva plays a critical role in the preservation of oropharyngeal health.

There is a desperate need for dental preventive strategies to be incorporated into long-term care to prevent or control the myriad dental problems and oral conditions experienced by residents. All long-term care residents would benefit from the expertise of oral health practitioners who specialize in or have experience in geriatric dentistry or gerondontology. Advocates have proposed that the approaches must include an assessment of the risk of disease; emphasis on early detection and prevention; external and internal remineralization therapy; use of a range of restorative materials; and surgical intervention only when required and only after oral disease has been controlled (Chalmers 2006).

Oral care provision

Dental professionals often believe that long-term care staff has little interest in the oral health of residents. In fact according to several studies, although 33% of

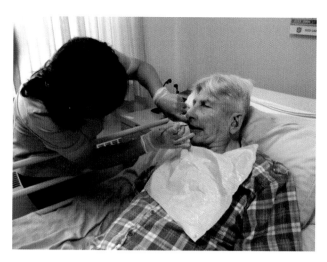

Figure 20-8 A staff member providing oral hygiene at the bedside with a resident upright. Courtesy of Lynda McKeown.

long-term care administrators requested help in improving the oral health of their residents, they had few oral health professionals express interest in attending to the long-term care population (MacEntee 1992; Weiss *et al.* 1993; Chalmers *et al.* 2001; Lewis 2001; MacEntee 2005; Turner and Ship 2007). Several studies, reviews, and reports confirm that dental service provision for nursing home residents is very low, and dentists preferred to provide treatment in their offices. Studies show that few dental hygienists were working in nursing homes due to restrictive legislation that imposed conditions such as supervision by, or an order from, a dentist (Chalmers *et al.* 2001; Lewis 2001; MacEntee 2005). Figure 20-8 shows a staff member providing bedside dental care to a resident.

In a 2010 review of long-term care homes, only 11% had a written dental care plan, 18% stated that a dentist had examined the resident on admission, and 19% had agreements for dental services and were mostly focused on emergency services. The greatest perceived barriers were the willingness of general and specialist dentists to treat residents within the long-term care home and/or in their offices, and financial concerns (Smith *et al.* 2010).

Oral health professionals site many reasons why they have no interest or do not provide services in long-term care including perceived apathy of staff and residents, uncooperative administrators, resident-related problems, lack of hands-on training for staff, financial constraints, inadequate clinical equipment, lack of portable dental equipment, and dental practice problems. There was also a lack of undergraduate education and clinical experiences related to geriatrics and the long-term care sector thus dentists preferred to provide treatment in their offices (Chalmers *et al.* 2001; MacEntee 1992; Weiss *et al.* 1993). Oral health professionals provided little educational assistance for nursing home staff, and were almost never involved in creating oral care policies or procedures (MacEntee 2005; Smith *et al.* 2010).

Currently, the level of awareness among citizens in general, as well as legislators, of the clear and direct relationship between oral health and general health is unfortunately low (CDA 2007). Not surprisingly then, the quality of oral health care (and access to it) varies greatly among Ontario's Long-Term Care homes (Haumschild and Haumschild 2009). Many long-term care homes, administrators, and staff, and oral health professionals are recognizing and beginning to address the oral care and dental treatment needs of residents. Many long-term care homes have arrangements with dental service companies, dentists, and/or dental hygienists to assist with screening, care coordination, treatment, and emergency services, along with denturists who provide denture services.

There are many barriers within the long-term care sector that help explain why oral health care is a low priority. The mix of long-term care staff from various cultural, educational, and professional backgrounds as well as the complexity of resident personal care and health issues compounds the problem of oral hygiene in long-term care. Long-term care staff members focus on promoting a strong sense of autonomy for residents, including those who are more dependent (MacEntee 2005). Respecting autonomy and choice can place the resident who repeatedly refuses oral hygiene care at greater risk for oral health problems. Poor oral hygiene can cause mucosal and gingival inflammation, caries, and periodontal disease, which can in turn cause substantial morbidity in long-term care residents (MacEntee 2005; Ettinger 2007). Poor oral hygiene and deficient oral care, combined with xerostomia, uncontrolled dietary sugar consumption, gingival recession, and the resulting root caries is often a challenge to treat and a care end point that can be avoided through an appropriate preventive care focus of long-term care staff (Terpenning 2005). See Figure 20-9 for an example of dental care by a team of staff members.

Other noteworthy challenges exist in long-term care settings such as the workload of staff and their perception of the value of oral health. Overworked staff may not have an understanding of basic oral hygiene activities and may react negatively to incorporating oral health activities into their daily responsibilities, so it is seen as one more thing they have to do in an already busy care shift. They also may not have had adequate education or training in oral health and hygiene practices (Coleman and Watson 2006; Glassman and Subar 2010). In addition, the lack of time and knowledge, protocols, and

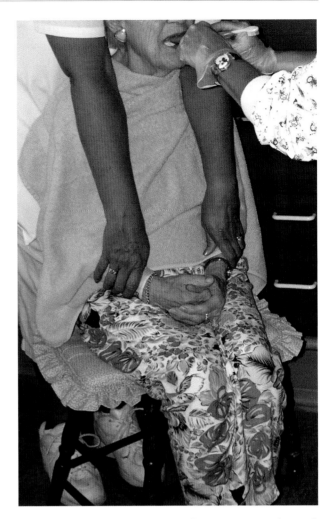

Figure 20-9 Team work: Two staff members providing safe and secure oral hygiene to a resident with dementia using the comforting hug technique.

regulations make oral hygiene care a low priority or render it unimportant. In some instances even when oral hygiene was deemed important, it failed because it was not implemented correctly or consistently, and adherence to standards was extremely low. When oral care was observed rather than self-reported, the observation rate of actual oral care provision was even lower than self-reported care provision by staff (Pyle *et al.* 2005; Coleman and Watson 2006; Shay 2007). Even when resident oral care needs were well described, staff did not perform effective oral hygiene consistent with the residents' needs (Frenkel *et al.* 2000). In some cases, nurses and direct care staff may view oral care assistance as more disagreeable than other nursing/personal care activities. Staff members do not necessarily dislike performing oral hygiene care but find it one of the most difficult personal care activities to provide for residents with dementia (Frenkel *et al.* 2000). Although registered nurses were found to have more positive attitudes toward oral care assistance than other direct care groups, they are seldom involved in the daily practice of oral hygiene care. The most common reason for not giving oral care is that the residents refused or did not want help (Wardh et al. 1997; Wardh et al. 2000; Wardh et al. 2003).

In a 2008 self-report survey, Administrator respondents of 47% of Ontario's long-term care homes reported that in their homes 90% had a relationship with oral health care professionals; 60% said all residents receive daily oral care; 30% had all residents receiving preventive, restorative, and urgent care services; 93% needed to transport residents externally for dental care services; 76% indicated lack of funds as the barrier to receiving oral health care services; 36% provided annual oral-health focused education to staff; and 45% identified challenging care behaviors such as resistance to oral care (ODA 2008). In many cases staff members attempt to provide oral hygiene care, but they have to deal with uncooperative, resistive, and physically aggressive residents, particularly those with moderate to severe dementia. Approximately, 72–84% of long-term care residents are unable to brush their own teeth effectively, 78–94% of denture wearers found it difficult or impossible to clean their dentures themselves, and 63% of residents who required assistance were resistive to care (Wardh et al. 2003; Coleman and Watson 2006; Chalmers and Pearson 2006). Residents exhibit high levels of behavioral issues in long-term care homes, and the most common oral health care difficulties of residents with behavioral issues are things such as residents biting the toothbrush, refusing care, and not opening their mouths (Wardh et al. 1997). Unfortunately, most residents who need help with their oral hygiene do not perceive that they need help (Frenkel et al. 2000). Effective toothbrush use requires a level of manual dexterity, tactile acuity, and visual ability that has likely diminished in long-term care residents who require assistance with personal care. Caregivers need to recognize when minimal standards of oral hygiene are not being achieved (Moynihan 2007). The Oral Hygiene Care Plan was introduced to Ontario long-term care homes in 2007 as a tool to assist staff in determining and recording each resident's unique oral hygiene care needs and to promote successful twice daily oral hygiene care especially in those residents with resistive-type behaviors when oral hygiene care is being attempted (Figure 20-10).

Nurses in managerial positions consider oral health an important and obvious, but neglected part of nursing. They express the wish to be updated in the relevant knowledge areas both for themselves and their personnel. Many managerial nurses see the need for standards for oral care, including documentation, which in many cases is considered to be necessary for successful implementation (Paulsson et al. 1999). The majority of direct care staff, upward of 98%, rank oral health care as very important to important (Wardh et al. 1997). Sadly, most training programs in nursing homes do not include adequate information about preventive oral health care that includes daily oral hygiene care. In-service training programs are often limited to one lecture a year or less and offer no opportunity to practice or apply the information under the supervision of an oral health professional (Jablonski et al. 2005). Furthermore, there is little integration of oral health education in the curricula of nursing programs. Nurses in long-term care need to know how to perform oral health evaluations as well as how and when to make appropriate referrals to oral health professionals (Wilder 2008).

Innovative oral care based on knowledge sharing

There is a need to implement every reasonable effort to prevent periodontal disease in long-term care residents (Boehm and Scannapieco 2007). Innovative service delivery models based on knowledge sharing, collaboration, and partnerships between oral health professionals and long-term care homes' staff are a necessary and successful approach to accomplish improved oral care in long-term care homes. Partnerships are fundamental to the provision of oral health care. The World Health Organization has promoted the "effective collaboration of partners from various disciplines and sectors of society" since 1978 and stresses that it can lead to "essential, practical and scientifically sound, accessible, appropriately delivered, coordinated and affordable health care" (WHO 1978). Two key reports out of the United States, the Surgeon General's Report on Oral Health in America (US Department of Health and Human Services 2000) and the National Call to Action to Promote Oral Health (Surgeon General 2003) emphasize the need for partnerships of key stakeholders to get involved in oral disease prevention (US Department of Health and Human Services 2000; Surgeon General 2003). Since 2006, the Canadian Oral Health Strategy (COHS) has been working to assist with the integration of oral health promotion with other health care services because a multifaceted approach may have a broader reach, thus being more effective than the traditional, independent approach that is viewed as being outside of mainstream health care (CDA 2006a). More recently, the Canadian Dental Association Committee on Clinical and Scientific Affairs (2009) emphasized that best practices for seniors' oral care that are shared along the continuum of care are necessary, along with an inter-professional approach that focuses on sharing of information and expertise among

ORAL HYGIENE CARE PLAN for LONG-TERM CARE

Resident: _____

Date: _____

Level of Assistance Required: ☐ Independent ☐ Some assistance ☐ Fully dependent

Assessment of Natural Teeth & Tissues:		
Upper (please circle)	Yes	No	Root tips present
Lower	Yes	No	Root tips present
General	*Indicate any other findings on chart below:*	

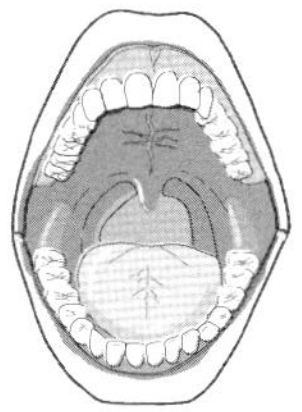

Assessment of Dentures: *(please circle)*			
Upper	Full	Partial	Not worn	No denture
	Name on denture:	Yes	No	
Lower	Full	Partial	Not worn	No denture
	Name on denture:	Yes	No	

Interventions for oral hygiene care:
(check all that apply and indicate frequency as needed)

- ☐ Regular large handled toothbrush ☐ am ☐ pm
- ☐ Use 2 toothbrush technique ☐ am ☐ pm
- ☐ Suction toothbrush ☐ am ☐ pm
- ☐ Regular fluoridated toothpaste ☐ am ☐ pm
- ☐ Do not use toothpaste
- ☐ Interproximal brush/ floss/ end tuft ☐ am ☐ pm
- ☐ Dry mouth products _____
- ☐ Other: _____

- ☐ Brush mouth tissues & tongue ☐ am ☐ pm
- ☐ Scrub denture(s) with denture brush ☐ am ☐ pm
- ☐ Soak denture(s) over night in **1** part water/**1** part vinegar solution
- ☐ Scrub denture cup & lid weekly with detergent & water
- ☐ Dry mouth products as needed
- ☐ Identify denture(s)
- ☐ Other: _____

Regular Barriers to Oral Care or Dental Treatment *(check all that apply)*

- ☐ Forgets to do oral hygiene care
- ☐ Can't remember how to do oral care
- ☐ Refuses oral hygiene care
- ☐ Won't open mouth
- ☐ Bites toothbrush
- ☐ Can't or doesn't follow directions
- ☐ Can't swallow properly (dysphagia)
- ☐ Can't rinse or spit
- ☐ Swallows all toothpastes or liquids

- ☐ Responsive behaviors:
  - ☐ Pushes away ☐ Hits
  - ☐ Turns head away ☐ Bites
  - ☐ Spits ☐ Swears
  - ☐ Other _____
- ☐ Constantly grinding / chewing
- ☐ Won't take dentures out at night
- ☐ Difficulty getting dentures in or out

- ☐ Head faces downwards
- ☐ Head is constantly moving
- ☐ Dexterity or hand problems / arthritis
- ☐ Can do some oral care but not all
- ☐ Tired, sleepy or poor attention
- ☐ Requires financial assistance for dental treatment
- ☐ Other: _____

Completed by: _____

2007 Halton Region's Health Department *modified with permission Chalmers (2004)*
Available for download: www.halton.ca

Central South Best Practice Coordinators in Long-Term Care Initiative
Available for download: www.rgpc.ca

Figure 20-10 Oral Hygiene Care Plan. Reprinted with permission from the Regional Geriatric Program Central.

Tip Box 20-6 Oral health in LTC

Oral health is a complex issue in long-term care homes that involves an interaction between, and combination of, resident, oral health, medical and functional health staff, organizational, oral health professionals, and other factors. Long-term care staff are generally poorly educated in oral health issues and poorly trained in oral hygiene care techniques. Oral health may be an unrecognized or a low care priority in long-term care homes.

---

dental providers, physicians, nurses, pharmacists, dieticians, social workers, and others (CDA 2009).

Research has documented that problems with inter-professional collaboration can have adverse effects on health care. In a recent Cochrane review that included dentists, dental hygienists, nurses, and other health care providers, one conclusion was that poor inter-professional collaboration can negatively affect the delivery of health services and patient care. Inter-professional care interventions that address inter-professional collaboration problems have the potential to improve professional practice and health care processes and outcomes (Zwarenstein *et al.* 2009). In a survey of 50 general physicians concerning dental collaboration, 94% of respondents agreed it was essential, and some of the beneficial outcomes of inter-professional collaboration noted by the respondents included improved standard of care, earlier detection and diagnosis, effective investigation and treatment, improved patient management, increased understanding of professional roles, and improved collaboration (Williams *et al.* 2003). Similarly, in a survey of 504 nurse practitioners, physician assistants, and nurse midwives, Thomas *et al.* (2008) found that 95% agreed that they should collaborate with dental professionals but only 20% agreed that their periodontal knowledge was current. However, 100% agreed that they should be taught about periodontal disease (Thomas *et al.* 2008).

The ability to work with professionals from other disciplines to deliver collaborative, patient-centered care is considered to be a critical element of professional practice (Canadian Health Services Research Foundation 2006). Oral health is a care issue that transcends professional boundaries, and long-term care provides a unique opportunity for collaboration and sharing knowledge. The "knowledge-to-action" cycle is a foundational and guiding framework developed to assist health care organizations and practitioners to move evidence into practice (Figure 20-11) (Graham *et al.* 2006). Knowledge is created or sought as a result of problem identification and need for a solution. Often evidence-based knowledge

never is used in the practice setting, or information from one discipline is never used by another discipline.

In the long-term care setting, oral health professionals are critical for improvement of the oral health status and care of residents. Sharing of knowledge will more readily promote both acceptance and integration of oral health knowledge as well as demand for practitioners within long-term care. Figure 20-12 shows how a knowledge-sharing approach between oral health professionals and long-term care staff could promote the development of innovative service delivery models. Sharing knowledge includes the two key knowledge-sharing activities of knowledge dissemination and knowledge mobilization. Oral health professionals as consultants and educators to long-term care can provide valuable knowledge regarding basic oral health, screening and assessment, practical skills, dealing with specific health conditions such as dysphagia, cariogenic foods, and other topics.

This knowledge is transferred through education and consultation encounters targeting the long-term care staff members that are most involved with the provision of oral care such as nurses, personal support workers, health care aides, dietary staff, speech language pathologists, volunteers, and family. This new knowledge could then be then used in the creation of new roles such as oral care aides and oral nurse clinicians. The new roles occur within new service delivery models that mobilize and reinforce the connectivity between long-term care and oral health care such as new government-funded programs, mobile field teams, innovative contract arrangements, and academic center partnerships.

Some examples of how knowledge can be shared to improve oral care in long-term care include dental examinations being supplemented with oral health assessments and screenings by trained nurses and care providers to monitor residents' oral health, evaluate oral hygiene care interventions, act as a trigger to call in an oral health professional when required, assist with residents' individualized oral hygiene care planning, and assist with triaging and prioritization of residents' dental needs (Chalmers and Pearson 2005a). In addition, the training of long-term care staff in the form of a comprehensive practical-oriented program addressing areas such as oral diseases, oral screening assessment, and hands-on demonstration of oral hygiene techniques and products is likely to have a positive impact on the management of oral hygiene care within residential aged care facilities (Pearson and Chalmers 2004). In fact, several studies have found that targeting oral health education to direct caregiving staff in nursing homes not only improved the resident's oral health but also improved staff member's knowledge, attitudes, and oral health care performance on functionally dependent

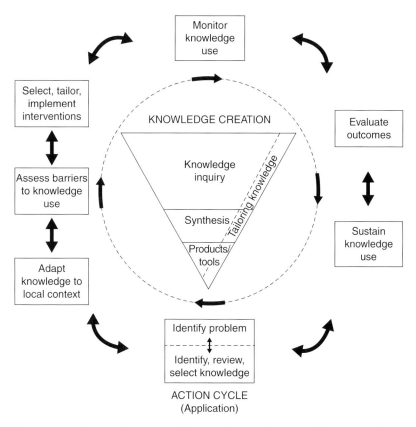

Figure 20-11 The knowledge-to-action framework. Reprinted from Graham *et al.* 2006, with permission from the Canadian Institutes of Health Research.

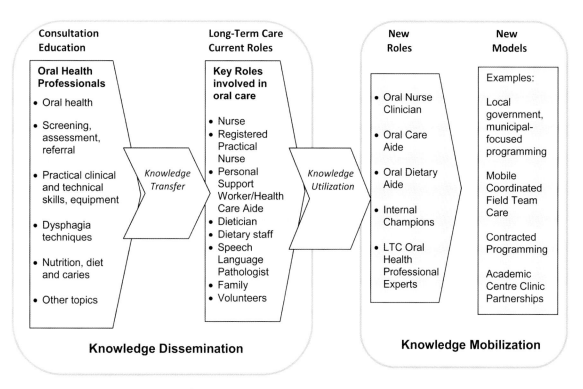

Figure 20-12 Innovative Service Delivery Models.

Table 20-5 SHRTN's Oral Health Community of Practice for Long-Term Care and Frail Older Adults. Samples of Resources and Tools

Resource/tool	Description	Resource link
Oral Health Webinars	Online Continuing Education archived webinars	All of the resources can be found at these Web sites:
Oral Health Practice and Knowledge Reference Tools	Quick reference resources such as panel cards, power point slide presentations, assessment tools, screening tools, booklets, etc.	– www.rgpc.ca/resource/index.cfm
BP Blogger	Best Practices Newsletter	– www.halton.ca/hoho
The Pocket Dockets for Oral Hygiene	Smart care cards for frontline care providers	– www.shrtn.on.ca/oralhealth
		– http://ltctoolkit.rnao.ca/
Oral Health Best Practices Guidelines	Interprofessional oral health guideline	– www.rnao.org/bestpractices

residents (Frenkel *et al.* 2001; Frenkel *et al.* 2002). Developing nursing assistants and nurses aides into specially trained oral care aides is one beneficial education strategy that has proven to be successful in a study that demonstrated when oral care aides were in charge of oral care and felt responsible for the oral hygiene care that residents received, the oral care was vastly improved (Wardh *et al.* 2003).

Another model of knowledge sharing is within a Community of Practice (CoP). Communities of practice are groups of people who share a passion for something that they know how to do and who interact regularly to learn how to do it better (Wenger, McDermott, and Snyder 2002). CoPs act as a social structure that serves as a repository of knowledge. CoP members are stewards of tacit as well as explicit knowledge and assume responsibility to develop and share specific knowledge with others and bring value to learners. Members come together based on common ground and share a sense of common identity. They foster interactions, relationships, and learning.

For example, in Ontario the Seniors Health Research Transfer Network (SHRTN) Collaborative is a network of networks—a partnership that includes the SHRTN Knowledge Exchange, the Alzheimer Knowledge Exchange (AKE), and the Ontario Research Coalition (ORC) (Seniors Health Research Transfer Network [Ontario] 2010). SHRTN works to improve the health and health care of seniors in Ontario by linking caregivers, researchers, and policy makers. SHRTN sponsors the Oral Health CoP, which is co-hosted by two Ontario organizations, the Regional Geriatric Program Central at St. Peter's Hospital-Hamilton Health Sciences and Halton Region Health Department's Oral Health Program. This CoP operates as a trans-sectoral knowledge-based inter-professional social network, which enables the dissemination of evidence-based and clinically relevant oral health information to care providers

of frail older adults through interconnected methods of awareness-raising strategies. These methods include education and learning opportunities and collaboration and networking between general health care and oral health sectors. Membership is open to anyone interested in improving the oral health of long-term care residents and frail older adults and includes professionals from the oral health and health care sectors. This constant knowledge exchange was found to be a factor that characterized effective inter-professional teamwork (Gaboury *et al.* 2009). SHRTN is providing an exciting venue for the oral health and health care sectors to interface and collaborate more effectively and begin to promote a growing collection of resources and tools aimed at improving oral health knowledge and skills within long-term care homes. Table 20-5 provides a sampling of some of the resources and tools.

There is no doubt that poor oral hygiene is a complex issue for long-term care homes. Figure 20-13 depicts another model that effectively details and summarizes the many interacting influences on resident's oral health and shows why solutions need to be multi-faceted (Pyfferoen *et al.* 2007). In this model, four cycles (resident-medical, resident-dental, caregiver-nursing home, and dental care) intersect and interact with one another and can perpetuate poor oral hygiene care in long-term care homes. The four cycles in this model follow:

Cycle 1: Resident-medical shows the medical and oral health issues that impact long-term residents.

Cycle 2: Resident-dental articulates the oral health issues as a result of Cycle 1 and additional care provision issues that impact oral health.

Cycle 3: Caregiver-nursing home describes the internal nursing home issues that impact directly on care provision and resident's resulting oral health status.

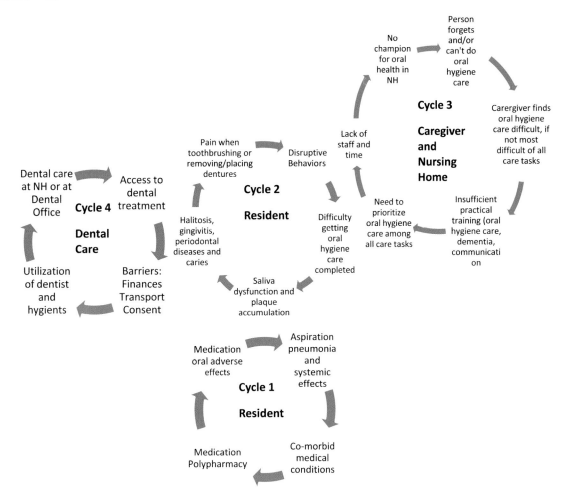

Figure 20-13 Model of cycles of poor oral hygiene in nursing homes. Reprinted from Pyfferoen *et al.* 2007, with permission from the author.

Cycle 4: Dental care highlights the dental care barriers and access issues that impact a resident's oral health (CDA 2010).

Oral health-related quality of life

Good oral health contributes to a resident's overall quality of life. Oral health, as defined by the Canadian Dental Association, includes the concept of well-being, not just the concept of absence of infirmity: "Oral health is a state of the oral and related tissues and structures that contributes positively to physical, mental and social well-being and the enjoyment of life's possibilities, by allowing the individual to speak, eat and socialize unhindered by pain, discomfort or embarrassment" (Pyfferoen *et al.* 2007). The Canadian Dental Hygienists Association emphasizes the integral link between oral health and general health in its statement "Oral health is essential for overall wellness" (Canadian Dental Hygienists Association 2010). The Canadian Oral Health Strategy reaffirms that

overall health and well-being cannot be achieved when an individual experiences oral disease (CDA 2006a). Achieving oral health requires an absence of disease and disorders in the oral, dental, and craniofacial tissues.

Oral disease and dysfunction can be extremely painful and can have an acute impact on quality of life of older adults, affecting their chewing, difficulties in eating, speaking effectively, self-esteem, as well as social interactions and relationships (CDA 2006a). In no segment of society are these domains of health more critical than in the older adult, for it is in this population that deficits in quality of life are the most devastating (Pyle 2002). There are significant associations between measures of oral health-related dysfunction, pain, and disability with psychological well-being and life satisfaction (Locker *et al.* 2000). Subjects who rated their oral health as poor had lower morale, more life stress, and were less satisfied with their lives. They concluded that oral health is an important contributor to the well-being of older adults. In those older adults who were financially disadvantaged, poor oral health had a great impact on their well-being. Similarly older persons who perceive that they have poor oral health also described diminished quality of life (Locker 1995). However, researchers have also observed that there is a degree of discordance between self-ratings of, and satisfaction with, both oral and general health status in the older adult population (Locker and Gibson 2005). The unexpected paradox was that some people who reported poor oral health or general health had high reported satisfaction. This may be because of the expectations concerning health in later life. People assess their health-related quality of life based on their expectations and experiences. In long-term care, the daily focus of care is promoting the best quality of life that is possible. Oral health needs to be a critical component of overall resident quality of life in long-term care homes.

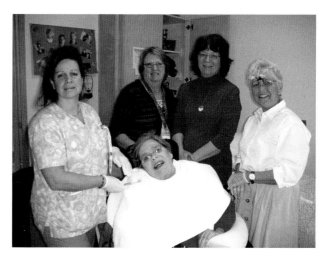

Figure 20-14 A dental hygienist working with the staff to provide a comprehensive oral care program. Courtesy of Lynda McKeown.

Challenges for oral care professionals

A great deal of information about long-term care has been presented in this chapter, and myriad significant barriers have been discussed regarding the provision of oral care (Figure 20-14).

By now the reader has concluded that long-term care homes rarely have space, let alone necessary dental equipment, to support dental treatments. In general most oral health providers have little or no experience delivering services outside the confines of a traditional dental operatory. In addition, oral health professionals are taught to provide quality care and optimal treatment for each client/patient, and the challenge of trying to meet this standard of care in a foreign environment such as long-term care can be very daunting. Compounding this is a significant lack of oral health knowledge and oral hygiene skills of staff in long-term care. Some staff may have received very basic training, but most have no education in, and do not recognize of the value of, daily oral hygiene care practices. If there is little support at the administrative level of the home and little or no legislation compelling a home to provide dental care and promote good oral health, then how likely are they to be receptive to oral health providers? Furthermore, if residents and their families fail to recognize the importance of good oral health then how likely are they to commit to receiving dental treatments?

Numerous articles have been published over the past 20 years describing models of care delivery for seniors and other special groups in long-term care sites, institutions, and community-based clinics. These models range from collaborative care networks, to mobile dental hygiene services, as well as dentist-owned mobile practices. Education-based models exist that are aligned with a faculty of dentistry and/or dental hygiene program,

community outreach programs, and even centrally based dental businesses that coordinate care using local contractors (Bowes and Hicks 1990; Crosson 1996; Heisterman 1998; Morreale *et al.* 2005; CDA 2006a; CDA 2006b). Despite the broad array of models presented in the literature, a consensus has not been met on what strategy is ideal, each model has its own set of challenges (Melanson 2008), and, perhaps even more startling, there is no consensus on the appropriate management strategy for improving the oral health care in residential settings (MacEntee 2009). What is constant and consistent in the literature is the repeated identification of the same challenges such as the lack of funding for dental care, absence of an effective dental care delivery system, need for appropriate education for all health care professionals, failure to appreciate the importance of oral health and logistics/administration of long-term care (Bonito 2002; Ontario Dental Association 2008). Challenges are not necessarily barriers but can and should be seen as opportunities for innovative approaches to both service provision and oral health improvement for long-term care residents.

In 2009 the Canadian Dental Association released a document outlining best practices for oral care in long-term care (CDA 2009), which can serve as a guide for oral health professionals to use when contemplating how to extend services into long-term care at a local level. The recommendations along with some additional descriptions follow:

1. Gain organizational support for the value of oral health. Organizational support can include government at all levels; professional colleges and training schools, long-term care organizations; long-term

care staff such as medical directors; administrators, directors of care, nurse practitioners, dieticians; professional associations; long-term care corporations; geriatric associations; and specialized geriatric services.

2. Use a multidisciplinary approach for the design. Help plan, implement, and evaluate the oral care program.

   Inter-professional collaboration and partnering is the key to understanding and adapting oral health services to the long-term care sector. Study each long-term care home closely, question and observe staff, and work with senior management to design a program that is appropriate and acceptable.

3. Ensure each home has an evidence-based policy on oral care. Long-term care homes prefer knowledge and care practices that are proven effective and that deliver positive outcomes. They need knowledge and assistance to develop appropriate policies and procedures that work within the constraints of the long-term care environment.

4. Ensure that a thorough oral examination, including an oral health history as well as an oral assessment, is conducted by a qualified dental health professional upon entry, and at regular intervals by trained nurses/caregivers. Long-term care would benefit from a refocus to a prevention and oral health promotion approach and shift away from emergency-style dental care. Sharing knowledge and training long-term care staff who interact daily with residents will promote a continuum of oral health services and increase cooperation, understanding, and appropriate use of oral health professionals.

5. Ensure an individual oral care plan is developed for each resident. Care and services must be individualized to each resident. Detailed yet easy-to-use oral hygiene care information entered into an oral care plan can promote twice daily oral hygiene and increase the success of oral hygiene care among residents with dementia, physical disabilities, and unique care needs.

6. Ensure that continuing education is provided for staff regarding appropriate oral health knowledge and skills. Many long-term care homes are void of oral health knowledge, assessment skills, and oral hygiene care skills. Oral health professionals have a tremendous amount of knowledge and skills to share with long-term care that is needed by direct care providers to improve the oral health of residents. Many college, university, and training programs for health care professionals and care providers include very minimal information on oral health and hygiene care techniques. Long-term

care has the knowledge on how to deliver care to their residents and what is possible within its environment.

A challenging case—how would you provide oral health services?

Case study

About 4 weeks ago I received a request from a nurse manager in a LTC facility to provide direction on mouth care for a new resident. She is not coping well in long-term care as she has been a fiercely independent person but could no longer cope in her own home. The resident is female, 76 years old with Parkinson's disease. She has tremors in both hands. Her dysphagia is worsening, and she has had many aspirations in the past and is known to be a "silent" aspirator.

I met with the new resident and the staff who care for her and demonstrated safe oral hygiene care. I recommended that toothpaste not be used. A toothbrush dipped in a fluoride mouthwash and tapped to remove excess liquid should be used instead in her heavily restored mouth. The staff are using "mop and go" or suction for all tooth brushing.

The resident and the family are upset that toothpaste is not being used. I am scheduled to return next week to follow-up.

What would be a satisfactory outcome? Factors to review and consider follow:

- Resident's current oral health status –plans for regular dental care, admission assessment
- Discuss with resident and family their understanding of oral health, hygiene care practices
- Resident's current health status—understanding Parkinson's disease
- The risk of aspiration, dysphagia with other activities such as eating and drinking
- Safe oral hygiene practices: mouthwash, toothpaste, mop and go, suction tooth brushing or other alternatives, proper positioning
- Resident's competency, decision-making capability, and resident's rights to choice
- Resident's wishes—realistic or not realistic
- Resident's physical capability for oral self-care, her past oral hygiene practices
- Staff experience with similar situations
- Inter-professional team—who has been involved in her care: physician, speech language pathologist, nurses
- Current research evidence or best practices
- Resident and family involvement in the decision—her preferences, her losses, her coping, her insistence, quality of life
- Documentation—oral care plan

Satisfactory outcome:

- Gather as much information as possible from as many sources as possible and include the resident and family, health care team members.
- Gather evidence-based information.
- Weigh the risks, benefits, and the resident's and family's wishes.
- Understand the resident's and family's perspective and reasons.
- Make recommendations and record in the resident's chart and oral care plan.

I met again with the Nurse Manager, collected and reviewed all information from the care team. I also reviewed the research evidence on dysphagia and met with the resident and family where they reiterated that it was very important to them to have her use toothpaste despite the risks. According to staff and the resident, the suction toothbrush was ineffective in dealing with the saliva. I suggested that the mouth rinse could be switched to a non-foaming type of toothpaste and a specialty toothbrush. I advised that staff should assist with her oral hygiene care and must always present. The resident is not allowed to do her oral hygiene care without a staff member present. The resident now feels her mouth and teeth are much cleaner. She and her family are very happy with the final care recommendation.

References

Accreditation Canada. (2010) *Accreditation Canada*. [online] available at http://www.accreditation.ca/accreditation-programs/.

American Medical Directors Association. (2010) *American Medical Directors Association website*. [online] available at http://www.amda.com

Avalere Health. (2008) *Long-Term Care: An Essential Element of Healthcare Reform*. [online] available at http://www.thescanfoundation.org/sites/default/files/ChartBook_121808.pdf.

Bassim, C.W., Gibson, G., Ward, T. *et al.* (2008) Modification of the risk of mortality from pneumonia with oral hygiene care, *Journal of the American Geriatrics Society*, 56, 1601–1607.

Boehm, T.K. and Scannapieco, F.A. (2007) The epidemiology, consequences and management of periodontal disease in older adults. *Journal of the American Dental Association*, 138, 26S–33S.

Bonito, A. J. (2002) Executive summary: dental care considerations for vulnerable populations. *Special Care in Dentistry*, 22(3) (Supplement), 53–10s.

Bowes, D. and Hicks, T. (1990) Provision of dental services to collective living centres: the Simcoe County experience. *Healthbeat. Ontario Public Health Association*. Summer 1990.

Butler, R. (2008) *The Longevity Revolution. The Benefits and Challenges of Living a Long Life*. Public Affairs: New York.

Canadian Dental Association. (2010) *Canadian Dental Association website definition of oral health*. [online] available at www.cda-adc.ca.

Canadian Dental Association. (2009) *Committee on Clinical and Scientific Affairs. Canadian Dental Association: Optimal Oral Health for Frail Older Adults: Best Practices Along a Continuum of Care*. July, Canadian Dental Association. Ottawa, Canada. [online] available at http://www.cda-adc.ca/en/dental_profession/ practising/best_practices_seniors/default.asp.

Canadian Dental Association. (2008) *Committee on Clinical and Scientific Affairs Canadian Dental Association Report on Senior's Oral Health*. Canadian Dental Association. Ottawa, Canada. [online] available at http://www.cda-adc.ca/_files/members/news_publications/member/pdfs/cda_seniors_oral_ health_report_may_2008.pdf.

Canadian Dental Association. (2006a) Federal, Provincial, Territorial Dental Director's working group. *A Canadian Oral Health Strategy*. Canadian Dental Association, Ottawa, Canada. [online] available at http://www.fptdwg.ca/assets/PDF/Canadian%20Oral%20Health%20Strategy%20-%20Final.pdf.

Canadian Dental Association. (2006b) Focus on Seniors' Programs. *Journal of the Canadian Dental Association*, 72, 385–590.

Canadian Dental Hygienists Association. (2010) Canadian Dental Hygienist Association definition of oral health. [online] available at www.cdha.ca.

Canadian Health Services Research Foundation. (2006) *Teamwork in Healthcare: Promoting Effective Teamwork in Healthcare in Canada*. Canadian Health Services Research Foundation. Ottawa, Canada.

Canadian Institute for Health Information. (2005) *Resident Assessment Instrument (RAI) MDS 2.0 and RAPs in Canadian Version User's Manual Second Edition March 2005 (Long Term Care Homes Common Assessment Project—RAI-MDS)* [online] available at https://www.ehealthontario.ca/portal/server.pt?open=512&objID=986&mode=2&in_hi_.

CBC News. (2007) *Canada's Nursing Homes National Statistics 2007*. [online] available at http://www.cbc.ca/news/interactives/map-nursing-homes/.

Chalmers, J.M. (2006) *Minimal Intervention Dentistry: Part 1, Strategies for Addressing the New Caries Challenge in Older Patients*. *Journal of the Canadian Dental Association*, 72, 427–433.

Chalmers, J.M, Carter, K.D., and Spencer, A.J. (2002) Caries incidence and increments in community-living older adults with and without dementia. *Gerondontology*, 19, 80–94.

Chalmers, J.M., Carter, K.D., and Spencer, A.J. (2003) Oral diseases and conditions in community-living older adults with and without dementia. *Special Care Dentistry*, 23, 7–17.

Chalmers, J.M. and Ettinger, R.L. (2008) Public health issues in geriatric dentistry in the United States. *Dental Clinics of North America*, 52, 423–446.

Chalmers, J.M., Hodge, D., Fuss, J.M., *et al.* (2001) Opinions of dentists and directors of nursing concerning dental care provision for Adelaide nursing homes. *Australian Dental Journal*, 46, 277–283.

Chalmers, J.M., King, P.L., Spencer, A.J., *et al.* (2005) The Oral Health Assessment Tool—Validity and reliability. *Australian Dental Journal*, 50, 191–199.

Chalmers, J.M. and Pearson, A. (2005a) A systematic review of oral health assessment by nurse and carers for residents with dementia in residential care facilities. *Special Care Dentistry*, 25, 227–233.

Chalmers, J.M. and Pearson, A. (2005b) Integrative literature review and meta-analyses: Oral hygiene care for residents with dementia: literature review. *Journal of Advanced Nursing*, 52, 410–419.

Cohen-Mansfield, J. and Lipson, S. (2002) The under-detection of pain of dental etiology in persons with dementia. *American Journal of Alzheimer's Disease and Other Dementias*, 17, 249–253.

Coleman, P. and Watson, N.M. (2006) Oral care provided by certified nursing assistants in nursing homes. *Journal of the American Geriatrics Society*, 54, 138–143.

Crosson, B. (1996). Mobile Oral Hygiene Services. *Probe*, 30, 1–4.

Cunha-Cruz, J., Hujoel, P.P., Nadanovsky, P. (2007) Secular trends in socioeconomic disparities in edentulism: USA, 1972–2001. *Journal of Dental Research*, 86, 131–136.

DiCenso, A., Guyatt, G., Ciliska D. (2005) *Evidence-based Nursing. A Guide to Clinical Practice.* Elsevier Mosby, Philadelphia, PA.

Ettinger, R.L. (2007) Oral health and the aging population. *Journal of the American Dental Association,* 139, 55–56.

Ettinger, R.L., O'Toole, C., Warren J. *et al.* (2000) Nursing directors' perceptions of the dental components of the Minimum Data Set (MDS) in nursing homes. *Special Care in Dentistry,* 20, 23–27.

Fernandez, N. and Spencer, B.G. (2010) The private cost of long-term care in Canada: Where you live matters. *Canadian Journal on Aging,* 29, 307–316.

Folse, G.J. (2001) National MDS and dental deficiency data reported by the US Health Care Financing Administration. *Special Care in Dentistry,* 21, 37–38.

Frenkel, H.F., Harvey, I., Needs, K.M. (2002) Oral health care education and its effect on caregivers' knowledge and attitudes: a randomised controlled trial. *Community Dentistry and Oral Epidemiology,* 30, 91–100.

Frenkel, H., Harvey, I., Newcomb, R.G. (2001) Improving oral health in institutionalised elderly people by educating caregivers: a randomised controlled trial. *Community Dentistry and Oral Epidemiology,* 29, 289–297.

Frenkel, H., Harvey, I., Newcombe, R.G. (2000) Oral health among nursing home residents in Avon. *Gerodontology,* 17, 33–38.

Gaboury, I.M., Bujold, M., Boon, H., *et al.* (2009) Interprofessional collaboration within Canadian integrative healthcare clinics: Key components. *Social Science & Medicine,* 69, 707–715.

Glassman, P. (2010) Creating and maintaining oral health for dependent people in institutional settings. *Journal of Public Health Dentistry,* 70, S40–S48.

Glassman, P. and Subar, P. (2010) Creating and maintaining oral health for dependent people in institutional settings. *Journal of Public Health Dentistry,* 70, S40–S48.

Gorovenko, M.R., Clark, D.C., Aleksej&ugraveuml;niene J. (2009) Over the counter xerostomia remedies currently available in Canada. *Canadian Journal of Dental Hygiene,* 43, 71–77.

Graham, I.D., Logan, J., Harrison, M.B., *et al.* (2006) Lost in Knowledge Translation: Time For A Map? *Journal of Continuing Education in the Health Professions,* 26, 13–24.

Haumschild, M.S. and Haumschild, R.J. (2009) The Importance of oral health in long-term care. *Journal of the American Medical Directors Association,* 10, 667–671.

Health Canada. (2008) *Canada Health Act: Annual Report 2007–2008.* [online] available at http://www.hc-sc.gc.ca/hcs-sss/alt_formats/hpb-dgps/pdf/pubs/chaar-ralcs-0708/2008-cha-lcs-eng.pdf.

Heisterman, B. (1998) Lest We Forget. *Probe,* 32, 1–3.

Institute for Clinical Evaluative Science. (2010) *Aging in Ontario. An ICES Chartbook on Health Services Use by Older Adults September 2010.* [online] available at http://www.ices.on.ca/file/AAH%20Chartbook_interactive_final_2010.pdf.

Interrai. (2010) Interrai Web site. [online] available at http://www.interrai.org/section/view/?fnode=29.

Jablonski, R.A., Munro, C.L., Grap, M.J. (2005) The role of biobehavioral, environmental, and social forces on oral health disparities in frail and functionally dependent nursing home elders. *Biological Research for Nursing,* 7, 75–82.

Leone, T. (2010) Measuring the quality of long-term care. *Eurohealth,* 16, 1.

Lewis, D.W. (2001) Alternative dental hygiene practice: access, cost and harm considerations. *Probe,* 5, 139–144.

Limeback, H. (1988) The relationship between oral health and systemic infections among elderly residents of chronic care facilities: a review. *Gerodontology,* 7, 131–137.

Locke, D. (1995) Xerostomia in older adults: A longitudinal study. *Gerondontology,* 12, 18–25.

Locker, D., Clark, M., Payne B. (2000) Self-perceived oral health status, psychological well-ageing and life satisfaction in an older adult population. *Journal of Dental Research,* 79, 970–975.

Locker, D. and Gibson, B. (2005) Discrepancies between self-ratings of and satisfaction with oral health in two older health adult populations. *Community Dentistry and Oral Epidemiology,* 33, 280–288.

MacEntee, M.I. (2005) Caring for elderly long-term care patients: oral health-related concerns and issues. *Dental Clinics of North America,* 49, 429–444.

MacEntee, M.I., Clark, D.C., Click, N. (1993) Predictors of caries in old age. *Gerondontology,* 10, 90–97.

MacEntee, M.I., Waxler-Morrison, N.E., Morrison, B.J., *et al.* (1992) Opinions of dentists on the treatment of elderly patients in long term care facilities. *Journal of Public Health Dentistry,* 52, 239–244.

MacEntee, M., MacInnis, B., McKeown, L., *et al.* (2009) *Dignity with a Smile. Oral Healthcare Report for Elders in Residential Care. A report for the Federal Dental Advisory Committee.* Summary Recommendation January 2009.

MacEntee, M.I., Wyatt, C.C., McBride, B.C. (1990) Longitudinal study of caries and cariogenic bacteria in an elderly disabled population. *Community Dental Oral Epidemiology,* 18, 149–152.

Melanson, S. (2008) Establishing a social dental clinic: addressing unmet dental needs. *Canadian Journal of Dental Hygiene,* 42, 185–193.

Morreale, J., Dimity, S., Morreale, M., *et al.* (2005) Setting up a mobile dental practice within your present office structure. *Journal of the Canadian Dental Association,* 71, 91.

Moynihan, P. (2007) The relationship between nutrition and systemic and oral well-being in older people. *Journal of the American Dental Association,* 138, 493–497.

Ness, J., Ahmed, A., Aronow, W.S. (2004) Demographics and payment characteristics of nursing home residents in the United States: A 23-year trend. *Journal of Gerontology: Medical Sciences,* 59A, 1213–1217.

Ontario Dental Association. (2010) *Oral Health and Aging: Addressing Issues and Providing Solutions. Ontario Dental Association Special Issue.* Oral health issues for Ontarians. Toronto: ODA. [online] available at http://www.oda.on.ca/ontario-dental-association-calls-for-help-for-the-frail-elderly.html Accessed November 29, 2010.

Ontario Dental Association. (2008) *Long-Term Care Access to Oral Health Care Summit. April 9, 2008. Ontario Dental Association, Ontario Dental Hygienists Association, Royal College of Dental Surgeons of Ontario. Final Report.*

Ontario Ministry of Finance. (2009) *Ontario Ministry of Finance Population Projections 2009–2036.* http://www.fin.gov.on.ca/en/economy/demographics/projections/. Accessed November 19, 2010.

Ontario Ministry of Health and Long-term Care. (2008) *People Caring For People Impacting the Quality of Life and Care of Residents of Long-Term Care Homes. May 2008. A Report of the Independent Review of Staffing and Care Standards for Long-Term Care Homes in Ontario.* [online] available at http://health.gov.on.ca/english/public/pub/ministry_reports/staff_care_standards/staff_care_standards.html.

O'Shaughnessy, C. (2010) *National Spending for Long-Term Services and Supports (LTSS).* [online] available at http://www.nhpf.org/library/details.cfm/2783. Accessed November 29, 2010.

Paulsson, G., Nederfors, T., Fridlund B. (1999) Conceptions of oral health among nurse managers. A qualitative analysis. *Journal of Nursing Management,* 7, 299–306.

Pearson, A. and Chalmers, J. (2004) Oral hygiene care for adults with dementia in residential aged care facilities. Systematic review. *JBI Reports,* 2, 65–113.

Peltola, P., Vehkalahti, M.M., Wuolijoki-Saaristo, K. (2004) Oral health and treatment needs of the long-term hospitalised elderly. *Gerondontology*, 21, 93–99.

Public Health Agency of Canada. (2010) *The Chief Public Health Officer's Report on the State of Public Heath in Canada, 2010: Growing Older—Adding Life to Years.* [online] available at http://www.phac-aspc.gc.ca/cphorsphc-respcacsp/index-eng.php.

Public Health Agency of Canada. (2006) *Healthy Aging in Canada: A New Vision from Vital Investment from Evidence to Action. September 2006. Background Paper Prepared for the Federal, Provincial and Territorial Committee of Officials (Seniors).* [online] available at http://www.phac-aspc.gc.ca/seniors-aines/alt-formats/pdf/publications/pro/healthy-sante/haging_newvision/vision-rpt_e.pdf.

Pyfferoen, M., Cody, K., Chalmers, J., *et al.* (2007) Observation of mealtime and oral hygiene cares for dementia residents. Abstract 955. In: The IADR/AADR/CADR 85th General Session and exhibition (March 21–24, 2007). New Orleans, LA.

Pyle, M. (2002) Changing perceptions of oral health and its important to general health: Provider perceptions, public perceptions, policy-maker perceptions. *Special Care Dentistry*, 22, 8–15.

Pyle, M.A., Jasinevicius, T.R., Sawyer, D.R., *et al.* (2005) Nursing home executive directors' perception of oral care in long-term care facilities. *Special Care Dentistry*, 25, 111–117.

Resident's First. (2010) Residents First Initiative Web site. Ministry of Health and Long-Term Care, Toronto Ontario. [online] available at http://www.ohqc.ca/en/ltc_prov_results.php.

Registered Nurses' Association of Ontario. (2010) Registered Nurses' Association of Ontario website. Nursing Best Practice Guidelines. [online] available at http://www.rnao.org.

Registered Nurses Association of Ontario. (2002) *Orientation Program for Nurses in Long-Term Care Workbook.* ISBN 0-920166-47-4. Registered Nurses' Association of Ontario, Toronto, Ontario.

Resident's Rights. (2010) *Resident's Rights Ontario Long-Term Care Homes.* [online] available at http://www.health.gov.on.ca/english/public/program/ltc/25_standards.html.

Rockwood, K., Fox, R.A., Stolee P., *et al.* (1994) Frailty in elderly people: an evolving concept. *Canadian Medical Association Journal*, 150, 489–495.

Sackett, D.L., Straus S.E., Richardson W.S., *et al.* (2000) *Evidence-based Medicine. How to Practice and Teach EBM.* Churchill Livingstone, London.

Scully, C. and Ettinger, R.L. (2007) The influence of systemic diseases on oral health care in older adults. *Journal of the American Dental Association*, 138, 7S–14S.

Seniors Health Research Transfer Network (Ontario). (2010) Seniors Health Research Transfer Network Web site (Ontario). [online] available at http://beta.shrtn.on.ca/.

Shay, K. (2007) Who is responsible for a nursing home resident's daily oral care? *Journal of the American Geriatrics Society*, 55, 1470–1471.

Sheiham, A., Steele, J.G., Marcenes, W., *et al.* (2002) The relationship between oral health status and Body Mass Index among older people: a national survey of older people in Great Britain. *British Dental Journal*, 192, 703–706.

Smetanin, P., Kobak, P., Briante, C., *et al.* (2009) *Rising Tide: The Impact of Dementia in Canada 2008 to 2038.* [online] available at http://www.alzheimer.ca/english/rising_tide/rising_tide_summary.htm.

Smith, B.J., Ghezzi, E.M., Manz, M.C., *et al.* (2010) Oral healthcare access and adequacy in alternative long-term care facilities. *Special Care Dentistry*, 30, 85–94.

Standing Committee on Public Accounts. (2007) *Standing Committee on Public Accounts. 2007. Long-Term Care Homes—Medication Management. Section 3.10 Annual Report of the Auditor General of Ontario.* [online] available at http://www.ontla.on.ca/committee-proceedings/committee-reports/files_pdf/img-Y181722-0001Eng.pdf.

Statistics Canada. (2010a) *Canadian Health Measures Survey Cycle 1 2007–2009 Table 40 Dental Status.* [online] available at http://www.statcan.gc.ca/cgi-bin/imdb/p2SV.pl?Function=getSurvey&SDDS=5071&lang=en&db =imdb&adm=8&dis=2.

Statistics Canada. (2010b) *Statistics Canada 2010 Minister of Industry. Residential Care Facilities 2007/2008 Catalogue 83-237-X Government of Canada.* [online] available at http://www.statcan.gc.ca/bsolc/olc-cel/olc-cel?catno=83-237-X&lang=eng.

Stevenson, D., Cohen M., Tell E., *et al.* (2010) The Complementarity of Public and Private Long-Term Care Coverage. *Health Affairs*, 29, 35–43.

Sullivan-Marx, E.M. and Gray-Micelli, D. (2008) *Leadership and Management Skills for Long-Term Care.* Springer, New York.

Surgeon General. (2003) *National call to action to promote oral health.* [online] available at http://www.surgeongeneral.gov/topics/oral-health/nationalcalltoaction.html.

Syrjala, A.M.H., Ylostalo, P., Sulkava, R.M., *et al.* (2007) Relationship between cognitive impairment and oral health: results of the Health 2000 Health Examination Survey in Finland. *Acta Odontologica Scandinavica*, 65, 103–108.

Terpenning, M. (2005) Geriatric oral health and pneumonia risk. *Clinical Infectious Diseases*, 40, 1807–1810.

Thomas, K.M., Jared, H.L., Boggess, K., *et al.* (2008) Prenatal care providers' oral health and pregnancy knowledge behaviours. Abstract 0725. The AADR 37th Annual Meeting and Exhibition. Dallas, TX.

Turner, M.D. and Ship, J.A. (2007) Dry mouth and its effects on the oral health of elderly people. *Journal of the American Dental Association*, 138 (9 supplement), 15S–20S.

University of Iowa. (2010) University of Iowa Geriatric Education Center Nursing clinical practice guidelines [online] available at http://www.healthcare.uiowa.edu/igec/publications/info-connect/default.asp.

US Department of Health and Human Services. (2000) *US Department of Health and Human Services Oral Health in America: A Report of the Surgeon General.* Rockville, MD: National Institute of Dental and Craniofacial Research, National Institutes of Health. [online] available at http://www.nidr/nih.gov/sgr/oralhealth.asp.

Wardh, I., Andersson, L., Sorensen, S. (1997) Staff attitudes to oral health care. A comparative study of registered nurses, nursing assistants and home care aides. *Gerodontology*, 14, 28–32.

Wardh, I., Hallber, L., Berggren, U., *et al.* (2003) Oral health education for nursing personnel: experiences among specially trained oral care aides: One-year follow-up interviews with oral care aides at a nursing facility. *Scandinavian Journal of Caring Science*, 17, 250–256.

Wardh, I., Hallberg, L.R.M., Berggren, U., *et al.* (2000) Oral health care: A low priority in nursing. *Scandinavian Journal of Caring Science*, 14, UI 137–142.

Weiss, R.T., MacEntee, M.I., Morrison, B.J., *et al.* (1993) The influence of social, economic, and professional consideration on services offered by dentists to long-term care residents. *Journal of Public Health Dentistry*, 53, 70–75.

Wenger, E., McDermott, R., Snyder, W.M. (2002) *Cultivating communities of practice.* Harvard Business School Publishing, Boston, MA.

Weyant, R.J., Newman, A.B., Kritchevsky, S.B., *et al.* (2004) Periodontal disease and weight loss in older adults. *Journal of the American Geriatrics Society*, 52, 547–553.

Wilders, R.S. (2008) Promotion of oral health: Need for interprofessional collaboration. *Journal of Dental Hygiene*, 82, 1–3.

Williams, F., Dowrick, C., Humphris, G. *et al.* (2003) Developing interprofessional collaboration in the care of dental patients with symptoms of anxiety and depression: the view from general practice. *Education for Primary Care*, 14, 39–43.

Winn, D.M., Brunelle, J.A., Selwitz, R.H., *et al.* (1996) Coronal and root caries in the dentition of adults in the United States, 1988–1991. *Journal of Dental Research*, 75, 642–651.

World Health Organization (WHO). (1978) Report of the international conference of primary care in Alma Ata, USSR. *WHO Chronicle*, 31, 409–430.

Wyatt, C.C.L, So, F.H.C., Williams, M., *et al.* (2006) The development, implementation, utilization and outcomes of a comprehensive dental program for older adults residing in long-term care facilities. *Journal of the Canadian Dental Association*, 72, 421–426.

Zwarenstein, M., Golmand, J., Reeves S. (2009) Interprofessional collaboration: effects of practice-based interventions on professional practice and healthcare outcomes. *Cochrane Database of Systematic Reviews*, 2009 (3), 1–148.

21

The effective preventive dental team

Ann-Marie C. DePalma and Shirley Gutkowski

Introduction (compare this to original for formatting)

Four-handed dentistry was developed during the 1960s to increase efficiency and productivity of dental teams. Four-handed dentistry involves the correct positioning of the operator and assistant, the organization of procedures and steps needed, and the use of appropriate equipment. This chapter will review the basics of four-handed dentistry and how they apply to preventive dentistry and how to achieve an effective preventive dentistry team. As the idea of minimally invasive dentistry and minimal intervention dentistry take hold, auxiliary health care providers will become more and more important. The medical model of diagnosis and treatment, with modifications, is the developing model of dentistry. Dental assistants and dental hygienists are gathering more and more patient information and providing increasingly more of the preventive care as prescribed by the dentist. The day of dentists drilling and filling are not gone; they may never be. However, the day of the dentist hunched over a patient/client all day every day is a thing of the past.

The four hands in dentistry may be the hands of the dentist and dental assistant or the dental hygienist and the dental assistant. The physical proximity of the people regardless of the title is the same (Figure 21-1).

The care provider, called the operator, and assistant work in the following four basic work areas:

- The operator's zone
- The assistant's zone
- The transfer zone
- The static zone

Each area or zone is represented by the face of a clock around the patient and the dental chair. The zones are dependent on whether the dentist/operator and assistant are right- or left-handed.

The operator's zone

The operator's zone is the area occupied by the operator seated and moving to various positions during the procedure using an operator's chair on rollers:

- Right-handed operators 7 to 12 o'clock position
- Left-handed operators from 12 to 5 o'clock

The assistant's zone

The assistant's zone is the area where the assistant is seated on a specialized dental assistant's stool on rollers, with access to a mobile cart, instrument tray, air-water syringe, and many other instruments and equipment that the assistant may use during a procedure:

- For right-handed assistants, from 2 to 4 o'clock
- For left-handed assistants, from 8 to 10 o'clock

The transfer zone

The transfer zone is the area where instrument and material transfer between the operator and the assistant occurs. The transfer zone follows:

- For right-handed operators from 4 to 7 o'clock
- For left-handed operators from five to 8 o'clock

It is imperative that the transfer zone be within easy accessibility for both the operator and assistant and does not occur over a patient's face for safety reasons.

Comprehensive Preventive Dentistry, First Edition. Edited by Hardy Limeback.
© 2012 John Wiley & Sons, Ltd. Published 2012 by John Wiley & Sons, Ltd.

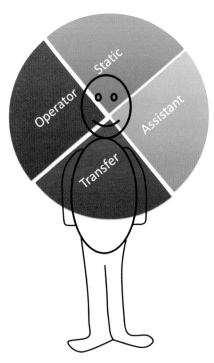

Figure 21-1 Arrangement of the working space surrounding the patient lying in the dental chair.

The static zone

The static zone is directly behind the patient from the 12 to 2 o'clock positions. This zone may contain handpieces, air/water syringes, portable equipment, or countertop space. During dental procedures, the operator and assistant function through each of the zones to achieve maximum efficiency and patient care while maintaining proper ergonomics. The operator and the assistant work in partnership to create optimum care for the patient while maintaining an optimum work environment for themselves. This partnership can then involve the patient to create an effective preventive team.

Preventive dentistry involves a program of patient homecare education; use of fluoride, xylitol, or other remineralizing agents; the application of dental sealants; dietary and tobacco product counseling; and any other patient-specific needs to prevent oral disease. Preventive dentistry targets oral diseases such as caries, periodontal disease, oral cancer, and salivary dysfunction. Preventive dentistry is accomplished to prevent or arrest early stages of oral disease. Preventive dentistry begins early in life, as the American Academy of Pediatric Dentistry recommends, by age 1. Preventive dentistry continues through various life stages encompassing preschool- and elementary-aged children, to adolescents, to young adults, through pregnancy, to middle-adulthood, and finally to the elderly and/or home- or institutional-bound patient. Preventive dentistry is a

(a)

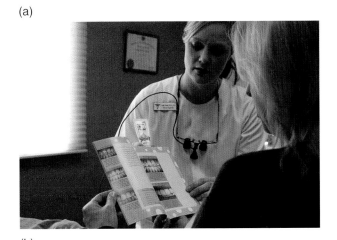

(b)

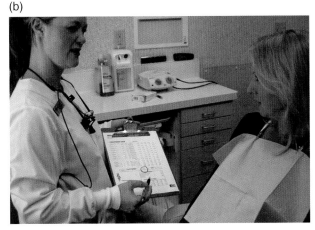

Figure 21-2 Patient education by a dental assistant. A dental assistant plays an important role in the education of oral conditions to the patient (a). The assistant could also be responsible for reviewing treatment plans, risks and benefits as well as the expected fees and recording the discussions in the chart (b).

combination of teamwork between dental professionals, including assistants, hygienists, dentists, and business support team members working with the patient to achieve optimum health.

As dental professionals, dental assistants may be involved in patient education. Patient education is an essential component of the preventive dentistry appointment. Dental assistants must be able to connect with people and provide instruction at a level that is appropriate for each individual. They are looked at as a translator of 'dental-ese' and are often called upon to assist the dentist in communicating with the patient/client and to bridge gaps in discussing fees (Figure 21-2).

As part of the overall dental health team, dental assistants can assist patients with the following tasks:

- Gathering diagnostic data
- Explaining pre- and post-operative care instructions
- Understanding of the role of biofilm

- Properly maintaining their oral hygiene
- Dispensing homecare products

Dispensing products from the office can be a wonderful or challenging experience. Many practice owners think that selling products from the office is unprofessional or complicated. They may feel comfortable giving away a couple of products or samples before crossing that threshold into selling. Others like the idea of selling products from the office because they can give their patients/clients the products and brands that they have researched and found to be the best answer for the person's unique needs. Monitoring these products as inventory may be a part of the dental assistant's job. An ordering system can make having all of these products on hand very easy. Many practice software systems include ordering systems that follow a product in the door, in the inventory, and out the door without much fuss. Dispensing free goods or selling products from the dental office is a choice best made by the practice owner. In many jurisdictions, the licensing bodies stipulate that the dental office can only add a reasonable office handling fee to the wholesale price of the product.

With the enormous amount of products available to the consumer today, a new business model may develop. A dental hygiene store owned by a dental hygienist, staffed by a dental hygienist who can offer advice and teach people how to use the dental hygiene products that fits customers' distinctive needs may be possible, depending on the jurisdiction. Or, this store may also work by prescription from another dental hygienist or dentist. A variety of products can be available to the variety of patients that can be recommended to this store. This marketing campaign can evolve around the essentials of any homecare routine—brushing and interproximal cleaning.

Manual brushes or power brushes are available for patients and should be recommended by the clinician with the patient's dexterity, comprehension, and motivation in mind. Dental practices may offer patient/clients "free" manual toothbrushes. The practice information may be imprinted on the handle as a marketing tool.

Power brushes are often sold from the office as a service to the patients and to provide the practice with an additional source of revenue, unless the state board prohibits making a profit from selling oral care products. Interdental cleaning products ranging from floss, to interproximal brushes and tips, to water irrigators, are valuable adjuncts to brushing. These are recommended to patients based on need and the patient's ability to perform procedures routinely. Dental professionals should take care not to overwhelm patients with products; one or two products that a patient uses effectively are more appropriate than several things done incorrectly.

In addition to patient homecare products and education, the dental professional may offer patients a variety of preventive measures in the dental office.

Preventive procedures in the dental office or for home use

Fluoride is applied topically in the office as a professional service or at home via month rinse, paste, or gel. An auxiliary preventive team member can be in charge of administering professional fluorides in the office or providing topical fluorides for home care, as prescribed by the dentist. Over the past several years, other products have been introduced that enable dental professionals to expand beyond fluoride and provide additional benefits for patients. These products may be dispensed or sold to help patients maintain oral health of the teeth or mucosa. Specialized ingredients in pastes, creams, or mouthwash may be offered as a service to the patient/clients.

Dental sealants

The application of dental sealants is an example of an in-office preventive procedure that in most jurisdictions can be applied by dental auxiliaries. (See Chapter 17.) The dentist will evaluate the risk for each person in the practice and prescribe the need for sealants and will choose the material to use. The following sealants may be used:

- High Risk: glass ionomer
- Medium Risk: glass ionomer or hydrophilic resin or resin containing ACP
- Low Risk: typical resin sealant or no sealants

After caries diagnosis and caries risk assessment have been completed, the dentist may assign the task to an auxiliary team member. As discussed in Chapter 17, obtaining a dry field is essential for resin-based sealants. Thus, four-handed dentistry improves the ability to maintain this dry field. Glass ionomer cements are more forgiving to fluid contamination and could be placed by a single operator without the aid of an assistant.

Protocols for sealant placement vary depending on the product and manufacturer. The provider should review manufacturer's directions prior to sealant placement.

Patient counseling

The following patient counseling could be assigned to a professional auxiliary (certified dental assistant or dental hygienist):

- Dietary counseling: Counseling a patient following a dietary analysis or recommending dietary changes prompted by admission by a patient of inappropriate sugar intake can be done on a one-to-one basis using teaching aids. Dietary advice can also be given to those patients susceptible to dental erosion (Chapter 13). Dietary counseling can be as simple as having a work sheet available for patients to complete. This work sheet can ask the patient what they had for breakfast, lunch, dinner, and any snacks that day or the previous day. The assistant or hygienist can break this worksheet into columns representing the food groups and have the patient check off each one for all of the foods consumed the day in question. The dental team member can review and inform the patient on any highs or lows in any area and use this as a starting point for further discussions. More elaborate nutritional counseling information sheets can be obtained from local nutritionists for further collaboration.

- Post-treatment advice: Advice on caring for an extraction socket or any dietary restrictions following oral surgery or orthodontics represent two examples where the auxiliary team member can be very helpful.
- Smoking cessation: Patients often see dental professionals more frequently than medical professionals. Therefore, it is the dental team member's responsibility to counsel patient/clients on health-related issues that, at first glance, may seem more appropriate for a medical office. However, as mentioned before, tobacco product abuse is the one etiological factor affecting all dental diseases (caries, periodontal disease, and oral cancer). Dental professionals are on the front lines to examine and counsel patients regarding habits that could increase their risk of developing these diseases.
- Oral injury prevention: Counseling families on the benefits of mouthguards for themselves or their children is another example of duties that can be assigned to the other dental team members.
- Medical updates and blood pressure: As an added patient benefit, blood pressure and other appropriate vital signs may be taken by dental team members with proper training and knowledge. In particular knowing the blood pressure is important before any major dental procedure. If an emergency should arise, first responders/EMTs will want to know the blood pressure before the emergency transpired. Taking a patient's blood pressure is good practice-building activity, and many dental health care providers have found patients who are extremely ill by taking this vital sign as a routine before any other procedure is embarked upon. Advice to the patients regarding any hypertension discovered (for example, referral to a medical doctor) can even be a life-saving gesture.

Diagnostics in periodontal disease

Dental hygienists and dentists perform routine examinations of the bone and gingival tissues including periodontal probing. Any increase in probing depth may signal disease processes. The dental assistant is an important team member in assisting the hygienist and dentist in diagnosing and treating periodontal disease.

Often periodontal probing numbers are charted to monitor changes in bone levels around the teeth. There are a variety of probes available to measure bone loss each with markers calibrated in millimeters and having either blunt or rounded tips. During the periodontal evaluation, the dentist or the hygienist will take six measurements around each tooth; mesial-buccal, buccal, disto-buccal, mesial-lingual, lingual, and disto-lingual. A complete charting will also include Clinical Attachment Loss (CAL) and recession. CAL and recession provide the clinician with a true measurement of bone loss around the tooth.

Charting is a complex procedure that is best performed by two people—one writing, the other measuring and commenting on tissue color and response to tissue manipulation. The assistant may record all information in either the computer or paper chart for the hygienist or dentist. Another approach to charting is to use voice activation software instead of a second person. The limitation to accurate data compilation with voice-activated charting involves the quality of the microphone. Accuracy is essential in charting, and using a higher quality microphone can achieve better results.

Charting is not early detection of a periodontal infection. Although still popular and potentially important, periodontal charting is late detection, and gives no feedback on whether the disease is in the active state or dormant. The presence of bleeding upon probing is also noted as a potential indicator of periodontal infections; however, causes for bleeding can range from operator error to diabetes and blood dyscrasias. New products support minimal intervention with respect to diagnosis. Saliva testing for oral pathogens can let the clinician know what types of bacteria are present, whether they will be susceptible to non-surgical treatments, or which or if any antibiotics will be helpful in the treatment of this silent disease. A dental assistant needs to be knowledgeable on all areas of periodontal management, whether she/he is charting information, assisting in surgery, or providing patient education.

Research continually implicates periodontal disease as a role player in cardiovascular disease, diabetes, pre-term low-birth-weight babies, respiratory diseases, and some cancers. Periodontal disease is an inflammatory process that has systemic implications. Dental professionals have the obligation to educate and inform patients about how their oral health impacts their entire health.

Polishing or desensitizing teeth

As part of dental hygiene procedures, polishing brings about a satisfying end to the appointment. On occasion dental assistants may be in a position to

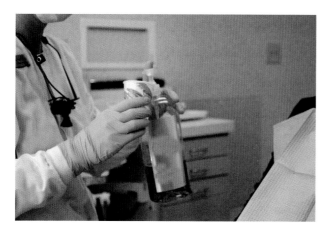

Figure 21-3 Providing a patient an antiseptic pre-rinse before the appointment. Rinses may be commercial or freshly made ozonated water. The rinse is then evacuated with the saliva ejector to keep pathogens at bay in the suction system.

polish teeth of their patient/client. This topic is explored in greater detail in the literature, but, a brief overview is appropriate here.

In a preventive dentistry practice, air polishing is appropriate. It has been found that using a bioactive glass polishing agent is the least damaging to enamel (Banerjee *et al.* 2010). Reports have shown decrease in enamel damage when using bioactive glass as compared to sodium bicarbonate or calcium carbonate. Bioactive glass has restorative properties as a calcium phosphate product. It can and does heal the enamel by providing building blocks to facilitate the healing.

Bioactive glass is the only air slurry polish that should be used on the root surface, because the root surface is softer than enamel and does not heal as quickly. If a regular pumice-based polish is used with a webbed cup and a slow-speed handpiece, the root should not be polished at all (Christensen and Bangerter 1987).

Although tempting, polishing should only be attempted on teeth with no biofilm accumulation. At the beginning of the appointment, a pre-procedural rinse will help cut down on the bioburden in the aerosol created by the air polisher (Figure 21-3), which is a benefit to the patient/client and the clinician.

In some instances, the patient/client may be sensitive to instrumentation used during a procedure. The patient/client can be made comfortable before any treatment by providing a desensitizing treatment to the teeth. Smart polishes are a good choice for this treatment. Preventive dentistry also encompasses preventing dental phobia. Absence of dental pain during the appointment can divert this reaction.

The word phobia is accurate in people who suffer a fear that is unfounded. Most people who suffer a dental phobia usually have earned it. In the case of persons over 50, the common practice of slapping children or The Velvet Glove technique for managing children was very pervasive. The Velvet Glove technique had the clinician hold their hand over the child's mouth and nose until they started to panic and remove the hand letting the child know "who was in charge." This technique is no longer practiced; however, memories of this technique and the fear developed from it are far from groundless. This fear is often passed onto the adult's children and manifests as overprotection or insistence on being in the room. A policy to allow parents into the treatment room should be written and given to each new mother or caregiver. (See Chapter 19)

Minimally invasive dentistry

Preventive dentistry includes a new area of treatment, minimally invasive dentistry. With the importance of systemic health and its relationship to the oral cavity, dental team members must have a significant understanding of the role that minimally invasive (MI) dentistry plays. Minimally invasive dentistry is defined by Fontana *et al.* (2010) as follows:

Minimally invasive dentistry is supported by the emerging evidence and international consensus; it has an international focus, from, for example, the FDI World Dental Federation and others, and continues to be built on. The Minimal Intervention approach stresses a preventive philosophy, individualized risk assessments, accurate, early detection of lesions, and efforts to remineralize noncavitated lesions with the prompt provision of preventive care to minimize operative intervention. When operative intervention is unequivocally required, typically for an active cavitated lesion, the procedure used should be as minimally invasive as possible.

What is not supported by the evidence or international consensus, but which is sometimes mislabeled as minimally invasive, is clinical activity in which small, early, and inactive/arrested lesions are sought out and prematurely or unnecessarily subjected to operative intervention.

Minimally invasive dentistry (MID), minimal intervention (MI), and caries management by risk assessment (CAMBRA) are relatively new terms developed in response to scientific advances in the field. The terms are used interchangeably by some, and by others as a source of debate as to which is the most proper term. For example, CAMBRA does not stop at prevention and chemical treatments; it includes evidence-based decisions on when, and how, to restore a tooth to minimize structural loss. In addition, MID and MI stand for much more than conservative cavity preparation.

The term MI was endorsed by the FDI World Dental Federation in a 2002 policy statement and is globally recognized. The terms CAMBRA and MID are in 100%

agreement with the FDI statement on MI. Thus, the authors support the interchangeability of all 3 terms and recognize the importance of local preferences as well as global collaboration (Fontana *et al.* 2010).

In particular, the definition of Minimally Invasive Dentistry is not creating smaller holes in teeth; it is about not removing tooth structure at all. Dental assistants, dental hygienists, and dentists play new roles in this paradigm. Not only is the dental assistant charged with mixing cements and passing instruments, the dental assistant may be asked to gather diagnostic information (under the supervision of a dentist), administer caries risk tests, and help the dentist develop treatment plans for dental interventions. Dental hygienists will also assist conducting diagnostic tests that supply information for better treatment options and as a result, better prognosis.

Photography as diagnostic tool

Photography is an important element in the patient educational process and is an important part of the diagnostic tools for intra and extra oral structures. Photography allows the patient and the dentist to visualize actual problems and better communicate patient needs and treatment objectives. The role of the dental assistant in photography encompasses a variety of skills, in taking and recording photographs, and having appropriate supplies, instruments, and forms available for the dentist or hygienist to proceed with the photographic session. Digital photography has greatly enhanced the ease of the case presentation process, and assistants may be invaluable contributors in the process.

Dental assistants should have the following equipment available for digital photography:

- Camera with charged battery and ring flash as needed
- Mouth mirror
- Photographic mouth mirrors (warmed under warm water to prevent fogging)
- Lip and/or cheek retractors
- Notebook to record patient name and type of photographs for later downloading to computer if not immediately printed for or shown to the patient

Photography of hard and soft lesions usually falls on the shoulders of the dental assistant once the team becomes proficient at it. Intraoral photography has its own rules and qualities. Color and light reflection and refractions have important meaning when taking photographs.

Intraoral photography

Using an intraoral (I/O or IO) camera is like using a wand (Figure 21-4).

The camera eye is on the end of the wand and may be placed directly opposite the photographic target. Once visible on the computer or television monitor, the

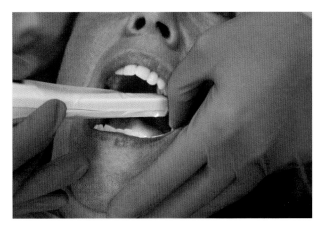

Figure 21-4 Using an intraoral camera for charting. The camera is held opposite the target, in this case the lower left premolar.

"shutter" is activated by a foot switch. This type of photography is often used for showing patient/clients what they cannot see in a hand mirror. IO photography is often of a low resolution and not adequate for publication or projection. Photographical targets are usually one or more of the following:

- Inadequate or decaying margins
- Broken cusps
- Soft tissue damage from biting or disease

After the photo is taken and shown on the screen, a dialogue is started with the patient/client. When she/he can see the rough margins of an old amalgam, or a lesion on her/his cheek, she/he may understand the restorative conversation better and will be more willing to accept treatment recommendations.

Extraoral photography

Extraoral photography is important in documenting treatment. This kind of photography is of very high quality and suitable for publication. As research from clinical practice takes on a new importance, photography becomes more important too. Photographic treatment sequencing of novel approaches to new or old procedures can explain more than mere words. In MID, photography can show the healing of an enamel lesion after topical treatments. It can also document hard and soft tissue lesions allowing the clinician a better view and potentially aid in diagnosis.

Extraoral photography requires cheek retractors, and a ring flash or other type of lighting that will allow the natural color of the teeth to show and minimize shadows. Timing is also important, because a newly cemented crown may often stimulate edema or abrasion of the soft tissue. A return visit is usually desired for photography. Dental practices with a focus on esthetics may have a photo studio for taking before and after patient portraits. Some dental practices even have a standing relationship with a spa that will include a facial or makeup for the after-treatment photo.

Lasers

Surgical lasers

In recent years and with the advent of MI dentistry, lasers have gained a prominence in treatment of periodontal disease, oral surgery, and caries detection. Laser is short for "light amplification by stimulated emission of radiation." A laser beam is a highly concentrated beam of light. At different wavelengths a laser has the ability to cut, vaporize, or cauterize both hard and soft tissue. Lasers are used to remove benign and malignant tumors or excess gingiva. Lasers are effective in releasing frenum attachments and control bleeding in highly vascular areas. There are a number of advantages to laser usage over conventional excisional surgery:

- Sites heal faster.
- Bleeding is controlled.
- Surgical area is easily maintained.
- Patients experience less trauma.
- Post-operative swelling and pain are significantly reduced.

Disadvantages of laser usage include the following:

- The patient and professionals must wear eye protection and never look directly into the laser.
- Specific instruments are needed.
- Non-target tissues (areas not being treated but that are close to the treated area) must be protected.
- High volume evacuation (HVE) is needed if tissue vaporization occurs since the cloud produced may be infectious.

It is the last point where four-handed dentistry becomes almost essential. One does not want the patient (or operator) smelling tissues that are being cauterized.

Lasers for caries detection

For caries detection, lasers are less traumatic to tooth structure than the use of conventional dental explorers. Explorers may cavitate the pseudo intact layer of an early caries lesion turning a small healable lesion into one that cannot respond to saliva or calcium phosphate products.

The term laser is accurate, however, a better term is fluorescence laser (DIAGNOdent and others, see Chapter 2). A dental hygienist can use these instruments after properly cleaning the tooth surface and then record the readings in the chart. The diagnosis as to whether caries is present, arrested, or active (which may require more than one reading on separate occasions) is made by the dentist, and a prescription for a sealant or remineralization therapy (see Chapter 18) can then be made.

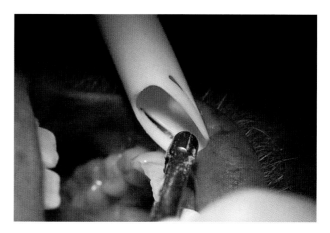

Figure 21-5 Polishing with an air abrasion unit and bioactive glass powder. Notice all that is required is high volume suction using a vented tip provided by the dental assistant.

The dental team can use this information to help the patient/client understand the caries process. Reporting the findings to the practitioner will assist in treatment planning and determining the prognosis for the treatment. The dental assistant will also likely be charged with maintaining this type of equipment. Disposables such as sleeves that cover the wand will need to be kept on hand. The dental assistant will also be choosing the appropriate disinfectant for the cables and housing of the unit. Building a relationship with a company who repairs dental equipment is also necessary. A person who repairs dental equipment is a critical part of the dental team who is hopefully never needed and never far from the office.

Air abrasion

Air abrasion is second in the short line of processes that claim to be a minimally invasive technique. A number of abrasives are used at high pressure and directed at the damaged enamel. The intention is to remove only the weakened enamel and proceed no further. This technique is often used in pit and fissure decay removal and also to prepare the tooth for a sealant. The traditional abrasives used for this type of treatment have metal shavings. In 2009 a new abrasive was introduced to the marketplace (Paolinelis *et al.* 2008). The new product has some very unique abilities due to its composition. It is a bioactive glass, and, although it will remove damaged enamel, it will also 'heal' enamel that is repairable. Bioactive glass is the preferred material for use in an air-polishing unit or an air abrasive unit before placing a resin-based sealant (Figure 21-5).

Ozone

Ozone is a true minimally invasive procedure. Ozone is a gas produced by electrifying air or pure oxygen. The ozone is applied as a gas to carious enamel to stop progression of the infection and in early lesions may be the only treatment necessary. The gas is applied with a small hose, syringe, or suction hose. If used without the suction hose, the procedure is performed with high volume suction.

Ozone gas is safe when used in this way, particularly when made with pure oxygen. Ozone is applied prior to placing a filling material, and can save the clinician from having to remove carious enamel that approaches the pulp horns. A remineralizing solution may be applied to the enamel, and it may heal if the damage is shallow enough. More information on ozone is located in Chapter 11.

Tray setups for lasers, air abrasion, and ozone include the device, along with two mirrors and an explorer. High volume evacuation (HVE) tips are also included and come in different configurations depending on operator preferences. HVE tips are found either as short or long, but the tips for these procedures are usually the 1-cm variety with beveled ends. They may or may not be vented. The vented tips are often thought to be easier to use and will not catch the soft tissue.

As with other uses of HVE, the evacuator (Figure 21-5) is positioned prior to the dentist beginning the procedure. The tip is placed on the surface of the tooth closest to the assistant, close to the tooth/tissue being treated, with the bevel of the tip parallel to the working area, and the edge of the tip slightly away from the area being treated. The assistant can hold the HVE in either hand with a thumb-nose grasp or pen-grasp while the other hand is free to hold the air-water syringe or exchange instruments during the procedure.

Ozone gas is heavier than air and when applied by the dentist or dental hygienist can be evacuated from the floor of the mouth. The HVE tip need not be directly adjacent to the tooth.

Ozone gas may also be delivered via a syringe. The dental assistant will fill the syringe with the gas from the generator and hand it over to the dentist or the dental hygienist (if the hygienist is permitted to apply ozone in her/his jurisdiction). Applying ozonated oils to a surgical site can decrease healing time. The dental assistant may be charged with created the oils for use in this application. The dental assistant may also be charged with mixing ozonated water throughout the day. Ozonated water in some offices is made in the morning and afternoon over the lunch hour. In the offices that use ozone for many procedures, it may be necessary to have a system that continually manufactures ozone water throughout the day.

For periodontal disease treatment applications, ozone may be used as a topical gas using a custom tray, or injected into the sulcus using a blunted cannula tip. The dental hygienist may also use fresh ozonated water as the lavage in the ultrasonic unit. Because ozone is readily released from water proportional to the temperature of the water, it's important to use water as cold as practical. The water will be a comfortable temperature as it exits the handpiece. The ozonated water need not be augmented with iodine or chlorhexidine.

The hygienist may also use ozonated oils to disinfect the periodontal probe between pocket readings. This diagnostic procedure will simultaneously treat pockets by disinfecting them and stop iatrogenic spread of the disease by disinfecting the vector.

Radiographs

As dentistry evolves from the traditional drill and fill mentality to the era of MID, radiography is moving from the traditional analog film-based diagnosis to digital radiography. Digital radiography allows the clinician the ability to capture diagnostic images quicker, with less radiation, and less exposure times. Digital radiography increases efficiency with less equipment/product cost. Although the initial cost for new radiology equipment may seem expensive, the long-term return on investment (ROI) is considerable since there are no chemicals or films to purchase regularly. In a world where consciousness is raised over damages to the environment, digital radiography is an even better fit for practices following the minimally invasive dentistry approach.

There are two basic types of digital radiographic recording devices: sensors (wired or wire-less charged couple devices [CCD]) and phosphorus plates. For direct digital imaging, sensors are placed into the patient/client's mouth and exposed to radiation, and the image is sent directly to the computer. Phosphorus plates are indirect digital imaging. The plates, which are similar to analog film, are placed into the client/patient's mouth, exposed, and removed. The plates are then placed into a high-speed scanner connected to a computer where images are transferred (Figure 21-6).

A phosphor plate digital radiographic system allows light to interact with the phosphor plate without damaging the image. Plates are re-used after exposure to white light. Both sensors and plates are placed in either plastic wraps or plastic bags for infection control purposes. Techniques for taking digital radiographs are based on traditional analog radiography but are altered based on each manufacturer's specific directions.

All radiographs should be taken using some kind of aiming device. In preventive dentistry, the ability to line up X-rays year after year, and have them all at the exact same angle is important to follow the progress of healing therapies or damage (Figure 21-7).

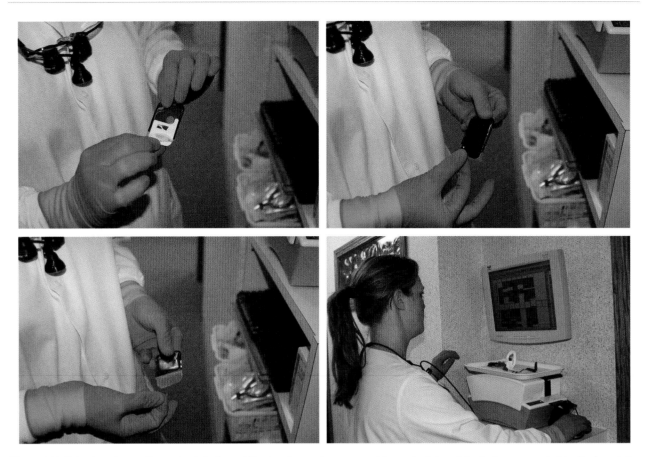

Figure 21-6 A phosphor radiograph plate for a bitewing image is processed by a dental assistant: the exposed side (*top*) and the opposite side are shown. The plate is uncovered (*bottom left*) and scanned into the computer (*bottom right*).

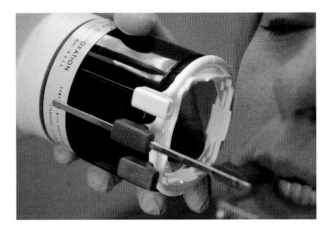

Figure 21-7 Device for achieving parallelism during radiography. This device is holding the radiographic sensors at 90 degrees to the line of the cone beam allowing repeatable angulation for serial evaluation of radiographs over time.

Digital radiography has advantages and disadvantages to traditional analog films. The advantages follow:

- Greater gray-scale resolution: The ability to distinguish minute differences of contrast and density is greater.

- Less patient radiation: Digital radiography has been estimated to be at least 50% less than E speed film.
- Increased speed of viewing images: Even with plates, time from exposure to processing is much less.
- Cost: The cost of processing and film is eliminated, along with it being better for the environment.
- Ease of use: Digital radiography is easily transferrable to referring dentists and insurance companies.
- Greener: It has a smaller environmental impact.
- Enhancement of images: The ability to create digital subtraction (gray scale is reversed so that normal black images appear white and white images appear black) can be useful when diagnosis is a challenge. Images can also be altered to change brightness, orientation, and color (although neither author has seen colorization in use clinically).
- Education: It makes increased patient education easier.

The disadvantages follow:

- Cost: The initial set-up costs are high.
- Image quality: Some still are not convinced of the true ability to detect early stage disease.

- Sensor size: Sensors are bulkier than traditional film and can be uncomfortable for the patient.
- Infection control: Use of sleeves is essential to prevent cross-contamination among patients.
- Legal issues: There is potential for image alteration and security issues.

In general, however, digital radiography is preferred to analog. Depending on provincial or state practice acts, dental assistants can take both analog and digital radiographs after completing a program on radiation health and safety.

Additionally, new digital technology, cone beam computed technology (CBCT), is entering the dental market. Traditional radiographs, both digital and analog, are basically two-dimensional images of three-dimensional beings. Distortions, overlaps, and magnification issues are common. CBCT uses a cone beam radiation source to acquire a 360-degree image of an area. This image is transferred to a computer where the image is displayed as three-dimensional. Better diagnostic abilities of both hard and soft tissues can been seen with CBCT, and their use is important in orthodontics, oral surgery, and implant therapies. The high cost of equipment and the question of patient safety are issues that must be resolved before their use is more widespread within dentistry. Currently CBCT units are found in dental school settings, radiology imaging centers, and some private dental offices where the dentist/owner "rents" the unit to local referring offices. Dental assistants and hygienists are important to the CBCT team since they can produce images and educate patients and referrers on the use of the technology. Offices that use this technology have a lower rate of failure in implants and lower complication rate in surgical procedures.

There is also a concern about the amount of radiation accumulated from dental X-rays. The number of dental X-rays should be kept to a minimum and follow a risk profile that the patient/client presents.

In dentistry, as compared to medicine, dental X-rays are taken to find early lesions, chronic abscesses, and a host of asymptomatic boney and soft tissue diseases and abnormalities. In medicine the problem is already manifested, for instance, a broken arm or a painful kidney stone. The dental professional should inform the patient/client of the risk versus benefit ratio of obtaining good quality, low radiation radiographs versus not imaging at all (Table 21-1).

The threat of thyroid cancer presents itself in nearly all discussions about radiography (Inskip *et al.* 1995; Memon *et al.* 2010). The concern has mainly centered in the patient; however, the clinician should be protected as well. Debates on who should wear the lead collar may eventually settle on the clinician wearing it. As scientists

Table 21-1 Radiation doses from various types of medical imaging procedures

Type of Procedure	Average Adult Effective Dose (mSv)	Estimated Dose Equivalent (No. of Chest X-rays)
Dental X-ray	0.005–0.01	0.25–0.5
Chest X-ray	0.02	1
Mammography	0.4	20
CT	2–16	100–800
Nuclear Medicine	0.2–41	10–2,050
Interventional Fluoroscopy	5–70	250–3,500

Source: The US FDA 2010. 10 http://www.fda.gov/Radiation-EmittingProducts/RadiationSafety/RadiationDoseReduction/ucm199994.htm#ft6a. Accessed January 2, 2011.

learn more about imagine radiation from a dental X-ray ricocheting after collision with skeletal tissues of the head, radiation just might be deflected downward into the thyroid, and then ricochet back after hitting the lead apron on the inside of the collar or skeletal tissue surrounding the thyroid. Scatter from the actual X-ray head is minimal, however, since the beam is highly focused.

The operator is in the room of bouncing X-rays multiple times a day, and may be better suited to wear the lead collar herself. A simple study to do on a quarterly basis in any practice is to tape a film to the outside of the lead apron with a penny or paper clip taped between the potential X-ray source and the dental X-ray film. After a day or a week, process the film to see if it had been exposed to the radiation. In some jurisdictions, radiation badges are still required by personnel administering X-radiation.

Practice settings

The world of dental hygiene offers a variety of intriguing opportunities. As laws within the provinces change, the importance of dental hygienists as contributors to patient systemic care is seen as vital. Alternative practice settings offer a new frontier for the adventurous dental hygienist to combine knowledge and skills of patient management with clinical skills and education.

The following examples of alternative practice settings are not all established. This is a new frontier in dentistry. Specialty practices can be set up anywhere people have teeth as the evidence linking oral and systemic health is swelling.

Hospital care

Hygienists have an opportunity with hospital care to enhance and improve patients' health needs. A variety of services within a hospital environment can offer the dental hygienist a new area to expand. A dental hygienist may be a valuable asset in the care of the surgical patient on a ventilator, to those who have respiratory disease, and to those who are in long-term care facilities.

Surgical care

Ventilator Associated Pneumonia (VAP) is a disastrous complication of any surgery. Oral hygiene care has been shown to decrease the chances of a hospitalized patient developing this hurdle to health (Ford 2008). The cost of VAP for both the hospital and patient is very high, however, the cost of oral hygiene care for hospitalized patients is very low. This demonstrates a high return on investment for the patient and hospital. The impact of a simple low-cost oral care protocol on ventilator associated pneumonia rates in a surgical intensive care unit has been found to provide a monetary savings resulting in a decrease of respirator days by 46% in 1 year (Sona *et al.* 2009). This study found that the cost for oral care was $2,000 US, and it is likely that this would have resulted in greater savings had the oral care services been provided by a dental professional. Less oversight would have been required from the nursing staff if dental professionals were used. Similar studies need to be performed and researched incorporating the dental sciences along with the medical information. More research based in dental science is needed under these conditions.

Respiratory care

A 2005 study noted that patients with respiratory infections can regain health by increasing their oral care (Okuda *et al.* 2005). Okuda found that as professional dental hygiene increased, oral microbiota decreased along with the incidence of aspiration pneumonia. Other studies have also demonstrated a reduction in respiratory infections with professional dental hygiene in the elderly (Abe *et al.* 2001; Adachi *et al.* 2002; Adachi *et al.* 2007). More research is needed at all levels for the dental hygienist to have other doors within hospital care open to them.

Long-term care

Positions for dental hygienists and dental assistants in long-term care facilities are beginning to develop. Many health care providers and facility administrators are becoming aware that the increased number of teeth in the facility brings about a unique set of problems that no one has been addressing. Nurses and nurses' aides are not prepared to take care of the oral cavity.

This is another venue that cries out for more research by dental professionals. (See Chapter 20.) Not only does a dental care professional need to provide education of oral care in the facility, the textbooks available for caregivers need to be evaluated (Bush and Donley 2002).

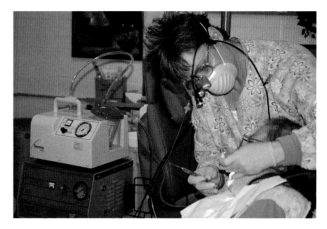

Figure 21-8 Dental hygienist with mobile equipment.

Currently dental care is relegated to the cosmetic section of textbooks; however, it should considered part of wound care.

The oral care does not need to be applied every single day by a professional dental hygienist. Once a week is sufficient to provide residents in long-term care facilities the benefits of oral care. This would be a great opportunity for dental hygienists to develop and organize a pilot program in a local facility. Oral hygiene care has also shown to affect the number two killer in long-term care facilities—influenza. Dental hygienists can and should be true partners and employees in adult care facilities to provide the utmost in care for residents (Abe *et al.* 2001; Abe *et al.*2006; Ishikawa *et al.*2008).

In Figure 21-8, the hygienist is cleaning the resident's teeth using mobile equipment. The resident is in a specialized upholstered wheel chair that reclines. The aid is with the resident and is instructed on how best to provide daily oral care for the unique needs of the resident.

Cardiac care

As the medical community begins to understand what the dental community has known for years (DeStefano *et al.* 1993; Joshipura *et al.* 1996), that the mouth is connected to the body, dental hygienists can play a crucial role in all aspects of medicine, including cardiac care (Wilder *et al.* 2009). Case management for all cardiac patients should include dental examination and treatment. Not all patients are prepared to consider dental care as part of their cardiac rehabilitation program. If a dental visit was included in the protocol, we may see an increase in life expectancy after a cardiac event. Most patients don't know that cardiac disease is bound tightly to the inflammatory process, or that the most common unchecked inflammation in the human body is in the periodontal space (Frisbee *et al.* 2010a; Frisbee *et al.* 2010b).

Pediatric offices

The dental hygienist employed in a pediatric office is a natural fit. Application of fluoride varnish by a dental hygienist is part of the role, but a larger role can be in the provision of anticipatory guidance. Anticipatory guidance helps parents understand their child's dental development, reassuring them as questions arise, and supporting dentists from the well-child visits in the first 36 months of life. Providing the parent and child with a "dental home" could be increased if a dental hygienist were to practice alongside a pediatrician.

The dental hygienist in this practice setting can provide the following services:

- Evaluate eruption pattern for normalcy
- Educate parents on topical fluoride applications
- Apply topical fluoride applications
- Discuss mouthguards
- Educate parents on xylitol and nutritional balance to support healthy dentition
- Encourage parents to find and maintain a dental home for the family
- Provide input to protocols for case management of childhood diseases such as cancers, asthma, and other diseases

The problem is summarized by dela Cruz *et al.* (2004). Many children do not have adequate access to dental care, and often pediatricians are forced to make dental decisions without adequate understanding of the implications of such decisions on the child's overall oral health and care. "Finally, pediatric primary health care providers can provide oral health promotion and disease prevention activities, thereby eliminating or delaying dental disease and the need for treatment at a very young age. However, effective and appropriate involvement of pediatric primary care clinicians can be expected only after they receive the appropriate training and encouragement and problems with the dental referral environment are addressed" (dela Cruz *et al.* 2004). The dental hygiene workforce is already in a position to provide that much needed support and bridge the gap.

Oncology

A dental hygienist can be an integral part of cancer patients' treatments helping to guide patients through the oral manifestations of cancer treatment. Oral health care providers can monitor oral conditions and support oral care when a patient/client is unable to do so.

The dental hygienist can provide palliative treatment of oral lesions, place temporary fillings as necessary, and manage the oral biofilm to support proper patient nutrition. All of these steps can contribute to the life-saving treatments that are rendered to the patient in the medical clinic setting. Hygienists can refer to dentists when the patient's condition warrants treatment beyond their scope and can support the patient, medical provider, and dentist in providing total care for the patient and family at a cost savings.

Endocrinology specialties

Patients with diabetes have an enormous amount of focused dental hygiene issues. Glucose management is more difficult in the presence of an untreated infection, and often that infection is a periodontally focused one. A dental hygienist practicing in an endocrinology practice will see patients who are seeking treatment and management of their diabetes. Nutritional counseling, oral hygiene care, and providing dental hygiene services can be a part of the endocrinology dental hygienists' job description.

A motivated dental and dental hygiene team may want to partner with an endocrinologist to specialize in the treatment of people with the following conditions:

- Diabetes
- Osteoporosis
- Infertility
- Menopause
- Thyroid

The door is wide open for practice settings that do not include chairside dental hygiene or dental assisting practice. Although many find great joy in developing relationships and practicing with a focus on the oral cavity, others may find pleasure working in non-traditional settings. A private practice working on referrals can include orofacial myology.

Orofacial myofunctional therapy practice

Myofunctional therapy, or orofacial myology, is the treatment of an orofacial muscle imbalance, an incorrect swallowing pattern, TMJ muscle dysfunction syndrome, and/or the elimination of bruxing, clenching, or sucking habits. The main muscles of concern to the orofacial myologist are the temporalis, the masseter, and the internal and external pterygoids, the buccinators, the orbicularis oris and mentalis. Oral myofunctional therapy is a form of oral facial orthopedics. It involves exercises and stimulation designed to inhibit inappropriate oral behaviors and/or strengthen appropriate oral muscle functioning.

Resting postures of the tongue, jaw, and lips are very important in normal oral growth. When the tongue rests between the posterior teeth, they may not fully erupt, resulting in an open bite appearance. If the tongue rests against the maxillary anterior teeth, especially if the upper lip is short or weak, the teeth may begin to protrude too far forward. When the lips are not in a closed resting position most of the time, the growth and development of the mouth can be adversely affected by the pressure of the tongue.

Excessive non-nutritive or non-speech oral behaviors, such as clenching, bruxing, thumb or digit sucking, and nail biting, can also affect the condition of the teeth and health and functioning of the mouth, especially the jaw. When any oral behavior is excessive in intensity, duration, and frequency, the pressures or collision forces can have serious impact on normal facial appearance and orofacial health and functioning.

"Tongue thrust" refers to a pattern of swallowing in which the tongue pushes forward and/or sideways against or between the teeth during swallowing. Swallowing occurs hundreds of times each day with little to no conscious thought. When the tongue presses against or between the teeth during swallowing, the pressure can have adverse effects on the position of the teeth, bone growth, soft tissue condition, and mouth functioning. Some of the following symptoms occur with tongue thrust:

● Aerophagia
● Difficulty swallowing pills or firm foods
● The inability to wear dentures
● A residual effect on the hard palate from a digit habit
● Chronic mouth breathing
● Continued nasal stuffiness
● Orofacial muscle strain and imbalance
● Chronic headaches or facial spasms or pain

Additional types of patients the oral myofunctional therapist may treat include individuals with the following:

● High-arched hard palate
● Weak lip structure
● Facial grimace when swallowing
● Ankylosed lingual frenum
● Protrusion of the tongue when in repose
● Overdeveloped mentalis muscle

Upper airway infections and obstructions (enlarged tonsils and adenoids) are frequently identified as causes of oral myofunctional disorders, especially when these problems cause the mouth to rest open most of the time. Reduced oral muscle tone or poor orofacial muscle postures appear to negatively impact the growing mouth and facial structures. Long-term non-nutritive sucking habits can also malform the oral structure. Sometimes poor speech articulation patterns may indicate neurological or physical deficits. It is often difficult to determine why an oral myofunctional disorder exists. The behaviors can be the result of stimuli no longer fully obvious.

Regardless of cause, once inappropriate oral behavioral patterns are established, they tend to continue until some external stimulus or treatment alters enough of the patterns so that new behaviors can be learned. Sometimes changes of the oral environment by an orthodontist may bring improved oral functioning. However, oral myofunctional therapy may be necessary when there are indications that dental treatment or orthodontic treatment alone may not bring about the desired changes in oral behaviors. Adverse oral behaviors can often interfere with dental or orthodontic treatment and the stability and condition of the mouth.

Oral myofunctional therapy is a structured, individualized treatment for retraining and restoring normal oral functioning. It seeks to inhibit incorrect muscle movements and develop normal, easy functions of oral rest posture, oral stage of swallowing and speech articulation. Therapy may include any or all of the following:

● Elimination of damaging oral habits
● Reduction of unnecessary tension and pressure in the muscles of the face and mouth
● Strengthening of muscles that do not adequately support normal functioning
● Development of normal resting postures of the tongue, jaw, and facial muscles
● Establishment of normal biting, chewing, and swallowing patterns

The length and timing of therapy depends on the severity and nature of the oral myofunctional disorder. In most cases, therapy is a short-term process with the active stage of treatment lasting about 3 months. Follow-up visits may be required with decreasing frequency over a period of 6–12 months.

Orofacial myofunctional therapists receive specialty training to evaluate and treat a variety of myofunctional conditions and problems. Many orofacial myofunctional clinicians have additional professional training in speech/language pathology, dental hygiene, dentistry, or other health-related fields. Most are members of the International Association of Orofacial Myology (IAOM).

The IAOM regulates how orofacial myology is practiced. The beginning steps include the completion of an approved 28-hour introductory course or an approved 28-hour internship.

After completion of the didactic education or internship, an individual may open his or her own practice following the Scope of Practice outlined by the IAOM. The Scope of Practice reads as follows:

The overall goals of orofacial myofunctional therapy are to assist in the creation, restoration and maintenance of a normal and harmonious orofacial muscle environment.

The orofacial myologist is trained to evaluate and treat patients with a variety of oral and facial muscle dysfunctions.

Certified orofacial myologists or orofacial myologists that are in the process of becoming certified may also have additional training and education in speech/language pathology, dental hygiene or other health related fields that the International Association of Orofacial Myology (IAOM) has determined to be within the Scope of Practice of orofacial myology (www.iaom.com/).

The practice of orofacial myology includes the evaluation and treatment of the following:

- Non-nutritive sucking habits
- Other detrimental orofacial habits
- Orofacial rest posture problems
- Neuromuscular muscle patterns associated with inappropriate mastication, bolus formation, and deglutition
- Functional breathing problems
- Swallowing patterns
- Speech patterns (only if the orofacial myologist is a speech/language pathologist)

Certification is not required to practice; however, it is highly recommended. In addition to the initial training, certification requires the following steps:

- The applicant asks IAOM for an "application for certification form."
- The completed form, accompanying fee, and documentation are returned to the Executive Coordinator who in turn sends the information to the Board of Examiners Chairperson for approval.
- An open-book examination is taken with 6 months to complete.
- The completed examination is returned to the Board of Examiners Chairperson who forwards the test to anonymous members from the Board of Examiners for grading.
- An on-site clinical evaluation is scheduled with a passing grade on the examination.
- The on-site clinical examination supplements the didactic portion of the evaluation. A member of the Board of Examiners chosen by the applicant evaluates clinical techniques and client interaction at the applicant's clinical setting. Successful completion of this final step results in certification and privileges.

In a normal day, the clinician will see clients who have new dentures and who whistle when they speak, thumb- or digit-sucking children or adults, people with tinnitus, people who suffer sleep apnea, stroke victims, accident victims, ortho relapse cases, pre-ortho cases, and many other types of people and cases.

Other professional settings

- Research: There are many gaps in dental hygiene research. From chairside clinical case studies to full-blown lab and cohort studies, dental hygiene is not well represented in this arena. For a profession to be recognized as a profession, members need to provide evidence of research studies. For dental hygiene to grow into a true profession, more research done by hygienists for hygienists needs to be accomplished.
- Sales: Due to the lack of serious independent research, many companies support their own research to fill in the gaps that organized dentistry didn't realize existed. For example, if it were not for the dental sales industry, dentistry would still be trying to manage dental decay and salivary dysfunction with fluoride alone. Research by product manufacturers has shown the way for remineralization therapies that have revolutionized how decay and saliva are viewed. Dental hygienists and assistants are in unique positions to educate others on these new products.
- Writing: There is a potential opening for more writers in the dental field. As research is completed, someone needs to write up the results so that they are coherent and relatable. Compared to nursing, very few books and magazines are dedicated to the practice of dentistry, dental hygiene, or dental assisting. Technical writing of brochures, inserts, Web site content, and product reviews are just a few examples of writing opportunities.
- Speaking: Though not for everyone, speaking on behalf of different companies can be very exciting work. Speaking on a specific topic is also exciting. Traveling and meeting new people is part of this job. This avenue for assistants and dental hygienists, although, is not all glamour. Speaking and presenting programs are actual businesses that require hard work and dedication. It takes hours of research and preparation to remain current on any topic. Marketing yourself as a speaker is easier now with the advent of the Internet, but it takes an enormous amount of time. Many speakers began their careers as writers, so writing is a great way to break into the lecture circuit. Trade magazines are always looking for new talent to fill their pages, and experts on a particular topic are always in demand.
- Product educators: Companies often hire dental hygienists to act as product educators. These product educators may or may not have sales goals. Their main function is to make office visits or phone calls to explain the following:

○ How to use the product

○ How to charge for the product

○ Address other aspects of the customer product interface

- Educators: Much is written on this topic. Educational requirements for teaching vary from school to school and from province to province. Those who have an interest in education need to be willing to spend long hours in preparation and rigorous training to fully understand the materials taught. The future of the profession is dependent on one's ability to describe and translate often difficult concepts to those who will be entering the profession. Many educational institutions require long hours of teaching and researching or publishing in addition to the educational component. But the rewards of seeing students grasp the difficult concepts are amazing. As with writing and speaking, educators reach many more people with their teaching. The people they educate will each touch one person per hour, or so. And that's how change happens.

- Dental hygiene consultant: With experience this will be wonderful way for the dental hygiene career to evolve. After "paying your dues" and practicing on a number of different kinds of patients in different practice settings and learning the business of dentistry, this type of job may suit many hygienists. For whatever reason sometimes dental hygienists and dental assistants find that the rigors of their jobs are too much for them. Or they may not be challenged any longer. These talented people make excellent consultants. There are schools where one can become dental consultants, and where some current consultants can train in their methods.

- Public Health: This is a growth industry. The problems in dentistry and dental health are focused on the poor or those who live in rural areas. With public health dentistry, dental hygiene and dental assisting can make a huge impact on countless people. As is the case in education, those who are employed in public health must be willing to work in a bureaucratic system.

- Specialist within the practice: This is likely one of the easiest transitions. With the explosion in minimally invasive and minimal intervention in dentistry, caries management, periodontal management, or special medical needs management are all areas that need specialists in a general practitioner's practice. Referral sources can be physicians, chiropractors, herbalists, other practices, or others within the practice.

- Risk factor manager: This person in the dental practice does all data gathering and management. X-rays, saliva testing, blood testing, oral hygiene instruction, and any other non-clinical procedures are part of the management of all patients in a practice. The risk factor manager would see all patients/clients first to do the data gathering and send the patient/client to the dentist or dental hygienist with whom the person had an appointment.

- Mouthguard provider: This type of position can be very rewarding. Athletic mouthguards protect the athlete from damage to the teeth, temporomandibular joint injury, and concussion. Any sport that has the athlete using any type of gear from shin guards to helmets should also be protecting the teeth. A properly fitted mouthguard will last an entire season and has the potential to increase athletic ability. The cost of the mouthguard for children should not put parents and family into a position to gamble with their child's oral health. Boil-and-bite mouthguards are not adequate.

Each of these practice settings is new to the world of dental hygiene and dental assisting. With that comes the understanding that their effectiveness and viability have not been tested. With the increasing numbers of dental hygienists graduating with clinical skills, the traditional job market for dental hygienists will be oversaturated. The seasoned dental hygienist may make room for the new graduate without giving up the profession by investigating other career options that would best suit their talents and needs.

Many dental hygienists have transitioned into existing non-traditional options such as working abroad, developing and owning a dental placement service, starting a business to offer continuing education, becoming an inventor, working for the military, or combining their love of dentistry with a nursing degree. The sky is the limit in possibilities for the right person.

Integrating preventive dentistry into a general practice

The term minimally invasive dentistry has evolved over the years. Originally it was a term that was used to describe a practice where the dentist used specially designed burs or lasers to cut smaller and smaller holes in the enamel. For years, studies have shown that removing decay does not cure the person of decay in other sites. Every filling margin is a potential site for new caries.

Caries is a disease of infectious bacteria that metabolizes fermentable sugars resulting in he dissolution of tooth structure. Decay can be arrested by altering the biofilm environment. The current focus in dentistry is to rebuild damaged enamel and reduce or eliminate the bacterial infection that causes the disease. Minimally invasive dentistry describes this new dental reality.

Preventive dentistry involves the dental professional's understanding of the disease process and the mechanisms that can be used to prevent or arrest disease. For example, caries prevention involves early diagnosis, and salivary and dietary evaluations and controls. The dental 'team' can focus on managing caries before they develop.

What is a preventive dentistry dental team?

A team is a group of people organized to function cooperatively as a group to achieve a desired outcome. The dental health care team is comprised of individuals in the dental practice who are responsible for various aspects of patient care. The dental preventive team consists of the dentist, the dental hygienist, the dental assistant, and the administrative support professional. The dental team works on the following patient issues:

- Periodontal Disease: Periodontal disease prevention can involve salivary and bacteriological evaluation, complete periodontal charting and evaluation, and blood testing. Dental professionals have the responsibility with the increasing evidence of the systemic-oral connection to practice preventive periodontal treatment on all patients.
- Occlusion: Many patients complain of some type of occlusal disharmony. When patients suffer from frequent muscular headaches or chipped or broken teeth or restorations, these can be symptoms of occlusal dysfunction. The dental professional who practices preventive dentistry should be evaluating all patients for occlusal discrepancies and recommend myofunctional or other therapies to reduce or eliminate these problems.
- Oral Cancer: The incidence of oral cancer has risen greatly in the last several years. As is the case with periodontal disease, it is the dental professional's responsibility to exam all patients with an eye on oral cancer detection and treatment. Early detection means better prognosis and less invasive treatment options. All patients should be subject to an intraoral/ extraoral examination by the dentist or dental hygienist, and any abnormality or deviation from norm should be noted and explained to the patient. Additionally, salivary testing is becoming an important component of oral cancer screening as well as periodontal evaluation. Early detection is at the center of preventive dentistry. Intervening at the molecular level can't be accomplished unless the disease is noticed early. The best way to integrate preventive

dentistry into the practice is to continually research products that help the clinician detect disease early. The technology of early detection involving fluorescence and infrared lights to DNA testing is now available to all dental professionals. We can now detect lesions before they're visible to the eye, and in locations that, until now, we couldn't see at all. For example, decay that was hidden under previous restoration was considered to be a bomb waiting to destroy the tooth. Dentistry has the ability to prevent these bombs by detecting them before they become visible or cause greater tooth damage.

Periodontal disease detection is similar. Dentists, hygienists, and dental researchers in the past argued that bleeding on probing was an indicator of periodontal disease. We now know that bleeding on probing is not always an indicator of periodontal disease, but rather a sign of inflammation and can be an indicator of systemic conditions such as the following:

- Antiphospholipid Antibody Syndrome
- Blood and Marrow Stem Cell Transplant
- Diabetes
- Hemophilia
- Idiopathic Thrombocytopenic Purpura (ITP)
- Von Willebrand Disease

Technically, a dentist or hygienist can induce bleeding on probing because of incorrect technique or pressure, thus creating the appearance of disease where none existed. Some clinicians, due to physical disabilities such as carpal tunnel syndrome or thoracic outlet syndrome, alter their probing technique by unknowingly applying too much pressure. This can result in inaccurate assessment of the patient's periodontal status. Charting previous bone loss is only a historical narrative of the disease process. It does not present an accurate picture of present active disease. Sadly, it often is used as such. Dental professional teams need to be on the same page regarding the role that preventive dentistry and minimally invasive dentistry will play in a dental practice. Team meetings are the first step in achieving this process. Team members need to understand the goals of the preventive-oriented practice. Many are reluctant to "change" the way things have been done in the past because change brings about fear of the unknown and a general reluctance to embrace it.

The term *progress* is much easier for many team members to understand, and it is a more accurate term for this type of movement. The term *progress* implies a rich history of proven results where many mistakes have already been made and the resulting protocols and science are the fruit of that labor.

The first team meeting to discuss the progress of a practice to a preventive practice will be an important one. It sets the tone and stage for introduction to the new philosophy. The agenda needs to be set prior to the start, and all team members should have input before, during, and after the meeting. The dental team needs to have complete buy-in or the transition will fail. Unlike cosmetic dentistry where the doctor coordinates the sale and the procedure, the entire dental team will be involved in the preventive practice, including the use of expanded functions as permitted by provincial or state practice acts.

To facilitate an effective meeting, the organizer needs to have significant supportive evidence. This can be found in the scientific literature and in the practice statistics. This information will demonstrate to the team that there is a need for evolving and progressing the practice to one that either supports minimal intervention or maximum intervention using either minimally invasive or more aggressive interventions.

Since information and technology is changing constantly, a minimally invasive practice needs to designate a team member who will be responsible for evaluating product claims. This person should be knowledgeable about all aspects of science and dentistry. For example, a recent report highlighted xylitol and Strep viridans. It appears that xylitol is effective against this type of bacteria by interfering with the bacteria's ability to adhere to mucosa (Palchaudhuri *et al.* 2011). In the same search, *Streptococcus viridans* was mentioned as an isolate in rhinosinusitis complications (Hwang and Tan 2007). This may spark the minimally invasive dental practice to create a practice-based study to evaluate the effectiveness of xylitol on patients in the practice where caries and rhinosinusitis are common. Practice-based studies may intrigue a team member and will advance scientific research within that practice. The information may only solidify the use of xylitol in the practice. Either way, diligent constant attention to changes in science improves patient outcome.

As part of the information gathering prior to the meeting, the facilitator can gather information on how early diagnosis and treatment can affect current practice inconsistencies. For example, 0.01% of all Canadians will receive an oral cancer diagnosis annually. About 0.01% of patients in any dental practice will have oral cancer. If this information is not reflected in the number of biopsies performed or referred from the practice, an area for improvement has been revealed. In medicine, this is termed "quality improvement" and is defined as an approach to the study and improvement of the processes of providing health care services to meet the needs of clients. Dentistry can use quality improvement to increase positive patient outcomes too. Dental practice management software is an asset in gathering this information. The following example shows one system that is used to evaluate whether the practice statistics fit the national average for dental diseases:

- There are _____ patients in the practice.
  33,739,900 people live in Canada (www.worldbank.org).
  3,400 new oral cancer cases were discovered in Canada in 2009 (0.01%).
  We see _____ patients per week.
  We see _____ patients per month.
    We have referred _____ lesions for biopsy last year. _____%
  75% of adults have periodontal disease.
    We treated _____% of our adult patients for periodontal disease last year.
- There are _____ children in the practice.
- There are _____ adults in the practice.
- There are _____ unfinished caries cases on the books right now.
- There are _____ unfinished periodontal cases on the books right now.
- We have _____ patients in active orthodontic treatment.
- Administrative staff makes _____ reminder calls per month.
- We have _____ broken appointments in dental hygiene per month.
- We have _____ broken appointments on the dental side per month.
- Dental hygiene production averages $_____ per month.

  _____% periodontal treatment related
  _____% caries related
  _____% _____

- Dental assistant production averages $_____ per month.
- Dentist production averages $_____ per month.

  _____% restorative
  _____% cosmetic
  _____% orthodontic
  _____% recurrent decay
  _____% endodontic
  _____% emergency
  _____% _____
  _____% _____

- Collections are at _____% of production.
- How many patients have frustrating levels of decay or periodontal disease that you can't stop? _____

Who are they? Bring their charts to the staff meeting.

    ———

    ———

    ———

    ———

    ———

    ———

    ———

    ———

    ———

- How many patients are on long-term dental prescriptions?

Fluoride ———
Periostat ———
Pain ———
Saliva stimulants ———
Chlorhexidine ———
Other ———

- Responsibilities

Making appointments
    Restorative: ———
    Hygiene: ———
Reminder calls
    Restorative: ———
    Hygiene: ———
Web site: ———
Brochures: ———
Chart Audits
    Restorative: ———
    Hygiene: ———
    How often: ———

One of the under-appreciated members of the dental team is the office manager who often is responsible for reception, accounts receivable, bookkeeping, and day-to-day management of personnel, and peace keeper. This chapter is charged with representing all team members and their contribution to the practice. Office managers are key in gathering data and deciphering it. They are also in a gatekeeper position. In the MI practice, the office manager must be aware of billing procedures and the basics of the science of MI dentistry so they can explain it intelligently on the phone or to patients/clients in person. This type of practice is outside the status quo, and patients will need reassurances from all team members.

Weekly meetings should be scheduled to review progress. Production goals could also be discussed but in the context that the patients' needs outweigh the need for the dental office to generate a large profit.

Preventive practices can be productive and profitable for all. Loss of revenue is not part of any business plan; however, when a practice does not understand the importance of the numbers, it will be unprofitable. Patients have been hearing the brush/floss message their entire lives. Only a certain percentage of patients/clients will benefit from this message and gravitate toward it for life-long health. There are other people who hear the message, and it will fall on deaf ears. It is the dental team members' responsibility to ensure that patients/clients are receiving the message of the importance of oral health that the patients/clients can hear. By creating a positive message about minimally invasive preventive dentistry, a practice will continue to meet its expectations and often exceed them.

For example, a patient with Sjögren's Syndrome may not be able to brush or floss any better than they are currently. However, there is still biofilm and deposit present. Instead of blaming the patient for declining oral health, the dental professional can offer the patient remineralization options, including salivary substitutes and enhancements.

Dental team members need to be aware of the language that is used during discussions with patients. "Filling appointment" can be switched to "surgical appointment" to provide the patient with the need for the urgency and importance of treatment. In a minimally invasive practice, to "fill" a tooth is to surgically repair the tooth. Use words and descriptions that accurately state the procedure being performed, not downplay it for the patient/client. This will take a concerted effort on the part of the dental team since it may involve a progression from terms used daily to a new vocabulary.

Seasoned dental professionals may have a more difficult time achieving this transition than newer graduates. New graduates are taught that drilling and filling are things of the past, and the new paradigm in dentistry is more toward the medical model of early detection and treatment.

Seasoned professionals may see that they have built substantial practices around the non-compliant patient, while newer graduates see opportunities beyond the non-compliance. Some will welcome and embrace this new paradigm and will find that minimally invasive preventive dentistry can be as profitable, if not more so, than the habitual model of practice. The ability to prevent or arrest disease is beneficial for the patient and the practice in ways that were previously not considered. When dental professionals understand that it is better for the patient and the practice to manage infection rather than amputate the tooth, all will benefit.

Conclusion

The preventive dental team involves the dentist, dental hygienist, assistant, practice manager, and the patient.

The ability of the dental professional to achieve overall lasting oral health is achieved only with the understanding of the client/patient. Clients/patients must become co-therapists with the dental professionals in achieving healthy smiles to last a lifetime.

Acknowledgements

The authors wish to thank the contribution of Stephanie Wall, RDH, MS, MEd, for the section on myofunctional therapy.

References

Abe, S., Ishihara, K., Adachi, M., *et al.* (2006) Professional oral care reduces influenza infection in elderly. *Archives of Gerontology and Geriatrics,* 43, 157–164.

Abe, S., Ishihara, K., Okuda, K. (2001) Prevalence of potential respiratory pathogens in the mouths of elderly patients and effects of professional oral care. *Archives of Gerontology and Geriatrics,* 32, 45–55.

Adachi, M., Ishihara, K., Abe, S. (2002) Effect of professional oral health care on the elderly living in nursing homes. *Oral Surgery, Oral Medicine, Oral Pathology, Oral Radiology and Endodontics,* 94, 191–195.

Adachi, M., Ishihara, K., Abe, S., *et al.* (2007) Professional oral health care by dental hygienists reduced respiratory infections in elderly persons requiring nursing care. *International Journal Dental Hygiene,* 5, 69–74.

Banerjee, A., Hajatdoost-Sani, M., Farrell, S., *et al.* (2010) A clinical evaluation and comparison of bioactive glass and sodium bicarbonate air-polishing powders. *Journal of Dentistry,* 38, 475–479.

Bush, B.C. and Donley, T.G. (2002) A model for dental hygiene education concerning the relationship between periodontal health and systemic health. *Education for Health (Abingdon),* 15, 19–26.

Christensen, R.P. and Bangerter, V.W. (1987) Immediate and long–term in vivo effects of polishing on enamel and dentin. *Journal of Prosthetic Dentistry,* 57, 150–160.

dela Cruz, G.G., Rozier, R.G., Slade, G. (2004) Dental screening and referral of young children by pediatric primary care providers. *Pediatrics,* 114, e642–e652.

DeStefano, F., Anda, R.F., Kahn, H.S., *et al.* (1993) Dental disease and risk of coronary heart disease and mortality. *British Medical Journal,* 306, 688–691.

Fontana, M., Young, D.A., Wolff, M.S., *et al.* (2010) Defining dental caries for 2010 and beyond. *Dental Clinics of North America,* 54, 423–440.

Ford, S.J. (2008) The importance and provision of oral hygiene in surgical patients. *International Journal of Surgery,* 6, 418–419.

Frisbee, S.J., Chambers, C.B., Frisbee, J.C., *et al.* (2010a) Self-reported dental hygiene, obesity, and systemic inflammation in a pediatric rural community cohort. *BMC Oral Health,* 10, 21.

Frisbee, S.J., Chambers, C.B., Frisbee, J.C., *et al.* (2010b) Association between dental hygiene, cardiovascular disease risk factors and systemic inflammation in rural adults. *Journal of Dental Hygiene,* 84, 177–184.

Hwang, S.Y. and Tan, K.K. (2007) Streptococcus viridans has a leading role in rhinosinusitis complications. *Annals of Otology, Rhinology and Laryngology,* 116, 381–385.

Inskip, P.D., Ekbom, A., Galanti, M.R., *et al.* (1995) Medical diagnostic x-rays and thyroid cancer. *Journal of the National Cancer Institute,* 87, 1613–1621.

Ishikawa, A., Yoneyama, T., Hirota, K., *et al.* (2008) Professional oral health care reduces the number of oropharyngeal bacteria. *Journal of Dental Research,* 87, 594–598.

Joshipura, K.J., Rimm, E.B., Douglass, C.W., *et al.* (1996) Poor oral health and coronary heart disease. *Journal of Dental Research,* 75, 1631–1636.

Memon, A., Godward, S., Williams, D., *et al.* (2010) Dental x-rays and the risk of thyroid cancer: a case-control study. *Acta Oncologica,* 49, 447–453.

Okuda, K., Kimizuka, R., Abe, S., *et al.* (2005) Involvement of periodontopathic anaerobes in aspiration pneumonia. *Journal of Periodontology,* 76, 2154–2160.

Palchaudhuri, S., Rehse, S.J., Hamasha, K., *et al.* (2011) Raman Spectroscopy of Xylitol Uptake and Metabolism in Gram-positive and Gram-negative Bacteria. *Applied and Environmental Microbiology,* 77, 131–137.

Paolinelis, G., Banerjee, A., Watson, T.F. (2008) An in vitro investigation of the effect and retention of bioactive glass air-abrasive on sound and carious dentine. *Journal of Dentistry,* 6, 214–218.

Sona, C.S., Zack, J.E., Schallom, M.E., *et al.* (2009) The impact of a simple, low-cost oral care protocol on ventilator-associated pneumonia rates in a surgical intensive care unit. *Journal of Intensive Care Medicine,* 24, 54–62.

Sugihara, N., Maki, Y., Okawa, Y., *et al.* (2010) Factors associated with root surface caries in elderly. *The Bulletin of Tokyo Dental College,* 51, 23–30.

US FDA. (2010) White Paper: Initiative to reduce unnecessary radiation exposure from medical imaging. Available online at http://www.fda.gov/Radiation-EmittingProducts/RadiationSafety/RadiationDoseReduction/ucm199994.htm#_Toc253092889.

Wilder, R.S., Iacopino, A.M., Feldman, C.A., *et al.* (2009) Periodontal-systemic disease education in U.S. and Canadian dental schools. *Journal of Dental Education,* 73, 38–52.

22

The independent dental hygienist

Fran Richardson

Introduction

Prevention of disease is the primary goal of the oral health care professions. Although each of the various oral health professions (dentistry, dental hygiene, dental assisting, dental technology, dental therapy, and denturism) has a distinct role to play in treating the effects of oral disease, the dental hygiene profession was specifically created for the purpose of prevention. Numerous publications outline the history of the profession, therefore, that particular component is not being addressed in this chapter.

Dental hygiene is a rapidly evolving profession. It is now practiced in more than 30 countries around the world, and there is a vibrant international organization (International Federation of Dental Hygienists) that promotes excellence in dental hygiene care and treatment. Different countries are in a variety of stages regarding the evolution within the profession, but all dental hygienists have a common purpose: to educate the client in the provision and maintenance of their oral health.

The newest emerging component of dental hygiene practice, especially in North America, is that of the practitioner who provides direct clinical care to the client without the referral or intervention of another health care provider, usually a dentist. The term "independent practice" is now widely used, but it was not one that was developed by dental hygiene but by organized dentistry. The term today is widely used. An independent dental hygiene practice can take on many forms, and these will be further explored in the following pages.

No matter the style of practice chosen by the dental hygienist, there are rules and regulations that must be considered. However, there are also times when the dental hygienist, in the interest of the public, must advocate on behalf of the clients and work toward modifying those rules in order to provide more equitable care. Client advocacy is one of the dental hygienist's most important roles.

Regulation

Dental hygienists and dentists are educated, regulated, and licensed health care providers. Dental assistants, denturists, dental therapists, and dental technologists may also be regulated in a particular jurisdiction. Understanding the regulation of other oral health care providers in one's location is necessary in order to provide appropriate referrals and advice to clients.

Some jurisdictions no longer refer to "licensing" individuals but rather delineating controlled "acts" that the registered practitioner is authorized to perform; the concept is essentially the same. Under the *Regulated Health Professions Act, 1991* in Ontario, Canada, practitioners are no longer "licensed" but have a certificate of registration. There are "controlled acts" that are authorized. Regulation of a profession serves one primary purpose—to protect the public. There are many regulatory variations within the dental hygiene world, but they all have similar mandates and responsibilities. Regulatory bodies are quite different from professional associations in that they determine the educational requirements for registration, scope of practice, quality assurance, or continuing education requirements and investigate complaints from the public that may lead to disciplinary action, or in extreme cases, revocation of the practitioner's permission to practice (Table 22-1). Both dentists and dental hygienists must be registered with the appropriate

Comprehensive Preventive Dentistry, First Edition. Edited by Hardy Limeback.
© 2012 John Wiley & Sons, Ltd. Published 2012 by John Wiley & Sons, Ltd.

Table 22-1 Comparison of the functions of the regulatory body for dental hygienists versus an association of dental hygienists

Regulator Body	Association
Advocates on behalf of the public interest	Advocates on behalf of the dental hygienists
Public members are usually part of the decision making process	Concerned with the professional profile of the dental hygienist
Registration is mandatory to practice dental hygiene	Membership is usually voluntary
Develops regulations and guidelines for practice	Addresses employment concerns of dental hygienists and assists in providing professional development programs
Enforces standards of practice and conducts and monitors quality assurance and continuing education	Lobbies government on behalf of its members

regulatory authority in order to practice the profession. In contrast, professional associations are voluntary and in the business of advocating for their members.

In most cases it is the professional association that has lobbied government for changes to the legislation that governs dental hygiene practice.

Dentists have always had the privilege of self-regulation, a system whereby members of the profession and more recently members of the public, form the governing body for the profession. Historically, dental hygienists have been regulated by the same board/council that also regulates dentists. Sometimes dental hygienists may be represented on the dental board/council, but often that representation is not equal to the number of dentists nor is it proportional to the number of dental hygienists in that jurisdiction. Legislators in Canada have realized that it is a conflict of interest for the primary employer to also be the regulator. Therefore, as health legislation is provincially based, dental hygienists in Canada are now governed by boards/councils consisting of dental hygienists and members of the public. At the time of writing, the province of Newfoundland and Labrador (NL) had passed legislation to create a form of self-regulation for dental hygienists in conjunction with four other non-related professions. In the Province of Prince Edward Island (PEI), Canada's smallest province, the dental hygienists were in the early stages of applying for self-regulation. All professions are regulated by the government in the three Territories.

The Dental Hygiene Committee of California (2011) is the first of its kind in the United States that registers and licenses dental hygienists directly. The difference

from the Canadian system of self-regulation is that in California, there is a dentist on the Committee along with public members and dental hygienists. These dental hygiene regulatory authorities have the same responsibilities, privileges, and obligations as dentists do in their regulatory structure.

As regulated health care practitioners, dental hygienists and dentists must always practice to the letter of the law. If a statute or regulation requires amending in order to better facilitate the preventive needs of the clients they serve, then that must occur through the appropriate legislative channels. A regulated health care practitioner who operates outside of their scope of practice or "flaunts" the rules of their regulatory body will soon find themselves the subject of disciplinary action.

Protection of the public from unregistered practitioners is also the responsibility of the jurisdictional regulator. Persons holding themselves out to be dentists or dental hygienists may cause harm to the public though improper sterilization of instruments, undetected oral disease, and damage to the oral cavity through incompetence. Dealing with illegalities is also a matter of prevention because the victims of illegal practitioners usually require attention and treatment from a registered/licensed health care provider after a problem has occurred.

Registration

The registration of a health care practitioner is the responsibility of each respective governing body. Before a practitioner can be registered, she or he must provide the authorities with information related to her or his school of graduation, provincial/state/national exam certificates, past history in another jurisdiction, and usually proof of professional liability coverage. A fee will be charged. In some areas new registrants are required to take a clinical examination, but nearly all jurisdictions require the applicant to have an understanding of local jurisprudence. Most jurisdictions require an annual renewal of the license/certificate and an indication that the practitioner is remaining current through a quality assurance or continuing education program.

Complaints and discipline

A major focus of the regulatory process is to investigate complaints from the public about the conduct of a particular registered practitioner. Depending on the nature of the complaint and the results of the ensuing investigation, the practitioner may be referred to a disciplinary panel that will hear arguments from both sides. If the panel has determined that a particular action was of such a nature that the practitioner is no longer safe to practice, registration/licensure may be revoked. In less serious cases, a penalty may be imposed that includes successful completion of required courses, fines, and possible suspension from practice for a designated period of time.

How is dental hygiene legislation and prevention of oral disease connected?

Legislation dictates not only what a dental hygienist may practice but also how and in what form that practice may occur. Therefore, legislation also dictates from whom a member of the public may receive oral health care, in what setting that may occur, and the restrictions placed on the client's ability to receive care directly from a dental hygienist without the intervention of another health care provider, usually a dentist.

Example A

Ms. X lives in a seniors' residence. She is very shy and moderately mobile but exhibits anxious feelings when she goes for appointments outside of home. Consequently, Ms. X prefers to see the chiropodist, physician, and physiotherapist that regularly see clients in her residence. The staff dietitian observes that Ms. X appears to have "gone off her food" and is not eating. The dietitian makes a number of changes to Ms. X's diet, but there is no change in Ms. X's eating habits. The dietitian brings the issue to the weekly staff conference. The diet is modified again. In the meantime a dental hygienist has offered to make visits to the residence. Being accustomed to in-house visits from other health care providers, Ms. X willingly agrees to an oral assessment. The dental hygienist discovers that Ms. X has a broken upper denture that is impeding on her tissues making eating painful. The dental hygienist checks Ms. X's chart and notes that there have been no oral assessments since Ms. X moved into the residence 5 years previously. The dental hygienist called a denturist who made house calls, and Ms. X received a new denture, thereby permitting her to resume her normal diet.

In Example A, Ms. X was fortunate to live in a jurisdiction where the legislation permitted the dental hygienist to provide intra-oral assessments for clients in their place of residence. Many jurisdictions do not. In other places, the dental hygienist would only be permitted to assess Ms. X's oral condition if a dentist was present or at least physically on the premises. Not only did the intervention by the dental hygienist resolve the oral problem, but it prevented the consequences that could have occurred from poor nutritional uptake and aspiration of oral bacteria (Limeback 1998; Stein and Henry 2009).

Example B

Mr. Y is a relatively young man who suffered a motorcycle accident. He is bedridden, has a complete dentition, and limited use of both arms. Prior to the accident, Mr. Y went regularly to his dentist for annual recall appointments. He was proud of his smile and wanted to maintain his oral health as part of his rehabilitation. Mr. Y lives at home with his brother and caregiver. His dentist of record does not make house calls.

In Example B, we have a situation where an individual's quality of life is dependent on care by others. Mr. Y wishes to maintain his oral health and he is mentally capable of making his own decisions. Due to his physical restrictions, and possible susceptibility to respiratory problems, Mr. Y would benefit from preventive interventions on a regular basis. The ideal would be for oral health care personnel to attend to Mr. Y in his home and to only transfer him to a dental facility for procedures that were not possible to conduct offsite. In many jurisdictions in North America it would be possible for a dental hygienist to attend to Mr. Y in his residence. However, many more jurisdictions restrict the practice of dental hygiene to when a dentist is present or provides direction (different terms are used in different jurisdictions such as prescription, order, delegation) thus making it almost impossible for a client such as Mr. Y to receive preventive oral health care unless he is transported to an external facility. If quality of life is the issue and prevention of further health problems is the goal of maintaining a healthy mouth, then the regulation of, by whom, what, and where preventive oral health care may be obtained and delivered is an important consideration.

If Mr. Y does not live in a jurisdiction that permits a dental hygienist to treat him in his home, then there are other alternatives that can be explored. The first is to ensure that Mr. Y has a thorough oral assessment. This can be done in his residence by a dentist who operates a mobile practice, or Mr. Y can be transported to a dental clinic equipped with facilities to accept clients with special needs. Following the oral assessment all clinical interventions should be completed to ensure that Mr. Y is in optimum oral health before a maintenance plan is developed. Both Mr. Y and his caregivers should be involved in the planning and decision making. An oral health care regimen is developed and the caregivers provided with the appropriate training. Mr. Y is to be encouraged to do as much for himself as possible. In this situation, it is imperative that the need to transport Mr. Y externally for his oral health care be kept to a minimum.

Advocacy for clients such as Mr. Y is as important for him as is the physical act of brushing his teeth. If Mr. Y is unable to obtain preventive oral health care within a reasonable timeframe and with minimum disruption to his daily living activities, then being able to obtain his oral care in his residence would be the ideal. Regulated health care practitioners' primary responsibility is to the public, and advocating for public access to health care services falls into that category. Not all regulators would agree with that statement, but those who do agree have been able to advance access to preventive oral health care in meaningful ways.

Anti-competition

In the early part of the twenty-first century, agencies charged with ensuring that there was a competitive element within the health care system began looking into the restrictive practices prevalent in the oral health care field. The Competition Bureau of Canada (Scott 2007) advocated for the self-regulation of dental hygiene in provinces where dental hygienists were still regulated by dental boards/councils. In the US, the Federal Trade Commission determined that it was anti-competitive for the state dental board to restrict dental hygienists from treating children in schools without the presence of a dentist (Federal Trade Commission 2010). In Europe the Organization for Economic Co-operation and Development (OCED) (2005) called for a reduction of costs and increased access to preventive oral health care through lifting restrictions on where and with whom dental hygienists could practice.

There have been instances where dental hygienists have tried to provide preventive oral health care services, primarily to underserved populations, without the direct control of dentistry thus challenging the right of one profession to interfere in the practice of another profession. In the US, many state dental boards now permit dental hygienists to provide local anesthesia, to work under general supervision, and to provide direct services to underserved populations. The evolution of the dental hygiene profession has not been without its stressors, and in many cases organized dentistry has gone to great lengths to thwart any progressive practices by dental hygienists. While the reason most often put forward by organized dentistry is that of "patient safety" or the need for a "comprehensive dental exam," the reality of the situation is that when dentistry controls the practice of dental hygiene, it also controls the revenue generated by dental hygienists.

In jurisdictions where dental hygienists are permitted to own and operate their own practices independent of a dentist and to provide direct services to the clients, the clients who access dental hygiene practices are those who for one reason or another, for example, financial, mobility, fear, or geography, are unlikely to have been regular dental office clients in the first place. When the clients

are firmly established with a dental hygienist for preventive maintenance, she or he will refer the client to a dentist for restorative treatment. If financial resources are considered to be a barrier to receiving dental treatment, the dental hygienist may be able to assist the client in locating alternative treatment options such as those provided through nearby dental schools or through accessing publicly funded outreach programs.

Choosing a practice setting

working for others

There is nothing inherently unprofessional in being employed by another person or organization. It does not matter whether your employer is a registered health practitioner (for example, a dentist), a private business, or government agency, a hospital, a residential care facility, or non-profit agency. What does matter is that professionalism is maintained at all times and the employer's position on a issue does not interfere with the maintenance of dental hygiene standards.

However, there are challenges in working for others. Dental hygienists must manage those challenges in an ethical and professional way. Fortunately, the vast majority of employers have high professional standards, and these issues either never arise or are easily resolved. Occasionally difficulties do arise and must to be addressed appropriately.

Within the private dental practice setting, ownership of client records and what can be told to clients about a departing dental hygienist are often the most common areas of dispute. This issue becomes particularly controversial if the dental hygienist is moving to a competing dental practice or is opening her or his own practice within the same general geographical area. Often employees have a contractual duty to avoid soliciting clients of the previous practice when moving to the new one. In addition, the regulations governing both dentistry and dental hygiene may stipulate that solicitation of clients is professional misconduct.

The client's interests come first

One issue is whether the client will be able to receive continuity of care at the previous practice. If there will be no dental hygiene care available then the client should be advised of this. Even where dental hygiene care remains available, clients should have a choice of whether to continue to receive it in the previous practice or to move with the dental hygienist to the new practice. Dental hygienists who are contemplating moving practices should consult with a lawyer before taking any action.

At a minimum there is a duty on those remaining at the previous practice to advise clients who ask where the dental hygienist has gone. In many circumstances it would also be appropriate for the departing dental hygienist and/or the previous practice to advise clients that the dental hygienist is leaving and provide the clients with the choice to stay or to transfer their care to the new practice of the dental hygienist. However it is handled, the communications, whether verbal or written, must be professional. In today's society, clients expect to be involved in the selection of their health care provider. To be told that their preferred practitioner is unavailable and that they must remain in a practice when that provider is still available, albeit in another location, goes against freedom of choice, a position long held by the dental profession.

Working for yourself

Although the majority of dental hygienists practice within dental offices, dental hygienists in some jurisdictions are able to set up independent practices. The term *independent practice* is commonly used to describe a dental hygienist-owned practice. It does not mean that dental hygienists who own their own practices work independently from other dental care providers, especially dentists who must be consulted for diagnosis of oral disease and orders for specific tests and procedures. By nature, dental hygienists are collaborative practitioners who are motivated to be partners in client care by recognizing and working with all members of the health care team. As amendments to legislation enable this possibility, it is anticipated that more dental hygienists will explore this option as a means of addressing the needs of clients who are unable or unwilling to seek care from the traditional dental office.

Dental hygienists can choose from three main business structures:

- Sole proprietorship
- Partnership
- Health professional corporation

A lawyer and/or an accountant should be consulted before the practitioner chooses a structure that best suits her/his needs. No matter what business structure is chosen, regulated health care practitioners are accountable for their professional actions both to the client and to their respective regulatory authority. The business aspect must never override the care and duty to the health and safety of the client.

Sole Proprietorship

A sole proprietorship is where the practitioner is the sole owner of the practice. People deal with the owner or staff directly. There is no one else responsible for the practice.

However, there are certain business registration and tax requirements that need to be complied with in this situation. The Ontario government has some useful information at its Ministry of Consumer and Business Services Web site at www.cbs.gov.on.ca or check with the relevant authority in your jurisdiction.

Partnership

A partnership involves two or more people joining together to operate a business or other venture. Generally partners are responsible for each other's actions. Typically partners share the profits of the business or venture. Dental hygienists, who form a partnership, especially if the other partner(s) is not a regulated professional, are advised to maintain control over the standards of practice, client records, and financial practices.

Professional corporations

A corporation is a legal entity recognized by the government and the courts that is owned by its shareholders. It can make contracts, own land and other assets, earn income, and borrow money just like an individual. It also pays its own taxes. Laws vary in each jurisdiction. Therefore, dental hygienists interested in professional incorporation should check into their provincial/state legislation before considering professional incorporation.

Advantages

For some dental hygienists, there may be advantages to incorporating their professional practices. For example, some accountants have said that the following advantages may be available:

- Small business deduction. The professional corporation can benefit from the small business deduction. Small businesses are taxed at a lower rate than high-income individuals and, so long as the money is left in the corporation, it can be used for other purposes. This is only a tax deferral; when the remainder of the money is taken out of the corporation, the remainder of the tax is imposed.
- Income fluctuations. If one's income fluctuates from year to year, the person can even out his/her income by taking advantage of the lower tax brackets each year.
- Year end. The professional corporation can have a non-calendar year-end. This permits the deferral of additional taxes.
- Capital gains exemption. Depending on the jurisdiction, there may be a capital gains exemption on the sale of shares in the professional corporation. However, there may be a number of rules and restrictions for which expert advice is required.

- Other tax advantages. There may be some minor tax advantages in relation to employment insurance and tax installments during your first year of operation and a tax free "death benefit."
- Trade creditors. Only the corporation is liable to trade creditors (such as, suppliers of equipment, supplies and services to the practice). Shareholders are normally not liable for non-payment of those accounts. However, this protection does not apply to professional liability claims from clients.

Not all of these advantages apply to all dental hygienists or in all jurisdictions. For example, the small business deduction deferral does not benefit dental hygienists who use most of what they earn for living expenses. A dental hygienist needs to consult with an accountant and probably a lawyer to assess whether these advantages apply to their circumstances.

Disadvantages

There are quite a few disadvantages to incorporating a professional practice, including the following:

- Cost. Incorporation itself will almost certainly require the services of an accountant and a lawyer for which they will charge a fee. Filing papers with the government will cost, and the regulatory/licensing body may charge an application fee for processing the required papers. There may be an annual renewal fee, and annual accounting services will be required.
- Paperwork. Professional incorporation requires extensive paperwork. The corporation has to file a special income tax return that may be more complicated than what an individual currently prepares.
- Accounting disadvantages. There are some complex disadvantages that should be discussed with an accountant.
- Transition costs. Changing from the current practice to a professional corporation may result in some specific difficulties. Expert advice is needed to minimize or avoid these problems.
- Restrictions. Each jurisdiction will have rules and regulations that could make incorporation less worthwhile for dental hygienists.

Going it alone: advantages and challenges faced by dental hygienists who choose to operate their own businesses

As noted in the section on Choosing a Practice Setting, there are currently opportunities in some jurisdictions for dental hygienists to practice their profession in a manner that could be considered non-traditional. Dental hygienists in several US states and in many Canadian provinces are able to practice without the oversight of another oral health care practitioner. This is a trend that will continue as preventive oral health care is sought by members of the public who for many reasons are unable or unwilling to attend a traditional dental office. As dental hygienists increasingly avail themselves of alternative practice settings, the public will ultimately determine which venue works best for their particular situation.

There are several modes of service delivery for the entrepreneurial-minded dental hygienist, but the two most common are "store front" or stand alone and mobile. The store-front practice is similar to a traditional dental office but does not require as much equipment and may include one or more operatories. Figure 22-1 provides examples of a dental hygiene clinic. In some cases, the dental hygienist/owner may rent one of the operatories to a denturist, dentist, or another dental hygienist. The clients go to the office and are treated by the dental hygienist on-site. A mobile practice is one where the dental hygienist travels to the client's residence and provides the treatment in their home. Mobile equipment is required, and depending on the individual situation, the dental hygienist may or may not provide a portable chair. In many cases dental hygiene care is provided in the resident's chair or bed. This form of practice can be very rewarding but does include the transporting and setting up of equipment plus the added physical issues related to working in unconventional positions.

Why do dental hygienists want to open their own business?

The following quotes are from dental hygienists who opened their own business.

> "The time was right in my life and I had the support system I would need at home. I had always thought about it as a possibility in my career and knew the time was right. Also I felt that I had a wide variety of experience in my profession, which would allow me to practice independently with a solid background of past experience. I had worked in family practice and periodontal practice and we moved a lot so my range of experience was huge." RDH in Alberta

Another dental hygienist indicated that the dentist with whom she was practicing retired and the new owner had a very different philosophy of oral health care.

> "Long term clients were leaving the practice in high numbers. The way I had been encouraged and enjoyed providing dental hygiene care for my clients had changed. I wanted to continue to provide the expert care that I had always been able to do under the guidance of my previous employer." RDH in Ontario

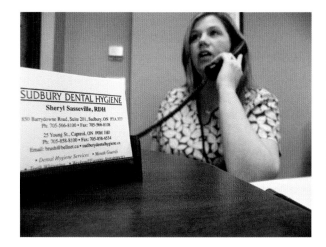

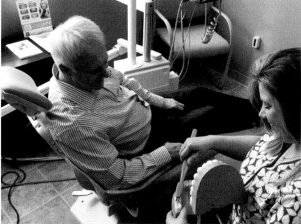

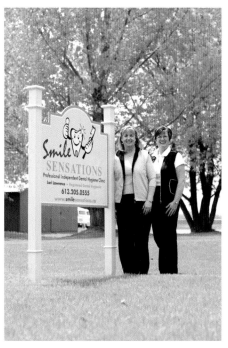

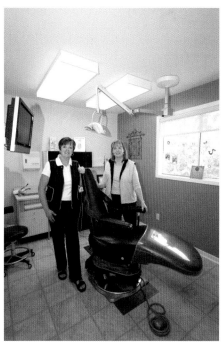

Figure 22-1 An example of an independent dental hygiene practice.

"My forte is dealing with 'difficult' people, plus I like to make big improvements—the 6 month R/C routine always left me feeling like I was doing an elite job for the wealthy, insured or already aware. My clinic focuses on lowering access barriers to dental maintenance, whether fear, physical or financial. Because I make deals, take assignment and don't balance-bill for people on income assistance, this clinic is growing in spite of economic meltdowns. It's what happens when you love what you do." RDH in British Columbia

Most dental hygienists choose to go it alone or in partnership with other dental hygienists because it provides them with the opportunity to control the hours they work, the physical environment in which they practice

and more importantly how they practice dental hygiene. Others choose to open a dental hygiene practice, either 'store front' or mobile because it provides the flexibility of treating clients who might not otherwise receive preventive oral health care. Others prefer the freedom of blending family considerations with being their own boss. For others it may be that they saw the inequity of working for someone else who they perceived reaped the profits of their labours.

"When I was up for a review by my last employer, he said that it was hard for him to justify giving me a $1/hour raise as I had only produced $200,000 for him the year before." RDH in Ontario

"I've been wanting to do this for almost 20 years. I'm very independent by nature. I was tired of working really hard to watch someone else build his dream on the fees I (he) was charging. I do not want to be dictated to as to how long it takes me to do a good job. Tired of feeling like a robot at the end of the day. I've done this in response to people being turned away from DDS offices who won't accept [government payments]. For those who cannot leave their home or long term care facility. For the person who hasn't been seen in decades do (sic) to bad experiences and fears at the hands of a DDS." RDH in Ontario

"I was becoming very discouraged working in private practice. In my personal experiences dentistry has become a 'money-machine,' where personal service and attention to detail have fallen by the wayside. The insufficient time that is assigned to perform the task of scaling and root planing teeth as well as the lack of education has created a society of misinformed clients with lingering subgingival calculus that they are unaware of, which is now leading to chronic periodontal disease. Eventually my conscience got the better of me and I realized that I was unable to perform to the level of my scope of practice and expertise without daily criticism from my employer. I was intending to leave my profession completely, until Bill 171 became law and another window of opportunity opened." RDH in Ontario

Not all dental hygienists will choose to provide full service dental hygiene care. One of the most common opportunities is that of providing custom made mouthguards for use by athletes in sporting venues. Those practitioners take portable equipment right to the arena or court, take the impressions, and return with the custom made mouthguard at a subsequent training session. By providing the service on-site, the athletes do not have to make the extra step of attending a clinic elsewhere.

"My son played house league hockey. In the dressing room I was amazed to see how many children were wearing store bought and or poor fitting mouthguards. Most coaches and parents think mouthguards are to protect damage to teeth only; several times I had to explain a mouthguard also provides protection to TMJ, gingival, and brain. I mentioned to my boss that we should provide a service and go to the arenas and take impressions for mouthguards. He was not interested so I decided to embark on my own. I asked one of my Level II D.A. colleagues if she would like to join me on this venture and she agreed." RDH who has a mouthguard clinic

However, all dental hygienists will agree that in reality there is no such thing as "independent practice" because clients with conditions beyond the scope of dental hygiene care must be referred to another health care practitioner for treatment. This may be a dentist, denturist, physician, dietitian, or any other regulated health care practitioner appropriate to treat the client's condition.

What are the advantages to the client in being treated directly by the dental hygienist?

There are many types of practice options. Dental hygienists who have store-front practices perceive that the clients prefer the relaxed atmosphere of having longer appointments that place a heavy influence on oral health education. There is also the ability to tailor the appointment times to the individual rather than to the schedule set by someone else. For those dental hygienists who have chosen the mobile route, there is the advantage of the client being treated in their own residence minus the inconvenience of having to travel to a traditional dental office. In those areas where dentists will also do house calls, the client is able to receive follow-up restorative treatment if required. Unfortunately, not all clients reside in areas where treatment is available in their place of residence, and they must leave their homes to receive restorative or surgical treatment.

Dental hygiene-only practices or those associated with multidisciplinary clinics may offer a non-threatening environment for clients who may be apprehensive about attending a traditional dental practice. The sights, sounds, and smells of the practice are different and may be less "clinical" in appearance thus easing the apprehensive client back into oral hygiene care.

"When people leave the dental hygiene clinic, they take away more than nice-looking teeth. They also have a renewed understanding, a plan, and tools to get there. It is money well spent, especially since it affects their overall health." RDH in British Columbia

Receiving preventive oral hygiene treatment in one's residence is not only for the aged or home-bound senior. Clients who with mobility challenges, several small children, or who live in a community residence may benefit from home-based care. Since preventive treatment can be done at the kitchen table, in an easy chair or at the bed-side, the dental hygienist can accommodate the needs of the client while providing a service that does not disrupt the client's household. For example, a mother and her three pre-school children could receive preventive oral health care in the home, thus reducing the need for the client to travel or to make arrangements for childcare. Another example would be for those clients who reside together in a group home due to mental or social concerns that make traveling to "strange" places uncomfortable for them. Preventive care is then accomplished in a familiar and comfortable setting.

"The clients where I go to their homes appreciate the convenience and privacy especially in cases when they suffer gag reflex. The embarrassment of accidents due to their gag reflex seems to be lessened in their home environment. A lot of would be gaggers can relax easier in their own homes and successfully endure the impression taking because of this." RDH who provides mouthguards

People who are in end-of-life care often experience oral discomfort due to their medications or therapy. A visit from a dental hygienist can not only provide the feeling of a clean mouth but also provide company to someone who may not receive many external visitors. While the dental hygienist may decide that it is not in the best interest of the client to proceed with debridement due to the client's frail tissues or contraindicating medical history, the dental hygienist may be able to provide daily/weekly basic plaque removal thus enabling the client to experience a relatively healthy oral cavity.

Surely there are also disadvantages to the client?

The primary disadvantage to the client who seeks or receives treatment directly from a dental hygienist is the fact that there may not be a dentist available to make a house call and the client will need to be transported to a traditional dental office or hospital facility to receive restorative of surgical dental care. While dental hygienists are aware that they must refer a client for treatment to the appropriate health care provider if the dental hygienist is aware that treatment required is beyond his or her competence, in some areas, other health care providers may be reluctant to accept referrals from dental hygienists. This will change as other health care providers become more aware of the interrelation of oral disease and adverse systemic conditions. In addition, there may still be some third-party payers who do not yet recognize dental hygienists as primary health care providers and refuse to pay insurance claims. Fortunately, this is changing as many third-party payers are realizing significant savings due to an increase in prevention rather than treatment.

Words of advice from dental hygienists who have chosen to "go it alone"

"Don't do it if you think you're going to get rich quick. But if you love what you do, you will find a way. We've come this far. We must stand and ensure our legal abilities continue to rise to the need of our clientele, so we can put the maintenance option to work. Client education has amazing effects on health. Because dental hygienists are the ones who spend the time with clients, we are in a unique position to educate clients on many more aspects of what they need to know to keep themselves and their families healthy than just brushing and flossing. Dental hygiene for a better world! That's what I am going for. Let's go there together!" RDH in British Columbia

"It is a very big undertaking that is not financially rewarding for a long time. Because it is still in its infancy, public awareness has not reached its optimum. I feel one day my practice will be where I hoped. However, after 18 months I'm still far from my goal." RDH in Ontario

"Do your research in demographics prior to opening. Consider sharing expenses with other health professionals. Keep it professional!" RDH in Ontario

"Yes—this type of practice is not for those that think they are going to make money right away. Too many practices have opened with that mentality and they rarely stay open more than a year or two. It is about loving what you do and preparing to stay in it for the long haul. The rewards are endless and job satisfaction is high but money needs not to be the motivator for getting one into independent practice." RDH in Alberta

"I believe that dental hygienists in independent practice must first and foremost be extremely competent and feel empowered to own their treatment and referrals. I feel that an experienced dental hygienist will be able to draw on her/his past experiences to be successful in business. The process of care must be easy for the client, and a dental hygienist who is very familiar and confident in their own process of care will have a greater chance of success. I also believe that you must not be motivated by the income potential but rather by the fulfillment of the independence of being the business owner. Learn as much about business as you can. Network with business owners and be a presence in your community so the public easily recognizes who you are and what you are about." RDH in Alberta

"Owning and operating a business can be challenging. It requires dedication, patience, and a variety of skills, and of course, money. Knowing how to handle the challenges of opening your own business and knowing yourself, is imperative to the success of your business. You must research it well, talk to your family, and take lots of time to do a complete business plan, before you make any decisions." RDH in Ontario

"Wait for slow and steady growth before expanding; i.e., start out small; don't take on too much debt at the beginning. Consider good quality used equipment versus brand new equipment. Don't invest in too much stock at the beginning—keep your overhead as low as possible." RDH in Ontario

Dental hygienists who are considering the option of practicing independently are advised to thoroughly research the prospect before leaving an employment situation. Unfortunately, most dental hygiene programs do not include a business course. This may change in the future as more and more dental hygienists with an entrepreneurial spirit venture out into the business world. Therefore, an individual contemplating owning and operating their own business would be wise to take a course at their local community college, university, or the varied offerings from private institutions and companies. Local governments often offer seminars on how to start a small business. It is also important to talk to others who are already operating their own practices.

Points to consider

Dental hygienists who want to start their own practice, should consider the following points:

- Develop a business plan.
- Know the rules and regulations in your area.
- Choose your mode of practice based on your strengths and resources.
- Choose a location based on client need.
- Start slowly.
- Purchase sturdy, good quality equipment; used equipment is fine.
- Make community contacts.
- Develop a relationship with the other health care providers in the areas.
- Be prepared to work long hours with little return on investment for a period of time.
- Put client care ahead of financial or personal gain.
- "Think long and hard before you do this, I wanted to help people and have more free time. I don't even know what free time is anymore but I sure am helping a lot of great people!"

Reflections

- *The adventure of independent dental hygiene practice has been extremely fulfilling. The financial rewards are slower in coming. However, I know that the small steps will eventually all pay off and the dividends will be exponentially rewarding—mentally and monetarily.*
- *Entrepreneur and small business development are vital to the success of economic development in any area. I believe that entrepreneurs are crucial for a thriving community and economy. The investments they create in your community are immeasurable. Our economic system is based upon free enterprise and the right of each person to take the risk, follow a dream, and open his/her own business.*
- *As risky as it was to open my own dental hygiene clinic, I wouldn't trade it for anything right now. To practice my profession of dental hygiene on my terms and within my scope is invaluable and I will enjoy my profession forever!*

- *Working as an independent provider in Long-Term Care has the advantage of a central location and one time equipment set up as opposed to visiting clients in the home setting. The equipment is set up right in the treatment room and the residents are easily transported to and from. Often times right in their wheelchairs or with the aid of a walker. All the safely protocols are there to make it easier, for example grab bars on the walls for support and call buttons for help. There is a physician on staff for consultations and RN's and Personal Support Workers available for assistance. It is a safe environment to work in and I love the difference I make for these residents. If my services were not available most of these residents would get little care at all. There is also the added advantage of being able to speak to the caregivers and staff and offer guidance and advise as it relates to each resident and their oral health needs.*

Success stories

"I have been totally overwhelmed by the support of my patients all are very proud of me and consequently have recommended me and in the 4 years I have been set up I have doubled my patient base. It's been a wonderful experience. I have also been lucky that I have some supportive dentist colleagues."

"I had a woman come in extremely scared and shaking to have her teeth cleaned. She did not smile. She had severe supra and sub calculus which made her think that her teeth were black with decay. I finished her cleaning, and showed her teeth in the hand mirror and she started to cry. She said that she never thought her teeth would look good again. She never wore lipstick in fear that it would draw people to see her teeth. She told me that from that day forward she is going to wear lipstick every day!!!!"

"The staff of a long-term care home was telling me how one resident, who was on my list of people to see, requested by his power of attorney, was not eating and was losing weight. I assessed the patient, and clinically saw an abscess. A dentist ordered an X-ray, the abscess was diagnosed, and the patient was brought to the dentist for treatment. The patient was able to eat well after and gained back his weight."

"One of my favourite success stories is about a lady that is in her 70's she had not seen a dentist in 30 years. She was too afraid. I took her to my operatory showed her how differently things were set up and that it was a relaxed atmosphere. I spent the time with her to get her comfortable, we did her treatment in two appointments and she was so happy that she will now keep up with her dental needs."

"I was involved with the *Gift from the Heart Day*. This is where several independent dental hygienists opened their doors and provided free service to those in need. I had over ten sheets of clients needing service unfortunately I was only able to see a very small fraction of the people requesting to be seen. It did open my eyes to the need for dental financial assistance."

Acknowledgments

The author of this chapter wishes to thank the dental hygienists who gave of their time to contribute their thoughts and experiences in an evolutionary way of meeting client needs.

References

Canadian Dental Hygienists Association. (2011) Self-employed vs. employee status. [online] available at http://www.cdha.ca/Content/NavigationMenu/Career/ACareerinDH/SelfemployedvsEmployed/Self_Employed_Vs_Emp.htm.

Dental Hygiene Committee of California. (2011) Department of Consumer Affairs, California USA [online] available at http://www.dhcc.ca.gov/index.shtml.

Federal Trade Commission, USA. (2010) South Carolina Board of Dentistry Settles Charges That it Restrained Competition in the Provision of Preventive Care by Dental Hygienists [online] available at http://www.ftc.gov/opa/2007/06/dentists.shtm.

International Federation of Dental Hygienists. (2011) [online] available at www.IFDH.org.

Limeback, H. (2008) Implications of oral infections on systemic diseases in the institutionalized elderly with a special focus on pneumonia. *Annals of Periodontology*, 3, 262–275.

Organization for Economic Co-operation and Development (OECD). (2005) Enhancing beneficial competition in the health professions. OAEC [online] available at http://www.oecd.org/dataoecd/7/55/35910986.pdf.

Scott, S. (2007) Reform of Dental Hygiene Profession. Competition Bureau of Canada [online] available at http://www.competitionbureau.gc.ca/eic/site/cb-bc.nsf/eng/02278.html.

Stein, P.S. and Henry, R.G. (2009) Poor oral hygiene in long-term care. *American Journal of Nursing*, 109, 44–50; quiz 51.

Steinecke, R. (2011) Complete Guide to the Regulated Health Professions Act, A, Canada Law Book, Toronto, Canada.

Index

abfraction, 221
abscess, 2, 334, 367, 386
acidulated phosphate fluoride (APF), 91, 252, 262, 264, 276, 298, 300
adenosine triphosphate (ATP), 160, 239
advertising, 134
air abrasion, 364, 365
alcohol, 2, 3, 10, 18, 20, 22, 62–9, 76–8, 85, 127, 138, 140, 146–8, 155, 164, 316, 318
alginate, 205
alveolar, 43–54, 100, 196, 196–9, 266
amalgam, 7, 9, 20, 70, 174, 219, 263, 293, 363
ameloblast, 272, 301
ameloblastin, 301
amino acid, 182, 227
amine fluoride, 259, 264
amorphous calcium phosphate (ACP), 15, 126, 215, 302–9
amylase, 10, 16, 106, 107
analytical, 71–3, 85
anaphylaxis, 151
anti-bacterial, 8, 18, 187, 264
antibody, 183, 373
APF *see* acidulated phosphate fluoride (APF)
aphthous, 126, 164
artificial sweeteners, 147
Aspartame, 146, 147
ATPase, 264
atrophy, 100, 132
asthma, 208, 214, 233, 324, 369
avulsion, 83, 196, 199, 201, 314

Bass technique, 121, 124, 131–3, 135
bicarbonate, 15, 126, 141, 154, 163, 303, 362
biofilm, viii, 18, 19, 25, 26, 51, 52, 58, 116, 119–21, 125–8, 130–135, 137, 138, 140, 141, 159, 165, 169, 175, 177, 185, 233, 241, 251, 253, 260, 264, 284, 293, 305, 313, 359, 362, 372, 375
biomarkers, 56–8, 76, 77
bis-GMA, 287, 290
bitewing, 27, 33
BioC, 166
Black, G.V., 6–8, 287
bond(ing), 164, 182, 186, 187, 219, 224–6, 229, 252, 283, 287, 288, 290, 292, 295, 307

breast milk, 265, 324
breast feeding, 86, 315, 317, 320, 324
brush(ing), 11, 17, 35, 49, 50, 104, 120, 121–35, 137–41, 150, 154, 159, 171–3, 208, 214, 215, 221, 222, 227–9, 255, 257–60, 264, 276, 284, 293, 294, 300, 303, 317, 318, 320–323, 326, 328, 346, 353, 354, 360, 375, 385
brushite, 55
Brushtest, 76
budget, 22, 337
buffering capacity, 1, 10, 26, 100, 103, 108, 154, 238, 240, 242, 244, 342
bruxism, 219, 229
burn(s), 70, 91, 138, 182, 184, 273, 274, 326
burnishing, 219, 224
business, ix, 134, 175, 352, 359, 360, 371, 372, 375, 378, 380–382, 385, 386

calcium, 3, 10, 15, 55, 100, 108, 111, 126, 140, 151, 153, 154, 160, 161, 163, 213–5, 224, 227, 229, 242, 252, 253, 249, 260, 262, 268, 270, 277, 290, 299, 300–307, 323, 324, 362, 364
calcium phosphate, 154, 161, 215, 299, 301–303
calculus, 10, 11, 38, 50, 53–6, 128, 221, 258, 304, 341, 384, 386
CAMBRA, 8, 140, 238, 362
cancer, viii, ix, 1–3, 20–22, 61–78, 87, 120, 121, 138, 165, 175, 306, 324, 332, 343, 359, 361, 367, 369, 373, 374
candida, 12, 117, 120, 125, 133, 181, 186
carbonate, 10, 15, 126, 127, 141, 154, 163, 214, 222, 225, 227, 242, 253, 299, 301, 303, 362
carcinogenic, 20, 21, 64, 68, 71
carcinoma, 20, 61, 63, 67–73
cariogenic, 3, 8, 10, 13–16, 86, 105–8, 111, 146–9, 154, 155, 160, 173, 182, 233, 234, 236, 238, 239, 242–4, 260–264, 294, 298, 299, 304, 313, 315, 316, 348
caries
  arrested, 1, 8, 25, 187, 191, 255, 256, 263, 284, 293, 306, 362, 364, 372.
  caries-free, 4, 9, 236, 243, 248

incipient, 1, 2, 12, 15, 20, 189, 235, 246, 253–8, 260, 263, 265, 272, 283, 284, 294, 299, 315
occlusal, 29, 31, 34, 37, 39, 40, 192, 283, 285–8, 291–5
reversal, 186, 187, 189, 191, 192
root, ix, 7, 16, 17, 21, 31, 32, 39, 100, 166–70, 176, 177, 187, 190–192, 243–7, 260, 264, 266, 267, 298–300, 303, 204, 340–342, 345, 362
white spot, 1, 10–12, 34, 187, 189, 190, 242, 253, 256, 263, 265, 270, 271, 284, 295, 302, 303, 306, 307
caries risk test (CRT), 239, 240
CarieScreen, 239
cariogram, 236, 238, 244, 245
casein, 215, 301, 303–5
cavitation, 6, 17, 29, 189, 253, 255, 263, 284
Cavitron, 187
cemento-enamel junction, 218, 226
Cervitec, 166, 187, 189
cetylpyridinium chloride (CPC), 138, 139, 164
cheese, 111, 115, 117, 214, 215, 319
chewing gum, 10, 104, 115, 117, 118, 126, 146–52, 154–6, 215, 235, 303, 305, 309, 325
chlorhexidine, 15, 47, 54, 119, 120, 124, 138, 140, 151, 152, 154, 155, 159–68, 172, 174–6, 187, 189, 208, 215, 235, 264, 315, 365, 375
client, viii, ix, 121, 124–6, 127, 128, 131–5, 138–41, 171, 333, 352, 358–87
Coca-Cola, 215
cohort study, 86, 88, 95, 103
Colgate, 227, 228, 259
concussion, 197, 198, 200, 206, 207
confounder, 3, 38, 93, 95, 96, 267, 268
connective tissue, 44–8, 50, 52, 53, 72, 121, 218
coronal, 16, 21, 45–7, 50, 54, 167, 168, 170, 173, 187, 243, 246, 266, 342
CPP-ACP, 126, 303–9
cracked tooth, 219–21
critical pH, 15, 17, 107, 108, 258, 259, 298, 299, 301
counseling, 1, 73, 77, 173, 315, 325, 337, 359–61, 369
cupping, 212

Comprehensive Preventive Dentistry, First Edition. Edited by Hardy Limeback.
© 2012 John Wiley & Sons, Ltd. Published 2012 by John Wiley & Sons, Ltd.